George H. Halse (07[illegible]0369)
0804359

Introduction to Clinical Medicine
a clerking companion

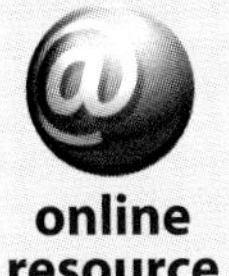

online resource centre

Online support

www.oxfordtextbooks.co.uk/orc/randall/

Go to the book's Online Resource Centre to access the following materials:

Downloadable PDFs of the pro formas provided throughout this book
You might find yourself wanting to clerk more than one patient presenting with the same condition; simply download and print out extra copies of the appropriate pro formas as required.

Large-size, annotated images
Due to the constraints imposed by the design of this book, many of the illustrations contained here lack the size and clarity of real life clinical images. To make the most of these features, please use the full-sized online images which are almost all presented as two-part slideshows with full annotation.

Sample charts
The Online Resource Centre also provides a sample drug chart, discharge summary, and fluid prescription chart. These can be printed off and used for the prescribing exercises in any of the questions in this book, as well as used on the wards to practice shadow prescribing. Every effort has been made to make it very clear that these are samples rather than proper drug charts. However, remember to keep these safe and not to leave them anywhere where they could cause confusion on wards.

Angiogram videos
A series of video clips are provided in the Online Resource Centre; they run in a sequence to follow an angiogram from a single patient.

These resources are available at no cost but are password-protected. To access the resources simply visit the Online Resource Centre at **www.oxfordtextbooks.co.uk/orc/randall/** and enter the following username and password:

Username: randall
Password: cobweb

introduction to clinical medicine

A CLERKING COMPANION

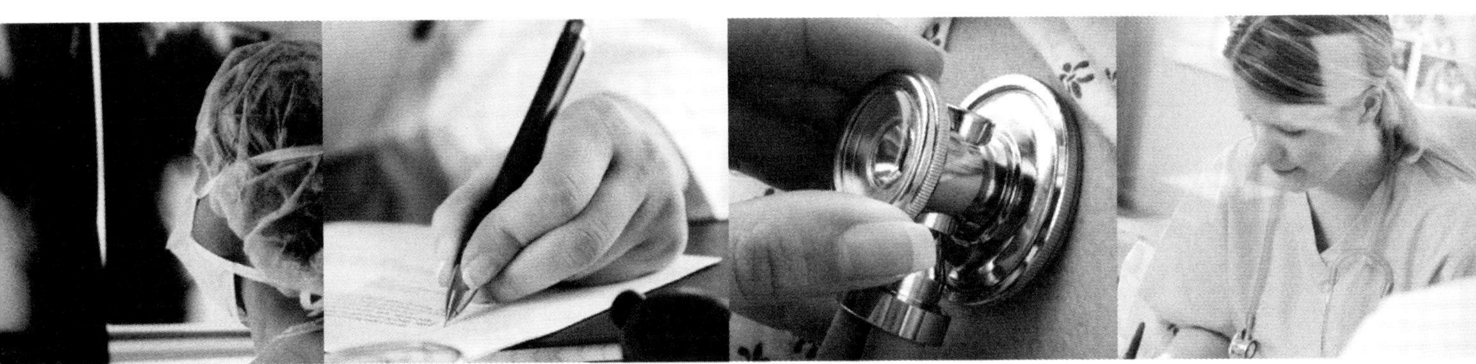

DAVID **RANDALL** MA, MBBS (London)

Queen's University Hospital, Romford

ADAM **FEATHER** FRCP

Barts and the London School of Medicine and Dentistry

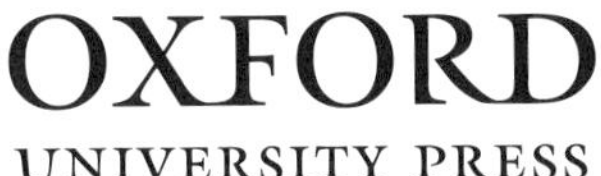

OXFORD
UNIVERSITY PRESS

OXFORD
UNIVERSITY PRESS

Great Clarendon Street, Oxford OX2 6DP

Oxford University Press is a department of the University of Oxford.
It furthers the University's objective of excellence in research, scholarship,
and education by publishing worldwide in

Oxford New York

Auckland Cape Town Dar es Salaam Hong Kong Karachi
Kuala Lumpur Madrid Melbourne Mexico City Nairobi
New Delhi Shanghai Taipei Toronto

With offices in

Argentina Austria Brazil Chile Czech Republic France Greece
Guatemala Hungary Italy Japan Poland Portugal Singapore
South Korea Switzerland Thailand Turkey Ukraine Vietnam

Published in the United States
by Oxford University Press Inc., New York

British Library Cataloguing in Publication Data
Data available

Library of Congress Cataloging in Publication Data
Data available

Typeset by Sparks—www.sparkspublishing.com
Printed in Italy
on acid-free paper by
L.E.G.O. S.p.A

ISBN 978-0-19-957437-7

1 3 5 7 9 10 8 6 4 2

To Abigail - with love

About the authors

David Randall studied medicine at Peterhouse, Cambridge, and then at Barts and the London School of Medicine and Dentistry. He then completed an academic foundation programme specialising in medical education and is now working as a junior doctor in general medicine at Queen's Hospital, Romford.

Adam Feather is Senior Lecturer in Medical Education at the Institute of Health Science Education, Barts and the London School of Medicine and Dentistry. Adam is a Lead for Clinical Skills with a particular interest in the teaching and learning of clinical examination skills. He is the co-lead for part 6a (written Finals) assessment with particular interest in the development of new and innovative written, computer-based, and clinical assessments.

Acknowledgements

We are grateful to Mr Tony Joy MBChB MRCS(Eng) DCH, Specialist Registrar in Emergency Medicine, St. Barts & The Royal London NHS Trust, for editing and suggesting helpful changes to the surgery chapter. Thank you to Dr Wade H. Gayed BSc (Hons) MBBS, Honorary Clinical Lecturer Queen Mary University of London, Specialist Registrar in Radiology, Barts & the London NHS Trust, and Dr Muaaze Ahmad MB ChB FRCR Consultant Radiologist, St. Barts & The Royal London NHS Trust, for supplying us with most of the X-rays included in the book. Thanks also to Dr C. Anwar A. Chahal BSc(Hons) MBChB MRCP (UK), Specialist Registrar in Cardiology & GIM, Barts and The London School of Medicine and Dentistry, for the angiogram and echocardiogram images, and to Dr Michael J. Reynolds BSc MRCP, Consultant Physician and Gastroenterologist, Basingstoke and North Hampshire NHS Foundation Trust, for the ERCP image.

Personal thanks for help in various aspects of writing and editing the book goes to Abigail Randall, Caleb Dixon, Richard Rance and various staff at Oxford University Press especially including Caroline Connelly, Jonathan Crowe, and Holly Edmundson. Thank you also to the students and lecturers who reviewed material from the book and for their helpful suggestions.

Anonymised images have been used with permission from a several NHS trusts including St Barts and The Royal London NHS Trust and Whipps Cross University Hospital NHS Trust: these remain copyright property of the Trusts in question.

Contents

Introduction

My method [is to] lead my students by hand to the practice of medicine, taking them every day to see patients in the public hospital, that they may hear the patient's symptoms and see their physical findings. Then I question the students as to what they have noted in their patients and about their thoughts and perceptions regarding the causes of the illness and the principles of treatment.

(Franciscus Sylvius, 1614-1672)[1]

Clinical medicine is very different from pre-clinical medicine. Whilst still having to learn large amounts of technical information one also needs to develop the professional skills, attitudes, and behaviours expected of a newly qualified doctor. Some of these skills can be learnt from books and the Internet or practised in simulated clinical areas such as clinical skills or simulation centres, but all good clinicians quickly find that they are best learnt at the patient's bed or chair side. As clinical students you will need to begin to develop the art of clinical diagnostic reasoning; the ability to assimilate information from the patient's history, examination findings, and the results of their investigations, in order to produce a list of clinical problems, diagnoses, and a subsequent management plan. This complex process is known as '**clerking the patient**'. This book has been written to try to help you acquire the fundamental skills necessary to clerk patients in a competent and professional manner.

Being a doctor is a privilege and an honour, and no other job can offer such satisfaction and reward. But becoming a doctor is a complex and challenging business! All doctors are expected to have a broad and diverse set of technical and interpersonal skills. You will need to be able to perform procedures such as phlebotomy and venous cannulation, and administer potentially harmful drugs. You will need to be able communicate important and sometimes difficult news to patients and their relatives, acting as their advocate in times of need. You will need to develop the awareness to work within the complex structure of modern healthcare systems. But above all you need to become the kind of trustworthy, honest, and compassionate person that you would want looking after one of your relatives or friends.

This book will give you the support you need for your first few bewildering months in clinical practice. It should enable you to take a full and relevant history, to make your examination focused and effective, review and make sense of relevant data from investigations performed, and help you draw up a management plan. It is not easy! Clinical medicine is learnt patient by patient. By observing, by practice, and by reading and reflecting on the cases that you see, you will slowly acquire the necessary skills to allow you to graduate and be called 'doctor'.

But always remember the patient is your first priority—help them get comfortable, ensure their consent, explain things where possible, and represent their concerns to the team. Although you may feel the least useful member of the medical team, you are the one with the most time to spend with patients. Make the most of this time to ensure that along with all the science, technology, and interventions you never forget to prioritize the patient as a person, not a disease, and show them the care and respect that they deserve.

We wish you many happy years in your chosen career. Happy clerking!

David Randall and Adam Feather

[1]Distlehorst LH, Dunnington G, Folse JR (2000) *Teaching and learning in medical and surgical education: lessons learned for the twenty-first century*. Lawrence Erlbaum Associates, Mahwah, NJ.

How to use this book

You can observe a lot by just watching

(Lawrence 'Yogi' Berra, 1925–present)

Hospital in-patients are usually looked after by a team of doctors at different levels of seniority. They will be assigned to the care of a consultant (or attending physician in the USA), who may see them only once or twice per week but who are responsible for the main, strategic decisions in their management. Day to day they will be seen by junior doctors, interns, and residents. The consultant (or attending physician) may also run out-patient clinics or perform operations or procedures (e.g. endoscopies) and have roles in hospital management, medical education, and clinical research. Middle grade doctors (registrars or residents) will split their time between the wards, the out-patient clinic, and learning technical skills such as operating, endoscopy, or bronchoscopy.

Time as a student is best spent divided amongst these activities. Make sure you accompany your patients to the procedures and investigations that they undergo. Observe the clinicians you are working with—watch and listen to the way they take histories, examine and communicate, support and care for patients. Do not miss important learning opportunities such as operating lists, clinics, and ward rounds; make sure you have something to contribute! The best way to get involved is to clerk new patients on the ward prior to the rounds and then present your clerkings to the person leading the round. Not only will they be impressed with you but you will also receive feedback on your performance, both directly and indirectly as you see how your senior's approach compares with your own.

This book is designed to help with clerking patients. Take it along with you each day and fill it in as you clerk patients. You can download additional forms as required from the website **www.oxfordtextbooks.co.uk/orc/randall/** using the log-in details provided at the front of this book. In order to achieve a broad portfolio of patients you will need to visit most of the clinical areas available to you, both in the hospital and the community. Think through the patients' presentations, your examination findings, and the investigation results. Together, these should lead you to a differential diagnosis and a management plan. Present and discuss the cases with seniors; once they have signed this off, you can place this and the other cases in your portfolio. Over time you will develop a good idea about your clinical strengths and weakness.

The **clerking pro formas** are restricted in size by the pagination and design of the book. The **History** box should be used to record the history of the presenting complaint (see p. 6), and any factors impacting on this condition i.e. a 'focused history'. You should also record risk factors, exacerbating and relieving factors. The rest of the history is vital and may be recorded on other areas of the page.

Similarly, the **Examination** boxes may not be large enough to record all your findings, so we recommend you use this box to record the relevant and essential clinical findings.

Once you have completed the clerking pro forma and presented the case to a doctor, using the **portfolio** section of the book, ask the doctor to sign that you have discussed the case with them. Reviewing this portfolio section gives you a clear idea of your strengths and weaknesses as well as providing evidence to your medical school or clinical supervisors of what you have achieved.

Approaching the patient

You will need to become accustomed to approaching patients and their carers. It is a good idea to discuss the suitability of patients to clerk on the ward or in the surgery/clinic with one of the nursing or medical staff. Especially at the beginning of your clinical career, you should try to clerk patients who are clinically stable and able to cooperate with your clerking. Your introduction should include your name, your role, and your intentions whilst you are with the patient. If patients or carers decide they would rather not participate with your clerking, thank them and move on, there are always other patients to see!

Four steps for getting the most out of this book

1. Clerk: Take a full history and examine thoroughly (described in the Introduction). Try not to read the notes and see what others have found—trust your own findings. Ask a doctor to for the relevant investigation results—they may need to log you in to the hospital computer system.

2. Evaluate: Work through the 'Evaluation' questions at the end of each clerking pro forma, writing your findings down as an 'Impression' and then deciding on a 'Plan'. Remember, patients may have several problems. A patient admitted with pneumonia may also have an unexplained iron-deficiency anaemia: if so, write this down under 'Impression', and include any investigations you will need to perform under 'Plan'.

3. Present: Whenever appropriate, try to present your patient clerkings to members of the medical team. Make sure you include your evaluation, differential diagnosis, and suggested management plan. You may find you will be expected to do this in classroom rounds with your colleagues; this may form the basis of case-based learning (CBL) or case-based discussion (CBD) evaluations. Note how junior doctors present very succinctly on business ward rounds, and try to imitate this when asked to present in this setting. Try to get feedback on your discussion and your presentation skills. If possible get the doctors to sign off your presentations.

4. Reinforce: Go to the hospital library or computer suite and research the condition you have just presented. To check your learning and understanding work through the questions at the end of the pro formas, each of which are based on typically encountered clinical scenarios. They aim to link what you have seen to the supporting basic science, as well as to the realities of modern hospital practice. Try to answer the questions yourself before turning over and reading the answers provided.

The 'Comment on...' boxes

All of the clerking pro formas in this book include, in each field, a box highlighting key points to comment on. So, for instance, when taking a history from a patient with an exacerbation of asthma, it is vital to comment on what their normal level of control is, how many times they have previously been admitted to hospital (or intensive care), and what regular medications they take. On examining them, it is vital to comment on signs of respiratory distress, on their baseline observations and on the presence of a wheeze on auscultation. On looking at their chest X-ray you should comment on the presence of consolidation or pneumothorax, when looking at their arterial blood gas analysis you should comment on the pO_2 and the pCO_2, and when reviewing their blood tests you should comment on evidence of infection. These 'Comment on...' boxes therefore bring out key points about each field—effectively, the reason why you bother asking questions, examining, or ordering investigations. These points should form the basis of your evaluation and presentation of the patient.

Chapter introductions

Each chapter is introduced by a short section designed to get you up to speed with the specifics of the specialty in question. This is necessarily brief, but gives tips on tailoring your history and examination skills towards the types of patient you will see in that specialty. At the end of these sections is a 'Medications' table, listing many of the common medications used in the specialty in question. Fill this in (or use a larger version available through the online resource centre) to familiarize yourself with the mechanisms, indications, contraindications and side-effects of commonly used drugs.

Glossary of abbreviations

ABPI	**Ankle:brachial pressure index**	The ratio of the systolic blood pressure at the elbow and at the ankle. A measure of the extent of peripheral vascular disease
ACE	**Angiotensin-converting enzyme**	An enzyme involved in blood pressure regulation. Serum level can be used as a marker for sarcoidosis
ACE inhibitor	**Angiotensin-converting enzyme inhibitor**	Angiotensin-converting enzyme produces angiotensin 2 from angiotensin 1, which then stimulates the release of aldosterone. The ACE inhibitors have important roles in the management of hypertension, heart failure, and chronic kidney disease
ACS	**Acute coronary syndrome**	An umbrella term for patients presenting with acute chest pain believed to be cardiac in origin. The initial presentation of unstable angina and myocardial infarction
ACTH	**Adrenocorticotrophic hormone**	Secreted by the pituitary, it stimulates steroid secretion by the adrenal gland
ADLs	**Activities of daily living**	Basic tasks it is essential that patients can perform in order to live alone and unassisted
AF	**Atrial fibrillation**	A dysrhythmia characterized by chaotic atrial activity causing irregular ventricular contractions
AIDS	**Acquired immunodeficiency syndrome**	Immunodeficiency caused by the HIV virus
ALP	**Alkaline phosphatase**	An enzyme found predominantly on the bile canalicular membrane of hepatocytes which rises significantly in biliary obstructions. It also rises in pregnancy and conditions causing raised bone turnover because of increased production of a different isomer of ALP
ALT	**Alanine transaminase**	An intracellular liver enzyme released in conditions causing hepatocyte death
AML	**Acute myeloid leukaemia**	A haematological malignancy
AMTS	**Abbreviated Mental Test Score**	A score out of 10 for rapidly assessing the level of confusion
ANCA	**Antinuclear cytoplasmic antibody**	An autoantibody particularly associated with systemic vasculitis
ANA	**Antinuclear antibody**	An autoantibody particularly associated with systemic lupus erythematosus
Anti-dsDNA	**Antidouble-stranded deoxyribonucleic acid**	An autoantibody particularly associated with systemic lupus erythematosus
Anti-GBM	**Antiglomerular basement membrane**	An autoantibody causing Goodpasture's disease
AP	**Anteroposterior**	Used in radiography to describe a radiograph taken with the X-ray camera in front of the patient and the film behind. AP chest X-rays are inferior in quality to PA chest X-rays since they cannot be used to estimate the heart size, though they may be easier to perform in an acutely unwell patient
ASOT	**Antistreptolysin-O-titre**	A measure of recent streptococcal infection
AST	**Aspartate transaminase**	An intracellular liver enzyme released in conditions causing hepatocyte death
ATLS	**Advanced Trauma Life Support**	A system for managing acutely ill patients after major trauma and prioritizing life-threatening injuries
AV fistula	**Arteriovenous fistula**	A connection made during a small elective operation between an artery and vein in the forearm to permit dialysis
AV node	**Atrioventricular node**	Part of the cardiac conduction system responsible for delaying impulses between the atria and the ventricles to coordinate the cardiac cycle

AVPU	**Alert, [responds to] Voice, Pain, Unresponsive**	The AVPU score is used to assess a basic level of consciousness (and is quicker to calculate than the Glasgow Coma Score)
AVRT/AVNRT	**Atrioventricular reciprocating tachycardia and atrioventricular nodal re-entrant tachycardia**	Two common forms of supraventricular tachycardia (SVT)
BCG	**Bacille Calmette-Guérin**	A live attenuated vaccine to protect against TB
bd	**Twice daily**	Medication schedule
BE	**Base excess**	The amount of base (alkali) which would have to be added to blood to return it to a normal pH. A measure of the metabolic component of acidosis or alkalosis
BiPAP	**Bilevel positive airways pressure ventilation**	A form of non-invasive ventilation (delivered by tightly fitting face mask) used in type II respiratory failure
BMI	**Body mass index**	Calculation based on the height and weight and used to assess overweight or underweight
BNF	**British National Formulary**	A book detailing all medicines licensed for use in the UK with their indications, cautions and contraindications, and doses
BP	**Blood pressure**	
bpm	**Beats per minute**	The measure of heart rate
CABG	**Coronary artery bypass graft**	Surgery for ischaemic heart disease where vein grafts are used to bypass areas of critical narrowing in the coronary circulation
CBG	**Capillary blood glucose**	A bedside test carried out with a lancet and blood glucose monitor to determine the serum glucose level
CCU	**Coronary Care Unit**	A specialist high-dependency unit for patients with acute cardiological problems with cardiac monitoring for all beds and specially trained nurses
CD	**Crohn's disease**	An inflammatory disease of the bowel
CK	**Creatine kinase**	An intracellular enzyme released when there is damage to skeletal or cardiac muscle
CKD	**Chronic kidney disease**	Chronically impaired renal function
CML	**Chronic myeloid leukaemia**	A haematological malignancy common in the elderly
CMV	**Cytomegalovirus**	Can cause significant disease in the immunocompromised
CNS	**Central nervous system**	The brain and spinal cord
COPD	**Chronic obstructive pulmonary disease**	A chronic lung condition caused by smoking which leads to irreversible airway obstruction and other abnormalities such as air trapping
CPAP	**Continuous positive airways pressure ventilation**	A form of non-invasive ventilation delivered by face-mask used for type I respiratory failure
CRP	**C-reactive protein**	A protein found in blood, the level of which rises significantly in response to inflammation, either as a result of infection or of a non-infective inflammatory condition
CSF	**Cerebrospinal fluid**	The fluid which bathes the brain providing support and nutrition
CT	**Computed tomography**	An imaging modality where images are produced by comparing the absorption of radiation passing through the patient's body from different angles
CTPA	**Computed tomography of the pulmonary arteries**	The gold standard investigation for pulmonary embolus
CURB-65		An acronym for calculating the severity of community-acquired pneumonia
CVP	**Central venous pressure**	A measure of the pressure in the right atrium, which corresponds to overall fluid status and cardiac filling pressures
CXR	**Chest X-ray**	
DHx	**Drug history**	A list of medications taken by the patient, and any drug allergies
DKA	**Diabetic ketoacidosis**	A severe hyperglycaemic complication of type 1 diabetes

DM	**Diabetes mellitus**	A disease caused by an inability to regulate plasma glucose levels
DOTS	**Directly observed treatment schemes**	To encourage compliance with long term medications such as anti-TB drugs or methadone
DVLA	**Drivers and vehicles licensing authority**	A UK government body for regulating the safety of drivers and cars
DVT	**Deep vein thrombosis**	Blood clot formation in the deep venous system, usually of the leg. Pieces of clot can break off to form pulmonary emboli
EAA	**Extrinsic allergic alveolitis**	A respiratory hypersensitivity disorder against environmental antigens
ECG	**Electrocardiogram**	A recording of the electrical activity of the heart, conventionally using 12 real or calculated 'leads'
EEG	**Electroencephalogram**	A measure of the electrical activity of the brain, used in the diagnosis of epilepsy
eGFR	**Estimated glomerular filtration rate**	A useful way of estimating kidney function
EBV	**Epstein–Barr virus**	Causes glandular fever and is linked to haematological malignancies including lymphoma
ERCP	**Endoscopic retrograde cholangiopancreatography**	A procedure for investigating and treating diseases of the biliary tract
ESBL	**Extended spectrum beta-lactamase-producing bacteria**	Gram-negative bacteria that have acquired resistance to a number of antibiotics commonly used to treat them, including penicillins and sometimes gentamicin
ESR	**Erythrocyte sedimentation rate**	A marker of inflammatory processes
ETT	**Exercise tolerance test**	A cardiac investigation where patients walk on a treadmill at increasing speeds according to the 'Bruce protocol', whilst their ECG is being monitored for changes (such as ST-segment depression) indicating myocardial ischaemia
FBC	**Full blood count**	A panel of tests usually performed by an automatic analyser, including measurements such as the serum haemoglobin concentration and some information about red cell size and structure, the white cell count and differential, and the platelet count
FEV_1	**Forced expiratory volume in 1 second**	The total amount of air breathed out in 1 second—reduced in obstructive lung disease
FHx	**Family history**	An enquiry into diseases suffered by members of the patient's family
FNA	**Fine needle aspiration**	A method for getting cells for cytology from a solid tissue mass
FSH	**Follicle-stimulating hormone**	A pituitary hormone with roles in stimulating the ovaries and testis
FVC	**Forced vital capacity**	The total amount of air that can be exhaled in one breath —reduced in restrictive lung disease
GCA	**Giant cell arteritis**	A large-cell vasculitis that causes severe unilateral headaches, with scalp tenderness and the potential to lose eyesight
GCS	**Glasgow Coma Score**	A measure of overall level of consciousness, ranging from 15/15 (fully alert) to 3/15 (unrousable)
G-CSF	**Granulocyte colony-stimulating factor**	Can be used to help the bone marrow recover after neutropenic sepsis caused by chemotherapy
GGT	**Gamma-glutamyltransferase**	A liver enzyme which is a particularly sensitive marker of increased alcohol intake. It rises along with ALP in biliary obstruction
GH	**Growth hormone**	A pituitary hormone with a role in stimulating tissue growth
GI	**Gastrointestinal**	
GORD	**Gastro-oesophageal reflux disease**	A disease producing dyspeptic symptoms caused by reflux of acidic stomach contents into the oesophagus because of an incompetent lower oesophageal sphincter
GP	**General practitioner**	A community-based primary care doctor

GRACE	**Global Registry of Acute Coronary Events**	A large international database of cardiac events including myocardial infarctions and unstable angina, from which a score has been developed to calculate the risk of death after a cardiac event
GTN	**Glyceryl trinitrate**	A drug which can be given intravenously or sublingually and in the body produces nitrous oxide, causing vasodilatation. Used in acute coronary syndrome and pulmonary oedema
HASU	**Hyperacute stroke unit**	Large centres to improve stroke management in the UK particularly thrombolysis provision
HAV/HBV/HCV/HEV	**Hepatitis A, B, C, and E viruses**	The commonest viruses causing viral hepatitis
Hb	**Haemoglobin**	Oxygen-binding protein in RBCs
HCC	**Hepatocellular carcinoma**	Primary liver cancer, often caused by viral hepatitis
HDL	**High-density lipoprotein**	A protein-lipid complex that transports lipids in blood
HDU	**High-dependency unit**	A unit for very sick patients, with high ratios of nurses to patients but not quite as well resourced as an ITU
HHS	**Hyperosmolar hyperglycaemic state**	A non-ketotic hyperglycaemic emergency of type 2 diabetes
HIV	**Human immunodeficiency virus**	The retrovirus that causes AIDS.
HLA	**Human leucocyte antigen**	A basis of intercellular communication with important roles in immunity
HONK	**Hyperosmolar non-ketotic state**	The older name for hyperosmolar hyperglycaemic state (see HHS)
HPC	**History of the presenting complaint**	The current medical problem experienced by the patient
HR	**Heart rate**	
IBD	**Inflammatory bowel disease**	An umbrella term for both Crohn's disease and ulcerative colitis, which are characterized by persistent bowel wall inflammation
ICU	**Intensive care unit**	*See* ITU
IF	**Intrinsic factor**	Cofactor for absorbing vitamin B_{12} from the gut. Decreased in pernicious anaemia
Ig	**Immunoglobulin**	Antibodies
IHD	**Ischaemic heart disease**	Heart disease caused by narrowing of the coronary arteries manifesting as a myocardial infarction, angina, or heart failure
INR	**International normalized ratio**	A way of measuring the clotting speed of blood in comparison with internationally agreed norms
ITU	**Intensive treatment unit**	A high-dependency unit with high nurse:patient ratios and the ability to offer intensive organ support such as haemofiltration or artificial ventilation
IV	**Intravenous**	A route of drug delivery using cannula or needle
IVDU	**Intravenous drug user**	
JVP	**Jugular venous pressure**	A clinical sign where flickering pulsation in the neck reveals the pressure (in mmH_2O) in the right atrium. Raised in right-sided or congestive heart failure
LAD	**Left anterior descending artery**	The main vessel supplying the anterior wall of the heart
LAD	**Left axis deviation**	An ECG abnormality where the mean flow of electricity through the heart is deviated to the left
LBBB	**Left bundle branch block**	An ECG pattern with widened QRS complexes and predominant downwards deflection in V_1 and predominant upwards deflection in V_6
LDH	**Lactate dehydrogenase**	An enzyme whose serum concentration rises in conditions causing raised tissue turnover, for instance after a myocardial infarction, in haemolytic anaemia, and in certain other cancers and infections
LDL	**Low-density lipoprotein**	A form of blood cholesterol associated with developing vascular disease

LFTs	Liver function tests	Tests of liver damage such as: ALP, ALT, AST, and tests of the liver's synthetic function
LOC	Loss of consciousness	
LTOT	Long term oxygen therapy	Oxygen delivered either by cylinders or by a small oxygen concentrator that the patient can use at home
LH	Luteinizing hormone	A pituitary hormone with roles in stimulating the ovaries and testis
LUTS	Lower urinary tract symptoms	Symptoms of bladder irritation or obstruction
LV	Left ventricle	
LVH	Left ventricular hypertrophy	Overgrowth of the muscle of the left ventricle, usually due to chronic heart failure
M,C&S	Microscopy, cultures, and sensitivity	Basic microbiological investigations which can be carried out on a range of specimens (e.g. urine, skins swabs, or pleural fluid), to investigate for bacterial infection
MCV	Mean corpuscular volume	The average volume of red cells, used to differentiate causes of anaemia
MDRTB/XDRTB	Multiple or extremely drug resistant tuberculosis	A growing public health problem producing severe disease resistant to most commonly used drugs
MI	Myocardial infarction	Cardiac ischaemia which has led to irreversible cell death
MMSE	Mini-Mental State Examination	A score out of 30 for assessing a patient's level of cognitive impairment
MPS	Myocardial perfusion scanning	Radioactive markers are used to assess areas of underperfused myocardium. Used in the diagnosis of acute myocardial infarction, or to diagnose ischaemic heart disease in patients presenting with troponin-negative chest pain, as an alternative to exercise tolerance testing in patients unable to walk on the treadmill
MRA	Magnetic resonance angiography	A recent non-invasive technique for imaging blood vessels (coronary, carotid, femoral, or elsewhere) without the need for invasive catheterization of the vessel in question
MRI	Magnetic resonance imaging	A radiation-free imaging modality where images are created by the differential activity of subatomic particles in materials of different kinds when they are held in a magnetic field. Excellent for imaging soft tissues
MRSA	Methicillin-resistant Staphylococcus aureus	A hospital-acquired organism that may simply colonize body sites or may produce invasive disease which is hard to treat because of antibiotic resistance
MS	Multiple sclerosis	A degenerative neurological disease with varying motor and sensory symptoms and signs that often remit and relapse over years
MSU	Mid-stream urine	Sent for microscopy, culture, and sensitivities
NASH	Non-alcoholic steatohepatitis	Swelling and inflammation of the liver not caused by alcohol often caused by obesity
NHS	National Health Service	The state-run provider of primary and secondary healthcare in the UK, financed by general taxation
NICE	National Institute for Health and Clinical Excellence	A UK body responsible for evaluating treatments offered by the National Health Service to determine indications for use and cost-effectiveness. Its produces evidence-based guidelines to govern the treatment of major conditions
NKDA	No known drug allergies	
NSAID	Non-steroidal anti-inflammatory drug	The work by inhibiting cyclo-oxygenase enzymes. Often used as analgesics
NSTEMI or non-STEMI	Non-ST-segment elevation myocardial infarction	A myocardial infarction where cell death does not extend through the full thickness of the myocardium
od	Once daily	Medication frequency
OGTT	Oral glucose tolerance test	A gold-standard test for diagnosing diabetes mellitus. Plasma glucose readings are taken after fasting overnight and again after ingesting a fixed quantity of glucose

OHCM	Oxford Handbook of Clinical Medicine	A pocket textbook of general medicine and surgery published by Oxford University Press
om	Once daily in the morning	Medication schedule
on	Once daily in the evening	Medication schedule
OSA	Obstructive sleep apnoea	A respiratory disease caused by obesity causing nocturnal desaturations and regular partial wakenings though the night
OSCE	Objective structured clinical examination	A practical examination used by all UK medical schools to assess students' ability in history-taking, physical examination, and practical procedures
PA	Posteroanterior	Used to describe a radiograph taken with the X-ray camera behind the patient and the film in front. PA chest X-rays are superior in quality to AP chest X-rays since they can be used to estimate the heart size
$PaCO_2$	Partial pressure of arterial CO_2	Crudely, this is a measurement of the CO_2 concentration in the blood, which rises in type II respiratory failure
PBC	Primary biliary cirrhosis	A chronic inflammatory disease of the liver resulting in cirrhosis
PE	Pulmonary embolus	A blood clot that becomes lodged in one of the pulmonary arteries, originating from a deep vein thrombosis
PEFR	Peak expiratory flow rate	The maximum rate at which air can be exhaled—reduced in obstructive airways diseases such as asthma
PEG tube	Percutaneous gastrostomy tube	For feeding in patients with an unsafe swallow (e.g. after a stroke). Inserted into the stomach through the abdominal wall
PEP	Post-exposure prophylaxis	Antiretroviral drugs to be taken in case of potential contact with HIV (e.g. after a needlestick injury on a ward), if there is a significant risk of HIV transmission
PMHx	Past medical history	
PND	Paroxysmal nocturnal dyspnoea	A symptom of heart failure where the patient wakes in the night acutely short of breath
pO_2	Partial pressure of oxygen	Crudely, the oxygen concentration of blood
PPI	Proton pump inhibitor	These drugs suppress gastric acid secretion and are used in acute upper gastrointestinal haemorrhage and gastro-oesophageal reflux disease
PR	per rectum	Route of drug administration, also used to describe a digital rectal examination
prn	As required	Medication schedule
PSA	Prostate-specific antigen	A protein produced by cells in the prostate gland that may be used as a marker of prostate cancer and which has a particular role in assessing response to treatment and disease progression in patients receiving treatment
PVD	Peripheral vascular disease	Atherosclerotic disease of the arteries of the legs, producing intermittent claudication, rest pain, and acute ischaemia
qds	Four times a day	Medication schedule
RA	Rheumatoid arthritis	A chronic inflammatory arthritis caused by immune complex deposition that also produces disease in e.g. the lungs
RAD	Right anterior descending artery	The main coronary artery supplying the inferior and posterior wall of the heart
RAD	Right axis deviation	An ECG abnormality where the mean flow of electricity through the heart is deviated to the right
RBBB	Right bundle branch block	An ECG pattern with widened QRS complexes and predominant upwards deflection in V_1 and predominant downwards deflection in V_6. Often associated with heart strain secondary to respiratory disease (cor pulmonale)
RF	Rheumatoid factor	An autoantibody particularly associated with rheumatoid disease
RRT	Renal replacement therapy	Either dialysis or renal transplantation
RR	Respiratory rate	

RTA	**Road traffic accident**	
SACD	**Subacute combined degeneration of the spine**	Degenerative disease of the spine caused by vitamin B_{12} deficiency
SBP	**Spontaneous bacterial peritonitis**	Spontaneous infection of ascites, caused by haematogenous (blood-borne) spread
SHx	**Social history**	An enquiry into risk factors for disease (e.g. smoking, foreign travel) and the patient's accommodation, employment, and degree of independence
SIADH	**Syndrome of the inappropriate secretion of antidiuretic hormone**	A relatively rare form of hyponatraemia, with many causes including atypical pneumonia or some lung cancers
SIGN	**Scottish Intercollegiate Guidelines Network**	An academic group in Scotland who draw up clinical guidelines
SIRS	**Systemic inflammatory response syndrome**	A systemic response to injury—such as infection, characterized by fever, tachycardia, tachypnoea, or other signs
SLE	**Systemic lupus erythematosus**	A chronic connective tissue disease producing a wide range of symptoms
SOAR		An acronym for calculating the severity of community-acquired pneumonia in the over-75s
STEMI	**ST-segment elevation myocardial infarction**	A myocardial infarction where cardiac ischaemia has led to cell death through the full thickness of the myocardium with a characteristic pattern seen on ECG
SVT	**Supraventricular tachycardia**	Used in a broad sense to refer to any tachycardia with an atrial pacemaker, or in a narrower sense to refer to atrioventricular node re-entrance and reciprocating tachycardias
T_3	**Triiodothyronine**	The more active of the two thyroid hormones, T_3 is formed from T_4 peripherally and acts on a wide variety of tissues to increase basal metabolic rate
T_4	**Thyroxine**	One of the thyroid hormones. Much more prevalent than T_3 in the blood, where much is bound to circulating protein. It is converted to T_3, and both produce a range of cellular effects including raising the basal metabolic rate
TACS, PACS, POCS, and LACS	**Total anterior, partial anterior and posterior circulation strokes, and lacunar strokes**	A way of describing different stroke syndromes according to the clinical signs present. This is known as the Oxfordshire Community Stroke Project (OCSP) or Bamford classification
TB	**Tuberculosis**	A chronic mycobacterial infection commonly affecting the lungs but which can involve any body tissue
TCC	**Transitional cell carcinoma**	The commonest type of cancer of the bladder and ureters
tds	**Three times a day**	Medication schedule
TIA	**Transient ischaemic attack**	Symptoms and signs of a recognized stroke syndrome which fully resolves within 24 hours
TIBC	**Total iron-binding capacity**	A blood test used in the investigation of anaemia
TIPSS	**Transjugular intrahepatic portosystemic shunt**	An artificial connection between the portal vein and the inferior vena cava, sometimes used in advanced cirrhosis to reduce the chance of catastrophic variceal haemorrhage
TNF-α	**Tumour necrosis factor-α**	A local hormone extensively involved in the inflammatory process
TNM	**Tumour-Nodes-Metastases**	A commonly used staging system for different types of cancer, based on appearances of the tumour and evidence of spread to the lymph nodes or distant sites
TSH	**Thyroid-stimulating hormone**	A hormone secreted by the anterior pituitary which leads to release of T_3 and T_4 by the thyroid gland
U&Es	**Urea and electrolytes**	Basic biochemical tests revealing information about renal function and electrolyte levels
UC	**Ulcerative colitis**	An inflammatory disease of the bowel
UTI	**Urinary tract infection**	Bacterial urinary infection
VF	**Ventricular fibrillation**	A chaotic heart rhythm, one of the causes or cardiac arrest, and incompatible with life. Requires electrical defibrillation

V/Q scan	**Ventilation-perfusion scan**	A nuclear medicine scan where lung ventilation (revealed by inhaled radiolabelled gases or aerosols) is compared with perfusion (revealed by intravenous contrast). Areas of mismatached ventilation and perfusion are suggestive of pulmonary embolism
V-P shunt	**Ventriculoperitoneal shunt**	For decompressing the forebrain in hydrocephalus
VSD	**Ventriculoseptal defect**	A hole through the intraventricular septum connecting the right and the left sides of the heart
VT	**Ventricular tachycardia**	A broad-complex tachycardia which may produce a pulse or produce cardiac arrest. If pulseless it requires electrical cardioversion, if associated with a pulse then either electricity or some drugs (such as amiodarone) can be used
WBC	**White blood cell [count]**	See WCC
WCC	**White cell count**	Part of the full blood count which measures the blood leucocyte concentration. Usually supplied along with a differential expressing the concentrations of different cell types
WPW	**Wolff-Parkinson-White syndrome**	A cardiac syndrome where an accessory pathway between the atria and ventricles causes early depolarisation of the ventricles, giving a shortened PR interval and delta-wave upstroke at the beginning of the QRS complexes

Table of normal values

Note – normal values differ by race, region, nationally, and internationally, and local 'normals' should always be checked.

Full blood count (FBC)		
Haemoglobin	Hb	Men 13–18 g/dL; women 11.5–16 g/dL
Mean corpuscular volume	MCV	76–96 fL
White blood cell count	WBC/WCC	(4–11) × 10^9/L
Platelet count	Plts	(150–400) × 10^9/L

Urea and electrolytes (U&Es)		
Sodium	Na^+	135–145 mmol/L
Potassium	K^+	3.5–5 mmol/L
Urea	Ur	2–6 mmol/L
Creatinine	Cr	70–110 μmol/L

Liver function Tests (LFTs)		
Bilirubin	Bili	3–15 μmol/L
Alkaline phosphatase	ALP	30–120 IU/L
Alanine transferase	ALT	5–35 IU/L
Albumin	Alb	35–50 g/L

Other tests		
Amylase	Amy	0–180 IU/dL
Creatinine kinase	CK	25–195 IU/L
C-reactive protein	CRP	<10 mg/L
Troponin T	Trop T	<0.04 μg/L
Total cholesterol	Chol	<5 mmol/L
Corrected calcium	CCa^{2+}	2.2–2.6 mmol/L
Thyroid-stimulating hormone	TSH	0.5–5 mU/L
Total thyroxine	T_4	70–140 mmol/L
Chloride	Cl^-	98–108 mmol/L
D-dimer		0.0–0.5 μg/mL
Erythrocyte sedimentation rate	ESR	Depends on age—conventionally worked out by: (age × 2)/10 mm/hour
Prostate-specific antigen	PSA	<4 ng/mL

Arterial blood gas (ABG)		
pH	pH	7.35–7.45
Partial pressure of carbon dioxide	pCO_2	4.5–6 kPa
Partial pressure of oxygen	pO_2	10–13 kPa
Bicarbonate	HCO_3^-	22–28 mmol/L
Base excess	BE	±2 mmol/L
Lactate		<2 mmol/L

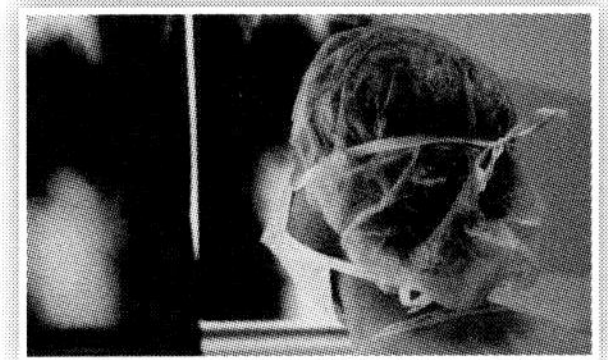
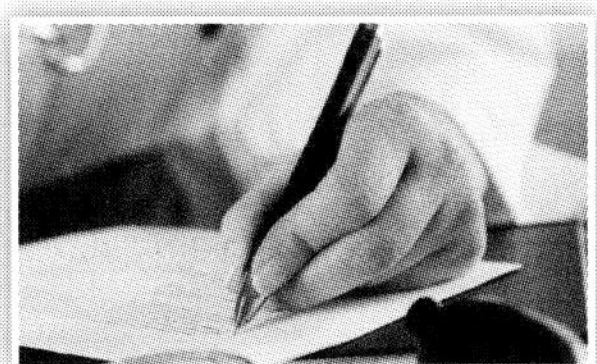
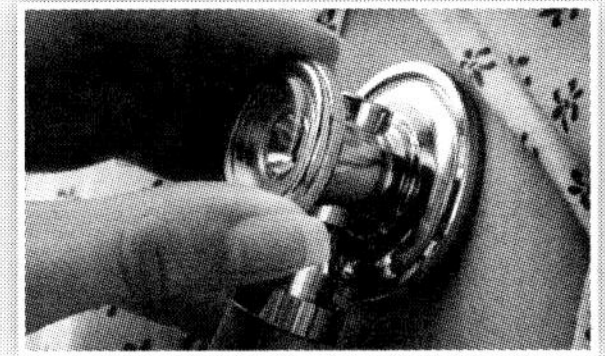
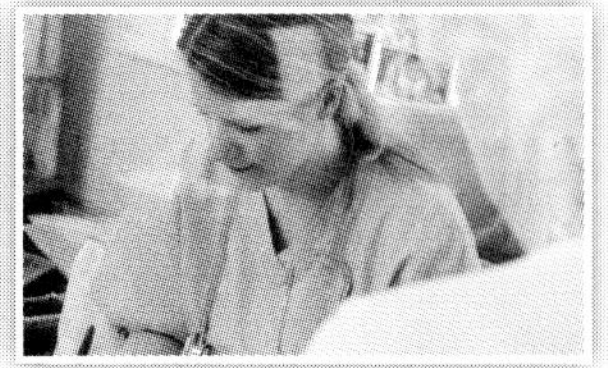

Introducing clinical medicine in practice

Recognizing and resuscitating the acutely unwell patient

'I grieve to tell you that I hear this morning that your mama is very ill'... 'She is very dangerously ill', she added... 'She is dead'

(Mrs Creakle to David Copperfield in *David Copperfield* by Charles Dickens)

Failure to recognize acutely unwell patients within hospital is a major cause of unnecessary death and admission to the ITU. The majority of cardiac arrests occurring in hospital are preceded by a period of clinical deterioration, offering a window of opportunity to intervene with prompt appropriate management to prevent a loss of circulation, which carries a very poor prognosis. Therefore although the majority of patients in hospital are clinically stable or improving, a proportion will be extremely unwell and require urgent resuscitation. As a student, if you go to see a patient who suddenly deteriorates or is acutely unwell on your arrival at their bedside you should immediately request that a doctor or nurse reviews the patient—patient safety is always the first priority in hospital. This section offers a brief guide to assessing and resuscitating patients based on an 'ABCDE' approach advocated by the resuscitation council in the UK.

Response

Always make a vigorous attempt to rouse any patient who appears collapsed. The AVPU score is used to assess a basic level of consciousness (and is quicker to calculate than the Glasgow Coma Score). The assessor works through the patient's level of consciousness from fully **Alert**, through to responsive to **Voice** (shouting 'open your eyes!'), to responsive to **Pain**ful stimuli (such as a vigorous sternal rub or pressure applied to a nailbed), to **Unresponsive** to any of these stimuli. Responses may be verbal (speech or verbal noises), eye responses (eyes opening to command), or motor (responds by lifting limb or hand):

- **A** Alert
- **V** Responds to **V**oice
- **P** Responds to **P**ain
- **U** **U**nresponsive

Patients who are unresponsive require rapid opening of the airway and assessment (for no more than 10 seconds) for signs of life—by **looking** for chest wall movements, **listening** for breath sounds, and **feeling** for a pulse. If there are no signs of life then this is a cardiac arrest and the cardiac arrest team should be summoned immediately whilst basic life support is initiated.

Airway

Assessment

No further assessment is necessary in a patient who is alert and talking.
Two groups of patients require urgent assessment and management of their airway:

1. Those who are obviously struggling to breathe, with signs of airway compromise include snoring, choking, stridor (a harsh upper airways noise heard during inspiration), abdominal breathing, and cyanosis.
2. Patients who are unresponsive. The reflexes which preserve airway integrity (against airway collapse or aspiration) are only maintained with a level of consciousness above 8/15 on the Glasgow Coma Scale. Below this patients need careful airway management to maintain their safety.

To assess the patient's airway, perform a head-tilt and chin-lift procedure, extending the neck, which will lift the tongue off the palate and maintain patency of the airway. Be very careful in patients with suspected cervical spine injuries—if there is any doubt about the stability of the cervical spine then get an assistant to hold the neck steady whilst performing only a jaw-thrust manoeuvre. Look in the mouth and use a suction device to remove any secretions. Use McGill's forceps to remove any foreign bodies if they are clearly visible.

Management

For an airway to be completely secured it must be both **maintained** (to protect it against collapse and allow breathing to continue) and **protected** (to prevent the oesophageal contents from entering the trachea). One or both of these aims can be achieved by:

- **Airway manoeuvres:** Simple head-tilt/chin-lift or jaw-thrust procedures can be used to maintain the airway. They are useful over short periods of time—for instance in general anaesthesia, after the patient is anaesthetized but before they are intubated. These manoeuvres maintain the patency of the airway but do not protect against aspiration and are obviously dependent on an experienced operator to maintain them.
- **Airway adjuncts:** An **oropharyngeal airway** (**'Guedel airway'**) or **nasopharyngeal airway** maintains the patency of the airway but does not protect it against aspiration. Oropharyngeal airways are poorly tolerated by patients with intermediate levels of consciousness, and often cannot be inserted into patients having tonic-clonic seizures whose jaws may be clamped shut, meaning that nasopharyngeal airways are often preferred. **Laryngeal mask airways** (LMAs) contain an inflatable cuff that maintains the position of the airway against the pharyngeal inlet but do not reliably protect against aspiration.
- **Definitive airways:** A definitive airway, which both allows easy respiration and protects against aspiration, is either an **endotracheal tube** or a **tracheostomy**, with the cuff of the device inflated within the trachea (preventing secretions or gastric contents from bypassing and entering the lungs). Endotracheal intubation is generally preferred, with tracheostomy only being performed when intubation is impossible (e.g. in the case of severe airway burns or a laryngeal foreign body), or where a protected airway will be required for a long period of time (for instance in patients in the ITU who will require prolonged ventilation). Endotracheal intubation can only be performed on patients who are either unresponsive (for instance in cardiac arrest) or in patients who are both anaesthetized and pharmacologically paralysed. Patients requiring emergency ventilation (for instance in severe asthma) therefore need to be both anaesthetized (often using a short-acting agent like propofol) and paralysed (using a short-acting paralytic agent like suxamethonium) within a short space of time—this is called **rapid sequence induction** of anaesthesia, which even when performed by an experienced anaesthetist carries a risk of aspiration.

Breathing

Assessment

Once the patient's airway is secured, assess their breathing. A brief assessment includes observation of:

- **Respiration rate:** The normal rate is 12–20 breaths per minute. **Tachypnoea**, a raised respiratory rate, is a sensitive but poorly specific marker of acute illness. **Bradypnoea**, a reduced respiratory rate, is a late, sinister sign in the acutely ill patient, and is also caused by opiate toxicity.
- **Oxygen saturations:** Normal oxygen saturations are 94% or above, but patients with chronic respiratory failure, for instance chronic obstructive pulmonary disease (COPD), may often have

saturations between 88 and 92%, and additional oxygen can cause them to retain carbon dioxide and become seriously unwell.

- **Pattern of respiration:** Look for signs of respiratory distress, including an inability to speak in sentences, use of accessory muscles, tracheal tug, cyanosis and sweating—patients displaying any of these features are likely to be extremely unwell and require rapid intervention.
- **Breath sounds:** Perform a rapid assessment of the patient's breathing—not a full respiratory examination but a quick check to ensure that breath sounds are equal throughout both lungs and to assess for wheeze and crackles. If you have a patient who is exhibiting signs of respiratory compromise this should be enough to suggest the likely underlying reason—for instance, tension pneumothorax, exacerbation of asthma, large pleural effusion, pulmonary oedema, or, in the absence of signs on chest examination, pulmonary embolus or a metabolic cause of breathlessness (e.g. diabetic ketoacidosis).

Interventions

Oxygen: Guidelines from the British Thoracic Society suggest giving oxygen therapy to acutely unwell adults only when hypoxia is present (see http://www.brit-thoracic.org.uk/clinical-information/emergency-oxygen/emergency-oxygen-use-in-adult-patients.aspx). Target saturations should be 94–98% in most patients, or 88–92% in those at risk of carbon dioxide retention. However, many resuscitation programmes still teach that high-flow oxygen is the first line of treatment for almost all acutely unwell patients and this approach is still widely practiced. Ventilatory failure is signalled by poorly correcting hypoxia, worsening hypercapnia, and acidaemia. These are the indications for assisted ventilation, whether that be invasive (via an endotracheal tube) or non-invasive (using a tight-fitting face mask—most commonly bilevel positive airways pressure ventilation (BiPAP), commonly performed on respiratory and acute care wards).

Other emergency measures: These include nebulizers and bronchodilators for severe asthma, chest drains or emergency needle decompression for pneumothorax (or effusions), and appropriate management for other conditions such as intravenous nitrates and diuretics for pulmonary oedema. An emergency (portable) chest X-ray and arterial blood gas analysis are almost obligatory at this stage.

Circulation

Assessment

Pulse: A normal heart rate is between 60 and 100 beats per minute. If the peripheral pulse is of low volume, then palpate a central pulse such as the carotid or femoral. The radial pulse is 'lost' at about 90–100 mmHg, the femoral pulse is difficult to palpate at pressures below 70 mmHg.

Blood pressure: Hypotension is a worrying sign in an acutely unwell patient, representing cardiovascular decompensation (usually vasoconstriction and tachycardia are used by the body to maintain blood pressure within a normal range). A normal systolic blood pressure may be as low as 90 mmHg in fit young people (especially women), with the definition of 'shock' being based on blood pressure inadequate to maintain tissue perfusion—for instance where there is confusion (cerebral hypoperfusion) or oliguria (renal hypoperfusion). A sudden drop in blood pressure may also be significant—if the patient's systolic blood pressure is usually 180 mmHg and now is only 110 mmHg this may still reflect that the patient is significantly unwell.

Capillary refill time: This is performed with the hand held at the level of the heart. The nail bed is pressed for 5 seconds and then the time taken for colour to return to it is assessed. This should usually be less than 2 seconds—a prolonged capillary refill time may be indicative of hypovolaemia.

Hands: These may be hot and sweaty in sepsis, cool in hypovolaemia, and cold and clammy in conditions raising sympathetic tone, for instance myocardial infarction.

Interventions

Venous cannulation: This is crucial in any acutely unwell patient. If it is likely that the patient will need large amounts of fluid (for instance if haemorrhage is suspected) then two large-bore cannulae should be inserted. Blood should be drawn for routine tests including full blood count, urea and electrolytes, liver function tests, clotting, glucose, and, if appropriate, group and save or cross-match.

Cardiac monitoring: Most modern defibrillators are able to monitor cardiac rhythm as well as offering DC cardioversion through the same pads. In acutely unwell patients these leads should be applied to the chest and the heart rhythm monitored on the screen. A rhythm strip can be printed off to examine the rhythm more closely, and at this point it may be appropriate to obtain a 12-lead ECG.

Intravenous fluids: These are often indicated when patients are acutely unwell, particularly if clinical assessment suggests they are shocked or hypovolaemic. Caution should be exercised if there is evidence of fluid overload (for instance crackles at the lung bases or a raised JVP), or if there is the potential for the heart being unable to cope with increased fluid loads—for instance, in acute myocardial infarction, in patients with known heart failure, or in patients with a dysrhythmia when the cardiac rhythm is assessed.

Other interventions: Algorithms exist for the assessment and treatment of tachy- and bradyarrythmias, using cardioactive medications (e.g. amiodarone or beta-blockers), or electricity (for instance DC cardioversion or electrical pacing). For detailed information on the use of these interventions see the Advanced Life Support algorithms available from the Resuscitation Council's website at http://www.resus.org.uk/pages/mediMain.htm.

Disability

Assessment

Level of consciousness can be assessed using the AVPU score explained above, or using the **Glasgow Coma Score (GCS)**:

Eyes	Voice	Motor
4 Opens eyes spontaneously 3 Opens eyes in response to voice 2 Opens eyes in response to pain 1 Does not open eyes	5 Orientated and appropriate 4 Confused conversation 3 Inappropriate speech—random words 2 Incomprehensible words—moans and groans 1 No verbal response	6 Obeys commands 5 Localizes to pain 4 Withdraws from pain 3 Abnormal flexor response to pain 2 Extensor response to pain 1 No response to pain

Pupils should be equal and reactive to light. There are various causes for fixed and dilated pupils including raised intracranial pressure, toxins, or direct pressure on particular cranial nerves. Pinpoint pupils may indicate narcotic overdose or a brainstem stroke.

A full examination of the **peripheral nervous system** will be impossible in an unresponsive patient. However, a brief assessment of tone, reflexes, and especially the plantar reflexes may suggest acute stroke as the cause in an obtunded patient.

Capillary blood glucose: Hypoglycaemia is a simply remedied cause of acute deterioration which should be considered in all patients. Intravenous or buccal glucose should be given without delay. The cause of hypoglycaemia should always be sought and corrected or removed.

Interventions

Care for the comatose patient: Comatose patients should be managed in the lateral position to prevent aspiration in the event of vomiting if their airway has not been secured. CT scanning of the head is indicated in all patients with an acute deterioration of level of consciousness unless a precipitating cause is obvious. Often a rapid assessment needs to made about the appropriateness of escalating care—for instance, in a 90-year-old patient who has been resuscitated following cardiac arrest after 40 minutes of CPR, and who has a GCS of 3/15 the probability of significant neurological recovery is slim. Rather than intubate and take the patient to ITU, a palliative approach may be more appropriate.

Exposure

Assessment

Full examination is a mandatory part of assessing an acutely unwell patient. Pull back the patient's bed-clothes and examine them from head to feet. Look for wounds, oedema, melaena, bleeding, ulcers, rashes, and signs of deep vein thrombosis.

Interventions

Ensure the patient is as comfortable as possible. Wrap them up again and keep them warm, maintaining their dignity. Patients with reduced consciousness require regular turning by nursing staff to prevent the development of pressure sores.

History taking

Listen to the patient. He is telling you the diagnosis

(Credited to Sir William Osler, 1849–1919)

Taking a history fulfils two fundamental functions. The first is to obtain a large proportion of the information necessary to make a diagnosis. The second is to build up a strong, working relationship between you and the patient—the 'clinical relationship'. By building rapport and trust with a patient, the clinician is able to ask intimate and difficult questions, perform examination and procedures on the patient, and negotiate therapeutic interventions. A poor relationship excludes any such negotiation or interventions.

It is said that as much as 70–80% of a diagnosis is based on the history. You will need to think of all the relevant differential diagnoses, and include and exclude them with your questioning. This is difficult for the novice but as your knowledge improves, you will find your line of questioning will also become more diagnostic.

As a trainee you should take every opportunity to strengthen your communication and clinical skills. Below we have tried to include some hints and aids to help you to take a history from the patient.

It is customary to divide the history under the following headings.

Presenting complaint (PC)

This should be summed up in as few words as possible, if appropriate adding a duration of time. Some are obvious, e.g. 'chest pain' or 'diarrhoea and vomiting', but some are more vague—'generally unwell for several weeks'. In very complex cases it is sometimes necessary to break the presenting complaint into several problems.

History of the presenting complaint (HPC)

The aim here is to get an accurate picture of exactly what has been happening, and what might be the underlying cause(s). There are several things that must be included here—in the acutely ill patient, we have found this opening to be a useful start to the HPC: 'So tell me when were you last well? How have things progressed since then?'

- **Exactly what has been going on:** What? How much? For how long? All the time or does it come and go? Is it triggered by anything?
- In the case of pain, the acronym SOCRATES ensures most things are covered (**S**ite, **O**nset, **C**haracter, **R**adiation, **A**lleviating factors, **T**ime course, **E**xacerbating factors, and **S**everity).
- Each system has its own individual set of questions that you will need to learn over time. These are included at the start of each unit. The best way of learning them and the questions that flow from them is practice!

By the end of the HPC you should have a differential diagnosis. The rest of the history will help you include or exclude these diagnoses. Over time you will find your approach to this part of the history will mature and change but we would highly recommend you follow this time-honoured approach until you are fluent in all of these areas.

Past medical history (PMHx)

Asking an initial question like 'Have you got any other medical problems', followed if necessary with 'Have you ever been admitted to hospital' or 'Have you ever had any operations', will usually generate a list of all of the patient's problems. Experience will help you decide where you need to ask a few more questions about particular illnesses to clarify their severity and their implications for the current problem. In particular, ask for more details about:

- **Diseases affecting the same organ system as the current problem:** If the patient presents with shortness of breath then it is necessary to take a full history of any cardiac disease and any respiratory disease. Acute shortness of breath in someone with no previous medical history is very different from acute shortness of breath in someone who has ischaemic heart disease or who has regular asthma attacks.

- **Chronic diseases:** Patients are commonly admitted to hospital with exacerbations of chronic diseases such as COPD or congestive cardiac failure (CCF). The following questions are useful to give an idea of the severity of the chronic condition and how it affects the patient:

> **Generic questions** to ask of a patient with a long-term condition, e.g. diabetes mellitus, epilepsy, ischaemic heart disease, or rheumatoid arthritis:
>
> (1) When, where, how, and why was it originally diagnosed?
>
> (2) How has it progressed since?
>
> (3) How is it normally controlled?—Who cares for you? Where? How often do you see them? How do you monitor the control? What medications do you take? Do you have any problems with them?
>
> (4) What is the best and the worst it has ever been? Have you ever been admitted to hospital? If so, have you ever been in intensive care?
>
> (5) How is your illness today compared with your best and worst?

- **Patients with a malignancy:** How has it been managed—surgery, chemotherapy, radiotherapy, or no active treatment? What were they told about the prognosis of the cancer? Are they being currently treated for it or monitored for recurrence? If so, by whom and where?

Drug history (DHx)

Ask about **regular medications**, including doses. Learn to use the abbreviations 'od', 'bd', 'tds', 'qds', and 'prn' (once, twice, three times, and four times per day, and 'as required', respectively). If it is relevant, ask about adherence—for instance, an exacerbation of an inflammatory disease like Crohn's disease may be caused by the patient having stopped their immunomodulatory medication.

Drug allergies: Ask what actually happens if the patient is given the medication . A clear history of serious symptoms, e.g. symptoms suggestive of anaphylaxis (such as facial swelling or difficulty in breathing) mean that the drug should never be given again. Mild symptoms such as nausea or a rash may not be a contraindication to giving the drug again, especially if it is vital to therapy. (Note: 'no known drug allergies' is shortened to NKDA.)

Family history (FHx)

A positive family history in first-degree relatives is important in many conditions, e.g. premature death in vascular disease, malignancies such as colonic cancer, or autoimmune disease, e.g. Graves' disease.

Social history (SHx)

This should give you a picture of the patient's normal quality of life and degree of independence. It should include any dependants, carers, and other support. This is vital when planning the patient's discharge, and is of particular importance with those who have significant disability, either on admission or as a result of their illness.

The social history should also include occupation and common lifestyle choices, e.g. cigarette smoking, alcohol consumption, illicit drug taking, exercise, and hobbies.

Social background

Who does the patient live with? What kind of accommodation is it? What is their usual level of mobility? Are they able to care for themselves? Do they have carers or family who help them with at home, and if so how often?

Risk factors

For all patients ask about:

- **Smoking**—quantify in terms of pack-years (1 pack-year is smoking on average 20 cigarettes per day for 1 year—if they smoke 40 cigarettes per day for 1 year they would have a 2-pack-years smoking history).
- **Alcohol**—work out the number of units drunk per week on average. To do this, find out the kind of drink they prefer to drink and their usual pattern of drinking—do they drink the same amount each day, or have heavy binges? Consult the table below, but remember to also ask about other types of drink too.

Drink	Quantity	Units
Beer/cider (4%)	Pint or 500 ml can	2 units
'Super strength' beer/cider (7–8%)	Pint or 500 ml can	4 units
'Alcopop' (5.5%)	Bottle (275 ml)	2 units
Wine (10–14%)	Standard glass (175 ml)	2 units
	Bottle (750 ml)	7–10 units
Spirits (40%)	Single measure (25 ml)	1 unit
	Bottle (1 L)	40 units

Recommended allowances: men less than 21 units per week; women less than 14 units per week.

If appropriate ask about **illicit drug use**, and whether they have ever used drugs intravenously. It may also be relevant to ask about **foreign travel**, particularly if the patient presents with potentially infective symptoms such as fever or diarrhoea. With other presentations, the patient's **occupation** may be relevant—for instance, a history of asbestos exposure is relevant in any older person presenting with breathlessness and weight loss.

Review of symptoms/systemic review (ROS)

Even in patients with single pathologies, e.g. asthma, it is important to make a brief systemic review. This includes bowels, micturition, weight, appetite, sleep, general well-being, and mood. In complex or non-specific presentations it is often necessary to ask a detailed set of questions in every system. In such cases this may be included in the history of the presenting complaint.

There may be **other issues**: for example , if a patient presents with features suggestive of an infectious disease (for instance HIV, TB, or acute viral hepatitis), then you may also need to ask about household contacts or sexual partners with similar symptoms.

Sum up and address concerns

Next you will move on to examine the patient, but before doing so, feed back to them what they have said. Summarize the information you have gained from them, and give them the chance to amend or correct any mistakes you have made. Ask how they are feeling and what worries they have.

If appropriate this may be a good place in which to take a **spiritual history**, especially if the patient is suffering from a serious, terminal, or very disabling condition. A spiritual history opens up how the patient is coping with their condition and how they fit the suffering they are enduring with their view of the world. Proceed sensitively and gently—your job is not to force your beliefs onto patients, but to give them the chance to talk about the impact of illness on their life if they want to do so.

We end this section by showing some useful styles to use within your clerking:

- **Use open questions at first:** 'So what has been the problem?'.
- **Empathize:** 'That must have been really scary'.
- **Make sure you have covered everything:** 'Have you noticed anything else that we haven't covered?'.
- **Sum up:** 'So for about a week you've noticed...'.

In the 19th century the TB physician Dr Edward Trudeau summed up the work of doctor as 'to cure sometimes, to relieve often, to comfort always'. Take time as a medical student not just to study diseases, but to engage with patients as individuals. You are often the only member of the healthcare team who has the time to sit down properly and talk with patients, so use the opportunity well. Try to develop into someone who can comfort as well as cure.

Examination

Observe, record, tabulate, communicate. Use your five senses. ...Learn to see, learn to hear, learn to feel, learn to smell, and know that by practice alone you can become expert.

(William Osler, 1849-1919)

Clinical examination is the first and primary way of obtaining objective information about the state of your patient's health. Any symptoms that they mention whilst taking the history are necessarily subjective. They will be influenced by your knowledge and communication skills, what the patient chooses to mention, how accurate they are at describing their problems, and what their ideas, concerns, and expectations are. Some patients will play down symptoms whilst others will be far more histrionic. The skill of a good clinician is to make sense of the information they have gathered, formulate a diagnosis, and then examine the patient to prove or refute their differential diagnoses.

In theory, clinical signs available through examination should be objective. In practice, the signs elicited may vary greatly due to the clinical environment and the technical skills and specialty of the examining doctor. Always bear in mind that the clinical condition of patients may change, and, as they do, their signs may alter greatly.

The aim of this section is to give a basic introduction to the skill of examination. It will introduce the components of a general examination of your patient. Each unit introduction will then give detailed information on how to perform particular examinations related to that speciality.

Aims

The aim of performing a clinical examination is not to produce an isolated list of findings. Rather, it is to produce a structured story by the end of which the doctor to whom you are presenting can say to you, 'so it sounds as if they have ...'. A good examination should fit tightly with the history you have just taken from your patient. For example, you may have taken a history from an elderly person complaining of fevers, breathlessness, and a productive cough, which have developed over the past week. You suspect a community-acquired pneumonia. Key items in the examination will then be:

- **Supportive evidence:** A full sputum pot by the bedside, a raised temperature, high respiratory and heart rates, and signs of regional consolidation in the chest.
- **Contradictory evidence:** No signs of infection, with a clear chest and no respiratory signs at all. Alternatively, signs of infection but evidence that it may be located in a different body system—for instance an obviously infected leg ulcer, or lower abdominal tenderness with a large palpable bladder.
- **Evidence of severity:** The patient may seem very well, have vital signs within normal ranges, and demonstrate only slight crackles at one of their lung bases. Alternatively, they might be very septic, tachycardic, and tachypnoeic, with evidence of dehydration and with extensive bilateral crackles and bronchial breathing.
- **Evidence of additional disease processes:** The patient may appear otherwise well. They may have evidence of neurological disease, suggesting aspiration as a potential cause for their pneumonia. There may be a hyperinflated chest with wheeze, suggestive of underlying COPD. There may be cachexia not explained by anything in the history, suggesting a possible lung cancer as a cause for the pneumonia.

The examination should be presented systematically, beginning with a general description of the patient and then proceeding to describe signs found in the different systems in an orderly way. Words like 'however...', or 'surprisingly...', can give the person you are presenting to an indication that what you are about to say does not quite correlate with what may be expected from the information you have already given.

By the end of your examination, you should be able to form an impression of what is wrong with your patient. This need not be a full diagnosis, and may include several differentials that require that results of investigations before a final decision. However, you should be able to gauge roughly how unwell the patient is and what kind of problems they are most likely to have.

Approaching the clinical examination

Medical schools initially teach students to examine each body system independently. Clinical assessments such as the **Objective Structured Clinical Examination** (OSCE), often assess students' ability to examine these systems (or parts of the system) in isolation. Once you have perfected the fundamental techniques within each system, it is important to try to join these individual system-based examinations together, in a holistic, comprehensive, and clinically relevant assessment.

Certain things must necessarily precede any useful clinical examination. You should be dressed appropriately for the clinical areas, with minimal jewellery, and look and smell clean! You should wash/clean your hands appropriately with soap and water or alcohol gel between each patient contact. You may need a chaperone if you are examining a patient of the opposite sex or performing an intimate examination, such as a digital rectal examination.

Get into the habit of performing these actions whenever you examine a patient on the wards and doing things properly and thoroughly every time:

- **Introduce yourself:** greet the patient, explain who you are and why you wish to examine them, explain what you will be doing, and obtain their consent.
- **Expose the patient:** first draw the curtains completely around the bed. Ask them to remove their shirt or hospital gown to reveal their upper body (women can generally leave their bra in place). Place a blanket or towel over their legs and lower abdomen to maintain dignity, and try if possible to ask them to expose only one part of themselves at a time. Cover the chest again before moving on to examine the abdomen.
- **Position the patient:** they should be initially positioned sitting back at 45° with their legs straight and uncrossed.
- **Adjust the environment if necessary:** ensure you have adequate lighting. Try to reduce noise and distractions on the ward if possible.

The general examination

We have used the following schema to help all novice clinicians through the complexities of the general clinical examination:

1. **Well or unwell?** What are your initial thoughts as you approach the patient? If unwell, are they seriously ill? Think more about this—why do you say they look unwell? Are they struggling to breathe? Are they confused? Always ask at this stage whether it is safe to continue or whether you should ask for help first.
2. **'Feet to face' assessment**—after introducing yourself and gaining consent, stand at the patient's feet. Take 30 seconds or so to observe the patient from their feet, their lower limbs, their abdomen, chest, and neck, up to their face. **'Seek and ye shall find'**—if you look for things, they will appear. If you just stare you will miss the possible clues that are staring you in the face.
3. **Vital signs**—look at the monitors and the charts at the end of the bed, and mentally record the vital signs. These include the blood pressure (BP), heart rate (HR), temperature (temp), O_2 saturations (sats), respiratory rate (RR), level of consciousness (the Glasgow Coma Scale may be used to objectively record the patient's level of consciousness; see Unit 6), and capillary blood glucose (CBG).
4. **'Clinical clues'**—look around both sides of the bed; take an interest in the infusions, the drug and fluid charts, the mobility aids, the drains and urinary catheter. Are there any inhalers or other medications on the bedside table? What's in the sputum pot? Are there any other charts, e.g. peak flow, capillary blood glucose, stool, dietary intake?

These four steps should take a minute or two at most but they may give you the important starting points on which to base the speed and content of your examination.

The general examination is something that will often given you a huge amount of information about the patient, but which can seem so obvious that people neglect to notice it. Always perform a full general examination, and *never be afraid to state the obvious*! After performing your four generic steps, the general examination traditionally starts at the hands working up the upper limbs, to the face and then down to the neck, chest, abdomen, and legs.

Hands

Look at the dorsum of the hands whilst supporting the patient's palms. Look at the nails. Are they abnormal? Is there clubbing, koilonychia, onycholysis? Are the nails dirty, painted, bitten, dystrophic? The nails are a useful source of information—ignore them at your peril!.

Ask the patient to turn their hands over. Look at the palms—is there wasting, palmar erythema, Dupuytrens' contracture? Are they cyanosed or pale?

Feel the patient's palms. Are they cold and clammy? This may suggest an increased sympathetic tone (causing vasoconstriction and sweating); a common cause of this is cardiac ischaemia. Are the palms hot and sweaty, due to vasodilatation, suggesting sepsis?

Pulse and blood pressure

At the radial pulse comment on the **rate**, **regularity**, **volume**, and **symmetry** between the left and right radial pulse. (The character of the pulse should be assessed at a central pulse). A strong, fast, bounding pulse may signify sepsis, carbon dioxide retention, or thyrotoxicosis. Low volume or poorly palpable pulses may be normal but may reveal shock, dehydration, or aortic stenosis. A systolic blood pressure below 90 mmHg (in an unwell patient) requires urgent attention and should be brought to the attention of a doctor.

Face

Does the patient have a classical facial appearance suggestive of a given condition, e.g. hypothyroidism, Cushing's disease, Down's syndrome, or mitral valve disease? What is the pattern and condition of their hair?

Look in and around the eyes. Is there evidence of xanthelasma? The sclera may reveal pallor or jaundice. Look for abnormalities of the pupils and eye movement. Are the corneas normal?

Check the mouth for the patient's dentition, evidence of oral ulceration, or of certain dietary deficiencies. Look at the tongue—is there evidence of candidiasis, ulceration, or tumour? Look under the tongue for evidence of central cyanosis.

Neck

There are for four key things to assess in the neck (a description of each can be found in the relevant units):

- the **regional lymph nodes**
- the **carotid artery**
- the **trachea**
- the **jugular venous pressure (JVP)**.

Where appropriate, assessment of a neck mass or goitre should also be undertaken.

Fluid status

Assessment of a patient's fluid status is an essential skill to master, especially in the acutely sick patient. A simple rule of thumb is 'what goes in, must come out'. As always a careful history, examination, and interpretation of investigation results should form the basis of your assessment:

- **History:** Thirst and poor urine output are useful symptoms of dehydration. Acutely ill patients may have had poor oral intake for several days; added to this they may have had further fluid loss through sweat (if pyrexial), vomiting, and/or diarrhoea. Post-operative patients will also lose fluid through wound drains and bleeding.
- **Examination:** Signs of dehydration or hypovolaemia include cool, poorly perfused peripheries, wrinkled skin with decreased turgor, axillary dryness, a reduced or 'absent' JVP, and dry mucous membranes (but beware mouth breathers who always have a dry mouth). Objective signs include hypotension, tachycardia, a reduced CVP, and oliguria/anuria. Signs of fluid overload include a high JVP or CVP, fine inspiratory crackles at both lung bases, and peripheral oedema.
- **Investigations:** Pre-renal impairment (as seen in dehydration and hypovolaemia) is signified by a high urea:creatinine ratio (see Unit 4). Likewise fluid overload may be apparent on a chest X-ray (see Unit 1).

Examinations of the individual systems are described in the relevant units, but, as previously stated, a clinically appropriate, holistic assessment should be attempted on each of the patients that you clerk.

Forming a clinical impression

Once you eliminate the impossible, whatever remains, no matter how improbable, must be the truth

(Sherlock Holmes in *A Scandal in Bohemia* **by Arthur Conan Doyle)**

Clinical diagnostic reasoning, i.e. how one arrives at a diagnosis, is a complex and multifaceted skill that takes most of us a lifetime to learn. It starts by being able to put together your initial clinical 'hunches' about a patient, the history and clinical signs you elicit, and their investigation results. Your 'clinical intuition' will be strengthened by reading around the patients and their pathologies, and by practising your clinical skills. But perhaps most importantly these are all informed by observation and feedback from peers, patients, and senior medical staff.

Clerking a patient should lead you to a '**clinical impression**'—what you think is wrong with the patient and why. Think about the facts. What diagnosis, or diagnoses, do they support? It is best to form this impression before looking in the clinical notes, and before reviewing the investigation results. Investigations should rarely make the diagnosis; they should confirm what is already suspected, or reveal the extent of problems.

Forming an impression involves working through the following steps:

- **Identify the main medical problem(s) leading to the patient's presentation:** This is often an expansion of the presenting complaint. Be aware that this may develop and change as the patient repeats and reflects on their problems.
- **Form a differential diagnosis:** In some cases there is an obvious, single pathology causing the patient's presentation, e.g. asthma attack, axillary abscess, or urinary tract infection. However, other presentations may be more complex and difficult to quantify, In these cases it may be more appropriate to write their symptoms and a differential diagnosis, e.g. 'chronic cough, fever, night sweats, and gross weight loss - ?TB, ?lung cancer'. This differential will become better informed the better your clinical knowledge, skills, and experience.
- **Identify severity:** Is this someone who needs to be rapidly assessed by a senior clinician or do you think they can go home? Do they need further investigations as an in-patient or an out-patient?
- **Identify other issues:** As well as multiple medical problems, patients may have important social issues that have an impact on their health and well-being; it is important to include any such issues in your problem list. For example, a 43-year-old man presents in the Emergency Department with a large upper GI bleed. He has known chronic alcoholic liver disease with tense ascites and a deranged INR. He is of no fixed abode. His problem list would include:

  (1) Upper GI bleed, ?oesophageal varices

  (2) Decompensated chronic alcoholic liver disease with tense ascites and impaired coagulation

  (3) Homeless—needs social services review

It is essential to revise and review your clinical impressions of the patient as more clinical facts become apparent, whilst not forgetting the initial problems and investigation results.

How to present patients to senior colleagues

There is no more difficult art to acquire than the art of observation, and for some men it is quite as difficult to record an observation in brief and plain language.

(William Osler, 1849–1919)

As a student you have to make the most of all learning opportunities. Always take opportunities to present formally to your seniors during quiet moments—sometimes consultants or other team members will arrange special teaching sessions for this purpose. The chance to talk through a history and examination, picking out important things, being asked to explain points, and then being challenged about future management of the patient is invaluable.

There are two types of case presentation. The '**teaching presentation**' is an all-inclusive presentation of the history, examination, and investigation findings, culminating with a well-constructed conclusion. You will be expected to utilize this type of presentation during teaching sessions. You need to present a comprehensive, chronological case report, trying to demonstrate to the audience your diagnostic reasoning, This kind of presentation is also used at academic meetings such as hospital grand rounds and conferences.

The second type is the '**business presentation**', utilized on busy ward rounds. The aim is to convey all the key points of the clerking in a few well-chosen sentences. If done well, the other members of the ward round are presented with a *fait accompli*, with which they should concur. This interaction is rapid and is learnt over many years on rounds. You will initially find it very difficult to master, but will improve with experience and knowledge. On business rounds listen to the way experienced doctors discuss cases. The good ones are focused, succinct, and quickly include and exclude relevant diagnoses with sharp and incisive comments. Try to get involved by clerking patients and asking to present them in this style. Presenting like this will force you to prioritize information and hone your diagnostic reasoning.

Both presenting styles share key principles :

- Always structure your presentation in terms of **history**, **examination**, and **investigations**, and conclude by outlining the current **management plan**. Finish one before starting the next and introduce the next section as you begin. 'This is a 43-year-old woman who presented with a history of .... On examination she had .... Blood tests revealed ... and chest x-ray showed .... She has been managed with ...'.
- Try to pack information into each sentence: 'a 24-year-old shop assistant presenting generally unwell with a 2-day history of pyrexia, dysuria, and now worsening flank pain'.
- Give people summaries of what is about to come next: 'examination was unremarkable, with a clear chest, normal heart sounds and soft non-tender abdomen'.

Example format for 'business' presentations

- **Demographics**: Age, sex, ethnicity, occupation.
- **Presenting complaint**: Just a few words needed.
- **Relevant background**: Any important factors from elsewhere in the history that directly impact on the presentation.
- **History of presenting complaint**: A few sentences. Only mention *relevant* negatives.
- **Past medical history**: Only dwell on conditions likely to affect diagnosis or management.
- **Drug history**: Often no need to read them all out. Mention key ones relevant to the presentation, e.g. warfarin or NSAIDs in a patient presenting with haemorrhage.
- **Family history**: Only if relevant.
- **Social history**: Give a one-sentence description of where the patient lives and how independent they are. Mention briefly tobacco and alcohol use.
- **Examination**: Mention how they look generally, and any specific positive findings. Sum up all the negatives where possible, e.g. 'little to find on examination except...'.
- **Impression**: Always try to form an impression.
- **Plan**: Mention what has been done already, and what your senior needs to decide upon.

The key to these presentations is *relevance*, something which is difficult to judge even with experience. Furthermore different seniors will have different preferences about how much information they wish to be told. If in doubt, the 'evaluation' sections of each clerking pro forma in this book should give a fairly clear idea of the questions your seniors will be asking themselves as you present, and should help guide you in knowing what is important and what is not.

Below is an example presentation of a very straightforward patient on a busy ward round. Making such a presentation is an excellent chance to be a part of clinical decision-making, though you may not have the chance to ask all the questions you would like to. Discussing the case thoroughly at a later date with a more senior colleague will mean you don't miss the teaching value of this case.

> Mr Luke Charles is a 19-year-old non-smoker who is studying English at university. He was admitted last night with acute shortness of breath, on a background of asthma that was diagnosed in childhood. He takes regular inhaled steroids and a long-acting beta-2 agonist as well as salbutamol when he needs it. He has had one previous serious attack 2 years ago for which he required admission for 48 hours. He has never been admitted to intensive care.
>
> On this admission he had been increasingly wheezy over the past 2 days, which he attributes to the cold weather. He has also had a cough and runny nose for several days. He has not produced any sputum or had a fever.
>
> On examination he was apyrexial, unable to speak in full sentences and had a respiratory rate of 30 breaths per minute at rest. Chest examination revealed a diffuse expiratory wheeze. His peak expiratory flow rate was 200 L/min, whilst his normal is around 400 L/min. Chest X-ray was unremarkable. His inflammatory markers were not raised.
>
> My impression was that this is a non-infective exacerbation of asthma possibly caused by the cold weather. He has received nebulizers, intravenous steroids, and magnesium sulphate. His peak flow is now 300 L/min and he is generally feeling better; however, on examination he is still quite wheezy. I feel that he should probably remain in hospital for another 24 hours of nebulizers, possibly going home tomorrow morning.

Writing in medical notes

The skill of writing is to create a context in which other people can think.

(Edwin Schlossberg, 1945–)

Good note keeping is vital in medicine. The medical notes are legal documents that form an essential record of the patient's medical and social issues. They are the principal method of communication between medical teams, allied health professionals, and the patient. In recognition of this, the Royal College of Physicians (RCP) has begun to explore the use of a national clerking admission pro forma (this can be accessed from http://www.rcplondon.ac.uk/clinical-standards/hiu/Pages/Medical-records.aspx).

As well as the patient's admission clerking, note keeping includes ward round entries, comment on investigation results, explanations to the patient of results and procedures, recording procedures (and complications), referral letters to other teams, and recording of specific events, e.g. a conversation between the consultant and a set of relatives. There are many opportunities for undergraduates to learn to how to write in, and use, the medical notes; just like prescribing, it is an essential skill that you will learn by practice. However, senior staff may vary in their opinion regarding students writing in their patients' notes, so check before you volunteer to be the scribe in a given clinical situation.

The aim of this section is to demonstrate the basic principles employed when writing in patients' notes, using examples of how different types of entry are structured. Local convention may vary, so you will need to adjust what we have advised in line with local practices. Think about making entries in the notes as if they were complex mathematical solutions; make sure you clearly state the problem as you see it, facts that help you with this problem, i.e. your reasoning, and your conclusions, i.e. the diagnoses. This in turn should lead to a management plan. In this way if another doctor has to review the patient, they can follow the line of diagnostic reasoning and work out what they should do.

General points on writing in patients' notes

- Write clearly and legibly in black ink—if others can't read what you have written then there is little point in writing it.
- Always begin with the date and time. If you are writing about something that happened several hours/days ago, write 'In retrospect' at the beginning.
- Write a title—for instance 'Dr Smith's ward round', or 'Discussion with patient's relatives'.
- Record facts (both positive and important negatives), not what you think or supposition. Personal comments about the patient should never be made.
- Make it clear who has written the entry—write your name and role, and add a bleep number or contact details at the end.
- Sign your entry.

Recording an initial clerking

This will often take several pages, and should be a comprehensive record of the history and examination you have just performed, along with any investigation results that are available. It should also include your impression of what is going on, along with your management plan.

When recording your clerking, you should use the subheadings discussed in the history, examination, and investigation sections. As you become more skilled and knowledgeable you will find the history of the presenting complaint will become an amalgamation of the relevant facts from each of the subsections of the history. However, until you reach this point we highly recommend that you use the structure suggested.

When recording examination findings, begin by recording a general impression of the patient before going into detail about particular systems. Record the vital signs—temperature, heart rate, blood pressure, oxygen saturations and respiratory rate, and capillary blood glucose. Use symbols to help describe your findings (see the examples below), and if necessary sketch a body part to give information, for instance, on the extent of a rash or inflammation.

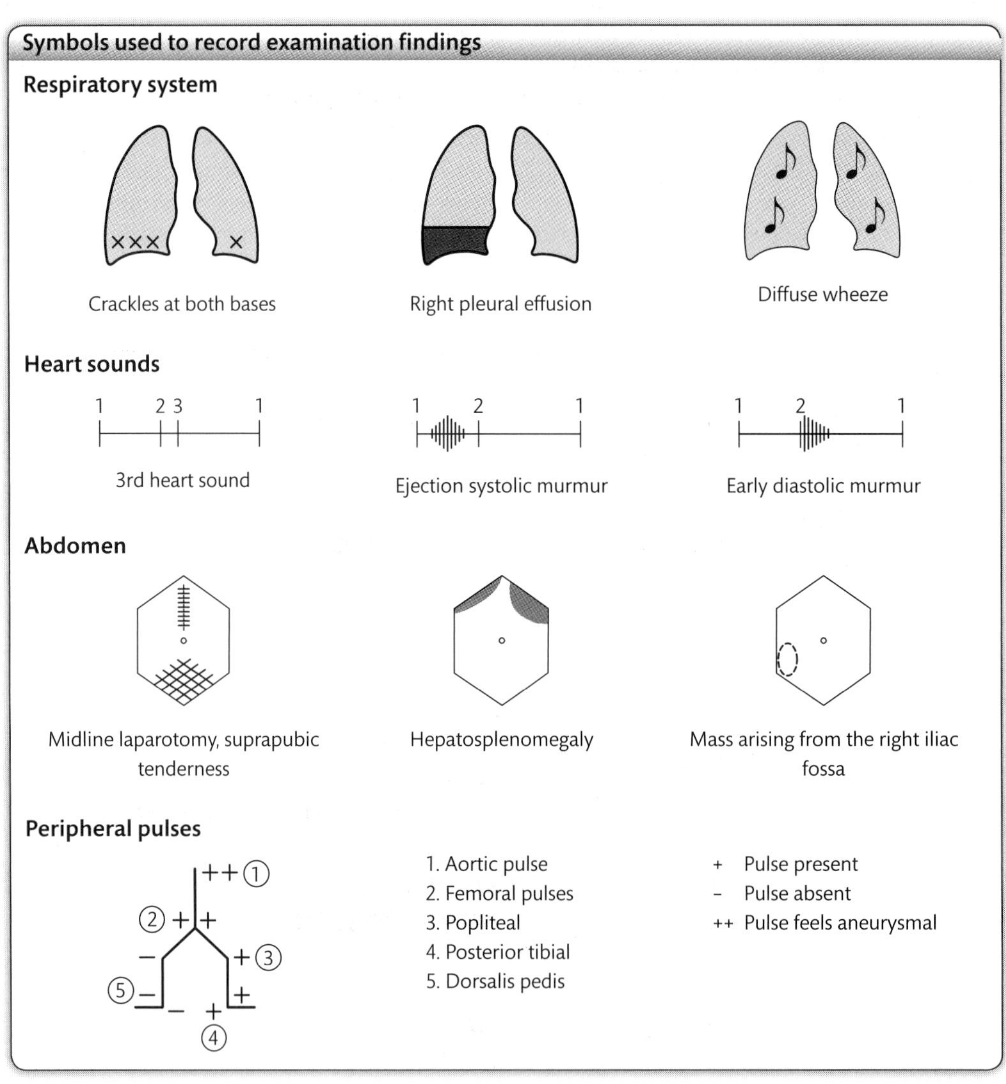

Finish by writing an impression (see the beginning of the section on 'How to present patients to senior colleagues' for information on what kinds of things to write, and how specific to be). Then write a plan, covering both management and investigations. Always sign at the bottom and write legibly who you are, what your role is and how you can be contacted.

Example of written clerking

28 May 2010, 10.00am

Medical clerking on the EAU (Emergency Assessment Unit)

Mr C, 68 y.o. Black-Caribbean male

PC: Breathlessness and increased sputum production

Background: Oesophageal cancer diagnosed October 2008
Resection November 2008 followed by chemotherapy – curative intent
PEG [percutaneous endoscopic feeding tube] inserted for feeding before the operation, nil by mouth since then
Copious upper airways secretions since then – suction machine at home
2 respiratory tract infections since the operation (in Jan and March), both requiring antibiotics

HPC: Unwell for 1 week
Copious sputum – white
Weak and dizzy on standing
Housebound for several days
Short of breath on walking 10 metres
Prescribed amoxicillin by family doctor 3 days ago – no improvement
No chest pain/palpitations/haemoptysis
No recent vomiting. PEG tube working well and patient not experiencing problems with it
No other symptoms except generally feeling weak and run down

PMHx: Oesophageal cancer and chest infections as above
Hypertension

DHx: Ramipril 2.5 mg od
Amoxicillin 500 mg tds for past 3 days
NKDA

FHx: Nil of note

SHx: Lives alone, generally independent, very supportive family who help out. Uses suction machine and arranges PEG feeding himself.
Gave up smoking 5 years ago – total history 25 pack years. Occasional alcohol.

On examination: Unwell; cachectic and lethargic.
Tachypnoeic
Fully alert and conscious
Producing large amounts of sputum/upper airways secretions – coughing ++
Clinically dry – decreased skin turgor, low JVP.
No clubbing/anaemia/cyanosis/jaundice

Observations: CBG 6.9 mmol/L, Temp. 37.8°C, BP 114/68 mmHg, HR 130 bpm, pO_2 94% on 10 L/min

Respiratory

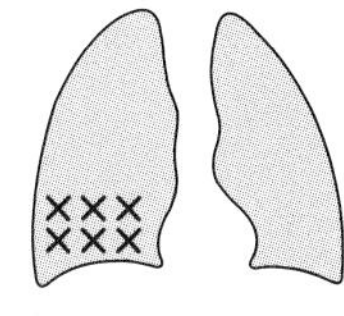

Tachypnoeic
Tracheal central
Expansion 2 cm bilaterally
Fully resonant to percussion throughout
Coarse crackles and bronchial breathing at the right base

Cardiovascular

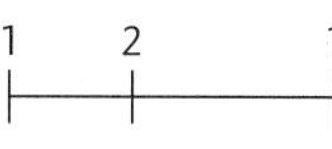

Heart sounds normal
No added sounds
No murmur; no signs of failure

Abdomen

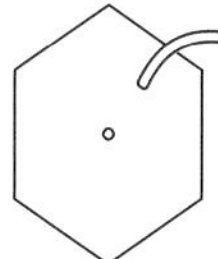

Soft, non-tender
No masses
PEG tube in situ – appears healthy
Bowel sounds present

Impression: Likely aspiration pneumonia
Dehydration

Plan: IV fluids – 1 L stat then regular maintenance
IV antibiotics to cover aspiration
Bloods and chest X-ray
Continue oxygen to keep sats >94%
Discuss with oncology team
Hospital dietician to arrange continued PEG feeding.

David Randall, Medical student

Writing in notes on a ward round

When you first start writing the notes on ward rounds you may think everyone is speaking at twice their normal rate just to upset you. This is because you are trying to record everything verbatim. As you become more discerning, and in possession of the full repertoire of medical shorthand, the entire experience becomes a lot easier! When you attend rounds try to make a recording in your own notebook of the exchanges that occur. Compare your entries with those made in the patient's notes. How much of the medical shorthand do you understand?

As with all entries, you need to record the date, time, ward round (WR) of the consultant, signature, and bleep number. Record the important clinical findings, changes in the patient's condition, and relevant investigation results. You should conclude with the lead clinician's impression (which can be simple statement, e.g. 'improving' or 'getting better'), and then their management plan. If you are unsure what is going on, or what the team want you to record, ask! It is your job as the scribe to bring important information to the attention of the team. Make sure they are aware of any previous investigation results, lines of reasoning, diagnoses, or social issues they have failed to address.

Below we have attempted to reproduce a typical junior doctor's ward round entry for the patient whose clerking is recorded in the box above the day after admission. Note the structure and the amount of medical shorthand utilized.

29/05/10 9am

WR DGR

68 yo

Asp pneumonia 5/7.

Resected Ca oesophus – 6/12 ago under Mr JT.

Day 2 – iv Ben pen and met

Today – feeling and looking better. Less sputum production. Still breathless.

Apyrexial since starting Abx

Now: BP 112/74, HR 95, pO_2 97% on 4L O_2 via nasal specs

On examination:

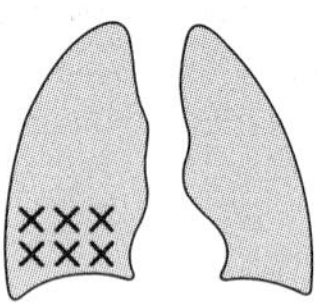

coarse right basal crackles – as before

Chest X-ray – RLL consolidation

Bloods – Na^+ 136, K^+ 4.6, Cr 110, Ur 13.2, CRP 143, Hb 12.4, WCC 14.1, Plts 218

Impression: Resolving pneumonia

Plan: Continue IV fluids as still looks clinically dehydrated. Convert antibiotics to oral. Physio to increase mobility. Speak to oncologist

Dr Randall, House Officer, Bleep 124

Writing other entries

It can be crucial to record things in the notes such as discussions with other professionals or discussions with the patient or their relatives. This allows other team members to understand what progress has been made in treating the patient, and what the patient understands; it can also act as a legal defence in proving what was done for the patient and when, and documenting the reasons why certain decisions were made.

Record the time and date, who you are, and then include a brief, legible, and comprehensive summary of what has been said, and if necessary any further results or plans. The two examples below show entries that could have been written in the notes of the patient outlined above.

29 May 2009, 15.30pm

Discussion with oncology consultant Dr Tyler

Details of Mr C's admission discussed. Mr C was due to have a CT scan as an outpatient next week to assess the success of his surgery and chemotherapy. Dr Tyler asks for this to be arranged during this admission, after which she will come and review the patient on the ward.

Plan: Arrange CT chest/abdomen, inform Dr Tyler of the results.

David Randall, Medical student

30 May 2009, 13.00pm

CT report: *No evidence of tumour recurrence locally or of any distant metastases.*

Right lower lobe consolidation

Full report filed in notes

Dr Tyler informed of the above – she will come to review tomorrow.

Discussion with patient: Mr C asked me for the results of the CT scan. Dr Jones (the registrar) informed him that the scan did not show any evidence of cancer, which was good news; however there is always the risk that small amounts of cancer may remain undetected by this scan. He was told that Dr Tyler will come tomorrow to see him to explain things more clearly and what his follow-up will be from an oncology perspective.

David Randall, Medical student

Prescribing skills

The art of medicine consists of amusing the patient while nature cures the disease.

(Voltaire, 1694–1778)

Remember: sample drug charts can be downloaded from the Online Resource Centre and used to practice shadow prescribing and to complete some of the questions in this book which require you to prescribe.

The report of the 2009 EQUIP study (http://www.gmc-uk.org/about/research/research_commissioned_4.asp) highlighted how poorly prepared medical students feel about their practical prescribing. Whilst it is relatively easy to learn the science, the art of prescribing is difficult for undergraduates. But once graduated you will be responsible for the prescription of many potentially harmful drugs. Of all hospital admissions, 1 in 10 patients will be harmed and 1 in 300 will die as a result of medical prescribing errors.

Learning to inform and negotiate with patients about their medications are vital skills if you wish to improve your patients' adherence to treatment. It is estimated that up to a third of prescribed medicines are not actually taken by patients, representing a considerable waste of resources as well as resulting in failure to achieve their desired therapeutic effect.

To become a proficient and safe prescriber you will need to get involved with the day to day prescribing on wards. By helping the team rewrite drug and fluid charts, you will endear yourself to the junior staff and will slowly learn drug doses, regimens, and common prescribing issues. Before graduation you should be able to write drugs on the once only (stat), as required (prn), and regular parts of the chart, and prescribe anticoagulation, oxygen, common fluids, and blood products.

Below we have produced an **undergraduate prescribing guide**. This should help you make the most of the prescribing opportunities and challenges you may face over the next few years.

Principles of prescribing

Benefits and risks: The last century saw the development of the majority of our medicinal armoury. Some drugs (such as antibiotics) can acutely change the course of an illness, saving life and assisting recovery. Others (such as analgesics) don't drastically alter prognosis but do improve the quality of life, whilst others (such as low-dose aspirin) may have no discernible immediate effects but have significant long-term benefit. All of their benefits must be weighed against their potential risks—the antibiotic may cause anaphylaxis if the patient is allergic, opiate analgesia can cause respiratory depression at high doses, and nausea and constipation at low doses, and aspirin predisposes to potentially life-threatening gastrointestinal bleeding. Get to know the benefits and risks of the commonly prescribed drugs. By doing so you can help your patients make informed decisions about their medications.

Interactions: Drug interactions are common! The British National Formulary (BNF) carries a list of all known interactions in its Appendix 1. The potency of a drug may be altered by changing its absorption, action, or excretion. Many medications are renally excreted after being hepatically metabolized by the cytochrome P-450 group of enzymes. These enzymes are affected by many classes of drugs; some make them more efficient (**enzyme inducers**) and some slow them down (**enzyme inhibitors**). Antibiotics (including the antituberculosis drugs), antiepileptics, and alcohol are commonly involved in such interactions.

Adverse effects: These may be **expected** (known, dose-dependent side-effects of medication, e.g. constipation with opiates) or **idiosyncratic** (non-dose-dependent and not experienced by all patients, e.g. anaphylaxis with antibiotics). If serious or life threatening, these effects need to be treated, and the drug should be stopped and an alternative started. Adverse effects should be reported by the yellow card system at the back of the BNF.

Monitoring: We clinically monitor all drugs through assessing patient adherence, response to treatment, and side-effects. On the wards daily 'drug chart reviews' should be performed, assessing the necessity of each drug on the chart. Some drugs, such as anticoagulants, or drugs with a '**narrow therapeutic window**', e.g. gentamicin or phenytoin, require formal monitoring by checking their blood levels.

Practising evidenced-based medicine versus tailoring therapies to individual patients: Whilst doctors need to practise evidenced-based medicine wherever possible, this evidence should never blind you to the patient sitting or lying in front of you. Patient preference, individual physiological and pathological differences, co-morbidities, and polypharmacy, should influence the choices and doses of any new therapeutic interventions.

Communication skills: Many factors influence the adherence of a patient to treatment plans, including the patient's trust in their doctor, their perception of their illness, and their views on what the medication does. Most of these factors can be addressed through good communication. When new medications are prescribed, it is a good idea to explain properly and appropriately to the patient what the medication does, what the benefits are, how long it will need to be taken, and what side-effects should be expected. This is especially true with medications that produce no immediate benefit but may reduce future problems or sustain remission. Remember, negotiation is always better than dictatorship.

Drug charts

Authentic copies of drug and fluid charts are available online at www.oxfordtextbooks.co.uk/orc/randall/

Any medication received by hospital in-patients must be recorded on their drug chart. But before the medications are noted down the patient's data needs to be recorded. This should include filling in the front and inside details including the patient's name, date of birth, hospital identification number, the responsible consultant and ward, drug allergies, a recording (or estimate) of their height and weight, and a clear documentation of the total number of charts for that patient (e.g. 1 out of 2).

Whilst most GPs now prescribe via electronic prescribing, hospital clinicians are still using hand-written charts. Perhaps more perplexing is that the formats of these charts still vary considerably across the UK. Despite this, most charts are subdivided into several common sections:

- **Once-off drugs:** This section allows once-off doses to be given, e.g. a single dose of sedation before a procedure, an enema for constipation, or bowel preparation ahead of a colonoscopy. If the drug needs to be given immediately, bring the prescription to the nurse's attention.

Drug	Dose	Route	Date	Time	Signature	Nurse	Signature
Phosphate enema	One enema	PR	18/6	15.30	GN	Watkins	CW
Midazolam	2 mg	IV	18/6	16.00	GN	Watkins	CW

- **Special Items—warfarin, insulin, and oxygen:** These therapies are often given specific areas on the chart. The warfarin section usually contains a guide to prescribing and monitoring the anticoagulant (e.g. a modified Fennerty regime), with space for writing in the INR and the doses. The insulin section facilitates different regimes of insulin to be prescribed, e.g. a long-acting insulin at night, with boluses of short-acting insulin after each meal. The oxygen section may include information for the rate of flow (in litres per minute), the concentration (if using the Venturi mask system), the route of delivery (nasal speculae or face mask), and the target oxygen saturations.

Warfarin Target INR: 2-3									
Date	15/6	16/6	17/6	18/6	19/6	20/6	21/6	22/6	23/6
INR	2.3	X	3.1	X					
Dose	4 mg	4 mg	3 mg	3 mg					
Time	18.00	18.00	18.00	18.00					
Signed	GN	GN	GN	GN					
Nurse	CW	DK	DK	CW					

- **Regular medications:** Both the patient's admission medications and any new therapies are written in this area. The generic name of the drug should be written clearly, along with the date started, the route of administration, and the times at which the drug should be given. Once-daily drugs are usually given at 08:00, twice-daily drugs at 08:00 and 18:00, thrice-daily drugs at 08:00, 14:00, and 22:00, and four-times-daily drugs at 08:00, 14:00, 18:00, and 22:00.

Drug: *Metformin*		**Instructions:** *With food*				**Signature:** *GN*					
Start: *17/6/9*	**Route:** *PO*	*15/6*	*16/6*	*17/6*	*18/6*	*19/6*	*20/6*	*21/6*	*22/6*	*23/6*	*24/6*
0800	*500mg*	*CW*	*DK*	*DK*	*CW*						
1800	*500mg*	*CW*	*DK*	*DK*	*CW*						

- **As required or 'prn' medication:** Drugs written in this area are only given 'as required', e.g. analgesia, sedation, antiemetics, or additional nebulizers. The indication should be documented, whether from the patient (e.g. 'pain'), or from the nursing staff (e.g. 'fitting'). If appropriate, document the maximum dose per day or the minimum amount of time between doses.

Drug: *Codeine phosphate*		**Date**	**Time**	**Nurse**	**Date**	**Time**	**Nurse**	**Date**	**Time**	**Nurse**
		15/6	*1000*	*CW*	*18/6*	*1000*	*CW*			
Dose: *60mg*	**Start:** *15/6*	*15/6*	*1700*	*CW*						
		16/6	*0800*	*DK*						
Route: *PO*	**Frequency:** *6 hourly*	*16/6*	*1400*	*DK*						
		16/6	*2000*	*DK*						
Indication: *Pain*	**Signature:** *GN*	*17/6*	*1200*	*DK*						
		17/6	*2200*	*DK*						

Discharge summaries

When a patient is discharged from hospital, a discharge summary is written. This gives details of their hospital management and their medications on discharge. This informs both the patient and community healthcare professionals what medications the patient should continue. This is known colloquially as the 'TTA' or 'TTO' ('to take away' or 'to take out'). The following abbreviations (with their basis in Latin, not English), are often used to describe the frequency at which medications should be taken:

- **od** once daily
- **om** once daily in the morning
- **on** once daily in the evening
- **bd** twice daily
- **tds** three times daily
- **qds** four times daily
- **prn** as required

The medication section of a discharge summary may look something like this:

Drug	Dose	Frequency	Duration (days)	Continue?
Aspirin	75 mg	od	14	Yes
Simvastatin	40 mg	on	14	Yes
Metformin	500 mg	bd	14	Yes
Ramipril	5 mg	od	14	Yes
Amoxicillin	500 mg	tds	7	No
Flucloxacillin	500 mg	qds	7	No

Opportunities to practise prescribing

Complete a sample drug chart after clerking and presenting a newly admitted patient: Download a sample drug chart from the Online Resource Centre. Discuss which new medications the patient needs, as well as writing up their regular medication (from the drug history part of the history). Remember to include 'as required' drugs—especially pain relief if appropriate. Look up doses in the BNF, and think about possible adverse reactions or interactions. You should annotate the chart with useful facts about each of the drugs and keep this in your portfolio.

Review drug charts: During your time on the wards, accompany the junior staff and/or the ward pharmacist on their rounds. Try to work through the rationale of the prescribed drugs, and where you are uncertain try to get clarification.

Reboarding drug charts: This is a chore that junior doctors will be glad for help with! Copy out all the patient details, allergy information, and then copy over all the drugs. Doing this you will become familiar with doses. Look up any drugs you are not familiar with, and keep an eye out for any interactions that may have been overlooked. Ask the junior doctor to check it through and to sign the medications off.

Complete discharge summaries: Copy the medications on the drug chart onto the discharge summary as above, using the abbreviated frequency notation. Ask the junior doctor to check and sign it. In many hospitals this is now a computer-based process and you will need to familiarize yourself with it.

Use the common medication tables: These are included in the introduction to each chapter and are available in a larger version online. Filling them in (and perhaps discussing them with a ward pharmacist) will familiarize you with commonly used medications.

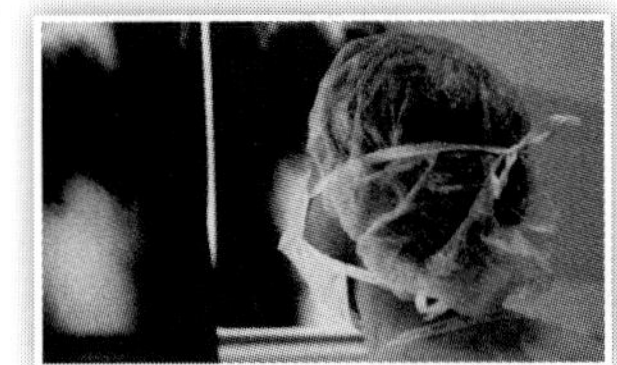
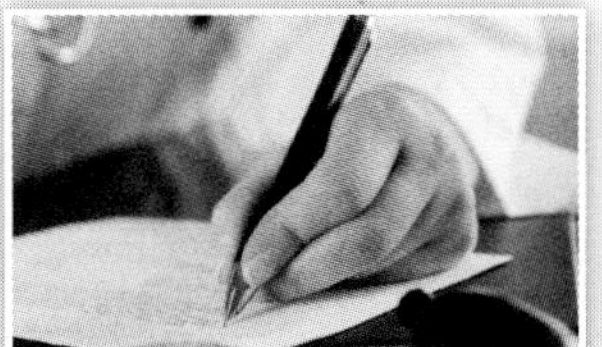
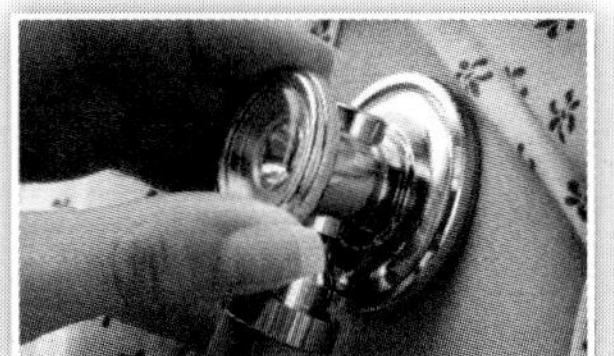
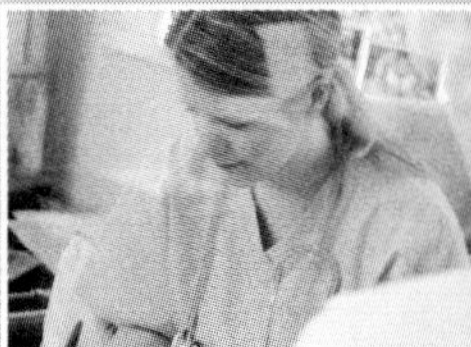

Unit 1
Cardiology

Key learning outcomes in cardiology include:

- **Taking a diagnostic chest pain history, determining the likelihood that the chest pain is cardiac in origin.**
- **Determining the severity of cardiac failure through history, examination, and investigations.**
- **Recognizing the common clinical signs of structural heart disease, especially valvular murmurs.**
- **Interpretation of common, basic abnormalities of the electrocardiogram (ECG).**
- **Initial management of acute coronary syndrome, pulmonary oedema, and common arrhythmias.**
- **Longer-term management of angina and heart failure and primary and secondary prevention of ischaemic heart disease.**

Tips for learning cardiology on the wards:

- Clerk patients presenting with acute onset of chest pain in the Emergency Department, Medical Admissions Unit (MAU), or the Coronary Care Unit (CCU).
- Write out the abnormalities of the ECGs from all the acutely unwell patients that you see. Ask a senior doctor to run through them with you.
- Attend the heart failure clinic; observe the consultations with the heart failure specialist nurse.
- Perform a full cardiovascular examination on several patients with known valvular heart disease. Ask junior and senior doctors to observe and feed back on your examination skills and technique.
- Attend the cardiac catheter laboratory at your local cardiac investigation unit. Observe the various procedures such as angiograms, electrophysiology studies, and pacemaker insertion.
- Attend your local cardiothoracic unit and follow a patient through their coronary artery bypass surgery.
- Watch several echocardiography procedures and ask how information from the scans will influence patient management.

History

The six building blocks of a cardiology history are shown below. Cardiac chest pain has a characteristic set of features and is associated with autonomic features, sometimes along with palpitations, dizziness, and collapse. Symptoms of fluid overload are suggestive of cardiac failure. Cardiovascular risk factors form the foundation of a cardiology history. As the number of risk factors increase, the likelihood of cardiovascular disease increases.

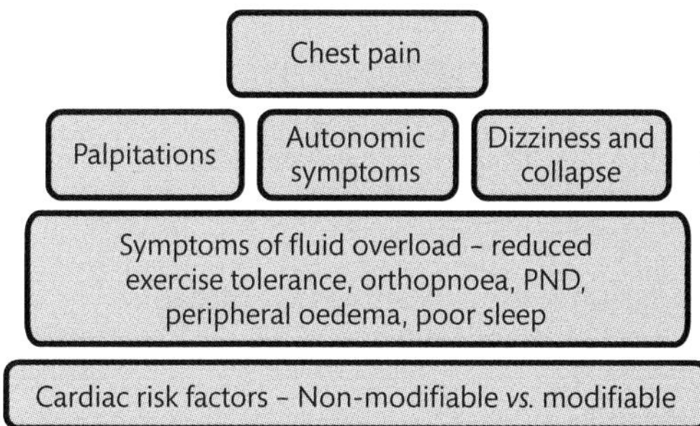

Cardiac risk factors

Cardiac risks factors are classified as non-modifiable or modifiable (see table below):

Non-modifiable	Modifiable
Increasing age	Smoking
Sex (women have a low risk until the menopause)	Diabetes mellitus
Race	Hyperlipidaemia
Family history—premature cardiovascular death	Hypertension
	Alcohol excess
Known atherosclerotic disease— ischaemic heart disease (IHD), stroke, peripheral vascular disease (PVD)	

When you record or come to present the patient's history to a senior include the risk factors at the start of the history. For instance, 'Mr Iqbal is a 58-year-old man from India with a history of hypertension, type 2 diabetes mellitus, and a long smoking history. He does not know if his cholesterol is raised. He has suffered with intermittent claudication of both legs for several years. He now presents with chest pain...'.

Cardiac symptoms

Chest pain: Heart muscle produces pain when it becomes ischaemic. When asking about cardiac pain, use the acronym 'SOCRATES' to ensure all the key points are covered:

Site of pain—classically in the centre or on the left side of the chest, felt 'deep inside'
Onset—the key question here is whether it was **at rest** or **whilst exercising**
Character—usually described as 'tight' or 'crushing'
Radiation—chest pain of cardiac origin may radiate to the left (or right) arm or to the jaw
Alleviating features—crucially, did the pain stop with **rest** or with **GTN spray**?
Time course—has the patient **had it before**? When did it begin? Is there **ongoing pain**?
Exacerbating features—less likely to be cardiac if associated with arm movement or inspiration
Severity—may be anything from very severe to a dull ache

One of the most important features of cardiac pain is the time course. This is crucial in determining when a troponin level should be taken (12 hours after the pain begins, or reaches its worst intensity), but may also suggest the underlying pathological process in the patient's coronary arteries:

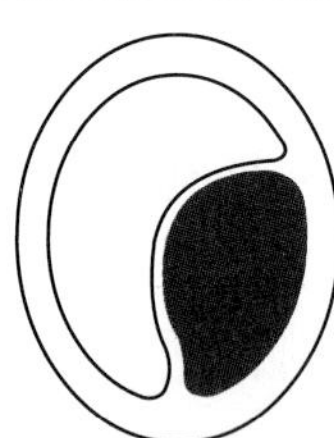	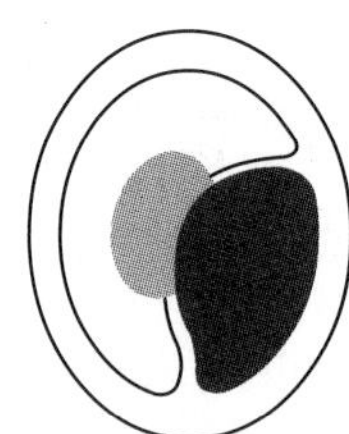	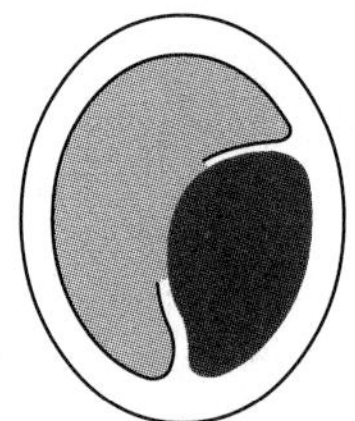
Significant atheroma (purple) forms a subendothelial plaque which may prevent adequate blood supply to the myocardium during exercise when requirements are high. This may cause pain which comes on during exertion and is relieved by rest or GTN—**stable angina**.	Rupture of the endothelial lining of this plaque may cause formation of a blood clot (pink), which may only partially obstruct the lumen of the vessel, causing a worsening of the severity, frequency, or duration of angina symptoms—**unstable angina**.	Alternatively, rupture of a plaque may lead to clot formation that completely occludes the lumen of the coronary artery. This will leave downstream myocardium completely ischaemic producing tissue death—a **myocardial infarction**.

Autonomic symptoms: Heart disease produces a powerful autonomic (sympathetic) response by the body. The presence of autonomic symptoms associated with an episode of chest pain suggests a cardiac origin for the pain, and likewise a patient with acute pulmonary oedema is also likely to display prominent autonomic symptoms. Ask the patient or a relative about:

- Vomiting
- Sweating
- Pallor
- Clamminess

Palpitations: Palpitations may occur in association with chest pain or independently. They are usually a symptom of an underlying arrhythmia and may precede dizziness, pre-syncope, and loss of consciousness. When taking the history of someone with palpitations, it is important to try to understand exactly what the patient is experiencing. When did the palpitations start? How often do they occur? How long do they last? Are they fast or slow, regular or irregular? Try asking the patient to tap the rhythm out on the table (although this may be a variable feast!). Are there any precipitants or exacerbating or relieving factors?

Dizziness and collapse: The term syncope ('fainting'), refers to episodes of loss of consciousness caused by inadequate blood supply to the brain. Syncope is often preceded by a collection of symptoms such as dizziness, muscle weakness, blurring of vision, tinnitus, and chest discomfort, which if not followed by loss of consciousness are called 'pre-syncope'.

The two big differential diagnoses for syncope or pre-syncope are **vasovagal syncope** (caused by an excess of vagal stimulation to the heart, as a result of stressful situations or by vigorous straining) and **cardiac syncope**, usually caused by a paroxysmal dysrhythmia. Ask about other cardiological symptoms—chest pain, palpitations, and shortness of breath.

Symptoms of fluid overload are highly suggestive of cardiac failure—the heart is unable to supply adequate oxygenated blood to tissues, and back pressure from a failing left or right ventricle may cause venous congestion in the lungs or peripheries, respectively. Shortness of breath may occur chronically with significant cardiac disease, but can also occur acutely, and may even be the only sign that the patient is having an acute ischaemic event or has developed an arrhythmia.

Another feature of fluid overload is **swelling of ankles and lower limb**—it is useful to note how far up the body 'pitting' can be felt (in severe cases there may be oedema all the way up the legs, over the sacrum and lower abdominal wall and also in the arms).

Breathlessness may be quantified by:

- When the patient feels short of breath—during exercise or at rest?
- Reduced exercise tolerance: How far can the patient walk along the flat? Can they climb a flight of stairs without stopping? How does the breathlessness affect their activities of daily living, e.g. washing or dressing?

Features suggesting chronic shortness of breath may be due to heart failure include:

- Orthopnoea: an inability to lie completely flat, because fluid re-distribution within the lungs causes worsening breathlessness. Defined by the number of pillows they sleep with; ask whether they can lie flat in bed.
- Paroxysmal nocturnal dyspnoea (PND)—do they wake up acutely short of breath during the night gasping for breath?

Examination

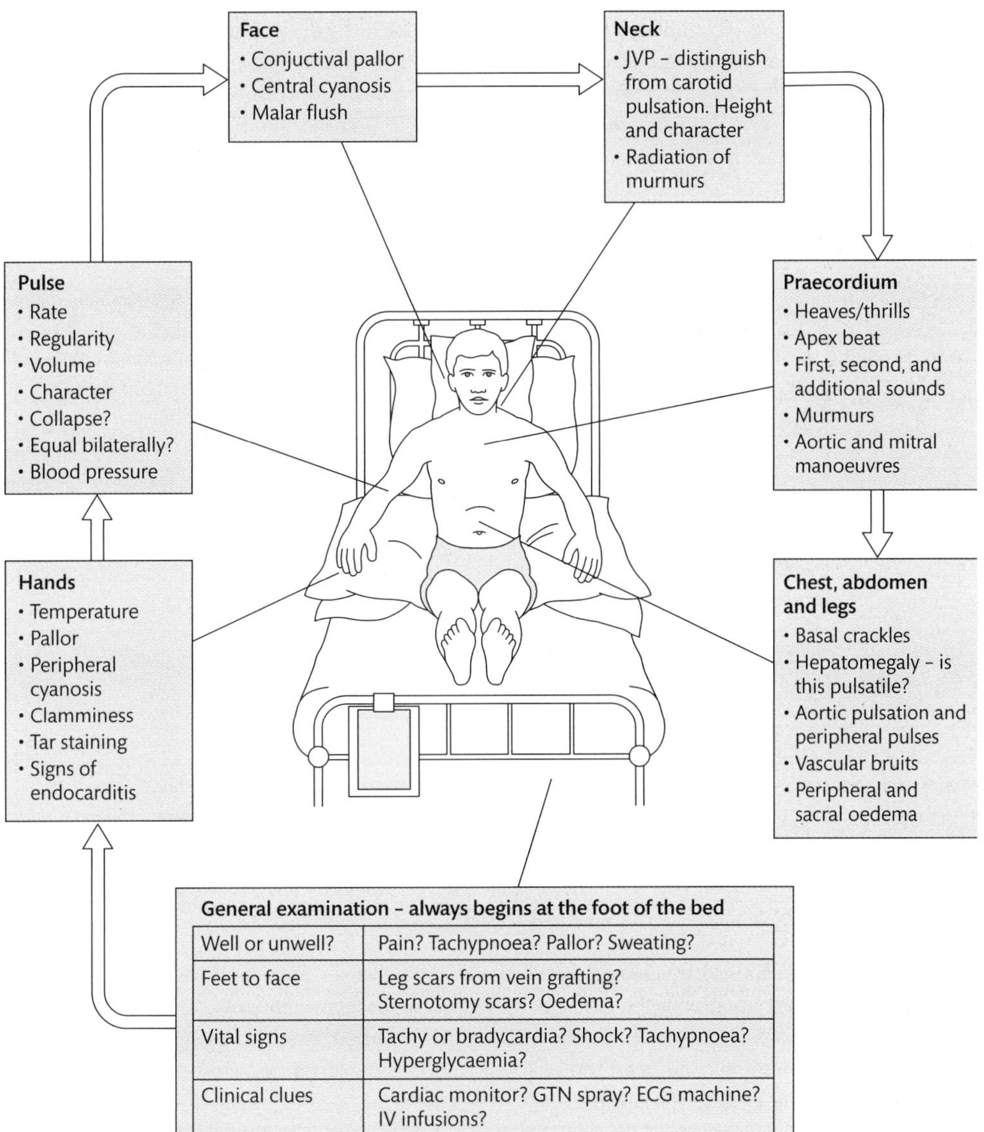

General examination – always begins at the foot of the bed

Well or unwell?	Pain? Tachypnoea? Pallor? Sweating?
Feet to face	Leg scars from vein grafting? Sternotomy scars? Oedema?
Vital signs	Tachy or bradycardia? Shock? Tachypnoea? Hyperglycaemia?
Clinical clues	Cardiac monitor? GTN spray? ECG machine? IV infusions?

Estimating the JVP and fluid status

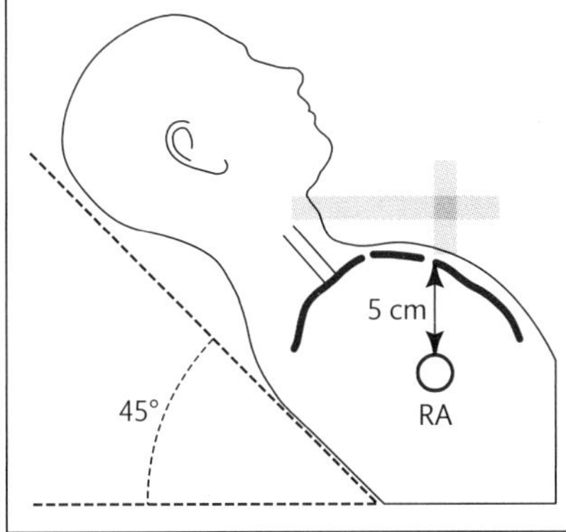

The JVP is measured with the patient lying at 45° to the bed (see diagram on the left; RA is right atrium). The course of the internal jugular runs just medial to the sternocleidomastoid muscle, and so the flickering of the JVP may be seen anywhere along here—from the base of the neck to the ear lobe. The height of the JVP is the vertical height above the angle of Louis.

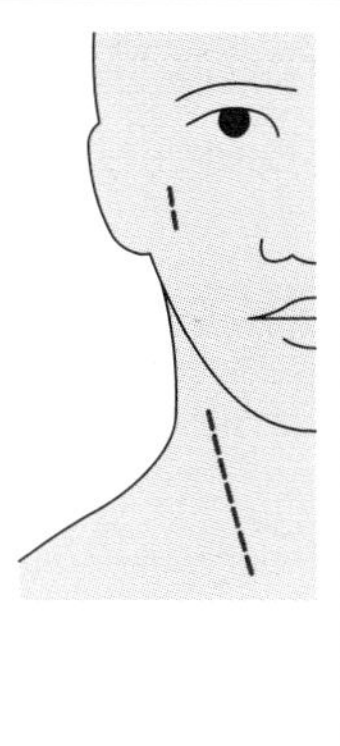

A key skill in evaluating a patient with heart failure is estimating their fluid status—in particular, looking for signs of fluid overload and ventricular failure:

Right ventricular failure	Left ventricular failure	Congestive cardiac failure
Raised JVP Ankle oedema Pulsatile hepatomegaly Ascites	Pulmonary oedema—leading to tachypnoea, hypoxia, and bibasal crackles Pleural effusions	Signs of both right and left ventricular failure

Auscultating the heart

Take your time when auscultating the heart. Make sure you can identify the first and second heart sounds and confirm these by timing against the carotid pulse. Are there any added sounds? A third sound (heard just after the second sound) is caused by rapid ventricular filling and is a sign of fluid overload. A fourth heart sound is a pre-systolic sound and represents pressure overload, e.g. due to aortic stenosis, hypertension, or coarctation of the aorta. Time any murmurs you hear with the carotid pulse. The three most important features for classifying a murmur are: (1) are they systolic or diastolic, (2) where on the chest are they loudest, and (3) which manoeuvres enhance them? See if your findings correlate with other clinical findings. The commonest murmurs are described in the table below:

	Murmur	Heard loudest	Other signs	Leads to...
Aortic stenosis	Ejection systolic 1 2 1	Aortic area, radiates to carotids	Slow rising pulse, narrow pulse pressure; heaving, hyperdynamic, apex beat	Syncope, angina, LVF, and then congestive cardiac failure
Mitral regurgitation	Pan-systolic 1 2 1	Apex, radiates to axilla	Normally a normal volume pulse, but signs of left- and right-sided failure and atrial fibrillation	Atrial fibrillation. Left-sided heart failure
Aortic regurgitation	Early diastolic 1 2 1	Aortic area	Collapsing pulse with wide pulse pressure, grossly displaced apex	Cardiac failure
Mitral stenosis	Late diastolic 1 2 1	Apex, accentuated with patient lying on their left side sternal edge	Malar flush, tapping, undisplaced apex beat	Atrial fibrillation. Pulmonary hypertension. Left- and right-sided heart failure

Remember: the heart sounds are created by the closure of the valves. Stenosis is the lesion of the 'open' valve whilst regurgitation is the lesion of the closed valve. If you remember these simple facts you should not confuse systolic and diastolic murmurs. For example in aortic regurgitation the aortic valve closes on the second heart sound; regurgitation is the lesion of a closed valve, so aortic regurgitation must be a diastolic murmur.

The nine signs of infective endocarditis

(1) Clubbing (subacute only)
(2) Splinter haemorrhages
(3) Osler's nodes
(4) Janeway lesions
(5) Roth spots
(6) New or changed murmur
(7) Splenomegaly
(8) Dipstick positive microscopic haematuria
(9) Fever

Investigations

ECG

ECG interpretation

The first key to interpreting ECGs is to have a clear scheme to work through so nothing is missed. The second key is practice, practice, and more practice! Whenever you see a patient, look through their notes and review their ECG. Write down what you think it shows and then ask a doctor whether they agree and whether you have missed anything.

A good schema for approaching ECGs is:

- Check patient details, date, and time—unlabelled ECGs should be thrown away!
- Speed of the paper (usually 25 mm/s), amplitude of complexes should be 1 mV/cm
- Rate
- Rhythm—regular or irregular, P wave or no P wave
- Axis—normal (−30° to +90°), left-axis deviation (<−30°), or right-axis deviation (>90°)
- P-wave morphology
- PR interval
- QRS complex—narrow <3mm, broad > 3mm
- If broad—is there bundle branch block?
- ST segments; T-wave inversion—these are potentially ischaemic features, particularly if found in several leads within a recognized vascular territory:
  - Inferior: II, IIII and aVF
  - anterior: V_1 and V_2
  - septal: V_3 and V_4
  - lateral: V_5 and V_6
  - high lateral: I and aVL
- Other changes—e.g. prolonged QT interval, U waves, peaked T waves—these may all be signs of global insults to cardiac function, for instance caused by drugs (may prolong the QT interval), hypothermia (produces bradycardia with U waves), or electrolyte imbalances (hyperkalaemia causes peaked T waves as well as broad QRS complexes and eventually cardiac arrest)

Specific points about the ECG

- **Rate and rhythm:** Calculate the rate by dividing 300 by the number of large squares between each QRS complex. Alternatively, count the number of QRS complexes in 30 large squares and multiply by 10.

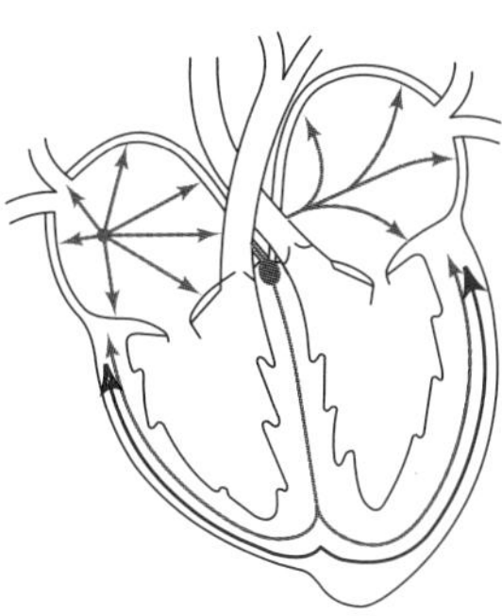

- **P waves** are caused by atrial depolarization after action potentials are generated in the sinoatrial node. Abnormally tall or broad P waves (>2 mm) may be caused by right or left atrial enlargement, respectively.

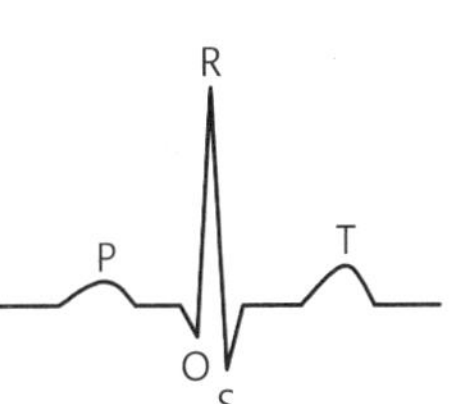

- The **PR interval** is caused by a conduction delay in the atrioventricular node. It should be <200 ms (<5 mm)—a longer delay is called first-degree heart block. In second-degree heart block, some P waves fail to pass the AV node at all, and in complete heart block no P waves conduct, and the atria and ventricles contract independently.
- The **electrical axis** of the heart reflects the overall average direction of electrical flow. To understand the axis, you must understand how the virtual leads I, II, and III act in relation to one another. Left-axis deviation causes the QRS complexes to be strongly positive in lead I and strongly negative in lead III, with the opposite in right-axis deviation.

- The **QRS complexes** are caused by ventricular depolarization. Broadened QRS complexes reflect delayed electrical conduction through the ventricles, often as a result of myocardial ischaemia. This is further divided into **right-bundle branch block** (widened QRS with prominent R wave in V_1 and prominent S wave in V_6), and **left-bundle branch block** (widened QRS with prominent S wave in V_1 and prominent R wave in V_6).
- The **ST segment** reflects the period before the ventricles have repolarized, and the **T wave** represents repolarization. Usually there should be no electrical flow during the ST segment (the tracing should follow the isoelectric line)—ST elevation may represent acute infarction and ST depression may represent ischaemia. Likewise the presence of inverted T waves is also a non-specific sign of ischaemia. ST-segment or T-wave changes may indicate ischaemia if they correspond to a vascular territory.

I	aVR	V_1	V_4
II	aVL	V_2	V_5
III	aVF	V_3	V_6

Inferior
Anterior
Septal
Lateral, high lateral

- ECG leads reflect the flow of electricity through the heart in a particular direction. So leads I, aVL, V_5, and V_6 all point towards the lateral (left) border of the heart. If they all show ischaemic features (such as T-wave insertion) then critical narrowing may be present in the circumflex artery that supplies this part of the heart.

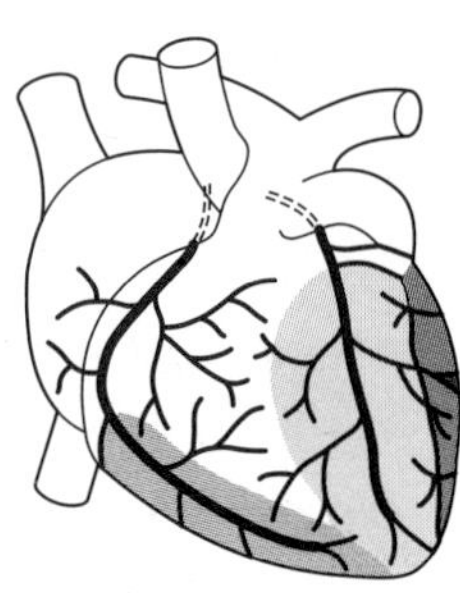

Chest X-ray

Two X-rays below show pulmonary oedema in two different patients, one in whom pulmonary oedema developed rapidly and one in whom there was a longer history of congestive cardiac failure.

Key signs of cardiac failure on chest X-ray include:

- cardiomegaly
- interstitial 'bat-wing' oedema
- fluid in the horizontal fissure (seen as a horizontal line midway up the right lung)
- increased vascular shadows in the upper zones
- pleural effusions, often bilateral

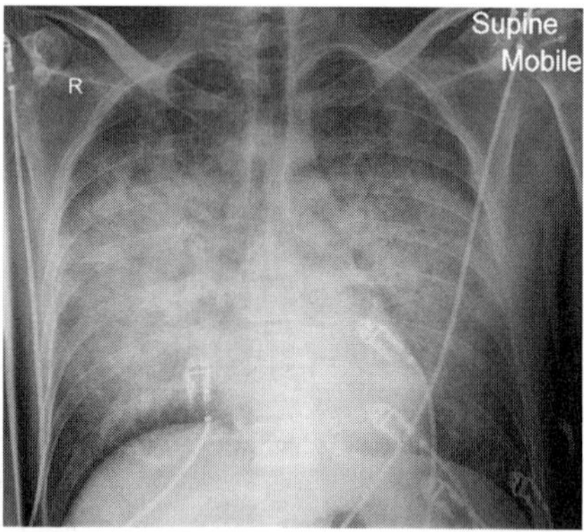

Acute pulmonary oedema

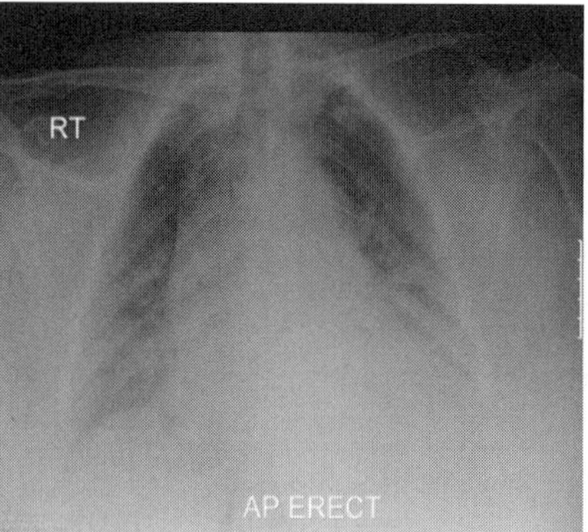

Chronic congestive heart failure

Remember that you can find large-size, annotated versions of many of the X-rays and ECGs that appear in this book on the book's web site at www.oxfordtextbooks.co.uk/orc/randall/

Markers of cardiac damage

The medical management of chest pain has been greatly changed by the introduction of rapid assays for the protein troponin, a component of cardiac muscle that signifies cardiac damage far more specifically than previous 'cardiac enzymes' such as CK or LDH. Troponin I or T levels peak 12 hours after a MI (though new guidelines emphasize the role of assessment of troponin as soon as a patient with chest pain arrives in hospital), but may remain elevated for several days.

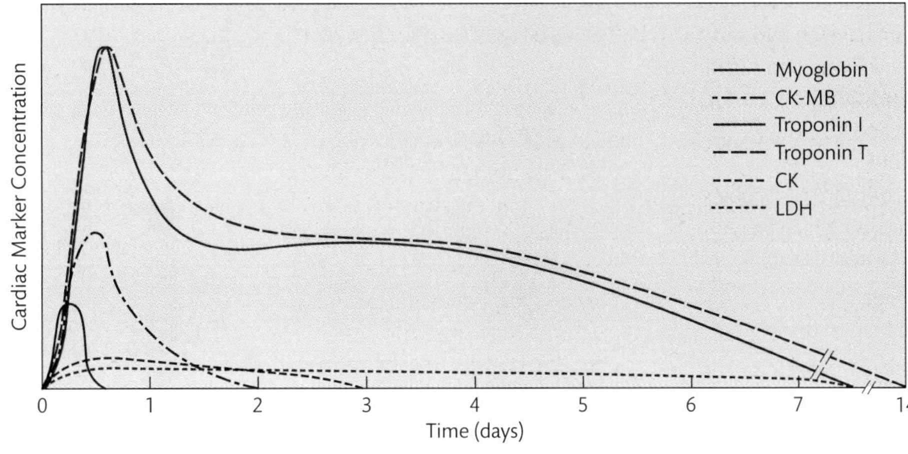

Together with the cardiac history (of new chest pain, or a change in the symptoms of normal angina), cardiac markers can help differentiate stable angina, unstable angina, non-ST segment myocardial infarction (NSTEMI), and ST segment elevation MI (STEMI)—the four commonest conditions that may present as acute coronary syndrome:

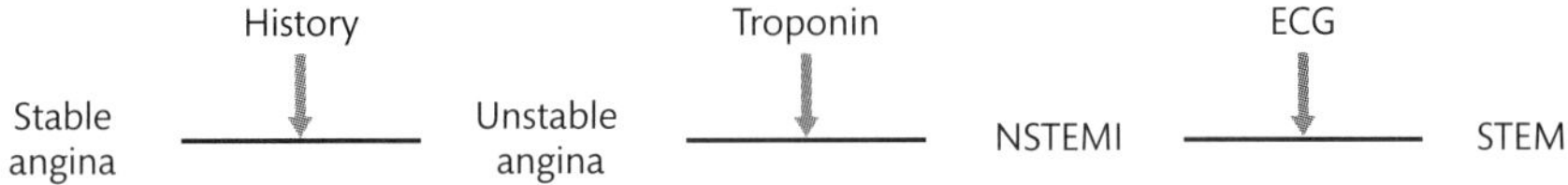

Echocardiography

A transthoracic echocardiogram, usually performed by cardiologists or cardiac technicians, is a relatively simple non-invasive test that can yield much information about cardiac function. Depending on the indications this may include:

- Size of the different chambers, including pathological enlargement and abnormal wall thickness
- Information about ventricular function and wall movement. The left ventricular ejection fraction is the most important, correlating well with prognosis in heart failure, and should be >55%
- Information about the valves, including narrowing (stenosis) and incompetency (regurgitation)
- Whether a pericardial effusion is present, and (if so) whether this is leading to tamponade

Angiography

A catheter is inserted into either the femoral or brachial artery that can then be manipulated into the different chambers of the heart or into the coronary arteries as required. Angiography can be used to visualize arterial patency or cardiac function, and can also be used therapeutically—most commonly for stenting blocked arteries or for ablating pathways of aberrant electrical conduction.

Interventions

Modifying cardiovascular risk

A 50-year-old Caucasian man attends his doctor's surgery because a workplace health check found that his systolic blood pressure, measured on three separate occasions, was persistently >160 mmHg. His doctor measures his blood pressure, which is found to be 168/104 mmHg. He has no other health problems, but does smoke. His fasting serum cholesterol is 4.1 mmol/L and his fasting serum glucose is 4.4 mmol/L.

The risk of him dying from cardiovascular disease in the next 10 years is high: 5–9%. All of his risk factors should be addressed:

- He should be encouraged to stop smoking and offered help to do so.
- He should be encouraged to exercise and lose weight.
- He should be commenced on a statin and an antihypertensive drug (according to hypertension guidelines, an ACE inhibitor if not contraindicated).

Men

Age	Systolic blood pressure	Non-smoker: Cholesterol (mmol/L) 4	5	6	7	8	Smoker: Cholesterol (mmol/L) 4	5	6	7	8
65	180	14	11	19	22	26	26	30	35	41	47
65	160	3	11	13	15	14	18	21	25	29	34
65	140	6	8	9	11	13	13	15	17	20	24
65	120	4	5	6	7	4	4	10	12	14	17
60	180	2	11	13	15	18	19	21	24	28	33
60	160	5	7	9	10	12	12	14	17	20	24
60	140	4	5	6	7	9	8	10	12	14	17
60	120	3	3	4	5	6	6	7	8	10	12
55	180	6	7	8	10	12	12	13	14	19	22
55	160	4	5	6	7	8	4	5	11	13	14
55	140	3	3	4	5	6	5	6	8	9	11
55	120	2	2	3	3	4	4	4	5	6	8
50	180	4	4	5	6	8	2	8	10	12	14
50	160	2	3	3	4	5	2	2	2	4	10
50	140	2	2	2	3	3	3	4	5	6	7
50	120	1	2	2	2	2	2	3	3	4	6
40	180	1	1	1	2	2	3	3	3	3	4
40	160	1	1	1	1	1	1	2	2	2	3
40	140	0	1	1	1	1	1	1	1	2	3
40	120	0	0	1	1	1	1	1	1	1	1

Key: 15% and over; 10%–14%; 5%–9%; 3%–4%; 2%; 1%; <1%

10-year risk of fatal CVD in populations at high CVD risk

See the NICE hypertension guidelines: http://www.nice.org.uk/CG034

Interventional cardiography

Primary angioplasty: This technique is used to visualize, unblock, and maintain (by stenting) coronary arteries which are occluded causing acute myocardial infarction. Primary angioplasty services are often provided 24 hours a day at regional cardiology centres. ECG indications for primary angioplasty include:

- ST segment elevation in two or more neighbouring leads
- New onset left bundle branch block
- True posterior myocardial infarction with anterior ST depression, tall R and T waves

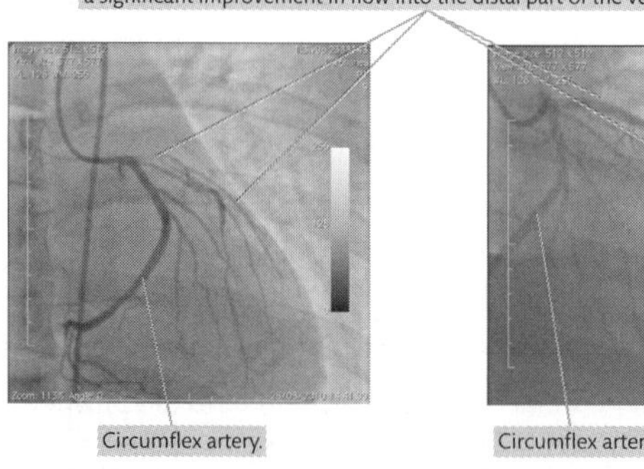

Implantable electrical devices: Pacemakers are used in patients suffering symptomatic bradyarrythmias (e.g. complete heart block) or with severe heart failure to maintain an adequate heart rate and coordinate ventricular contraction. Implantable cardiac defibrillators are used in patients who have suffered, or who are at risk of suffering, cardiac arrest. They are usually inactive but deliver an electrical shock if ventricular tachycardia or fibrillation develops.

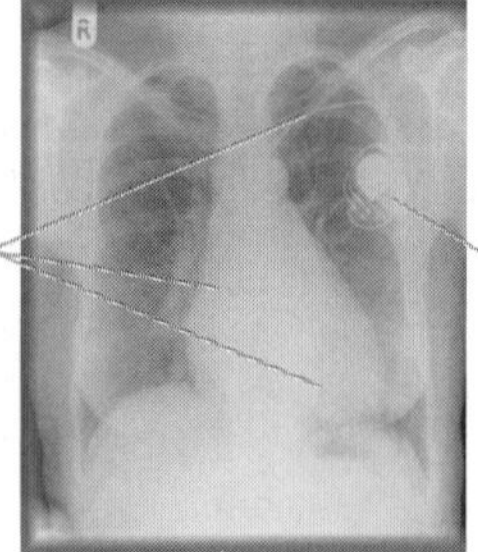

Cardiac ablation: This is used in patients with tachyarrhythmias to destroy accessory conduction pathways.

Coronary artery bypass grafting: An open operation in which a section of vein is used to bypass a narrowed portion of coronary artery. Used in extensive ischaemic heart disease or if atheromatous narrowing is not suitable for stenting.

Remember that you can find large-size, annotated versions of many of the X-rays and ECGs that appear in this book on the book's web site at www.oxfordtextbooks.co.uk/orc/randall/

Common cardiac medications

Class	Examples	Mechanism	Indications	Contraindications	Side-effects	Special notes
Antiplatelet drugs						
Oral anticoagulants						
Other anticoagulants						
Thrombolytics						
Thiazide diuretics						
Loop diuretics						
K^+-sparing diuretics						
ACE inhibitors and angiotensin receptor antagonists						
Dihydropiridine calcium-channel blockers						
Myocardial selective calcium-channel blockers						
Beta-blockers						
Alpha-blockers						
Nitrates						
Type 4 antidysrhythmics						
Cardiac glycosides						
Statins						

Acute coronary syndrome (ACS)

This section should be used to clerk patients presenting acutely with chest pain presumed to be cardiac in origin. You should attempt to clerk them in the first few hours after they present to hospital. The patient pathway leads from the Emergency Department to either the Angiography Suite, CCU, or Admissions Unit depending on the diagnosis and stability of the patient.

Learning challenges

- What key technological advances of the past 20 years have revolutionized the care of ACS patients?
- Why is speed of the essence in dealing with ACS?

History

Comment on

- Full chest pain history
- Associated cardiovascular and respiratory symptoms
- Previous episodes of chest pain
- Previous cardiovascular disease and coronary interventions
- Cardiovascular risk factors

Examination

Well or unwell?	Why?
Feet to face:	
Vital signs:	Temperature ___ Blood pressure ___ Pulse rate ___ Respiratory rate ___ O2 saturations ___
Clinical clues:	

Cardiovascular:

1 2 1

Respiratory:

Abdominal:

Neurological:

Other:

Comment on

- Well or unwell?
- Haemodynamically stable?
- Signs of complications, e.g. shock or pulmonary oedema
- Pulse—rate, regularity, volume, and symmetry
- Cardiac murmurs and vascular bruits
- Pain on palpation of chest wall
- Signs of co-morbidities—hypertension, diabetes, and hyperlipidaemia
- Fluid status and signs of heart failure

ECG

Comment on

- ST elevation or new left bundle branch block?
- Other ST segment or T-wave changes?
- Evidence of old ischaemia, e.g. Q waves, left bundle branch block, and left-axis deviation?
- Rate or rhythm abnormalities?

Chest X-ray

Comment on

- Evidence of pulmonary oedema?
- Evidence of chronic cardiac disease, e.g. cardiomegaly

Blood tests

Comment on

- 12-hour troponin
- Lipid profile
- Glucose

Evaluation

1. Is the patient stable or do they need resuscitation? Is there evidence of pulmonary oedema or fluid overload?

2. Does the initial ECG reveal a full-thickness (ST elevation) MI suitable for immediate angioplasty or thrombolysis?

3. Is the history suggestive of pain due to acute cardiac ischaemia rather than to musculoskeletal, respiratory (pleuritic), or gastrointestinal causes? If so, consider giving aspirin 300 mg and an antithrombin drug such as fondaparinux (dose according to bleeding risk).

4. What is this patient's 6-month risk adverse cardiac events (use a risk stratification tool such as the GRACE score available online at http://www.outcomes-umassmed.org/grace/)?

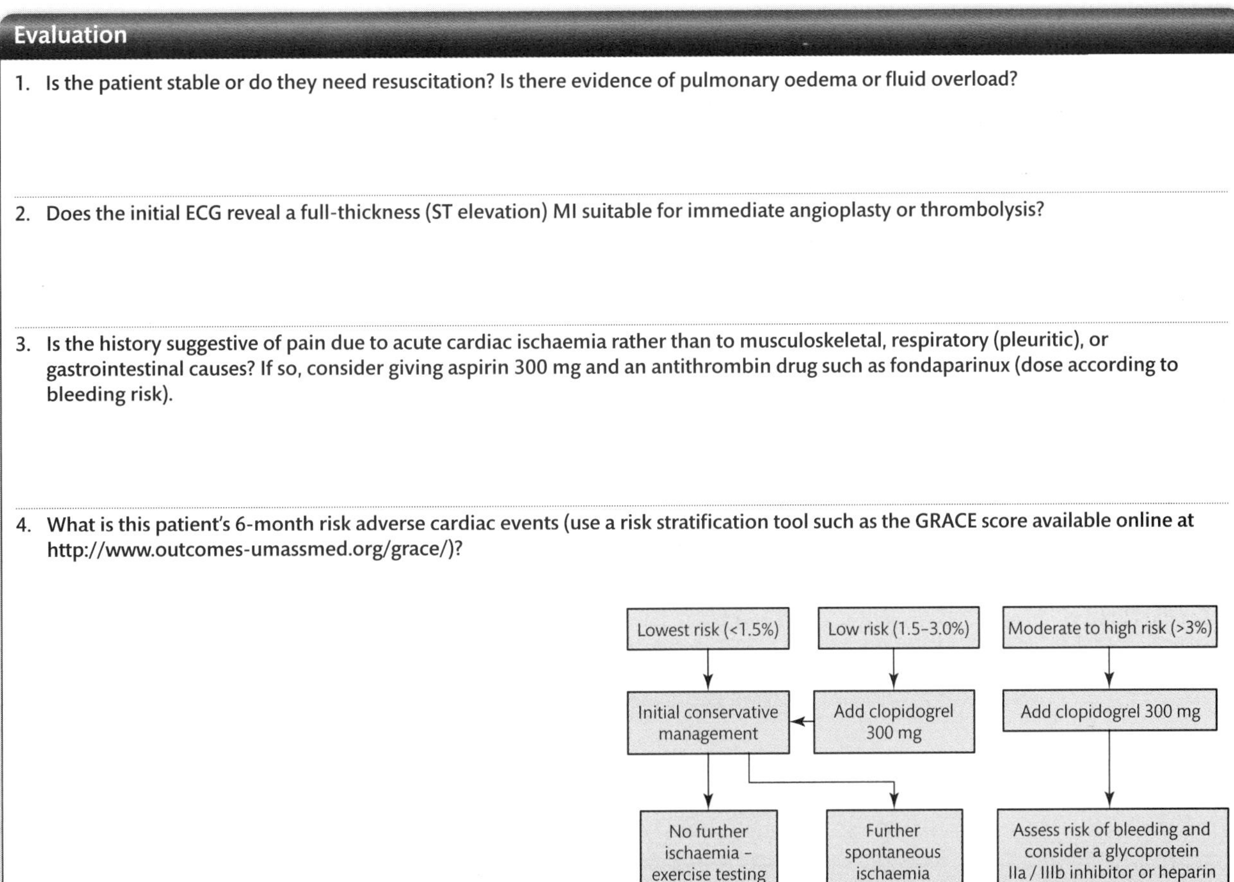

Questions

1. A 60-year-old man is admitted from the Emergency Department after suffering an episode of central crushing chest pain radiating down his left arm and into the left side of his neck. The pain came on suddenly that evening whilst he was walking his dog. It was associated with sweating and the patient vomited once. The pain gradually subsided, with the whole episode lasting 10 minutes. He had never experienced that type of pain before. He does not smoke but was recently diagnosed with diabetes mellitus. His father suffered angina from the age of 45 and had a myocardial infarction aged 48. On arrival at hospital he was pain free and his initial ECG was unremarkable. On examination his chest was clear. His heart rate was 64 bpm, blood pressure 134/85 mmHg, and his creatinine 87 μmol/L. He was managed as an acute coronary syndrome and received aspirin, fondaparinux, and clopidogrel. Twelve hours after the pain occurred his serum troponin level was measured at <0.04 μg/L, and repeat ECGs showed no changes compared with the first one. What would be the next steps in his management?

2. A 67-year-old man with type 2 diabetes mellitus, who has previously had coronary artery bypass surgery for ischaemic heart disease, presents to the Emergency Department with shortness of breath that has worsened considerably in the previous 2 days. He reports a feeling of tightness in his chest but no pain. His oxygen saturations are 88% on air. Examination reveals crackles at both lung bases extending to the mid-zones. His blood pressure is 114/76 mmHg, his heart rate 121 bpm, a baseline troponin is 0.78 μg/L, and his serum creatinine is 148 μmol/L. His ECG is shown below. Describe the abnormalities shown on the ECG and suggests what steps should be taken next.

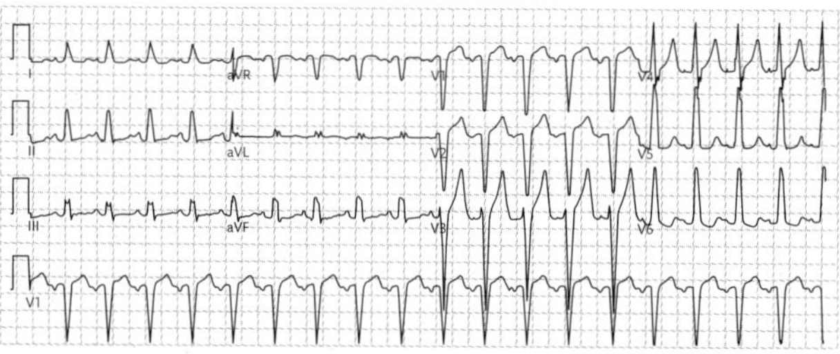

3. A 52-year-old man with hypertension and type 2 diabetes is brought into hospital by ambulance after having continuous chest pain for over an hour. The pain is in the centre of his chest and radiated to his left arm, and is accompanied by nausea and sweating. Physical examination is unremarkable.

(1) Describe the changes shown on his ECG below.

(2) What pathological process is likely to be occurring, and what is the correct management?

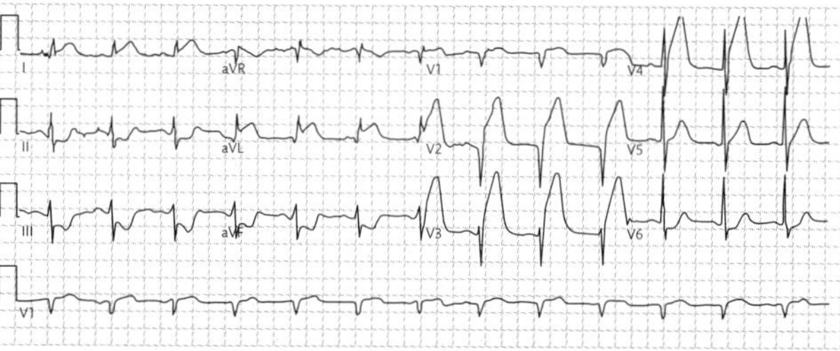

Presentation

Presented to | Grade | Date

Signed

Remember that you can find large-size, annotated versions of many of the X-rays and ECGs that appear in this book on the book's web site at www.oxfordtextbooks.co.uk/orc/randall/

Answers

1. This man has developed angina-like chest pain on the background of several major cardiovascular risk factors. His GRACE 6-month mortality is 2%, putting him in the 'low risk' part of the algorithm. He has not had a MI (his repeat ECGs and 12-hour troponin are unremarkable), so the initial diagnosis is unstable angina (sometimes patients presenting like this are described as having 'troponin-negative chest pain'). Until recently the next step would have been an exercise tolerance test (ETT), which involves the patient walking on a treadmill whilst being monitored by continuous ECG recording. The treadmill gets progressively faster and steeper every 3 minutes, whilst the patient and ECG trace are monitored for signs of cardiac ischaemia. Angina-like pain, or excessive exertional dyspnoea, associated with ST-segment depression, represents a positive test and confirms the diagnosis. Patients with a positive ETT should be referred for in-patient angiography. The new NICE guidelines suggest that those in moderate to high risk categories are investigated further with angiography and appropriate intervention within 96-hours of admission. Those in the low-risk group should be reviewed in a cardiology clinic with a view to assessment for alternative testing such as myocardial perfusion scanning. Newer scanning techniques, e.g. MRA, may make these other tests redundant in the near future.

All patients with ACS should receive:

(1) Antithrombotic therapy, e.g. aspirin and/or anticoagulants and/or clopidogrel.

(2) Antianginals, e.g. beta-blockers, nicorandil, or nitrates.

(3) Medications to reduce long-term cardiovascular risk, e.g. statins.

(4) Education around lifestyle changes, e.g. smoking cessation, exercise, and weight loss programmes (where appropriate).

2. This ECG reveals:

This ECG shows a classic 'left bundle branch block' (LBBB) pattern. This represents slowed electrical conduction through the ventricles, with the left ventricle depolarizing slightly after the right. Causes include acute myocardial infarction, extensive disease of the cardiac conduction system (e.g. extensive ischaemic heart disease) or a dilated or hypertrophic left ventricle

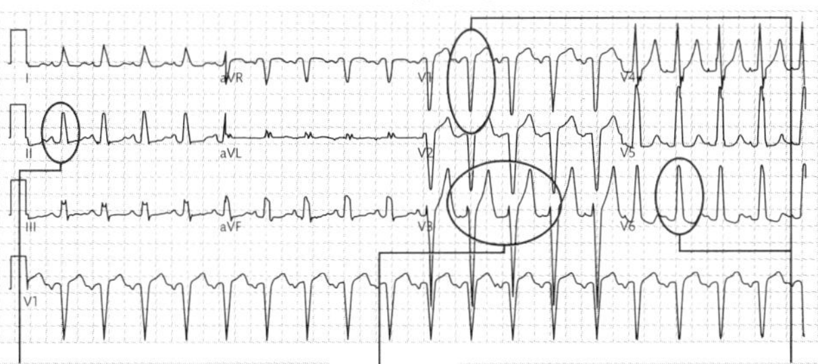

Note widening QRS complexes - wider than 3 small squares (120 ms).

LBBB has pronounced downwards deflections (S waves) in V_1 and pronounced upward deflections (R waves) in V_6. The reverse is true in right bundle branch block.

It may seem like there is ST segment elevation in leads V_2 and V_3. However, in LBBB it is impossible to comment on the ST segments in the chest leads.

In the context of ACS, new-onset left bundle branch block may be consistent with an acute MI, and is an indication for thrombolysis or primary angioplasty in the same way as ST elevation; however, given his previous cardiac history, the ECG changes may be old.

His shortness of breath is likely to be secondary to pulmonary oedema; an urgent chest X-ray should be arranged to assess for this and he should be treated appropriately for it. He should be managed for a non-ST-elevation MI (though the troponin result in this man should be viewed with a certain degree of suspicion because he has some degree of renal failure which can cause false-positive results). He should be treated in a high-dependency area, like a CCU, and serial ECGs should be taken. His GRACE 6-month mortality score is 25%, meaning that he should receive aspirin, fondaparinux, and clopidogrel. If an acute ischaemic event is strongly suspected (for instance if serial ECGs reveal dynamic ST-segment or T-wave changes), a risk assessment for bleeding should be carried out and then if appropriate a glycoprotein IIa/IIIb inhibitor such as tirofiban started. He should be reviewed by a cardiologist and an in-patient angiogram arranged as soon as possible, within 96 hours.

3. The ECG shows:

This ECG shows features of an acute ST elevation MI.

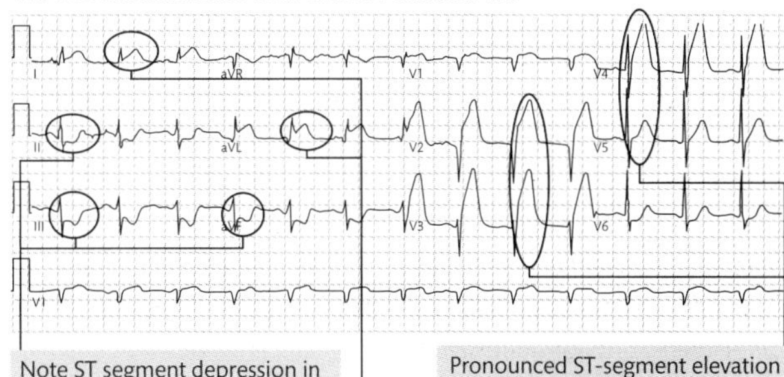

Note ST segment depression in leads II, III and aVF - the inferior leads. ST depression indicates myocardial ischaemia but not infarction.

Pronounced ST-segment elevation leads V_2 to V_4 consistent with an anterior STEMI. ST elevation is significant if more than 2 mm in the chest leads (V_1 - V_6) or more than 1 mm in the 'limb' leads.

This ECG also shows ST elevation in leads I and aVL, the 'high lateral' leads, showing that a large amount of myocardium has been infarcted.

An ST-elevation MI is a medical emergency. Immediate revascularisation is indicated, either by primary angioplasty (if available), or thrombolysis (if primary angioplasty is not available and there are no contraindications). In the meantime, the patient should be managed on a CCU or high dependency area, receiving oxygen (if appropriate), aspirin, clopidogrel, morphine (and an antiemetic), nitrates (sublingual, buccal or intravenous) and low molecular weight heparin or fondaparinux.

Within the 24 hours after admission, he should receive a beta-blocker and an ACE inhibitor, and secondary risk factors such as hyperlipidaemia and diabetes mellitus should be addressed.

This patient was transferred for emergency primary angioplasty, which he received only 90 minutes after presenting to the Emergency Department. A sequence of images taken during his primary angioplasty is shown below (see the book's website for video clips of the procedure being performed). After stenting of the left anterior descending artery the patient made a good recovery. This treatment greatly reduces the amount of myocardial damage caused by the acute myocardial ischaemia, leading to considerable reduction in morbidity and mortality.

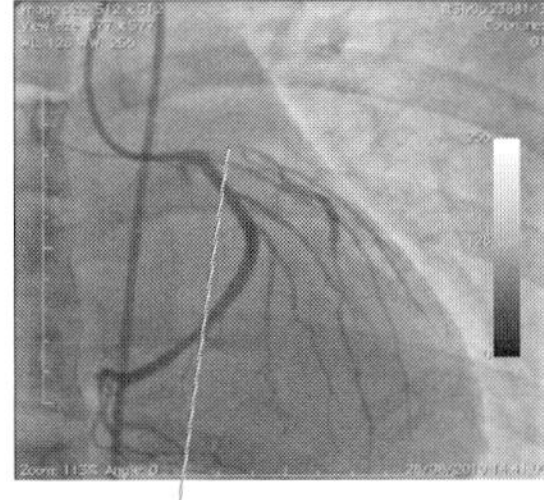

1. Partially occluded LEFT anterior descending artery.

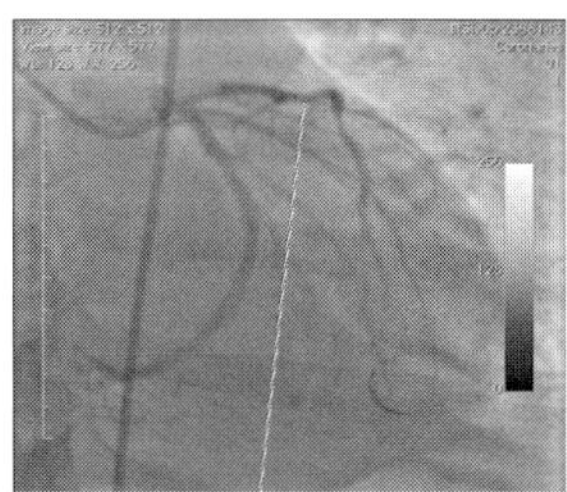

2. Using a guidewire to re-open the artery some flow has resumed.

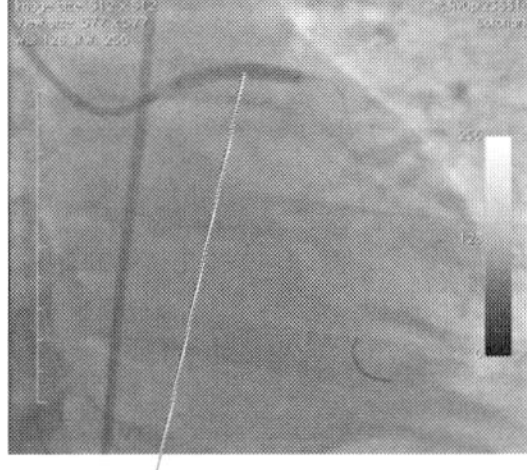

3. A stent being deployed.

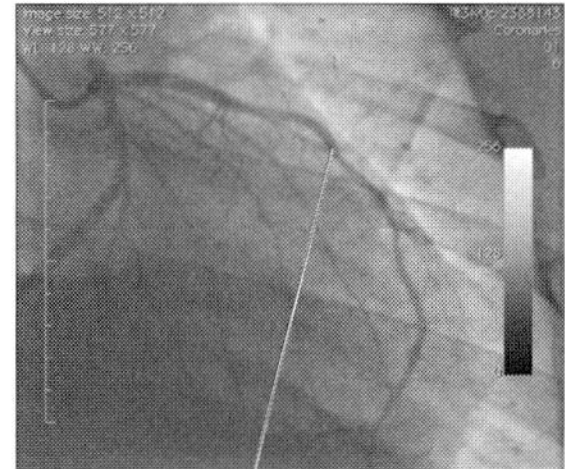

4. Good return of blood flow through the now unblocked artery.

Further reading

Guidelines: NICE guidelines for NSTEMI and unstable angina (http://guidance.nice.org.uk/CG94)

OHCM: 110–115, 148, 798, 808–810

Myocardial infarction (MI) and secondary prevention

Learning challenges

- What are the commonest causes of death as a complication of MI?
- How is a CCU different from a normal ward?

This section should be used to clerk patients who have been admitted to hospital with a MI. The focus is on managing complications and preparing for discharge. Patient journeys lead from the Emergency Department (via primary angioplasty in some cases) to the CCU, and then to a General Cardiology or Rehabilitation Unit. Today many patients presenting with STEMI or nSTEMI and complications are rapidly transferred to a local cardiac centre for primary coronary intervention.

History

Comment on

- History of the event leading to admission
- Cardiac symptoms since admission
- Level of disability in performing activities of daily living
- Cardiac risk factors
- Full social history for discharge planning

Well or unwell? Why?

Feet to face:

Vital signs: Temperature | Blood pressure | Pulse rate | Respiratory rate | O2 saturations

Clinical clues:

Cardiovascular:

Respiratory:

Abdominal:

Neurological:

Other:

Comment on

- Haemodynamic status
- Fluid balance and signs of overload
- Stigmata of hyperlipidaemia, and hypertensive or diabetic complications
- Murmurs

Serial ECGs

Comment on

- Signs of old myocardial ischaemia
- Signs of developing or resolving ischaemia
- Arrhythmias

Echocardiogram

Comment on

- Overall ventricular function
- Signs of complications, e.g. left ventricular aneurysm, valvular lesions

Chest X-ray

Comment on

- Evidence of fluid overload
- Cardiomegaly

Angiogram

Comment on

- Presence of significant arterial stenosis
- Suitability for stenting or bypass surgery

Evaluation

1. Is the patient haemodynamically stable? What is their fluid status?

2. What damage has been done to the heart (damage both to the contractile function and also the conducting system)? What is the prognosis?

3. How can the patient's risk factors be managed to reduce the chances of recurrence?

Lifestyle modifications:

Cardioprotective drugs:

4. Is there any significant disability preventing discharge or requiring rehabilitation?

5. Which other healthcare professionals have been involved in the patient's care? What are their roles?

Questions

1. A 62-year-old man with no known previous medical problems presents to the Emergency Department with an episode of chest pain lasting 20 minutes. The pain began at rest whilst watching television, was in the centre of his chest, radiating to his jaw, and resolved with oxygen and a single spray of sublingual GTN in the ambulance. He was pain free on arrival in the hospital, and subsequent clinical examination, ECG, and chest X-ray were unremarkable. He is haemodynamically stable (pulse 84 bpm, blood pressure 146/87 mmHg) and blood tests were all within normal ranges (creatinine 72 μmol/L). He was managed appropriately for acute coronary syndrome; however, his 12-hour troponin level is raised at 0.18 μg/L (normal <0.04 μg/L). He has been asymptomatic since. Which of these investigations are relevant and why?

Investigation	Relevant?	Why?
Repeat ECG		
Repeat chest X-ray		
Fasting glucose level and lipid profile		
Echocardiogram		
Exercise tolerance test		
Angiogram		
Cardiac MRI scanning		

2. A 78-year-old man is admitted to the CCU after suffering an inferolateral non-ST-elevation MI. His initial ECG revealed ST depression in leads II, III, and aVF which resolved along with his pain after intravenous morphine and GTN were given. Two days later, awaiting angiography, the patient is found to be bradycardic. He is pain free and feeling well, with a heart rate of 45 bpm, a blood pressure of 110/66 mmHg, and oxygen saturation of 98% on air. His ECG is shown below:

(1) What abnormalities are shown?

(2) What is likely to be causing this?

(3) What treatment should be initiated?

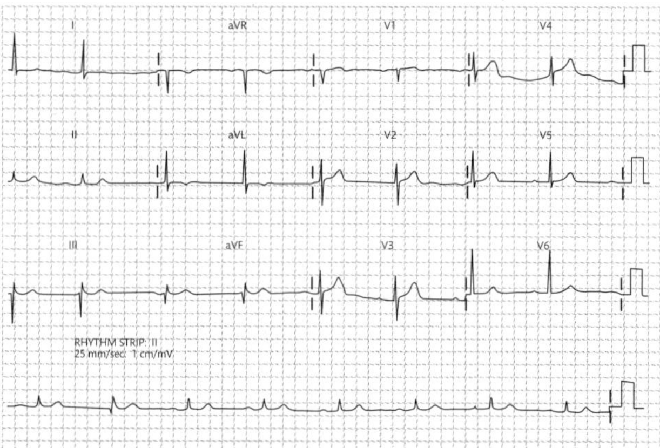

3. A 74-year-old woman was admitted 2 days ago with a large anterior ST-elevation MI. Because of delays in transfer to a local cardiac centre she received primary angioplasty 10 hours after the onset of pain, where critical stenosis was revealed in the left anterior descending artery, and two stents were inserted. She was making a good recovery on the CCU until she suddenly becomes acutely short of breath whilst sitting on her bed. Her blood pressure is 84/56 mmHg, pulse 118 bpm, and her oxygen saturation is 86% on air, rising to 94% on high-flow oxygen. On auscultation of her chest she has crackles extending from the lung bases to the midzones, and a loud pan-systolic murmur loudest at the apex, radiating to the left axilla. No-one has documented this murmur in the previous entries in the notes.

(1) List three essential, urgent investigations.

(2) How should she be managed in the meantime?

Presentation

Presented to ______ Grade ______ Date ______

Signed

Remember that you can find large-size, annotated versions of many of the X-rays and ECGs that appear in this book on the book's web site at www.oxfordtextbooks.co.uk/orc/randall/

Answers

1. This man has had a non-ST-elevation MI. His GRACE 6-month mortality is 4%. The purpose of keeping him in hospital is first to monitor for any acute complications which may develop, but secondly to investigate him fully to minimize the chances of him suffering further cardiac disease.

Investigation	Relevant?	Why?
Repeat ECG	✓	Repeat ECGs are carried out daily for several days after admission, to exclude ongoing or recurring ischaemia and to reveal developing arrhythmias
Repeat chest X-ray	✗	All patients admitted with acute coronary syndrome should have an initial chest radiograph. However, this only requires repetition if the patient's breathing becomes compromised or their oxygen saturations fall
Fasting glucose level and lipid profile	✓	Reducing cardiovascular risk is important in patients admitted with ACS, acute MI, or other vascular disease. Measuring fasting glucose and lipids, as well as monitoring the patient's blood pressure, allows previously undiagnosed diabetes, hyperlipidaemia, and hypertension to be picked up
Echocardiogram	✓	Should be performed routinely on all patients admitted with a MI. This allows the extent and severity of myocardial damage, valvular lesions, and deformities, such as ventricular aneurysms, to be identified. Poor ventricular function (for example, a left ventricular ejection fraction of <40%) is associated with a poor prognosis and significant heart failure
Exercise tolerance test	✗	This test is useful in confirming the presence of ischaemic heart disease in patients presenting with troponin-negative chest pain. It is not indicated in this man because he has had a proven MI.
Angiogram	✓	An in-patient angiogram should be performed on this man since he falls into the 'intermediate risk' category on the NICE guidelines for NSTEMI. This would look for areas of discrete critical narrowing in his coronary arteries. These are potentially treatable with angioplasty and stent insertion or coronary artery bypass grafting
Cardiac MRI scanning	✗	Cardiac MRI scanning is an advanced and expensive test for investigating structural heart disease which is not indicated in the initial investigation of ischaemic heart disease

2. The abnormalities shown on this ECG are illustrated below:

This ECG reveals first degree heart block

The heart rate can be calculated from an ECG either by dividing 300 by the number of small squares between each QRS complex (in this case, 300/6 = 50), or by counting the number of QRS complexes within 30 large squares and multiplying this by 10 (in this case, 5 x 10 = 50).

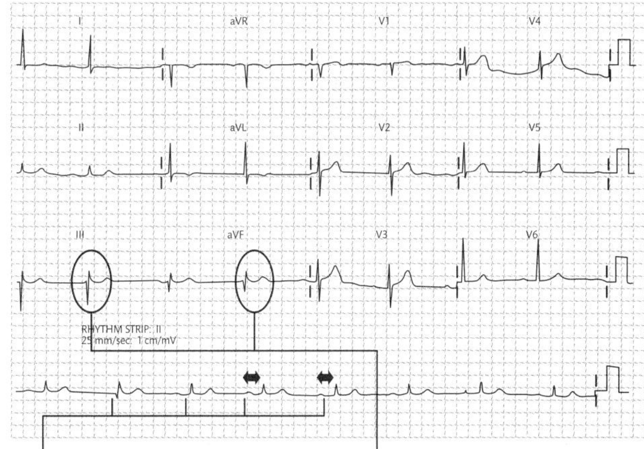

First degree heart block is defined by a PR interval (beginning of the P wave to beginning of the QRS complex), or greater than 200 ms (or 5 small squares). Here the PR interval is around 280 ms (7 small sqaures). Importantly, all P waves are followed by QRS complexes (in second degree block, some P waves fail to produce QRS complexes and in complete heart block none do).

Note Q waves in leads III and aVF – two of the three inferior leads, in keeping with this patient's previous MI.

The simplest explanation for this patient's bradycardia might be rate-limiting medications, since there is evidence to support starting all patients suffering an MI on beta-blockers (to prevent the development of tachyarrythmias), unless there are clear contraindications. However, inferior MIs are also frequently associated with disorders of cardiac rhythm, because they are caused by occlusion of the right coronary artery which in the majority of patients supplies the atrioventricular node.

If there is no evidence of haemodynamic compromise (as in this man), first-degree heart block does not require any treatment. Repeat ECGs should be carried out regularly since a proportion of patients will progress to second- and third-degree heart block. If there is haemodynamic compromise then the low rate may be increased by giving intravenous atropine (initially 600 micrograms, which can be repeated several times). Failure to respond to atropine is an indication for temporary cardiac pacing. Most bradycardias associated with inferior MIs are benign and spontaneously resolve within a few days or weeks.

3. Three crucial investigations are an ECG (to exclude a new dysrhythmia which commonly causes acute heart failure following an MI), chest X-ray to confirm that the respiratory compromise is due to fluid overload, and an urgent echocardiogram to determine the cause of this newly observed murmur.

This woman is in 'shock' (hypotensive and tachycardic), that initially must be assumed to be cardiogenic in origin. There is also evidence of respiratory compromise (probably secondary to pulmonary oedema given the examination findings), and a new systolic murmur. She is critically unwell and requires urgent assessment by a senior doctor. The likeliest cause for this deterioration is severe acute mitral regurgitation, which may complicate anterior and septal MIs. Such infarcts cause rupture of the papillary muscles, which anchor the leaflets of the mitral valve. A similar clinical picture may be produced by acute rupture of the intra-ventricular septum.

Treatment of cardiogenic shock should include management in a high-dependency area and invasive monitoring, and often requires inotropic and vasoconstrictive drugs. It is commonly complicated by multiorgan failure, including renal and respiratory compromise, and patients may need invasive ventilation and renal support. Acute, severe mitral regurgitation requires emergency valve replacement, so this patient's case should be discussed urgently with cardiothoracic surgeons.

Further reading

Guidelines: NICE guidelines for secondary prevention after MI (http://guidance.nice.org.uk/CG048)

OHCM: 114–117, 142, 808–810

Heart failure

This section should be used to clerk patients admitted to hospital with a worsening of heart failure. As a chronic disease, management is principally in the community; however, acute exacerbations may require admission to hospital. Typical patient pathways lead from the Emergency Department to the CCU and General Medical or Elderly Care wards.

Learning challenges

- What is the Frank–Starling law of the heart? How might this mechanism fail in heart failure?
- Why may a patient with stable heart failure suddenly decompensate?

History

Comment on

- Known cardiac disease
- Normal and present exercise tolerance; duration of change
- Orthopnoea, PND, and peripheral oedema
- Chest pain or palpitations
- Medications

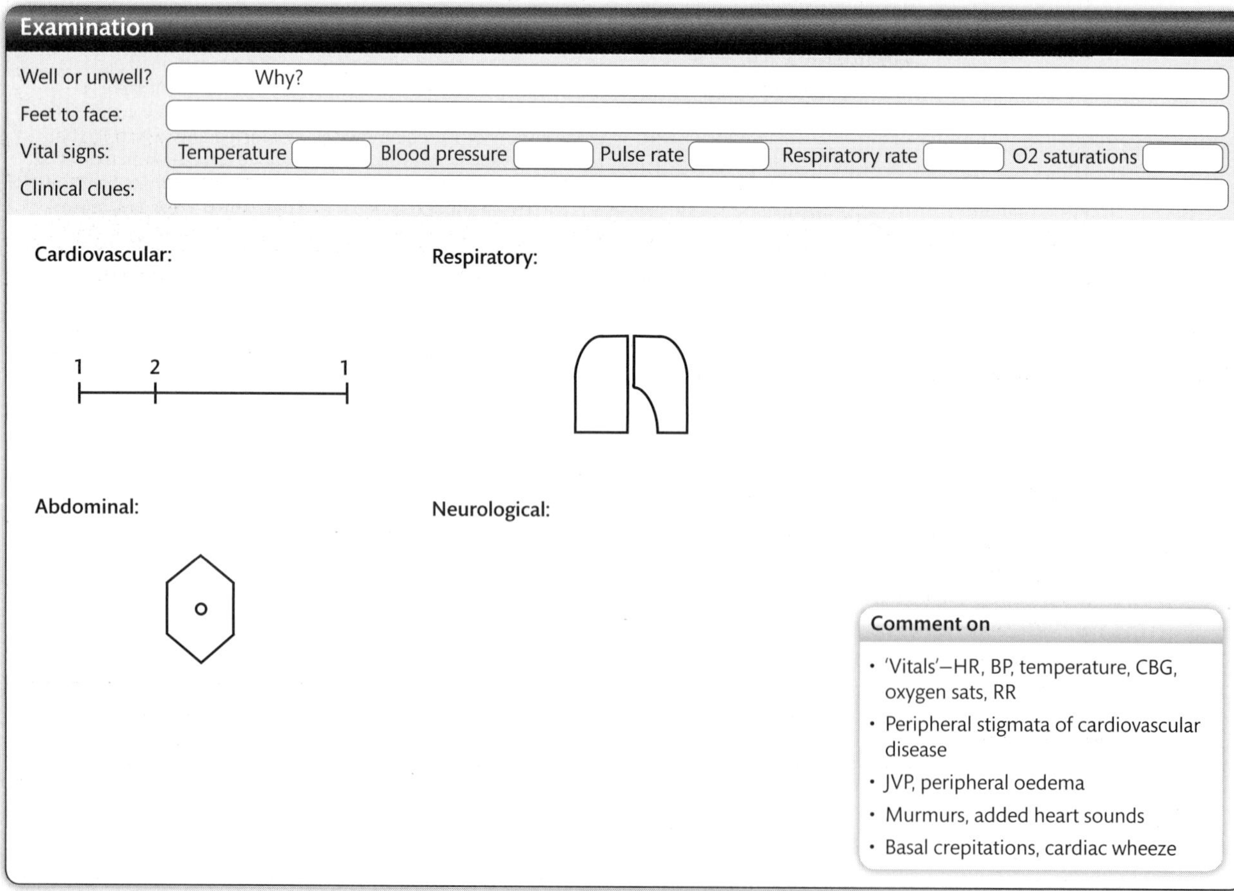

Comment on

- 'Vitals'—HR, BP, temperature, CBG, oxygen sats, RR
- Peripheral stigmata of cardiovascular disease
- JVP, peripheral oedema
- Murmurs, added heart sounds
- Basal crepitations, cardiac wheeze

Chest X-ray

Comment on

- Heart size—cardiomegaly?
- Pulmonary oedema; other signs of failure

Arterial blood gas

Comment on

- Respiratory failure? Type 1 or type 2?

Echocardiogram

Comment on

- Overall ventricular function
- Valvular lesions
- Ejection fraction
- End-diastolic volume

ECG

Comment on

- Ischaemic changes
- Chamber hypertrophy or strain
- Arrhythmias

Blood tests

Comment on

- U&Es
- Troponin
- Fasting blood glucose and lipids

Evaluation

1. Does this patient have acute pulmonary oedema? Are they on appropriate treatment for it? Do they need ventilatory support?

2. What is the likely cause of the patient's worsening heart failure?

3. What is the patient's baseline 'cardiac status'?

New York Heart Association grading of 'cardiac status'

- **Grade 1:** Uncompromised (no breathlessness)
- **Grade 2:** Slightly compromised (breathlessness on severe exertion)
- **Grade 3:** Moderately compromised (breathlessness on mild exertion)
- **Grade 4:** Severely compromised (breathlessness at rest)

4. Which management options are appropriate?

- Lifestyle measures:
- Increased medication:
- Invasive measures, e.g. surgery:

Questions

1. An 89-year-old man is brought into the resuscitation room of the hospital Emergency Department after becoming breathless with a significantly decreased exercise tolerance over the previous few days. He has a previous medical history of two MIs but until recently was able to walk around indoors without becoming breathless. Now he is breathless after only a few steps. He does not complain of palpitations or of chest pain, and says that that he has not experienced any other symptoms. On examination basic observations include pulse 110 bpm, blood pressure 145/88 mmHg, respiratory rate 24 breaths/min, and oxygen saturations 94% on high-flow oxygen. His JVP was measured at 18 cm and auscultation of his chest revealed fine crackles heard throughout inspiration in both lower zones. An X-ray is arranged, which is shown below.

(1) What features of heart failure does it show?

(2) What further investigations would you arrange?

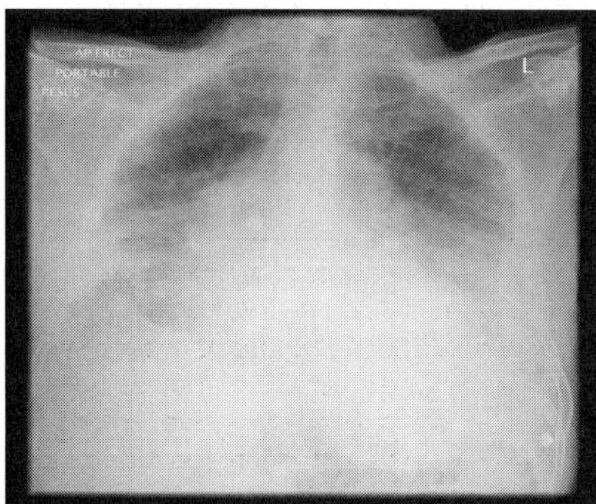

2. A 60-year-old man with congestive heart failure is managed in the community by the heart failure nurse. When she sees him on a home visit, he reports feeling much more breathless than usual, and has oxygen saturations of 82% on room air. She calls an ambulance and sends him to the Emergency Department for a fuller assessment. Initial triage reveals that he is extremely breathless, with a respiratory rate of 30 breaths/min and saturations on high-flow oxygen of 88%. His JVP is elevated, a third heart sound is heard, and crepitations are present bilaterally in the lower and mid-zones. His arterial blood gas analysis (taken immediately, with the patient on high-flow oxygen) is shown below.

- pH: 7.36
- pO_2: 7.65 kPa
- pCO_2: 5.45 kPa
- HCO_3^-: 23.2
- BE: 2.0

List 10 important immediate management steps, including therapeutic interventions, where the patient should be managed and what vital clinical observations you would monitor.

3. A 48-year-old man is admitted to a regional cardiology centre for primary angioplasty after suffering a large anterior STEMI. Several days later he is making good progress on the ward though he feels himself to be very short of breath on exertion, and unable to lie completely flat. An echocardiogram, carried out as part of his routine in-patient assessment, reveals an ejection fraction of 25% with significant left ventricular hypokinesia, normal diastolic filling, and no significant valve defects.

(1) What do these results mean?

(2) List the important management steps prior to his discharge.

Presentation

Presented to ______ Grade ______ Date ______

Signed

Remember that you can find large-size, annotated versions of many of the X-rays and ECGs that appear in this book on the book's web site at www.oxfordtextbooks.co.uk/orc/randall/

Answers

1. This chest X-ray shows many of the classic features of heart failure:

This x-ray shows many classic features of left ventricular failure and pulmonary oedema:

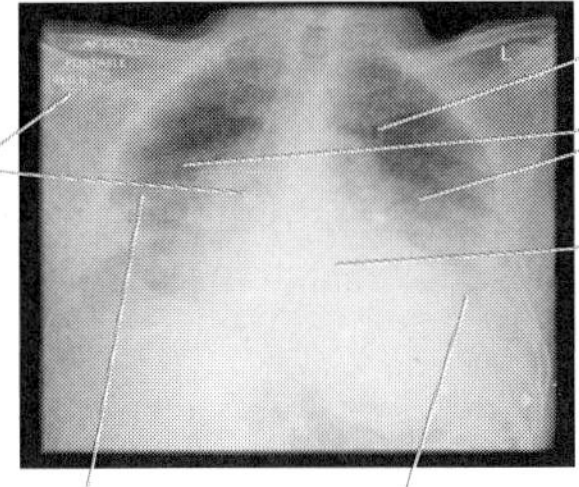

The most important investigations to perform acutely are those to determine how sick the patient is and why he has acutely deteriorated. Arterial blood gas analysis will determine the degree of respiratory failure, and guide oxygen therapy. An ECG will help determine whether this sudden decompensation in cardiac function may have been caused by an acute arrhythmia (such as atrial fibrillation) or by new cardiac ischaemia or infarction. Serum troponin will reveal whether the patient has had a MI, which may present only with pulmonary oedema in the elderly. Acute renal failure can also cause pulmonary oedema, so urea and creatinine levels should also be checked and compared with previous levels. In the next few days, an echocardiogram will confirm and quantify the degree of heart failure, as well as suggesting possible structural causes such as valve disease or cardiomyopathy.

2. This patient is in type one respiratory failure. He is considerably hypoxic even on high-flow oxygen. Pulmonary oedema can cause either type one or type two respiratory failure. Priorities for management of acute pulmonary oedema are:

1. Sit the patient up and maintain him on high-flow oxygen.
2. Obtain a chest X-ray to confirm the diagnosis of pulmonary oedema.
3. Perform blood tests, including renal function and a troponin level.
4. Manage him in a high-dependency area—either the Emergency Department resuscitation room or an acute or coronary care unit.
5. Monitor basic observations including, most crucially, the oxygen saturations.
6. Give intravenous GTN, reducing the pre-load and after-load on the heart. However, intravenous GTN produces hypotension and so can only be started if the systolic blood pressure is well maintained.
7. Give intravenous morphine, along with an antiemetic.
8. Give intravenous frusemide if there is good renal function, intravenously since oral absorption is likely to be limited by bowel wall oedema.
9. Review the patient shortly after these measures have been taken. Signs of improvement would include an improvement in breathlessness, oxygen saturations and respiratory rate, alongside improving blood gases—a rising pO_2 and pH and a falling pCO_2.
10. Consider ventilatory support if respiratory function worsens—either invasive ventilation with endotracheal intubation in the intensive care unit, or a trial of non-invasive ventilation.

3. This patient has echocardiological evidence of systolic heart failure, with the ventricle filling normally during diastole but with a low ejection fraction. This correlates with his symptoms of exertional breathlessness and orthopnoea. However, a phenomenon called 'myocardial stunning' has been observed where ventricular function can be severely decreased after a MI with subsequent reperfusion, improving significantly in the days or weeks afterwards.

Before leaving the hospital, this patient's cardiovascular risk should be addressed, with lifestyle advice and secondary prevention medications such as aspirin, a statin, and antihypertensives. He should be encouraged to take as much exercise as possible to try to improve and maintain cardiac function. Various medications are effective in heart failure (see the answer to Question 5), but loop diuretics (which improve symptoms but not prognosis) are often first line until the severity of the heart failure can be assessed.

Further reading

Guidelines: NICE guidelines for chronic heart failure (http://www.nice.org.uk/cg005)

OHCM: 128–130, 146, 812–814

Arrhythmias

This section should be used to clerk patients with brady- or tachyarrhythmias. Patient pathways for patients with arrhythmias vary: many patients with palpitations are not admitted to hospital but are managed in the Emergency Department and in out-patient clinics.

Learning challenges

- What is the differential diagnosis for a 'blackout' or 'funny turn'?
- What are the different types of cardiac pacing?
- What is endocardial ablation therapy?

History

Comment on

- Description of palpitations
- Syncope, autonomic symptoms
- Chest pain, breathlessness
- Duration of symptoms
- Previous history of cardiac disease, e.g. valvular heart disease or IHD

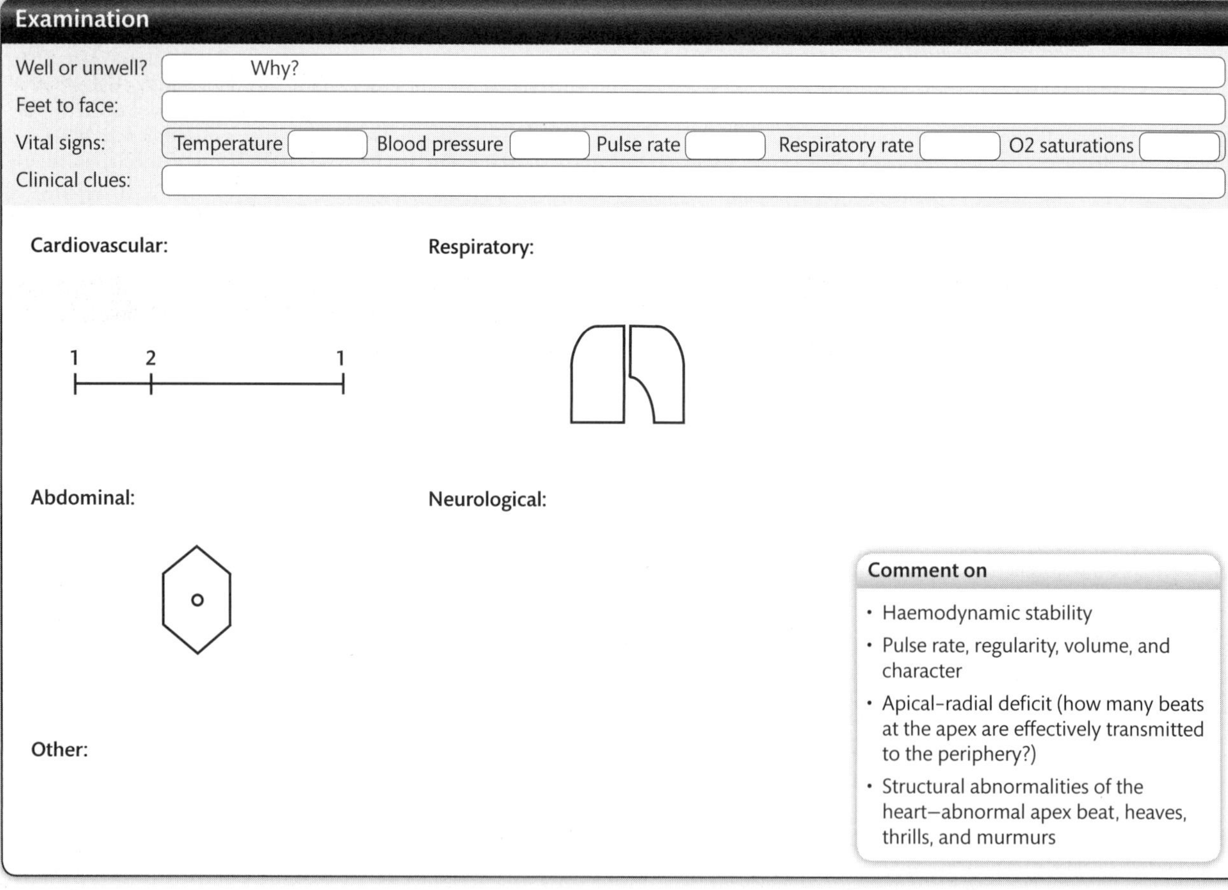

Examination

Well or unwell? Why?

Feet to face:

Vital signs: Temperature | Blood pressure | Pulse rate | Respiratory rate | O2 saturations

Clinical clues:

Cardiovascular:

1 2 1

Respiratory:

Abdominal:

Neurological:

Other:

Comment on

- Haemodynamic stability
- Pulse rate, regularity, volume, and character
- Apical-radial deficit (how many beats at the apex are effectively transmitted to the periphery?)
- Structural abnormalities of the heart—abnormal apex beat, heaves, thrills, and murmurs

ECG

Comment on

- Rate
- Rhythm—regular or irregular; presence/absence of P waves
- PR and QT intervals
- Width of QRS complexes (broad >3 mm)

Rhythm strip/serial ECGs

Comment on

- Response to vagal manoeuvres/drugs

Chest X-ray

Comment on

- Cardiomegaly
- Valvular calcification
- Signs of cardiac failure

Rhythm strip/serial ECGs

Comment on

- Structural heart disease

Blood tests

Comment on

- 12-hour troponin
- Electrolytes (K+, Mg2+, Ca2+)
- Thyroid function
- Evidence of infection

Evaluation

1. **Is this patient haemodynamically compromised? Do they need any emergency interventions?**

2. **Look for P waves, QRS complexes, and T waves. Which rhythm are they in?**

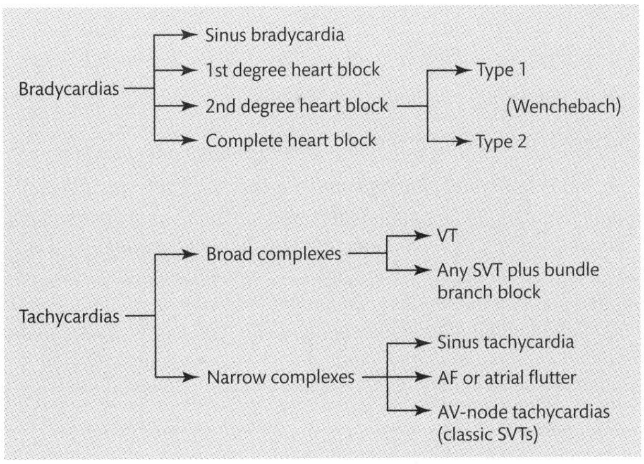

- Bradycardias
  - Sinus bradycardia
  - 1st degree heart block
  - 2nd degree heart block
    - Type 1 (Wenchebach)
    - Type 2
  - Complete heart block
- Tachycardias
  - Broad complexes
    - VT
    - Any SVT plus bundle branch block
  - Narrow complexes
    - Sinus tachycardia
    - AF or atrial flutter
    - AV-node tachycardias (classic SVTs)

3. **Is this acute, chronic, or paroxysmal? What is the likely cause?**

4. **What there a definitive treatment for this condition? Is it appropriate for this patient?**

5. **In the meantime, what other treatments are appropriate to improve symptoms and longer-term risks?**

Questions

1. A 64-year-old woman presents to the Emergency Department complaining of palpitations and shortness of breath which started several days before and have been gradually getting worse. She had never experienced palpitations before. She had otherwise been well, with no other symptoms, and had no significant previous medical history. On examination the patient was alert and conscious, with a respiratory rate of 20 breaths/min and oxygen saturations of 98% on air. Her pulse was irregularly irregular at a rate varying between 120 and 140 bpm, with normal volume and character. The blood pressure was 110/65 mmHg. Examination of the praecordium was unremarkable. Her ECG is shown below:

(1) What is the abnormality shown?

(2) What should be the priorities of management?

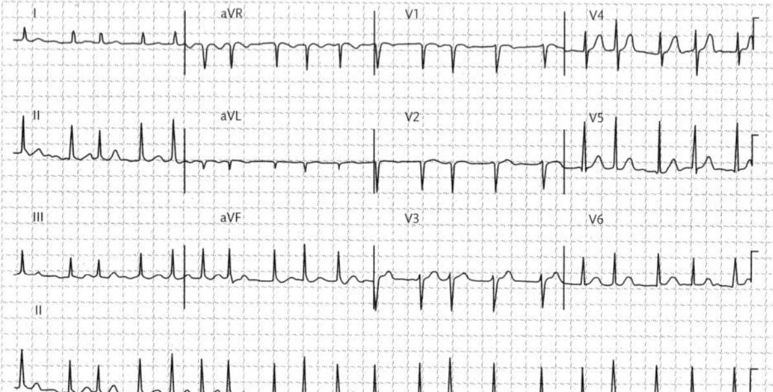

2. A 29-year-old man presents to the Emergency Department with an hour-long history of fast, 'heavy' palpitations. He is also experiencing 'chest tightness' and mild shortness of breath. He has had two similar episodes in the last couple of months, both self-terminating in less than a few minutes, and he did not seek medical advice. On examination he is pale and sweaty, with a heart rate of 200 bpm and blood pressure of 95/55 mmHg. The rest of the examination is unremarkable. The cardiac monitor reveals a regular narrow-complex tachycardia. The Emergency Department doctor asks the patient twice to attempt the Valsalva manoeuvre, but after this is unsuccessful gives a bolus of intravenous adenosine, after which the rhythm strip reveals a sinus rhythm with a rate of 90 bpm.

(1) What is the diagnosis?

(2) What is the Valsalva manoeuvre?

(3) The patient now feels completely better, and wants to go home. His heart rate is 90 bpm and his blood pressure is 122/78 mmHg. How should he be followed up?

3. A 77-year-old man is brought to the Emergency Department by ambulance after being found drowsy and breathless by his daughter. He had seemed completely well earlier in the day. Of note he suffered a non-ST-elevation MI a few months ago. On examination his GCS is 12/15 and he has a heart rate varying between 35 and 45 with a blood pressure of 74/38 mmHg. His ECG is shown below:

(1) What is the ECG rhythm?

(2) What immediate management is indicated?

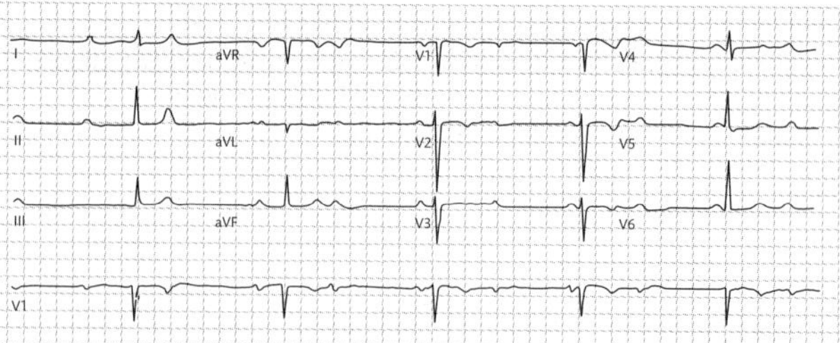

4. The alarms on one of the cardiac monitors on the CCU start to sound. The patient, a 58-year-old woman admitted several days before after suffering a non-ST-elevation MI, is sitting in a chair alert and oriented but complaining of palpitations and a tight feeling in her chest. Her blood pressure is 104/56 mm Hg.

(1) What is the rhythm shown on the cardiac monitor strip below?

(2) What treatment is indicated?

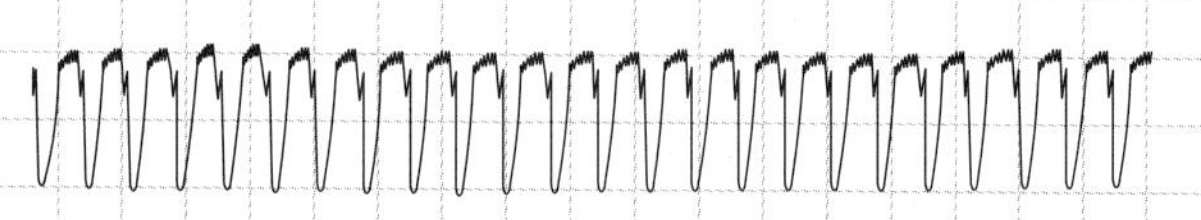

5. A 70-year-old woman visits her doctor complaining of left-sided chest pain which is worse on deep inspiration, shortness of breath on exertion, and a non-productive cough. These symptoms came on rapidly 1 week ago. Apart from this she has been generally well, though is receiving out-patient physiotherapy after suffering a fractured neck of femur a month before. On examination she has a pulse rate of 130 bpm (regular), a blood pressure of 112/56 mmHg, and oxygen saturations of 90% on room air. Her ECG, recorded on arrival in the Emergency Department, is shown below.

(1) Describe the ECG abnormalities.

(2) List the essential investigations.

(3) What is the management?

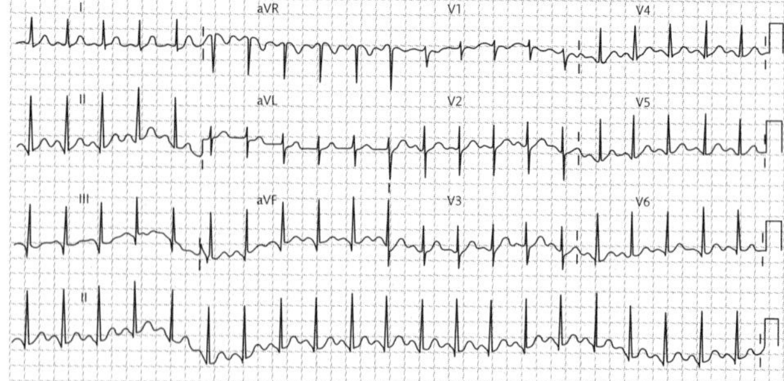

Presentation

Presented to | Grade | Date

Signed

Remember that you can find large-size, annotated versions of many of the X-rays and ECGs that appear in this book on the book's web site at www.oxfordtextbooks.co.uk/orc/randall/

Answers

1. The ECG confirms the clinical diagnosis of fast atrial fibrillation (AF), with a variable interval between each QRS complex (this can be confirmed by laying another piece of paper on top of the ECG, marking each QRS and then sliding the paper along the ECG), and absent P waves. However, despite a fast ventricular rate, the blood pressure is not compromised and the patient feels quite well.

In the absence of hypotension, the first priority of management will be to achieve control of the ventricular rate. This is usually achieved in younger patients with a beta-blocker , a rate-limiting calcium-channel blocker such as diltiazem, or with amiodarone (digoxin may be preferred in older patients or those with a history of heart failure). The next step is to search for an underlying cause of the AF, with basic tests such as:

- **Inflammatory markers**–rule out infection
- **Troponin**–rule out an ischaemic event
- **Echocardiogram**–rule out structural disease, especially mitral valve abnormalities
- **Thyroid function tests**–rule out thyrotoxicosis

A proportion of AF has no obvious cause and is termed 'lone' atrial fibrillation. This type of AF is often the most amenable to cardioversion. AF secondary to defined pathologies tends to relapse unless the precipitating cause is treated or removed.

Cardioversion should be carried out acutely only if it can be proven that the patient has been in AF for less than 48 hours. Otherwise the risk of stroke is too great and typically the patient should be anticoagulated for 6 weeks prior to elective cardioversion. So in this case the management could be:

(1) Rate control with medications

(2) Discharge (once rate control is achieved and symptomatically better) on warfarin

(3) Out-patient echocardiogram

(4) Elective cardioversion in 6 weeks

2. The differential diagnosis here is between different forms of supraventricular tachycardia (SVT). Since adenosine cardioverts the patient back to normal sinus rhythm, it is clear that that the AV node was involved in the process. In atrioventricular nodal re-entry tachycardia (AVNRT), or atrioventricular reciprocating tachycardia (AVRT), abnormal loops of conductive tissue allow action potentials to cycle around the AV node.

Management is based on slowing or blocking electrical transmission through the AV node. In the Valsalva manoeuvre the patient closes their glottis and strains hard–the resultant rise in intrathoracic pressure produces a reflex rise is vagal tone which slows AV node conduction. A similar effect is produced by carotid sinus massage. The drug adenosine produces complete block of the AV node for several seconds, which will terminate any tachycardia caused by an abnormal loop involving the AV node. Below is a rhythm strip showing (arrow) when a bolus of adenosine was given:

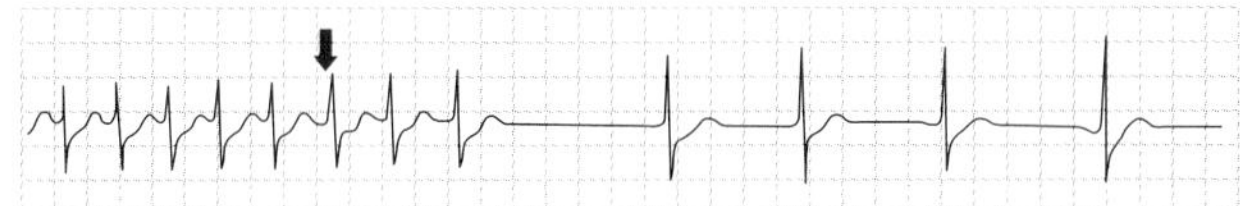

A repeat ECG should be performed once the patient has reverted back to sinus rhythm, looking for precipitating causes. A short PR interval, with early excitation of the ventricles (a slurred upstroke in the QRS complex) is indicative of Wolff-Parkinson-White (WPW) syndrome, one cause of AVRT and a cause of sudden cardiac death in young people. All AVRTs are caused by accessory pathways allowing action potentials to accelerate through the AV node; they can be cured by radiofrequency ablation where the accessory pathway is mapped out using various intracardiac probes and then destroyed.

3. This ECG reveals complete (third degree) heart block (CHB).

Note the complete dissociation between P waves (marked with a ⬇) and QRS complexes (marked with a ★). Here the ventricular rate is around 35 beats per minute (divide 300 by the number of large squares between each QRS complex, in this case 9)

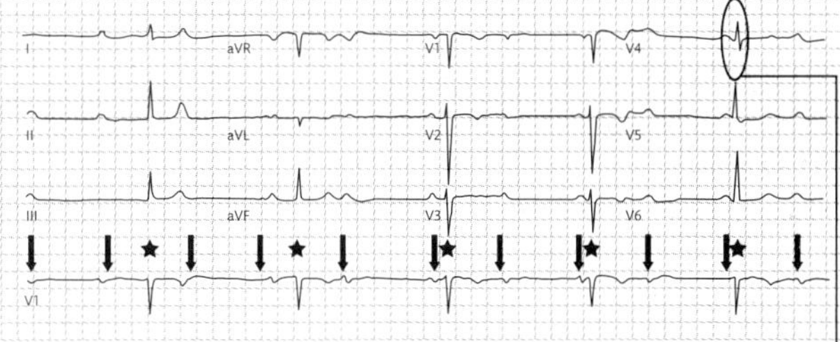

Urgent action is needed since this man is haemodynamically unstable. Atropine, which blocks the effect of the vagus nerve on the heart, may be successful in increasing the heart rate in complete heart block with narrow complexes, where impulses are being generated from fairly high up in the conducting system–perhaps the AV node itself, which is where atropine acts. Broad complexes imply a pacemaker lower down in the His-Purkinje system, or even in the ventricles themselves, which respond less well to atropine. If atropine is unsuccessful in correcting the bradycardia and hypotension, then this man will require pacing, which can be done either externally via defibrillator pads with the patient sedated, or internally with a temporary pacing wire inserted via one of the great veins. This provides a temporary solution before a permanent pacemaker is fitted.

4. This is a broad complex tachycardia. Since it is regular and all complexes are identical, this should be assumed to be ventricular tachycardia (VT). Although VT is one of the rhythms that cause cardiac arrest, it can also be accompanied by a pulse and well-maintained blood pressure. Either way, rapid cardioversion is required. This can be done either by electricity, with the patient sufficiently sedated, or pharmacologically. Since this woman is not hypotensive, an infusion of amiodarone could be given into a central vein, with electrical cardioversion attempted if the amiodarone fails. Longer term she will require an implantable cardiac defibrillator to deliver an internal shock or overdrive pacing should she develop VT outside hospital.

5. This ECG shows sinus tachycardia, with a normal 'P-QRS-T' rhythm. Sinus tachycardia is an abnormality of cardiac rate (not an arrhythmia), and usually does not reflect intrinsic cardiac disease. Rather it is usually an appropriate response of the heart to extrinsic pressure–for instance, all normal individuals experience sinus tachycardia during exercise.

In the hospital setting, in patients at rest, common causes of sinus tachycardia may include pain, pyrexia of any cause, haemorrhage, systemic inflammation (for instance secondary to sepsis), pulmonary embolism, or dehydration. In this woman, a history of hypoxia, pleuritic chest pain, hypoxia, and recent immobility mean that a pulmonary embolus has to be ruled out. In other patients, since hypovolaemia is a common factor in many causes of sinus tachycardia, a fluid bolus if often given to see if this helps control the heart rate.

Further reading

Guidelines: Resuscitation Council (UK) advanced life support algorithms (http://www.resus.org.uk/pages/periarst.pdf)

OHCM: 118-127, 816-818

Valvular and structural heart disease

This section should be used to clerk patients with any kind of valvular heart disease, whether it is causing symptoms, presenting as infective endocarditis, or simply picked up incidentally. Patient journeys begin when they present to the Emergency Department or their GP, and are then managed either on cardiology wards (or cardiothoracic surgery units) or are investigated as out-patients.

Learning challenges

- What is rheumatic fever? How does it damage the heart, and why is it so rare now in the developed world?
- How does the heart form in utero? What are the commonest congenital heart abnormalities?

History

Comment on

- Symptoms of heart failure. Syncope
- Previously noticed murmurs, or rheumatic fever
- Infective symptoms—sweats, shivers, malaise
- Risk factors for bacteraemia

Examination

Well or unwell? Why?

Feet to face:

Vital signs: Temperature Blood pressure Pulse rate Respiratory rate O2 saturations

Clinical clues:

Cardiovascular:

1 2 1

Respiratory:

Abdominal:

Neurological:

Other:

Comment on

- Peripheral or central cyanosis
- Peripheral stigmata of infective endocarditis
- Fever
- Breathlessness
- Pulse rate, regularity, volume, and character
- Apex beat and character, JVP
- Careful description of murmur
- Signs of heart failure

Echocardiogram (transthoracic or transoesophageal)

Comment on

- Nature and severity of valve lesion
- Effect on heart chambers
- Presence of vegetations

ECG

Comment on

- Signs of chamber enlargement or strain
- Dysrhythmias

Chest X-ray

Comment on

- Cardiomegaly, chamber enlargement, valvular calcification

Blood tests

Comment on

- Evidence of infection
- Blood cultures

Evaluation

1. **What are the main structural lesions identified? How severe are they?**

2. **How is the heart compensating? Is there chamber enlargement, pulmonary hypertension, or other valve lesions?**

3. **Are Duke's criteria for diagnosing infective endocarditis met?**

Major criteria	Minor criteria
Positive blood cultures—two or more with the same organism which is known to cause infective endocarditis Evidence of endocardial involvement—vegetations or abscess	Risk factors for bacteraemia or known valve lesion Fever Emboli Immunological phenomena (e.g. splinters) One positive blood culture or serology Other echocardiographic evidence of infective endocarditis
For diagnosis: Two major criteria One major and three minor criteria Five minor criteria	

4. **What short-term and long-term management options are available?**

Questions

1. An 84-year-old man without any significant health problems is brought in by ambulance after collapsing whilst running to catch a bus. Two onlookers described him stopping running, appearing very pale, and then collapsing, lying still for a few seconds on the ground with slight twitching of his left hand. He fully recovers within a few moments. He gives a history of feeling very breathless and dizzy on exertion for the past 2 months, with occasional chest pain on exertion accompanying these symptoms. On examination he appeared well, had pulses that were difficult to palpate globally, and had a murmur that was loudest in mid-systole, heard clearest at the right sternal edge in the second rib space, and that radiated to the carotids. What is the likely diagnosis and what are the next steps?

2. A 38-year-old man of Indian origin reports feeling much more short of breath over the previous 2 weeks, and complains of palpitations. He had suffered with rheumatic fever as a child but was otherwise well. When he is seen in the Emergency Department he is found to be extremely breathless, requiring high-flow oxygen to maintain oxygen saturations above 94%. Physical examination revealed a fast irregularly irregular pulse.

Later ECG confirmed fast atrial fibrillation, with a ventricular rate of around 140 bpm. Physical examination revealed an irregularly irregular pulse, a normal JVP, and a 'tapping' apex beat felt at the left parasternal edge. He had a rumbling mid-diastolic murmur heard loudest with the bell of the stethoscope held lightly over the apex of the heart. ECG confirmed atrial fibrillation, and his chest X-ray is below.

(1) What abnormalities are shown on the X-ray?

(2) What is the likely diagnosis and how is it managed?

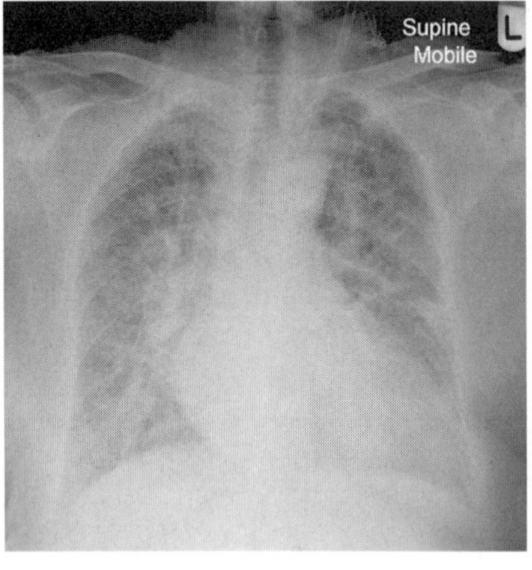

3. A 54-year-old woman known to have mitral regurgitation secondary to a connective tissue disorder attends for her 6-yearly review. Physical examination reveals a loud pan-systolic murmur loudest at the apex and radiating to the axilla, along with a thrusting apex beat felt in the sixth intercostals space in the anterior axillary line. She has an ECG (shown below) and is due to have an echocardiogram. In view of the examination findings and ECG, what would you expect the echocardiogram to reveal?

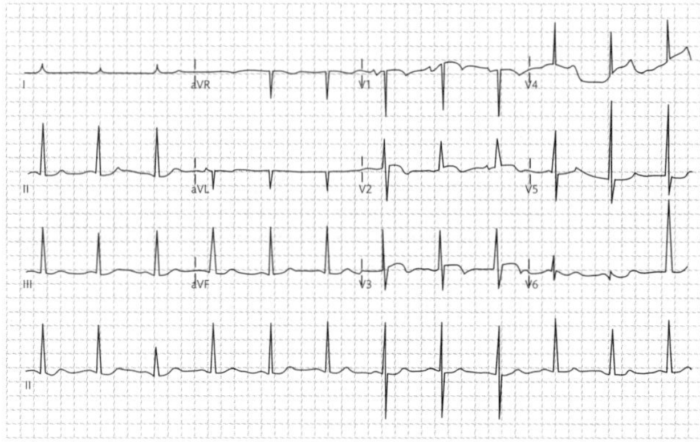

4. A 34-year-old man who injects heroin intravenously presents with a week-long history of worsening shortness of breath and feeling generally unwell. He has been feverish and had a productive cough. On examination he has a temperature of 38.9°C, no peripheral stigmata of infective endocarditis, a raised JVP with a prominent V wave, a pan-systolic murmur at the left sternal edge, and a tender, pulsatile liver with some ankle oedema. His chest X-ray is below. What does it show, and how would you proceed?

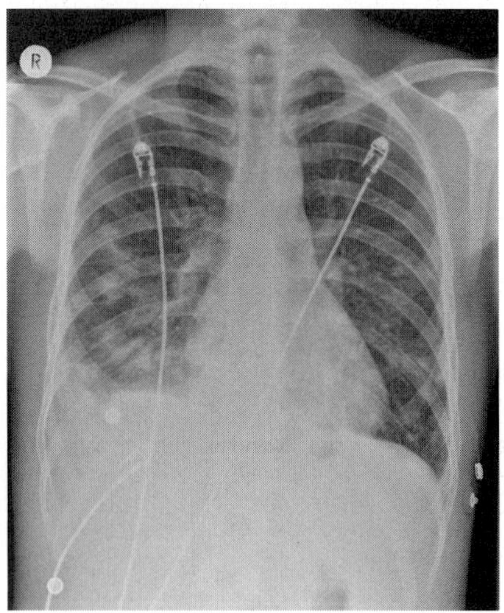

Presentation

Presented to | Grade | Date

Signed

Remember that you can find large-size, annotated versions of many of the X-rays and ECGs that appear in this book on the book's web site at www.oxfordtextbooks.co.uk/orc/randall/

Answers

1. The diagnosis of blackouts is difficult and requires a careful description of events from bystanders who observed what happened. The history here is suggestive of syncope, especially given that he has a longer history of feeling dizzy and breathless on exertion. The signs found on physical examination are suggestive of aortic stenosis, with an ejection systolic murmur radiating upwards from the aortic area to the carotids. The classic 'slow-rising pulse' can in practice simply feel difficult to palpate—remember this before questioning your examination technique!

Aortic stenosis is a common finding in older people, caused most commonly (in the developed world) by age-related calcification. It limits the amount by which cardiac output can rise during exercise. This produces exertional syncope, where the blood pressure falls due to the generalized vasodilatation caused by exercise and inadequate cardiac compensation. Aortic stenosis can be confirmed and quantified by echocardiogram. ECG may show signs of left ventricular hypertrophy. All symptomatic patients should be offered valve replacement if they are fit enough to survive and benefit from surgery.

2. This x-ray shows:

Note various features of pulmonary oedema, including redistribution of blood to the upper lobes ('upper lobe diversion'), general interstitial shadowing, bronchial wall thickening (due to oedema) and Kerley 'B' lines (interlobular septal oedema) seen best at the right base.

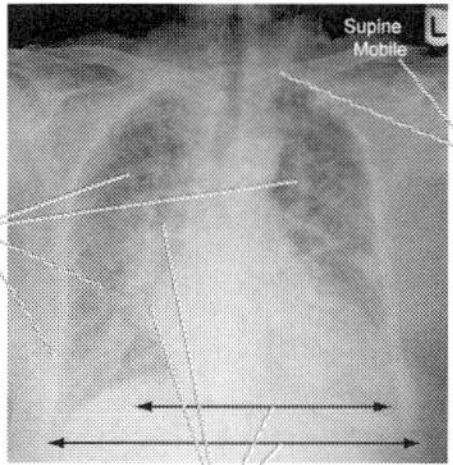

This is a classic 'resus film' taken of an acutely unwell patient in the resuscitation room of the emergency department. Notice the oxygen tubing, that it is a mobile film and was taken with the patient supine (therefore it will be an anteroposterior film). The first thing to do to help this man is to sit him up!

Look at the heart. The first thing to say is that it appears enlarged; although cardiomegaly should only be diagnosed on postero-anterior films (because antero-posterior films make it look artificially large), it is likely nevertheless that this man's heart is enlarged (on this film, the width of the heart is clearly >50% of the maximum internal diameter of the rib cage). There is also a prominent bulge of the right heart border, suggesting right atrial enlargement. This, together with bulky appearances of the hila, suggests pulmonary hypertension with right heart strain.

This patient's pulmonary oedema is likely to be due to his going into fast atrial fibrillation, and priorities for management are rate control and management of pulmonary oedema along standard lines.

Signs found on physical examination of this man are in keeping with an underlying diagnosis of mitral stenosis—a tapping, non-displaced apex beat accompanied by a rumbling mid to late diastolic murmur heard at the left sternal edge. Just as aortic stenosis causes a fixed outflow obstruction leading to hypertrophy of the left ventricle, so mitral stenosis causes a fixed outflow obstruction and enlargement of the left atrium. Almost all mitral stenosis is caused by rheumatic heart disease, which may often be encountered in patients who grew up in the developing world.

As mitral stenosis progresses, the following complications may develop:

- **Left sided heart failure**, causing symptoms of exertional breathlessness and orthopnoea.
- **Atrial fibrillation**, caused by distension of the left atrium, as in this man. The development of atrial fibrillation may cause palpitations, and cause a rapid worsening of symptoms. It also predisposes to embolic phenomena, e.g. strokes.
- **Pulmonary hypertension** caused by persistently raised pulmonary venous pressures—this leads to worsening dyspnoea and recurrent chest infections.
- **Right-sided heart failure** ('congestive' heart failure)—causing peripheral oedema, hepatomegaly and ascites.

Mitral stenosis is initially treated with diuretics to relieve the symptoms of heart failure. If atrial fibrillation develops, the patient may require rate control and anticoagulation. Surgery, either valvuloplasty to open up the valve or complete valve replacement, is needed if pulmonary hypertension or right-sided failure is beginning to develop.

3. The most obvious abnormality on this ECG is left ventricular hypertrophy:

This ECG reveals left ventricular hypertrophy as well as (more subtly) left atrial enlargement

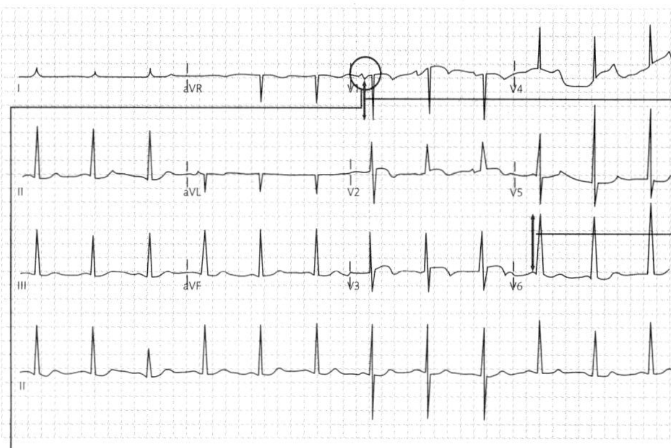

This ECG also reveals evidence of left atrial (LA) enlargement - a common consequence of mitral valve disease. An enlarged LA produces a P wave broader than two small squares, often with a bifid appearance, seen here most clearly in V_1 and called P-mitrale. Right atrial enlargement in contrast produces P waves that are more than two small squares in height, called a P-pulmonale.

One of the voltage criteria for left ventricular hypertrophy involves adding the heights of the S wave in V_1 and the R wave in V_6. Here that gives over 15 mm + 25 mm which adds up to just over 40 mm - a sensitive but poorly specific marker of LVH.

This woman's echocardiogram may be expected to show left ventricular enlargement, in keeping with the ECG findings and the laterally displaced apex beat. Symptoms develop late in mitral regurgitation, and patients who are asymptomatic can be managed conservatively with regular screening by ECG and echocardiogram. Development of either dysrhythmias or chamber enlargement (as in this woman), even in the absence of symptoms, is an indication for early surgical intervention.

4. This chest X-ray shows:

This x-ray shows multiple patchy opacities in both lungs (though especially the right). The differential diagnoses for these are broad, including infection (e.g. an atypical pneumonia), non-infectious inflammatory exudate (e.g. in acute lung injury), pulmonary haemorrhage or metastatic cancer. However, in the context of a suspected right-sided endocarditis the likely diagnosis is lung abcesses caused by an infected emboli from an infected heart valve.

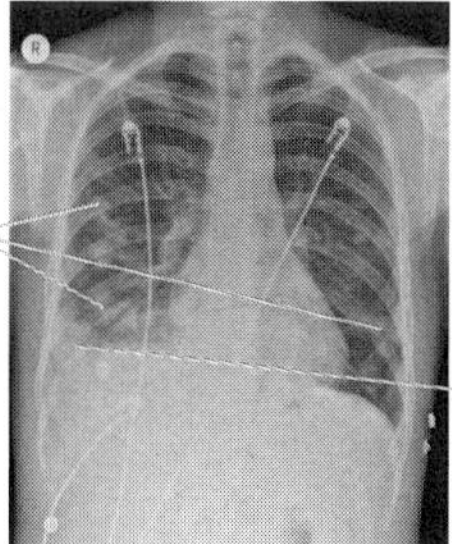

Lung abcesses may appear like this, or they may cavitate, where the radiolucent ('dark') central area appears within a patch of what appears to be consolidation. They may even show a fluid level (a horizontal line) if they contain a significant amount of pus. This man has a right-sided pleural effusion. Unilateral effusions are often caused by infective or malignant disease within the corresponding lung, where bilateral effusions are often caused by systemic disease.

The patient has signs of right-sided heart failure, and a pan-systolic murmur along with a raised JVP implies tricuspid regurgitation.

Intravenous drug users are particularly prone to right-sided infective endocarditis, and skin pathogens are commonly to blame. This man needs an urgent echocardiogram—if available, a transoesophageal echocardiogram which is more accurate in revealing vegetations. He also needs a minimum of three sets of blood cultures, taken at different times (whenever he is found to be pyrexial) and from different sites. This man grew *Staphylococcus aureus* from four of the six blood culture bottles taken, and the images from his transoesophageal echocardiogram showed tricuspid valve vegetations. Despite intravenous antibiotic therapy with flucloxacillin and vancomycin, his tricuspid regurgitation progressed and he required valve replacement.

Further reading

Guidelines: European Society of Cardiology guidelines on infective endocarditis (http://www.escardio.org/guidelines-surveys/esc-guidelines/Pages/infective-endocarditis.aspx)

OHCM: 106, 136–142, 144–145, 150–151

Falls, faints, and funny turns

This section should be used to clerk patients presenting to hospital with episodes of collapse, dizziness, or unresponsiveness, or who have fallen after feeling dizzy or faint. There should be a high suspicion of pathological falls in the elderly—'young people trip, old people fall'. Such patients can be found on Admissions Units or Elderly Care wards.

Learning challenges

- What are some of the dangers of polypharmacy? Which drugs are commonly linked with falls in the elderly?
- What is a tilt test and how is it performed?

History [try to get a corroborative history]

Comment on

- PRE episode—feeling well or unwell; pre-warning symptoms—dizziness 'pre-syncopal', chest pain, palpitations, sweaty, clammy, loss of colour
- DURING episode—patient's recall of events; loss of consciousness, features of seizure—limb jerking, shaking, frothing of the mouth, tongue biting, urinary incontinence
- POST episode—patient's recall of events; memory loss, 'when did you next feel back to your normal self?'
- Features of stroke—higher functions—speech, comprehension, vision; weakness of limbs or face
- Injuries/pain
- Previous similar episodes or falls
- Recent health—symptoms of infection of other illness
- General mobility—including exercise tolerance and walking aids
- Medications—especially medications causing cardiotoxicity, postural hypotension, bradyarrhythmia

Examination

Well or unwell? Why?

Feet to face:

Vital signs: Temperature | Blood pressure | Pulse rate | Respiratory rate | O2 saturations

Clinical clues:

Cardiovascular:

1 2 1

Respiratory:

Abdominal:

Neurological:

Other:

Comment on

- Level of consciousness, confusion
- Obvious injuries/deformities to face, head, limbs
- Evidence of a 'long lie' on the floor—eschars and pressure wounds to limbs, face, buttocks
- Cardiovascular stability—BP (lying and standing if able), HR; murmurs (particularly significant aortic stenosis)
- Evidence of infection—vasodilation; temperature; chest, abdomen, urine
- Evidence of neurological deficit
- Mobility, gait

ECG

Comment on

- Arrhythmia—bradycardia including evidence of heart block and significant pauses; tachyarrhythmia including fast AF or VT.
- Evidence of new or old IHD including LAD, LBBB, ST-segment and T-wave changes

Blood tests

Comment on

- FBC, clotting
- U&Es, CBG, calcium, magnesium
- CK (if long lie)
- Troponin (if indicated by history and ECG)
- Blood and urine cultures (if appropriate)

Lying/standing blood pressure

24-hour ECG

Comment on

- Significant bradyarrhythmia and long pauses
- Tachyarrhythmia—AF and VT

Echocardiogram

Comment on

- Valve defects
- Impaired contractility

Tilt testing [when appropriate]

Comment on

- Positional collapse

Evaluation

1. **Does this fall/funny turn have features suggestive of a cardiovascular cause (e.g. dizziness, palpitations, ECG abnormalities. or postural hypotension)?**

2. **Are there any obvious injuries caused by the fall? Is there evidence of rhabdomyolysis?**

3. **What are this patient's risk factors for falling?**

Area of potential concern	Risk factors
Gait	
Home environment	
Cognition/behavioural factors	
Medication	
Sensory impairment	

4. **How can this patient's cardiovascular risk factors for falling be addressed?**

5. **Would this patient benefit from in-patient rehabilitation/physiotherapy/occupational therapy input?**

Questions

1. An 87-year-old woman is admitted to hospital after a fall. She says that she had been feeling dizzy for several days, with a productive cough, and then fell over just after getting out of bed that morning. She complains of severe pain in her left hip. On examination she is fully alert and conscious. Her left leg appears shortened and externally rotated. She is pyrexial (temperature 38.2°C) and tachycardic (heart rate fluctuating between 120 and 150 bpm, irregularly irregular), with a blood pressure of 156/76 mmHg. Initial blood tests reveal CRP 135 and white cell count 14.2 × 10^9/L, with urea 8.9 mmol/L and creatinine 136 μmol/L. A pelvic X-ray reveals a left-sided fractured neck of femur. Her chest X-ray and ECG are below.

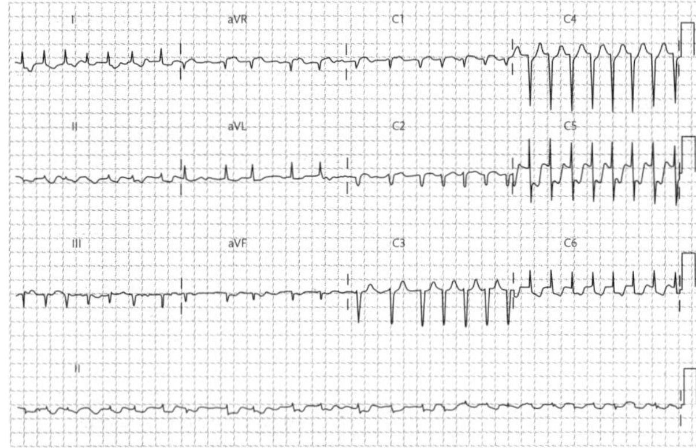

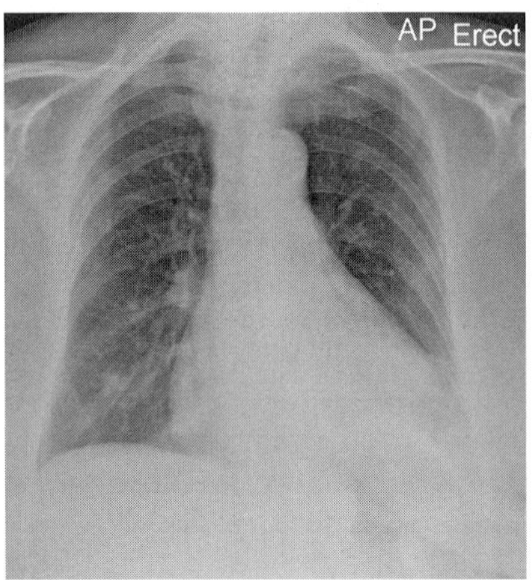

(1) Write a clinical problem list.

(2) List the members of the medical and allied health professional team you would involve in her care.

(3) List five essential therapeutic interventions in this case.

2. An 86-year-old man is brought in to the Emergency Department by ambulance. His neighbour had called the ambulance after not seeing the patient over the last 48 hours. He was found alert but slightly confused, sitting on the floor of his bedroom. He said that he had tripped over on the rug as he was walking to the toilet in the middle of the night and had been unable to get up again. He denies any sinister cardiovascular or neurological symptoms. The ambulance crew report that the house was generally very dirty and untidy. The patient's previous medical history includes a stroke 6 months previously, after which he was left with a residual mild right-sided hemiparesis. His regular medication includes aspirin, slow-release dipyridamole , simvastatin, perindopril, and amlodipine. Examination is unremarkable, with all basic observations within normal ranges. The patient scores 6/10 on an abbreviated mental test score. His ECG reveals normal sinus rhythm with a rate of 80 bpm and no ischaemic changes. Chest X-ray, urine dipstick, and blood tests are all unremarkable.

(1) How would you proceed if you were the Emergency Department doctor?

(2) What other information may you want to know before making any decisions around his future management?

3. A 72-year-old woman is brought to hospital by ambulance after an episode of near-collapse which occurred when she tried to rise from the sofa that morning. She reports that for the past several days she has been feeling dizzy, especially when standing up or after walking for a few minutes. She also reports dysuria and lower abdominal pain over this period of time. Her past medical history includes hypertension, type 2 diabetes, depression, and angina. On examination she is alert, oriented, and not confused. Basic observations include temperature 37.2°C, heart rate 65 bpm regular, blood pressure 145/95 mmHg on lying and 112/84 mmHg on standing, and saturations 95% on air, CBG 7.9 mmol/L Examination is normal except for mild suprapubic tenderness on palpation of the abdomen. Blood tests are within normal ranges except for a mild raised CRP (32 mg/L) and white cell count (12.2 × 10^9/L). Urine dipstick is positive for nitrites and leucocytes. Her list of medications is below.

Medications:

- Aspirin 75 mg once daily
- Bendroflumethiazide 2.5 mg once daily
- Atenolol 10 mg once daily
- Isosorbide mononitrate 60 mg twice daily
- Simvastatin 20 mg each night
- Ramipril 5 mg once daily
- Amitriptyline 50 mg twice daily
- Gliclazide 80 mg once daily

(1) Given the history and examination findings, list the most likely cause of her funny turn.

(2) List three other possible causes of falls/funny turns in this patient.

(3) List the essential steps in the management of this patient.

Presentation

Presented to		Grade		Date	
Signed					

Remember that you can find large-size, annotated versions of many of the X-rays and ECGs that appear in this book on the book's web site at www.oxfordtextbooks.co.uk/orc/randall/

Answers

1. This woman's chest X-ray reveals evidence of consolidation at the left base. A clinical problem list would therefore include:

- Fracture of the left neck of femur
- Fast AF
- Community acquired pneumonia
- Mild renal impairment

Fractures of the femoral neck carry a 10% in-patient mortality and 30% 1-year mortality, often as a result of coexisting medical problems (which may have contributed to the initial fall). A multidisciplinary approach is needed to maximize the chances of a good recovery. Key professionals to involve early in her management include:

- An orthopaedic surgeon—early surgery enables early mobilization to avoid the risks of prolonged bed-rest.
- Anaesthetists—to make surgery safe, the patient should be optimized medically before going to theatre. In particular, control of heart rate by fluids and possibly rate-controlling drugs is important to allow the body to cope with the physiological effects of anaesthetic agents.
- Elderly care physicians—once surgery is completed, these patients may still be very unwell medically and require good quality in-patient medical management—in many hospitals, patients are jointly cared for by orthopaedic surgeons and by elderly care physicians.
- Nursing staff—patients with femoral neck fractures are very prone to developing pressure ulcers without good nursing care and regular turning.
- Allied health professionals—once the fracture is repaired then mobilization is necessary with the support of physiotherapists, and discharge can be planned safely (based on the level of mobility the patient can achieve) by social workers and occupation therapists.

2. There is lots that we do not know about this man, such as whether his confusion is acute or chronic, whether he has any carers helping him at home, and how he has been getting on at home generally. Phoning the patient's relatives or GP may be helpful in gaining this information.

Most falls in elderly people are multifactorial. Confusion can be an important contributor, leading to risky behaviour and an unsafe environment. Environmental factors such as untidiness, fraying slippers, or a lack of hand-holds make the home a dangerous place to live. Chronic problems with mobility (such as limb weakness, peripheral neuropathy, or parkinsonism) predispose to falls, as can medications, visual impairment, or intercurrent illness. Some of these 'falls risk factors' cannot be modified (for instance the patient's hemiparesis in this case) but others can be (for instance, unnecessary medications can be stopped, infections can be treated, houses can be tidied, and simple modifications like hand-rails added to houses).

If there are serious concerns about this patient coping at home then he should be admitted for in-patient assessment by the multidisciplinary team, and proper discharge planning.

3. This woman is feeling dizzy, and has suffered episodes of pre-syncope as a result of postural hypotension—her body lacks the ability to maintain an adequate blood pressure when she is erect. There can be a number of causes for this (those affecting this woman are in bold), of which the easiest to amend is medication. Postural hypotension from an irreversible cause (e.g. diabetic autonomic neuropathy) is often very difficult to manage, with strategies including maintaining an upright posture (e.g. a head-up tilt whilst asleep) or by use of fludrocortisone.

Hypovolaemia	Haemorrhage
	Dehydration
	Diuretics
Impaired autonomic function	**Diabetes**
	Tricyclic antibiotics
	Adrenaline receptor blockers
Impaired vasoconstriction	**Calcium-channel blockers**
	Nitrates
	Infection
Cardiac deconditioning	Prolonged bedrest

Further reading

Guidelines: European Society of Cardiology guidelines on syncope (http://www.escardio.org/guidelines-surveys/esc-guidelines/Pages/syncope.aspx)

OHCM: 13, 26, 35, 152, 464

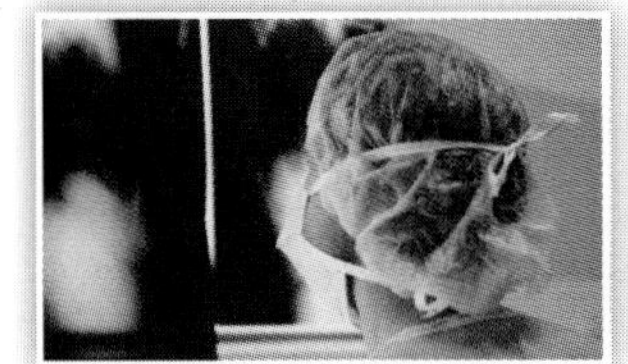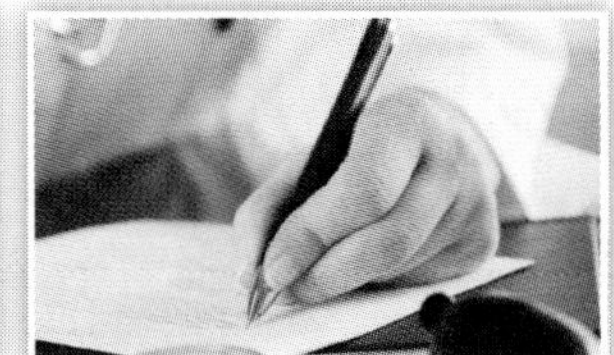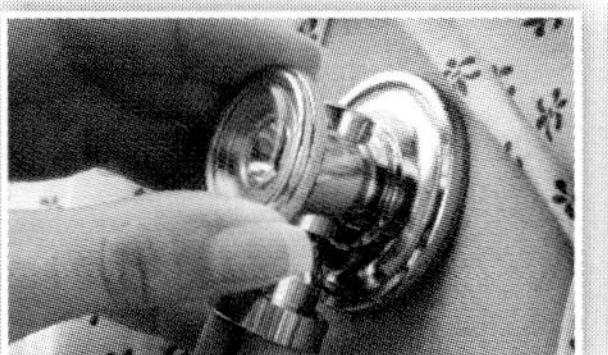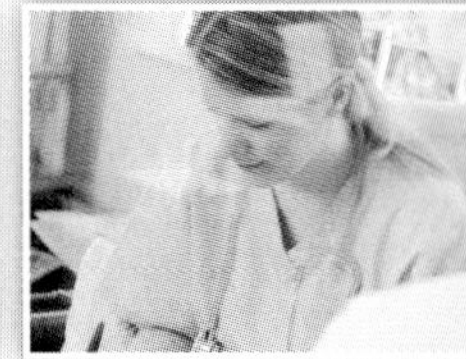

Unit 2
Respiratory medicine

Key learning outcomes in respiratory medicine include:

- Defining and quantifying symptoms such as breathlessness, cough, chest pain, and haemoptysis.
- Detailed enquiry about environmental causes of respiratory disease including smoking, occupation, and pets.
- Detection and description of clinical signs such as tracheal deviation, reduced expansion, dullness to percussion, and abnormal breath sounds.
- Interpreting relevant investigations such as chest X-rays, CT scan of the chest, arterial blood gas analysis, and spirometry.
- Initial and longer-term management of asthma, COPD, pneumonia, pneumothorax, and pulmonary embolus.
- Appreciation of strategies used in treating lung cancer.
- Management of the long-term breathless patient in the community.

Tips for learning respiratory medicine on the wards:

- Clerk any new patients with respiratory conditions in acute areas such as the Medical Admissions Unit.
- Compare the clinical signs you elicit with those presented by the senior members of the medical team on ward rounds; if they are different, try to go back and re-examine the patient.
- Attend lung cancer multidisciplinary team meetings.
- Learn how to perform and interpret arterial blood gas sampling and spirometry.
- Regularly review the drug charts of respiratory patients—you will quickly learn the common therapeutic interventions used in this group. Look them up in the BNF, a textbook, or a pharmacology website.
- Review patients on non-invasive ventilation—look at their blood gas analyses and determine their type and degree of respiratory failure.

History

Patients with respiratory disease present with three major symptoms—cough (and associated sputum production), breathlessness, and chest pain, classically pleuritic in nature. The building blocks of this history should also include whether they have a known respiratory disorder, a well-defined smoking history, and enquiry about environmental factors, such as occupation, and furry or feathered pets.

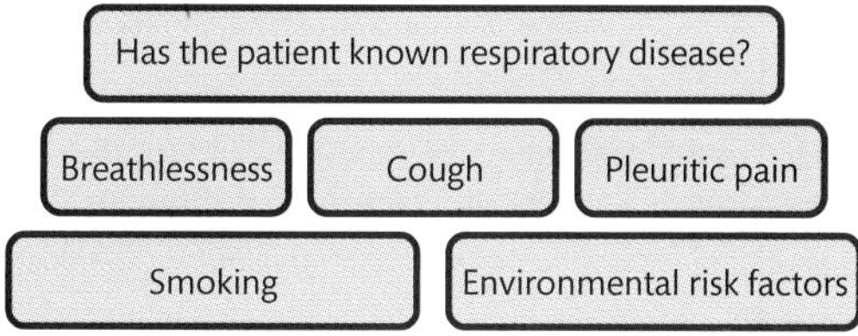

These key building blocks need to be covered in the history of ALL patients with respiratory disease. They are covered below in an order moving from the presenting complaint to the social history.

Breathlessness: If patients have signs of moderate to severe respiratory distress (see box below), then a rapid history whilst performing a clinical assessment is indicated. If the patient is less distressed or stabilized a full history can then be obtained.

Signs of respiratory distress

Tachypnoea	Tracheal tug
Inability to complete sentences	Intercostal and subcostal recession
Use of accessory muscles	Pulsus paradoxus
Nasal flaring	

Similar to many histories, the first thing to establish is the duration and severity of the symptoms. Shortness of breath is best quantified in terms of the patient's functional limitations (and how they have changed over time). One way to get a good feel for their level of breathlessness is to ask what they are able to do at the moment (on the scale below), what they could do 1 month ago, and what they could do 1 year ago.

A functional grading system for shortness of breath

- Walking unlimited, able to run
- Can walk to the shops, stopping occasionally
- Can get out of the house just about (e.g. into the car)
- Can get to other rooms in the house (e.g. the toilet)
- Can only walk across the room
- Can only walk a few steps
- Gets breathless even just washing or changing position

A combination of the speed of deterioration, other associated symptoms, and risk factors for developing specific conditions should help you make a diagnosis of the likely causes for the patient's breathlessness:

Common causes of acute shortness of breath	Common causes of chronic shortness of breath
Pulmonary oedema Asthma exacerbation Pneumonia COPD exacerbation Pulmonary embolus Pneumothorax	COPD Congestive cardiac failure Pulmonary fibrosis Pleural effusion of any cause Sarcoidosis

Cough: Coughing is a physiological mechanism to remove debris from the airways. It is triggered by airway irritation, so almost all lung disease may produce coughing; however, different types of cough are produced by different underlying diseases. Key questions to ask are:

- Whether it is acute or chronic.
- Whether it is productive of sputum. If so:

- what the sputum is in terms of volume, colour, consistency, and frequency,
- whether there is blood mixed in, or separate from, the sputum.

The answers to these questions can help you start to describe different types of cough:

	Productive	Non-productive
Acute	Possible lower respiratory tract infection (especially if sputum is green, yellow, or brown)—may require antibiotics and hospital admission if severe	Atypical pneumonias and upper respiratory tract infections may produce dry, tickly, or wheezy coughs
Chronic	Smokers' cough (if carbon-stained sputum), COPD, or possible long-term suppurative lung disease (e.g. bronchiectasis). Requires investigation	Consider malignancy, TB, asthma, sarcoid, or laryngeal nerve palsy. Requires investigation, urgently if there are any worrying symptoms (e.g. weight loss)

Pleuritic chest pain: The lungs have no pain receptors, but their pleura do. Pleuritic chest pain is localized to one particular region of the chest wall, and is said to 'catch' on deep inspiration: ask the patient to take a 'deep inspiration' and see if the pain is reproduced. Pleuritic pain suggests disease of the pleura (e.g. a pneumothorax) or lung disease reaching to the peripheries of the lung (such as a large lobar pneumonia or a pulmonary embolus with subsequent lung infarction).

Smoking: Tobacco use is by far the single biggest risk factor for developing lung disease and exacerbating pre-existing disease, and so it has been isolated from other risk factors and mentioned independently because of the critical importance of taking a good smoking history from a patient with respiratory disease. Ask:

- Do you smoke now?
- If not, have you smoked in the past? When did you start and when did you quit?
- How many do you (did you) smoke every day?
- Have you ever tried to quit? Would you like to quit?

The amount that a patient smokes should be quantified in **pack-years**: someone who has smoked 1 pack-year has smoked 20 cigarettes (one pack) every day for 1 year, or 10 cigarettes per day for 2 years.

Always encourage patients to stop smoking, in a friendly, encouraging, and non-judgemental way. This might be the most significant thing that can be done to help them! Repeated suggestions from health professionals are one of the most effective ways of encouraging patients to give up. Most hospitals have a smoking cessation counsellor who will be able to help patients give up and arrange nicotine replacement if the patient wants this.

Environmental risk factors: Environmental factors cause many severe lung diseases, and may also prove a trigger for asthma. Asking about environmental risk factors is especially important in patients presenting with chronic shortness of breath, where occupational or environmental lung diseases should always be considered. Ask about:

Occupation: Take a full occupational history (all jobs that the patient has ever done), looking for evidence of exposure to:

- asbestos: building trade, demolitions, ship-building
- mineral dusts: mining, smelting, ceramics, sand-blasting
- cotton dust: textiles industry
- fungus: farmers, bird-keepers

Pets: furry pets, e.g. cats, may cause exacerbations of asthma. Birds are the risk for contracting *Chlamydia psittaci* (psittacosis) infection.

Travel: Always think about tuberculosis and atypical pneumonia.

Sexual history: Think about HIV risk factors: *Pneumocystis jiroveci* (previously called *P. carinii*) pneumonia is common.

Drugs: Many can cause pulmonary fibrosis, notably cancer chemotherapy , amiodarone, and nitrofurantoin.

Examination

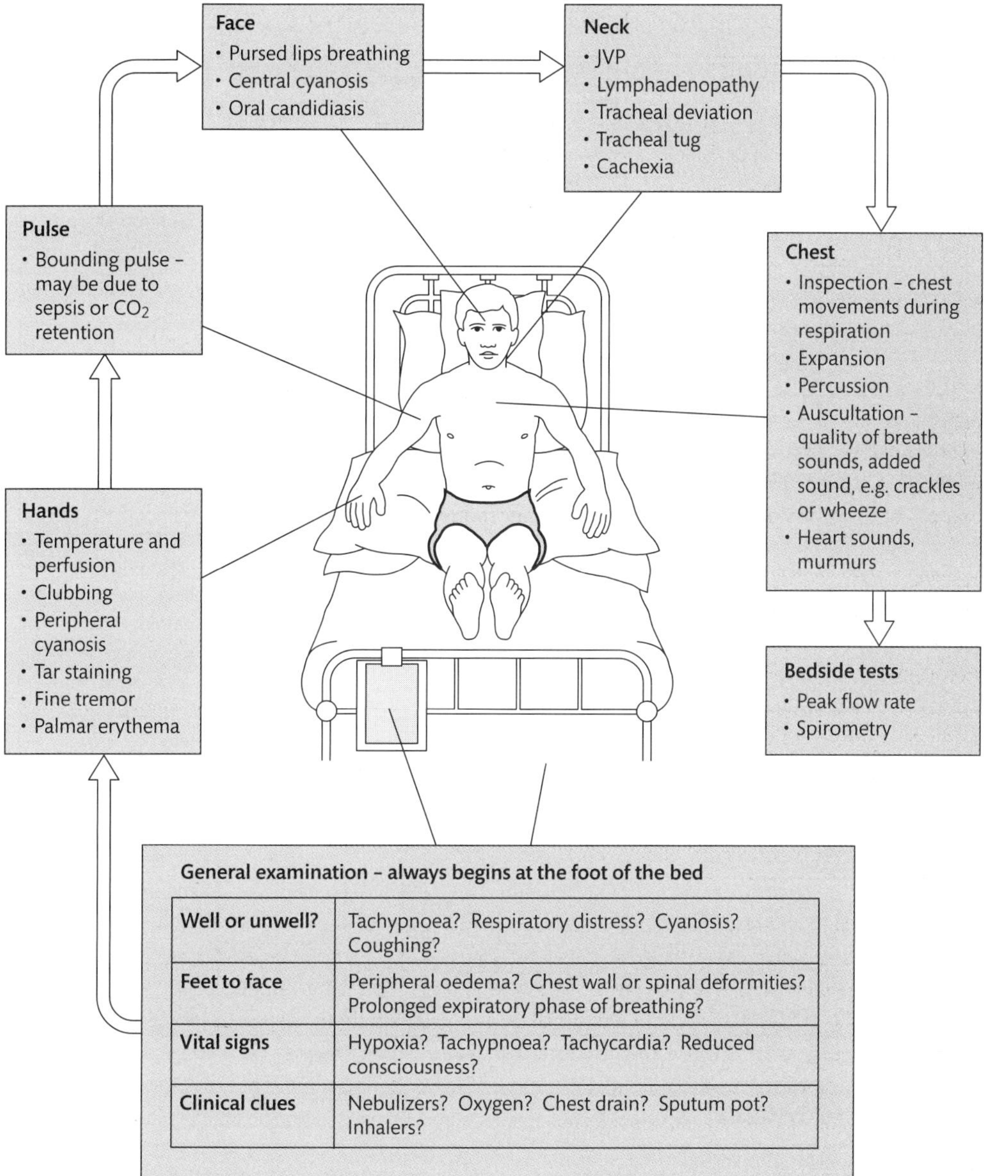

Well or unwell?	Tachypnoea? Respiratory distress? Cyanosis? Coughing?
Feet to face	Peripheral oedema? Chest wall or spinal deformities? Prolonged expiratory phase of breathing?
Vital signs	Hypoxia? Tachypnoea? Tachycardia? Reduced consciousness?
Clinical clues	Nebulizers? Oxygen? Chest drain? Sputum pot? Inhalers?

Clubbing

Look for loss of the nail bed angle, fluctuation and softening of the nailbed, increased convexity of the nail with increased shininess, and generally thickening of the distal part of the digits.

Respiratory causes:

- Chronic suppurative lung disease—abscess, empyema, bronchiectasis, tuberculosis, cystic fibrosis
- Malignancy—primary and secondary lung cancers, mesothelioma
- Fibrotic lung disease—primary and secondary pulmonary fibrosis

Cardiac causes: Chronic infective endocarditis, congenital cyanotic heart disease

Abdominal causes: Inflammatory bowel disease, upper abdominal malignancy, cirrhosis

Others including: Idiopathic, thyroid acropachy

Common patterns found on chest examination

	'Normal' examination	Consolidation	Effusion	Pneumothorax
CT appearance				
Effects on examination findings	Beware of thinking that a 'normal' examination means no lung disease! A centrally-located lung tumour may produce no signs on examination of the chest. Better to say that examination was '**unremarkable**'	Consolidation (e.g. produced by a lobar pneumonia) will produce localized crackles. It may also caused increased transmission of high-frequency breath sounds—'**bronchial breathing**'. Consolidation to the peripheries may cause **pleuritic chest pain**	A pleural effusion disrupts the mechanics of the chest wall (affecting expansion) and also reduces sound transmission. The trachea is **pushed away** from an effusion	Air in the pleural space (a pneumothorax) causes reduced chest expansion by affecting the mechanics or breathing. The trachea may be pushed away from the affected area, and blood flow restricted causing a **raised JVP**
Expansion	Normal	Normal or reduced	Reduced	Reduced
Auscultation	Normal	Crackles, bronchial breathing	Reduced breath sounds	Reduced breath sounds
Percussion	Normal	Normal or reduced	'Stony dull'	Hyperresonant
Vocal fremitus	Normal	Increased	Reduced	Reduced

Crackles and wheezes

Crackles are caused by small airways, which were closed off by fluid, exudates, or local collapse, suddenly 'popping' open. Coarse crackles often occur in consolidation or bronchiectasis, whilst fine crackles (late in inspiration) occur in pulmonary oedema and pulmonary fibrosis	Wheeze is produced by the walls of airways vibrating as a result of turbulent flow through narrowed airways. Diffuse airway narrowing (widespread wheeze) is common in asthma or COPD, whereas localized wheeze can be caused by an obstructing tumour or foreign body

Remember that you can find large-size, annotated versions of many of the X-rays and ECGs that appear in this book on the book's web site at www.oxfordtextbooks.co.uk/orc/randall/

Investigations

Arterial blood gas analysis

There are two elements to the arterial blood gases: the pH, reflecting acid-base balance, and the $PaCO_2$ and PaO_2, reflecting respiratory function. You should consider each element in isolation as shown below. We have chosen to start with acid-base balance.

1. Consider the pH (normal 7.35–7.45) Is there an acidosis or an alkalosis?

According to the Henderson-Hasselbalch equation:

$pH \propto bicarbonate/PaCO_2$

Thus the pH is proportional to bicarbonate and inversely proportional to the $PaCO_2$.

We will consider the bicarbonate as the **metabolic** element and the $PaCO_2$ as the **respiratory** element.

If there is an acidosis present (a low pH) it follows it must be metabolic if the bicarbonate is low or respiratory if the $PaCO_2$ is high. It is a mixed acidosis if these conditions occur together.

Causes:

- **Metabolic acidosis**—DKA, lactic acidosis, renal failure, salicylate poisoning.
- **Respiratory acidosis**—compatible with type II respiratory failure (see below).

If there is an alkalosis present (a high pH) it is a metabolic problem if the bicarbonate is high and a respiratory alkalosis if the $PaCO_2$ is low.

Causes :

- **Metabolic alkalosis**—commonly due to gastrointestinal bicarbonate losses, e.g. in diarrhoea or vomiting. May be due to alkali overdose or some drugs.
- **Respiratory alkalosis**—compatible with hyperventilation ("blowing off the $PaCO_2$"). Note that hyperventilation secondary to hysteria is a diagnosis of exclusion, and serious underlying pathologies including hypoxia (e.g. a pulmonary embolus) and DKA should be excluded before this is accepted as the diagnosis.

Is there any compensation?

Compensation is only present if the two elements (bicarbonate and $PaCO_2$) are moving in the same direction, i.e. synchronously increasing or decreasing.

If the pH is normal, despite abnormalities of the bicarbonate and $PaCO_2$, this is regarded as a fully '**compensated system**'.

If the pH is abnormal, any compensation occurring is '**attempted compensation**'.

Thus, the compensation of a metabolic acidosis seen in DKA is a respiratory alkalosis with Kussmaul breathing—blowing off the carbon dioxide.

The compensation of a respiratory acidosis is a metabolic alkalosis classically seen in patients with type II respiratory failure. The kidneys compensate the chronic $PaCO_2$ retention by retaining bicarbonate, buffering the acid.

Having completed the acid-base components, you should now move on to the respiratory components.

2. Is there respiratory failure?

This is defined by the presence of hypoxia (i.e. PaO_2 less than normal, <10 kPa) with or without hypercapnia. A PaO_2 of <8 kPa defines severe respiratory failure. If hypoxia is present then one must ask is the respiratory failure **type I** or **type II**? This is determined by the $PaCO_2$: if this is <6 kPa then there is type I respiratory failure, if it is >6 kPa there is type II respiratory failure.

Type I respiratory failure is caused by failure of oxygen to diffuse across the alveolar space into the pulmonary capillary bed. By definition the pO_2 is low, whilst the pCO_2 is normal or low.

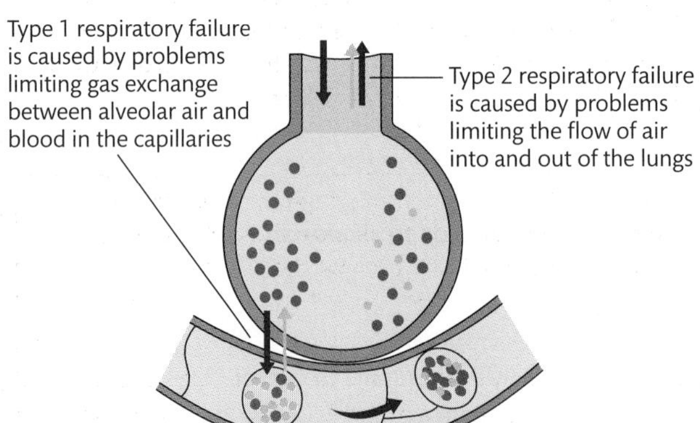

Causes of type I respiratory failure

- Asthma
- Pneumonia (classically atypicals)
- Pulmonary embolus
- Pulmonary fibrosis
- Pulmonary oedema
- Pulmonary haemorrhage

In type II respiratory failure the hypoxia is accompanied by a rise in pCO_2. Type II respiratory failure is caused by ventilatory failure, i.e. the inability to effectively ventilate the lungs. Thus not enough oxygen gets in and not enough CO_2 gets out.

Causes of type II respiratory failure

The commonest cause by far is COPD; the others may be divided by anatomical layers

- Skin—severe scarring, e.g. burns
- Fat—obesity hypoventilation syndrome
- Skeletal—congenital deformities of the chest wall; flailed chest
- Neuromuscular—Guillain-Barré, polio, tetanus, motor neurone disease
- Lungs—COPD
- Extrathoracic—problems affecting the respiratory centres of the brainstem, e.g. opiate overdose, brainstem stroke

All causes of type I respiratory failure may present with type II. This is a late and very sinister sign. It is a sign the patient is very ill and requires urgent ventilatory support.

Spirometry

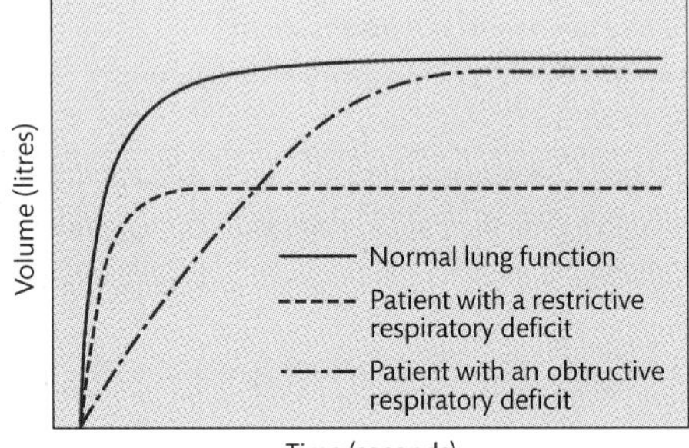

Spirometry assesses the effectiveness of **ventilation**. It measures the forced vital capacity (FVC; the amount of space available for gas transfer in the lung) and forced expiratory volume in 1 second (FEV_1; a measure of how quickly air can enter and exit the lungs).

Restrictive pattern (dotted red line)—lung volume has been lost so there is less space left for air to fill—seen in pulmonary fibrosis, pneumonia, and others. There is a reduced FVC but a normal FEV_1.

Obstructive pattern (dot-dashed red line)—lung volumes are normal, but air cannot get in and out of the lung effectively—seen in asthma, COPD, and neuromuscular conditions affecting chest wall movement. The FVC is normal but the FEV_1 is greatly reduced.

The chest radiograph

Check:

- **Patient details**—which patient, how old, when was this image taken?
- **X-ray details**—PA or AP? Rotation, adequate penetration, adequate inspiration?

1. Trachea	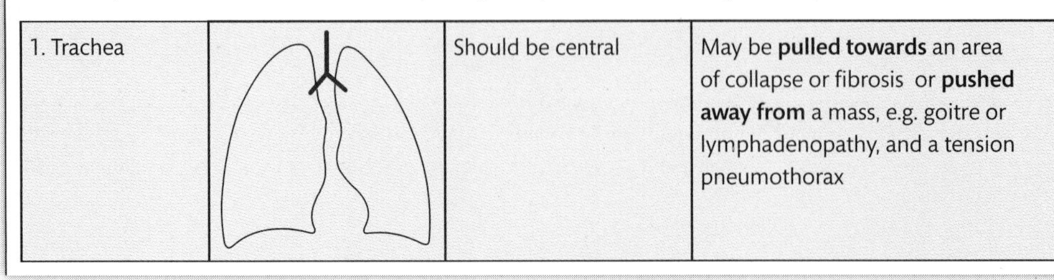	Should be central	May be **pulled towards** an area of collapse or fibrosis or **pushed away from** a mass, e.g. goitre or lymphadenopathy, and a tension pneumothorax

2. Mediastinum	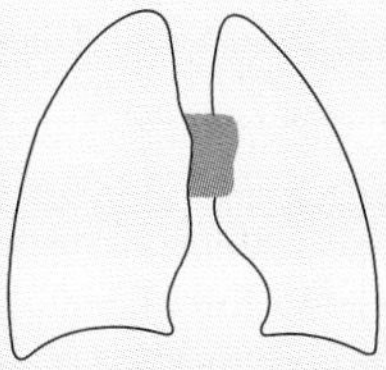	Aortic notch should be just visible. The left hilum should be slightly higher than the right	The mediastinum is **widened** by lymphadenopathy, masses such as thymoma, and an aortic aneurysm. The hila may be pulled up or down by collapsed lobes
3. Heart size	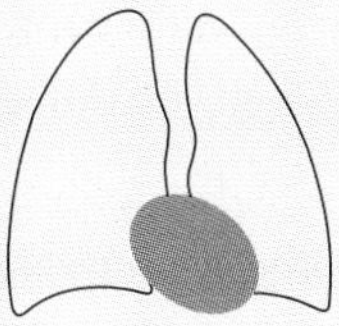	Heart size should be less than 50% of the thoracic width on a PA chest film.	Cardiomegaly may be caused by hypertension, valvular disease, or cardiomyopathy
4. Diaphragm	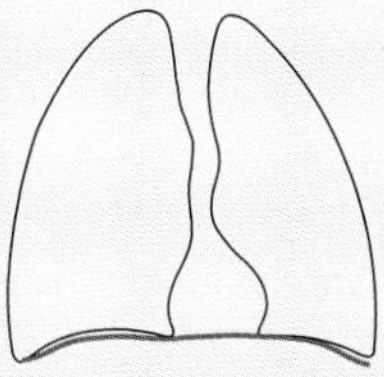	Look for air/gas under the diaphragm and for elevation of the diaphragm on either side	Air under the diaphragm indicates a perforated abdominal viscus. A hemidiaphragm may be raised from above by lobar collapse, or from below by a large mass
5. Bases	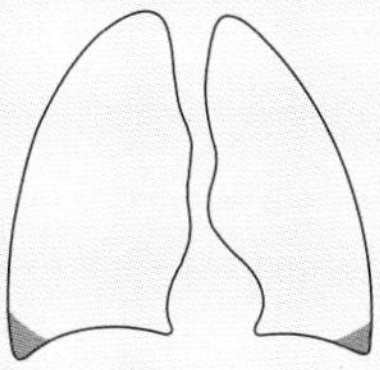	The costophrenic angles should be clearly definable. Sometimes very large effusions can 'white out' an entire lung	Bilateral effusions often have systemic causes. Effusions on one side may be due to local lesions, e.g. malignancy or pneumonia
6. Consolidation	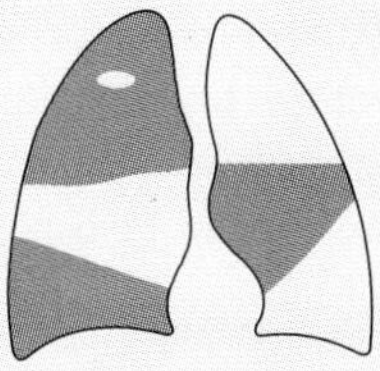	Upper lobe (stops at horizontal fissure), middle lobe/lingula (heart edge unclear) or lower lobe (diaphragm unclear)?	Caused by pneumonia. You may see an air bronchogram (airways outlined) or evidence of cavitation
7. Pneumothorax	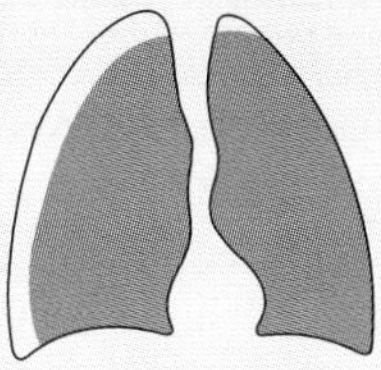	Look for lung markings extending all the way to the chest wall	Look for evidence of underlying lung disease or trauma, e.g. rib fractures and surgical emphysema
8. Round shadows	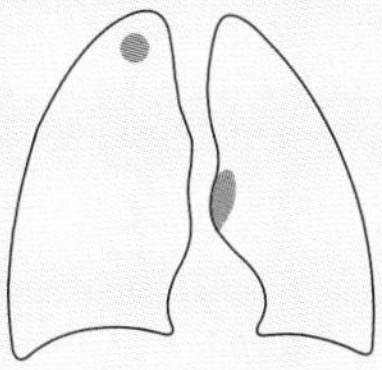	Look peripherally and at the hila. Look for pleural thickening	May be cancer (primary or metastatic), TB, fungal, or sarcoid
9. Interstitial shadowing	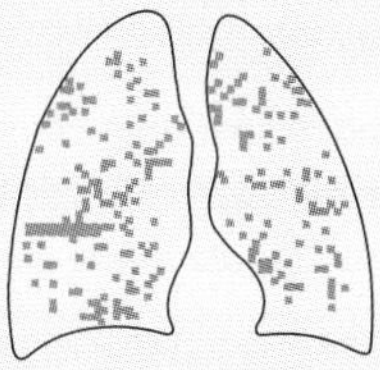	May be fluid overload pattern, or streaky (reticular), lumpy (nodular) or with small dots (miliary)	Fluid overload is seen in pulmonary oedema. Fibrosis gives a streaky appearance. Diffuse TB gives miliary mottling
10. Bones	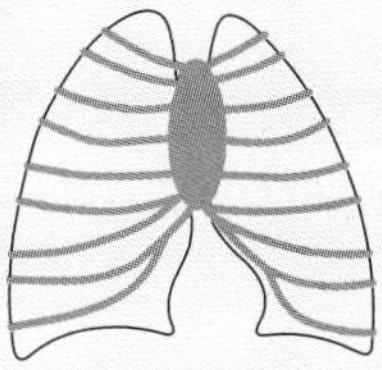	Rib fractures? Faint bones (osteopenia)? Are there lytic lesions?	Think of systemic diseases—osteoporosis, cancers

Interventions

Prescribing oxygen

Oxygen gas is vital in maintaining oxygen saturations in patients with respiratory failure. A simple rule of thumb is 'hypoxia kills you, hypercapnia makes you drowsy and unwell'. The treatment of hypoxia is supplemental oxygen; the treatment of worsening hypercapnia is ventilatory support.

The British Thoracic Society guidelines (2009) for treating patients with supplemental oxygen therapy places the emphasis on target oxygen saturations rather than fixed percentages of oxygen. Put simply, patients with type I respiratory failure should have enough supplemental oxygen to maintain their oxygen saturations at 94–98%; patients with or at risk of developing type II respiratory failure should receive enough oxygen to maintain their oxygen saturations in the range 88–92%. In type II patients, a poorly correcting hypoxia and/ or a rising CO_2 (and especially with worsening acidaemia) are indications for ventilatory support. This may be non-invasive or invasive ventilation, depending on the clinical context.

When prescribing oxygen on the drug chart one should document:

- The route: either nasal speculae, Venturi fixed concentration masks , or non-rebreathe masks.
- The concentration: expressed either in litres per minute, or better as the percentage of oxygen.
- The target saturations.

For instance, a patient with an exacerbation of COPD may present to hospital with saturations of 85% on air, a pH of 7.31, a pCO_2 of 7.1 kPa, and a pO_2 of 6.8. If they are given high-flow oxygen via a non-rebreathe mask (effectively 85% oxygen), then an hour later they may have oxygen saturations of 98% but a pH of 7.11, a pCO_2 of 11.8 and a pO_2 of 20.3—in other words they would be oxygenating well but retaining CO_2 and consequently becoming acidotic.

Such a patient should instead be prescribed lower concentrations of oxygen. An appropriate prescription would be 24% oxygen via a Venturi mask (which allows fixed concentrations of inspired oxygen to be administered), aiming to maintain the oxygen saturations at 88–92%. If this is not achieved with 24% oxygen then the next Venturi mask up can be used, delivering 28% oxygen or if necessary 35% or 40%.

Non-invasive ventilation

Sometimes patients simply cannot maintain adequate oxygen saturations because of severe lung disease, for instance pulmonary oedema or a COPD exacerbation. They develop either type I or type II respiratory failure, with severe hypoxia despite oxygen and possibly rising pCO_2 levels with a respiratory acidosis. Options to provide further respiratory support include invasive ventilation (which requires sedation, intubation, and management on a ventilator on the ITU) and non-invasive ventilation. This is delivered in high-dependency wards or specialist respiratory wards using a tight-fitting face mask connected to a machine which blows air triggered by the patient's own breathing.

There are two forms. In **continuous positive airways pressure ventilation** (**CPAP**) the patient breathes in and out against a fixed pressure (the machine blows air at the patient during inspiration and expiration), which acts to hold open small airways which would otherwise collapse. This increases the number of alveoli which are available for gas transfer, and therefore increases the pO_2. CPAP is used in type I respiratory failure. It is described as like trying to breathe in a wind tunnel or with your head stuck out of a the window of a speeding car.

In **bilevel positive airways pressure ventilation** (**BiPAP**) air is blown towards the patient during both expiration and inspiration but the pressures are adjustable in the two phases. The settings are relatively high in Inspiration (e.g. 15 mmH_2O) and lower in expiration (e.g. 5 mmH_2O). This arrangement increases tidal volume, reduces the work of breathing and allows CO_2 to be blown off. Therefore BiPAP is used for type II respiratory failure. If COPD patients who retain oxygen are given high-flow oxygen and become very acidotic then BiPAP may be required to drive down their pCO_2 and improve their pH.

Common respiratory medications

Class	Examples	Mechanism	Indications	Contraindications	Side-effects	Special notes
Oxygen	Modes of delivery:					
Short-acting beta agonists						
Long-acting beta agonists						
Inhaled corticosteroids						Combination inhalers:
Oral corticosteroids						Duration of treatment:
Anticholinergic agents						
Leukotriene antagonists						
Theophyllines						
Magnesium sulphate						
Mucolytics						
Oral anticoagulants						Duration of treatment:
Other anticoagulants						
Penicillins (for respiratory infections)						
Macrolides (respiratory infections)						
Antituberculous antibiotics						Duration of treatment:

Acute asthma

This section should be used to clerk patients suffering an acute exacerbation. Many patients are discharged home from the Emergency Department for community follow-up, other patients require brief periods in the Admissions Ward or even a Respiratory Ward until they have recovered sufficiently to go home.

Learning challenges

- What are the short-term and longer-term effects of abnormal inflammation in asthma? Why do people with asthma respond abnormally to benign stimuli?
- Do you feel comfortable setting up a nebulizer?

History

Comment on

- Previous asthma history (see generic questions for a long-term condition on p. 7)
- Regular medications
- Known environmental triggers
- Any infective symptoms?
- Smoking; occupational history; furry or feathered pets

Examination

Well or unwell? Why?

Feet to face:

Vital signs: Temperature | Blood pressure | Pulse rate | Respiratory rate | O2 saturations

Clinical clues:

Cardiovascular:

1 2 1

Respiratory:

PEFR

L/min

Abdominal:

Neurological:

Other:

Comment on

- Respiratory rate, oxygen saturations
- Speaking in sentences? Using accessory muscles?
- Wheeze? Localized consolidation? Pneumothorax?
- Patient's usual (or expected) PEFR versus present PEFR

Chest X-ray

Comment on

- Focal consolidation?
- Lobar collapse?
- Pneumothorax?

Arterial blood gas

Comment on

- pCO_2—low, normal, or raised?
- Hypoxia?

Blood tests

Comment on

- WCC and differential (evidence of infection?)
- Microbiology—blood and sputum cultures

Evaluation

1. How severe is this patient's asthma attack?

	Moderate exacerbation	Severe exacerbation	Life-threatening exacerbation
PEFR	>50% of expected	33–50% of expected	<33% of expected
Appearance	Breathless with more symptoms than usual	Unable to speak in complete sentences, respiratory distress	Feeble respiratory effort. Cyanotic. Pre-morbid
Baseline observations	Within normal limits	High respiratory or heart rate	Hypotensive, bradycardic, severely hypoxic
Chest auscultation	Wheeze	Wheeze	Silent chest

2. What initial management is indicated?

3. Is this patient improving with the management that has been started?

4. If failing to improve, does this patient require treatment on the Intensive Care Unit? Do they require admission to hospital? Are they well enough to go home?

5. How should the patient's regular medications be changed in view of this exacerbation?

Questions

1. A 28-year-old woman who is known to suffer from asthma presents to the Emergency Department after becoming wheezy and short of breath. She is stable enough to allow you to take a full history. List five questions you should ask to establish a clear picture of the history of her asthma.

2. On examination, the patient in Question 1 is relatively comfortable and is able to speak in full sentences. She is not using accessory muscles of respiration. Her respiratory rate is 22 breaths/min and her heart rate is 96 bpm. Her oxygen saturations are 98% on room air. Auscultation of the chest reveals a diffuse polyphonic wheeze. Her peak expiratory flow rate (PEFR) is 300 L/min (she is 160 cm tall); she does not know what her usual PEFR reading is.

(1) How would you categorize her present asthmatic status? (Use the peak flow chart below.)

(2) List five essential steps in her management.

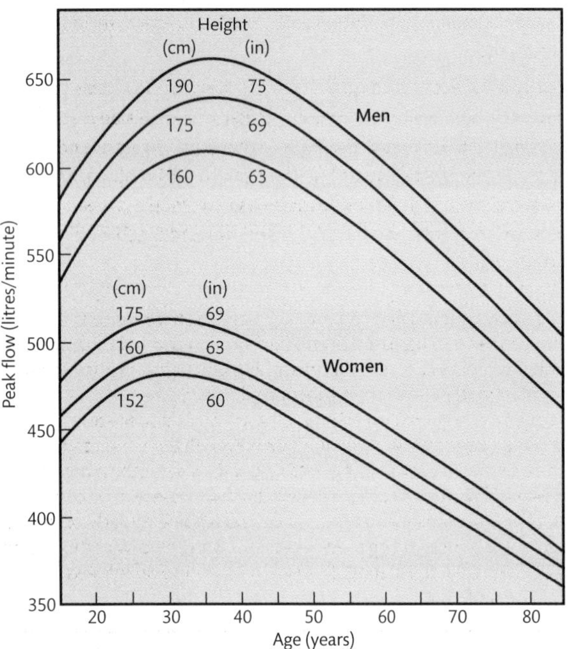

3. A 19-year-old woman attends her family doctor complaining of feeling breathless with a dry cough which seems worst after exertion, especially when the weather is cold. She has also been sleeping poorly due to a nocturnal cough. She has no other medical problems are does not take any medication. Physical examination is unremarkable. The doctor instructs the patient in how to use a peak flow meter and tells her to record her PEFR at different times during the day. She returns a week later.

(1) What does the chart show?

(2) How should this patient be managed?

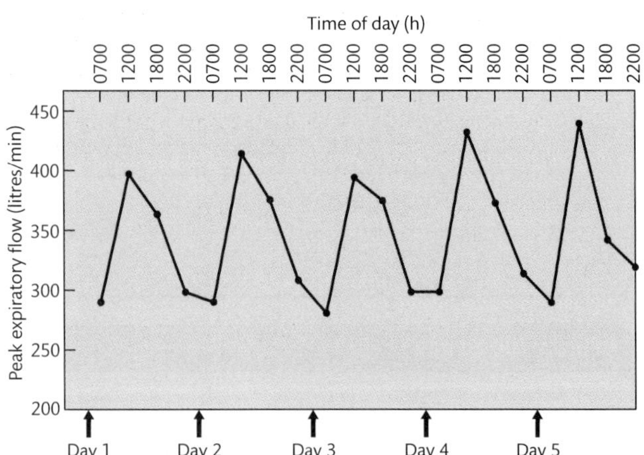

4. A 22-year-old woman is brought into the Emergency Department by ambulance after becoming short of breath over the preceding 2 hours. On initial assessment she is agitated and not completing sentences—gasping 'you've got to help me' with each breath. She is using accessory muscles in her neck and shoulders to help her breathe. Her basic observations include respiratory rate 32 breaths/min, heart rate 114 bpm, blood pressure 112/78 mmHg and oxygen sats 92% on 6 L/min (driving a salbutamol nebulizer). The patient appears flushed and sweaty. Auscultation of the chest reveals a diffuse polyphonic wheeze with air entry heard equally throughout the chest and no crackles heard. She is unable to perform a peak flow recording. The nurse asks whether more salbutamol should be given since the current nebulizer has run out.

(1) What is your initial 'triage' assessment of this patient?

(2) List the next steps you would take in managing this patient—including the location where they should be managed and when additional help should be requested.

5. A 20-year-old man has been newly diagnosed with asthma. He has been started on a salbutamol inhaler for use as required and a steroid inhaler to be used each morning and evening. He is also given a peak flow meter to record his PEFR at home. Describe how would you teach him to use the inhalers and peak flow meter.

6. A 29-year-old woman has suffered with asthma for many years, though has never been admitted to hospital. She usually takes a steroid inhaler twice a day, but over the last few weeks has been needing to use her salbutamol inhaler up to 10 times per day to relieve symptoms of cough and breathlessness. She attends her family doctor to ask for advice on achieving better control of her symptoms.

(1) What things is it important for the doctor to check with the patient?

(2) What additional management options exist?

Presentation

Presented to ________ Grade ________ Date ________

Signed

Answers

1. Whenever a patient with an acute exacerbation of a chronic condition comes into hospital it is important to get a feel for how the condition generally affects them and how well it is controlled. Generic questions (such as those listed in 'History Taking' in the Introduction, p. 7) can be adapted to fit each individual condition—those below would provide a clear picture of the history of this patient's asthma:

1. Where, when, and why was it first diagnosed?
2. How has it progressed since then?
3. Control:
   - What maintenance therapy does she take regularly?
   - Does she monitor her peak flow rate?
   - Which medical staff and allied health professionals are involved in her care?
4. Worst its ever been:
   - Has she ever been admitted to hospital?
   - Has she ever needed treatment on an ITU?
5. How is it now (today)?

2. This woman has an expected PEFR of 480 L/min but is only achieving 300 L/min, roughly 60% of expected. Based on the table in the 'Evaluation' section for this condition she has a moderate exacerbation of asthma.

In the Emergency Department, the key components of management are:

- nebulized salbutamol (using an oxygen-driven nebulizer)
- oral prednisolone—usually 40 mg is given

If she improves and feels she is well enough to go home, then:

- she can be discharged
- she should receive a short course of oral prednisolone (e.g. 40 mg/day for 5 days)
- she should be seen by her GP within 48 hours and should have her regular medications increased.

3. A dry cough, worse at night, on exertion, or in cold weather, is a common presentation of asthma in children and young adults. The chart shows diurnal variation in PEFR, lowest in the morning, which is characteristic of asthma. A diagnosis of asthma is based on 20% variability if airway obstruction—this variation may be discovered (as here) by monitoring of peak flow readings, by 20% improvement after treatment (e.g. after a nebulizer), or by 20% deterioration after a known trigger (e.g. exercise).

This patient should be started on a salbutamol inhaler for use as required—whenever she is breathless. Inhaled corticosteroids may also be started (e.g. beclometasone 200 micrograms each morning) because she is getting regular symptoms. (See the 'asthma ladder' in the answer to Question 6.)

4. This patient has a potentially life-threatening attack of asthma—she is clearly working extremely hard and yet is still notably hypoxic despite significant oxygen therapy. She requires immediate attention and should not be placed into the queue of patients waiting to be seen. Key management priorities include:

- Management in a high-dependency area—she should be moved into the Emergency Department resuscitation room for one-to-one nursing.
- Continued oxygen-driven salbutamol and ipratropium nebulizers.
- Rapid arterial blood gas analysis—a normal or high pCO_2 implies that the patient is tiring and should lead to consideration of intubation.
- Chest X-ray—to exclude a pneumothorax.
- Steroids—these can be given either orally or intravenously (e.g. 200 mg intravenous hydrocortisone), though both forms will take hours to produce an effect.
- Intravenous magnesium sulphate.
- Consider intravenous salbutamol, intravenous aminophylline, or subcutaneous adrenaline.
- Repeat arterial blood gas analysis since this patient is likely to tire unless her airway obstruction improves considerably.
- Involve the intensive care team early if the patient may require intubation.
- Antibiotics if there is convincing evidence of infection.

5. Instructing patients in using inhalers or peak flow meters is a common communication skills station in practical medical school exams, partly because poor inhaler technique is a common reason for poorly controlled asthma.

Inhaler technique: Hold the inhaler ready and breathe out as far as possible. Hold the inhaler to the lips forming a tight seal around the mouthpiece. As you begin to breathe in, press the button. Take a steady, deep breath in and then hold the breath with the lungs fully expanded until you have counted to 10 in your head. Then breathe out slowly.

Using a Volumatic (spacer): These clear plastic chambers help those who struggle to coordinate breathing in with pressing the button on the inhaler. The two halves of the spacer should be slotted together and the inhaler mouthpiece should slot easily into one end. The button on the inhaler is then pressed, releasing the contents of the inhaler into the spacer. The patient then takes five deep breaths in through the other end of the spacer, holding their breath with the lungs expanded at the end of each—this allows all the aerosolized drug to enter the lungs efficiently.

Peak flow meter technique: Assemble the peak flow meter if necessary and ensure that the sliding gauge on the side is set to zero. Hold the meter making sure that your fingers are not touching the sliding gauge. Stand up, take a full breath in, and then breathe out as fast as possible—as if blowing out a candle on a birthday cake. Repeat this three times and the PEFR is the highest number achieved.

6. The doctor should first check this patient's adherence to the treatment plan she has been prescribed—and in particular her inhaler technique. There is no point in prescribing additional medication if the current medication is being incorrectly used.

Chronic management of asthma is based on a 'ladder'—an abbreviated version is given in the box below. Patients can begin at any step on the ladder, moving up a step if their symptoms are poorly controlled. If symptoms are then well controlled they can move down again after 3 months. The woman in this question is already on step 2, so beginning a long-acting beta-2 agonist is indicated. A combination inhaler—for instance Seretide 250, which combines an inhaled steroid and salmeterol—is often used.

Step 1	As required short acting beta-2 agonist (e.g. salbutamol)
Step 2	Regular inhaled steroid (e.g. beclomethasone) + step 1
Step 3	Regular long-acting beta-2 agonist (e.g. salmeterol) + steps 1 and 2
Step 4	A 6-week trial of a leukotriene receptor antagonist (e.g. monteleukast) **or** an oral theophylline + steps 1, 2, and 3.
Step 5	Regular prednisolone tablets + steps 1, 2, and 3

At each step the doctor should check adherence to medications, inhaler technique, smoking cessation, and environmental factors.

Further reading

Guidelines: British Thoracic Society asthma guidelines (http://www.brit-thoracic.org.uk/clinical-information/asthma/asthma-guidelines.aspx)

OHCM: 172–175, 820

Chronic obstructive pulmonary disease (COPD)

This section should be used to clerk patients presenting acutely with exacerbations of COPD, or recovering afterwards on the wards. Patient pathways lead from the Emergency Department through the Admissions Unit to the Respiratory Ward, with community care being offered by GPs assisted by hospital out-patient appointments.

Learning challenges

- What is the difference between a 'pink puffer' and a 'blue bloater'?
- What is lung volume reduction surgery and what is the rationale behind it?

History

Comment on

- Breathlessness
- Cough, sputum, haemoptysis, wheeze
- Regular medications
- Exercise tolerance (baseline, on this presentation and the rate of decline)
- Previous hospital admissions

Examination

Well or unwell? Why?

Feet to face:

Vital signs: Temperature | Blood pressure | Pulse rate | Respiratory rate | O2 saturations

Clinical clues:

Cardiovascular:

1 2 1

Respiratory:

PEFR

L/min

Abdominal:

Neurological:

Other:

Comment on

- Respiratory distress
- Signs of CO_2 retention, e.g. tremor
- Pattern of breathing, shape of chest
- Wheeze, crackles
- Signs of right heart failure

Chest X-ray

Comment on

- Hyperexpansion, bullae
- Focal consolidation; lobar collapse
- Malignancy

Arterial blood gas analysis

Comment on
- Type I or II respiratory failure

Spirometry

Comment on
- Obstructive deficit
- Degree of reversibility

Blood tests

Comment on
- Evidence of infection (WCC and differential)
- Polycythaemia (raised Hb and haematocrit)

ECG

Comment on
- Arrhythmia, e.g. atrial fibrillation
- Signs of ischaemic heart disease—new and old
- Signs of right heart strain (RBBB, RAD, P pulmonale)

Echocardiogram

Comment on
- Cor pulmonale

Evaluation

1. Is this patient in respiratory failure? How much oxygen can they safely be given? Do they need non-invasive ventilation?

2. What other treatment might they require for an acute exacerbation of COPD?

3. How could this patient's regular medications be modified in view of their baseline level of symptoms?

Smoking cessation advice
- Stage 1: Short-acting inhaled beta-2 agonist or antimuscarinic agent
- Stage 2: Longer-acting antimuscarinic bronchodilator
- Stage 3: Consider oral theophylline or inhaled steroids
- Stage 4: Consider need for regular oral steroids

Also consider:
- Yearly influenza and pneumococcus vaccinations
- Mucolytic drugs to help with cough
- Packs or 'rescue medication' with steroid courses and antibiotics to treat early exacerbations

4. Does this patient meet the criteria for home oxygen? Would they be a candidate for surgery?

Questions

1. A 59-year-old woman with a 40 pack-year smoking history (20 cigarettes/day for 40 years) presents to her GP complaining of worsening exercise tolerance and shortness of breath. During the last three winters she has coughed up copious amounts of greenish sputum and in the summer had a chest infection that took almost 2 months to recover. After examining her, the GP refers her to the respiratory out-patient clinic, which requests lung function tests (the results of which are shown below).

(1) What do these tests demonstrate?

(2) List the essential steps in her management.

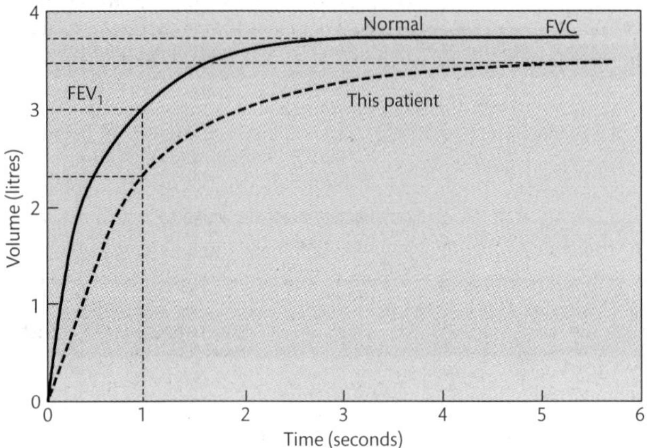

2. A 58-year-old woman with known COPD is assessed in the Emergency Department with severe shortness of breath. Her husband had called an ambulance after her breathing had become increasingly laboured over the preceding few days. On examination she is barrel-chested and obviously distressed. She is tachypnoeic (respiration rate 36 breaths/min) and breathing through pursed lips. She is tachycardic (104 bpm), pyrexial (38.2°C), hypoxic (saturations 92% on air), and is unable to speak in full sentences. The examining doctor notes that the time she takes to exhale is considerably longer than the time she takes to inhale. Her chest X-ray is shown below.

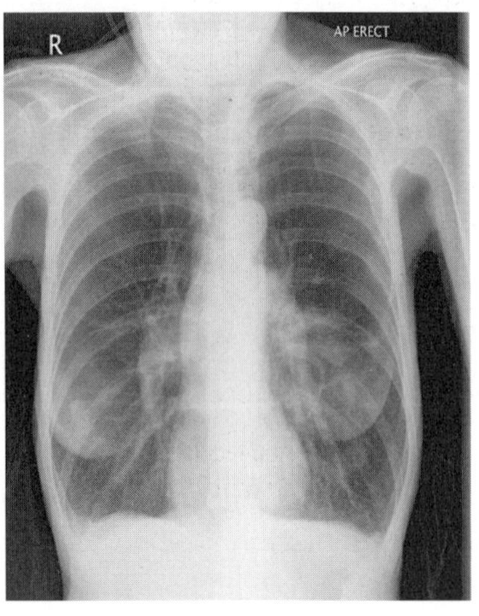

(1) What are the radiological abnormalities shown?

(2) List the other essential investigations you would arrange, with a reason for each.

(3) List the essential management steps.

3. A 74-year-old man with long-standing COPD is brought to the Emergency Department by ambulance. He has become increasingly short of breath and wheezy, and has been unable to get out of bed over the last few days. When the paramedic crew arrived at his house, he had been short of breath at rest, very anxious, with a respiratory rate of 28 breaths/min, and oxygen saturations of 86% on air. He was placed on high-flow oxygen in the ambulance, but during the 30-minute journey to hospital he became increasingly drowsy. On arrival at the Emergency Department his GCS is 11/15, his oxygen saturations are 94%, and he is observed to be taking only around 14 shallow breaths per minute. Arterial blood gas analysis is performed and the results are below. What has happened, and what management is urgently required?

- pH: 7.09
- pCO_2: 10.65 kPa
- pO_2: 10.86 kPa
- HCO_3^-: 34.4 mmol/L

4. A 68-year-old woman is ready for discharge from a respiratory ward after having recovered from a severe exacerbation of COPD. She reports that even at her best she is extremely breathless at home, struggling to wash and dress herself. She asks about the possibility of taking an oxygen cylinder home with her to improve her ability to function. Describe how you would assess this patient for home oxygen therapy.

5. A 42-year-old man unwillingly attends his GP surgery with his wife. She tells the GP she gets very anxious at night because he snores very loudly and then suddenly appears to stop breathing for several seconds, before noisily snoring again. This pattern is repeated throughout the night. On closer questioning he reveals that for the last 6 months he has been much more drowsy than usual during the daytime and has been struggling to get through all of his office work because he feels so sleepy. Physical examination is unremarkable except for pronounced obesity.

(1) What is the likely diagnosis?

(2) List your management steps.

Presentation					
Presented to		Grade		Date	
Signed					

Remember that you can find large-size, annotated versions of many of the X-rays and ECGs that appear in this book on the book's web site at www.oxfordtextbooks.co.uk/orc/randall/

Answers

1. Spirometry reveals that this patient has an obstructive breathing deficit, with a near-normal forced vital capacity (FVC) but the ability only to blow out around 60% of this in the first second (FEV_1). The FEV_1:FVC ratio is a key concept in spirometry, with obstructive deficits being revealed by the ratio of FEV_1:FVC being less than 70%, and restrictive defects having a normal ratio but reduced FVC (i.e. the reduction in FEV_1 matches that of the FVC). Spirometry can also be used to differentiate COPD from asthma. Whilst asthmatics may show a similar obstructive respiratory deficit, their FEV_1 should improve by more than 20% with the use of inhaled bronchodilators, whilst COPD shows responsiveness of less than 20%.

COPD is a diagnosis commonly made on history and examination, confirmed by spirometry. Patients have often had a chronic 'smokers' cough' for many years, but then suffer repeated chest infections with excessive sputum production. Symptoms are worse during the winter months, exacerbated by the cold, damp weather. As the disease progresses, breathlessness becomes a more prominent feature with an associated reduction in exercise tolerance, wheeze, and laboured respiratory movements.

Management of COPD

- **Smoking cessation**—including support from a smoking cessation counsellor. This will considerably improve her chances of symptomatic improvement, and slow the rate of progression of her airways disease.
- **An inhaled bronchodilator** (e.g. salbutamol) may improve symptoms of breathlessness.
- **Prompt treatment of exacerbations** with steroids (and possibly antibiotics) prevents hospital admission.
- The early addition of an inhaled, **long-acting antimuscarinic agent** (tiotropium), alongside the beta agonist, has been recommended to slow the rate of progression.

2. This chest radiograph demonstrates many of the classic radiographic features of COPD:

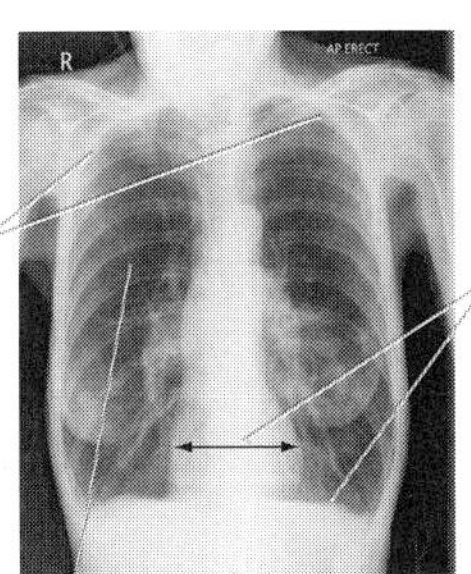

This woman requires treatment for an acute exacerbation of COPD:

- Arterial blood gas analysis is essential here, to exclude CO_2 retention and to guide oxygen therapy. Persistent type I respiratory failure can be treated with increased oxygen, but type II failure may require reduced oxygen or even non-invasive ventilation.
- Steroids form the mainstay of management for COPD exacerbations—typically 40 mg of prednisolone is given daily for 5 days, though if the patient is particularly breathless 100 mg hydrocortisone can be given intravenously.
- Nebulized salbutamol will relieve breathlessness.
- If the WCC and CRP are raised, especially in the presence of fever, then antibiotics are indicated—according to hospital's antibiotics policy, with doxycycline commonly used.

This woman's pattern of breathing is typical of COPD. Because the lungs lose their elastic recoil, expiration is prolonged and sometimes forced (leading chronically to a barrel-shaped chest in some patients). Small airways tend to collapse during expiration, so the patient breathes out through pursed lips to try to raise the pressure in the upper airways and prevent this from happening. This patient is likely to be too unwell for discharge from the Emergency Department, and will benefit from in-patient care until her breathing improves.

3. The arterial blood gas analysis demonstrates severe type II respiratory failure with a significant respiratory acidosis and relative hypoxia (given that the patient is on high-flow oxygen). The patient is drowsy and has dropped their respiration rate because of the effect of hypercapnoea and acidosis on the central nervous system, producing narcosis. This patient is critically unwell and will soon develop respiratory arrest without prompt treatment. He requires urgent non-invasive ventilation with biphasic positive airways pressure (BiPAP). BiPAP is so called because it has an inspiratory phase, where the air/oxygen is literally forced into the lungs, and an expiratory phase that provides resistance on expiration, holding open the small airways and preventing their collapse. Constant pulse oximetry and repeat arterial blood gases in 30 minutes will monitor the effect of treatment.

CO_2 narcosis may develop in any patient with chronic type II respiratory failure who is given high-percentage oxygen. This paradoxically reduces their respiratory drive by correcting the arterial hypoxaemia. Rising arterial CO_2, worsening or poorly correcting hypoxia (despite oxygen therapy), and worsening acidosis (reducing pH and bicarbonate) are all signs of worsening ventilatory failure, and are indications for BiPAP.

4. Long-term home oxygen therapy (LTOT) improves symptoms and life expectancy in advanced COPD. Careful evaluation is needed to confirm that the patient meets the criteria. Most essentially they must agree to stop smoking. If this criterion is met, then they should be assessed by arterial blood gases once they have made a complete recovery from any acute exacerbation, i.e. when they are clinically stable. The criteria for home oxygen are below:

- PaO_2 (on air) < 7.3 kPa or
- PaO_2 < 8 kPa with evidence of secondary complications, e.g. polycythaemia or cor pulmonale

Oxygen may be given by oxygen cylinders that are delivered weekly to the patient's house, by an oxygen concentrator (a small machine that produces concentrated oxygen from room air), or by small portable cylinders that can be carried by the patient when they go out. To derive any prognostic improvement they must wear their oxygen for at least 15 hours/day, and to reduce mortality patients must wear the oxygen for >19 hours/day. Other oxygen therapies include:

(1) **short burst therapy**, to allow patients who do not qualify for LTOT, to deal with episodes of acute breathlessness

(2) **ambulatory oxygen** for those who desaturate with exercise.

5. This man and his wife are describing the symptoms of obstructive sleep apnoea (OSA). This is a condition that occurs most commonly in obese middle-aged men. It is caused by decreased tone in the muscles of the pharynx, leading to pharyngeal obstruction during sleep. During each night the patient may regularly 'lose' their airway and stop breathing, being woken from deep sleep by rising pCO_2 which stimulates forceful respiration and reopens the airway. Such patients never get enough deep sleep and so are permanently tired; they are also at high risk of vascular disease because of their chronically raised pCO_2 whilst asleep. Other symptoms include headaches on waking in the morning and daytime somnolence.

This man should be referred for sleep studies. Pulse oximetry may reveal cyclical desaturations, with OSA being diagnosed if there are more than 15 desaturations in any hour-long period. Patients are greatly helped by continuous positive airways pressure (CPAP) non-invasive ventilation, which improves symptoms of tiredness as well as long-term cardiovascular risk.

Further reading

Guidelines: NICE guidelines on COPD (http://guidance.nice.org.uk/CG12)

OHCM: 176–177, 180, 194, 822

Deep vein thrombosis (DVT) and pulmonary embolism (PE)

Learning challenges

- What is Virchow's triad and how does it aid identification of patients at high risk of DVT/PE?
- Why might the D-dimer blood test be unhelpful in certain situations?

This section should be used to assess patients presenting to the Emergency Department with symptoms of PE or DVT, or for assessing patients on any ward who develop sudden breathlessness or hypoxia, in whom PE is always a concern. Pathways for patients with suspected PE lead from the Emergency Department via radiography to respiratory wards and then out-patient anticoagulant clinic appointments.

History

Comment on

- Leg swelling
- Pleuritic chest pain, breathlessness
- Major risk factors: surgery, pregnancy, immobility, malignancy, previous DVT/PE
- Minor risk factors: cardiovascular disease, oral contraception, long-haul travel, obesity

Examination

Well or unwell? Why?

Feet to face:

Vital signs: Temperature | Blood pressure | Pulse rate | Respiratory rate | O2 saturations

Clinical clues:

Cardiovascular:

1 2 1

Respiratory:

PEFR

L/min

Abdominal:

Neurological:

Other:

Comment on

- Haemodynamic status—BP, pulse, temperature
- RR, oxygen sats, signs of respiratory distress
- Leg swelling (measure diameters), skin changes
- Chest examination
- Signs of right heart failure
- Wells score (see p. 77)

Arterial blood gas analysis

Comment on

- Type I respiratory failure/type II failure (in severe cases)

Chest X-ray

Comment on

- Usually clear

ECG

Comment on

- Often normal or sinus tachycardia
- Right ventricular strain—classically a prominent S wave in lead I, with a prominent Q wave and T-wave inversion in lead III

D-dimer (is this indicated?)

Lower limb venous Doppler ultrasound scan/ CT pulmonary angiography or ventilation-perfusion (V/Q) scan

Comment on

- Evidence of DVT or PE

Evaluation

1. Based on history, risk factors, and physical examination, what is the clinical probability of DVT/PE?

Wells score for DVT/PE probability

DVT	PE
Active cancer: +1	Clinically suspected DVT: +3
Difference in calf circumference >3 cm: +1	Alternative diagnosis less likely: +3
Superficial (non-varicose) veins: +1	Tachycardia: +1.5
Unilateral pitting oedema: +1	Recent surgery or immobility: +1.5
Swelling of entire leg: +1	Previous history of DVT/PE: +1.5
Localized pain in deep venous system: +1	Haemoptysis: +1
Paralysis, paresis, or plaster cast: +1	Active cancer: +1
Recent surgery or immobility: +1	
Alternative diagnosis equally likely: -2	

DVT: 0–1 low probability, 2+ high probability.
PE: 0–3.5 low probability, 4+ high probability.

2. How should this patient be investigated and managed based on their pre-test probability?

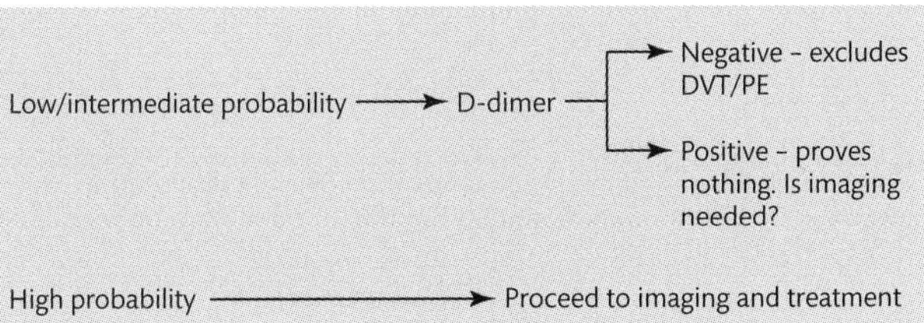

Despite negative investigations, with a strong clinical suspicion empirical anticoagulation could be started. Remember PEs kill!

3. What is the appropriate treatment option?

4. For how long should the patient be treated? Is further investigation needed to determine why this patient has suffered a DVT/PE?

Questions

1. A 78-year-old man presents to the Emergency Department with a swollen right leg, which has worsened over the previous week. He is generally fit and well, but he is obese and has type 2 diabetes mellitus. On examination the diameter of his right leg is 46 cm (measured 10 cm below the tibial tuberosity) compared with 38 cm round the left leg. There is pitting oedema to the mid-calf on the right side, and the skin is red and thickened, and hot to touch. There is generalized tenderness and engorgement of the superficial veins. His temperature is 37.5°C and blood tests reveal a CRP of 14 and a white cell count of 8.9 × 10^9/L. D-dimers were 0.6 ng/mL (normal 0–0.5).

(1) What is the differential diagnosis?

(2) Describe the next steps in his management.

2. An 87-year-old patient who is recovering after major lower limb surgery 2 weeks previously, is noted to be acutely short of breath whilst having his physiotherapy. His oxygen saturations on room air are 88%, when earlier they had been 96%. His heart rate is 106 bpm and his blood pressure 156/87 mmHg. The patient does not complain of any chest pain. He does not have a history of any cardiac or respiratory disease. Chest examination is unremarkable. He is placed on high-flow oxygen via a non-rebreathe mask and then arterial blood gas analysis is performed, the results of which are below.

(1) What is the abnormality shown on the blood gas analysis?

(2) Describe the next essential management steps.

- pH: 7.49
- $PaCO_2$: 3.85 kPa
- PaO_2: 9.04 kPa
- HCO_3^-: 24 mmol/L
- Base excess (BE): +1.2 mmol/L

3. A 54-year-old woman is being treated with warfarin for a right lower limb DVT. She is otherwise well and has no significant past medical history, though her mother and brother have both suffered with recurrent DVTs. She presents to the Emergency Department with sudden-onset breathlessness and right-sided pleuritic pain. CTPA revealed extensive bilateral pulmonary emboli with a right-sided pulmonary infarction. Describe the investigations and management to reduce the risk of her condition worsening.

4. A previously fit and well 32-year-old man is found to have a right above-knee DVT after having open reduction and internal fixation of a complex ankle fracture. He is otherwise well, taking no regular medications, and weighs 80 kg.

(1) Download a sample drug chart from the Online Resource Centre and prescribe warfarin for this man, using the modified Fennerly nomogram below. His INRs for today and the next three days are 1.0, 1.4, 2.2, and 2.8. Also prescribe enoxaparin, a low-molecular-weight heparin, to provide anti-coagulant cover until the INR is therapeutic.

(2) List five medications which may interfere with this man's INR levels after he has achieved a steady state on a stable warfarin regime.

Oral anticoagulant:
Target INR:
Duration of treatment:

Date									
INR	1.0	1.4	2.2	2.8					
Dose									
Time									
Signed									
Nurse									

Modified Fennerty nomogram

Day	Morning INR	Warfarin dose	Day	Morning INR	Warfarin dose
1	<1.4	10 mg	4	<1.4	10 mg
2	<1.8	10 mg		1.4–1.5	8 mg
	1.8–2	1 mg		1.6–1.7	7 mg
	>2	0		1.8–1.9	6 mg
3	<2	10 mg		2–2.3	5 mg
	2–2.2	5 mg		2.4–3	4 mg
	2.3–2.5	4 mg		3.1–4	3 mg
	2.6–2.9	3 mg		>4	0
	3.0–3.2	2 mg			
	3.3–3.5	1 mg			
	>3.5	0			

Presentation

Presented to ______ Grade ______ Date ______

Signed

Answers

1. The two most likely diagnoses in this man are DVT and cellulitis. Both may present with swelling, redness, and a low-grade pyrexia. Cellulitis is especially likely in this man given that he is diabetic (and therefore predisposed to skin and soft-tissue infections); however, the significant oedema and venous engorgement also make DVT a possibility.

His Wells score is +1 (+1 for each of the disparity in circumference, the superficial veins, and the oedema, −2 for the alternative diagnosis), making DVT unlikely. The weakly positive D-dimer result is unhelpful: whilst a negative result would rule out DVT, a weakly positive result is consistent with either DVT or cellulitis. However, the lack of significantly raised inflammatory markers counts against (but does not exclude) cellulitis.

The best test to differentiate between DVT and cellulitis is lower leg venous Doppler ultrasound. In most hospitals this can be arranged within a few hours, but if there is a delay, it would be fair to treat the patient both with a low-molecular-weight heparin and antibiotics to cover both possibilities. If no clot is visible then the swelling and redness would be expected to settle with antibiotics.

2. There is a high pH and low pCO_2 (respiratory alkalosis), consistent with hyperventilation. However, the more alarming measurement is the mild hypoxia despite treatment with high-flow oxygen via a non-rebreathe mask. This should elevate the PaO_2 to a far higher level than 9.04. Thus there is type I respiratory failure with a mild respiratory alkalosis, which would be consistent with any pulmonary disease process affecting gas exchange—including PE.

The most relevant investigation in this man will be a plain chest X-ray, to exclude a different cause of hypoxia (for instance pulmonary oedema or pneumonia, though both are unlikely given the unremarkable examination). This man's Wells score is 6 (high probability of PE), suggesting that a D-dimer test may be unhelpful. A V/Q scan should be performed to exclude PE. Hypoxia this significant requires an explanation, so CT may be preferred since it would also diagnose other possible aetiologies (e.g. consolidation not picked up on X-ray). Therapeutic low-molecular-weight heparin should be commenced as soon as the diagnosis of possible PE has been reached, before the scan is performed. A slice from this man's CTPA is below. He was commenced on warfarin and maintained on low-molecular-weight heparin until his INR was therapeutic (2–3).

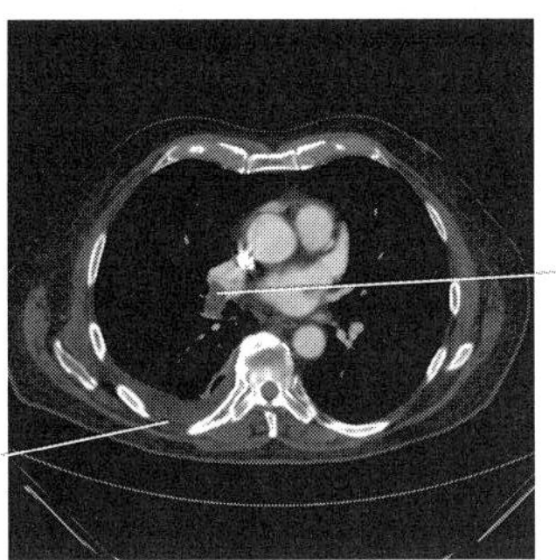

Large pulmonary embolus within the right main pulmonary artery.

Small right-sided pleural effusion, probably caused by the pulmonary embolus.

3. Recurrent DVT and PE whilst on warfarin is unusual and requires investigation. In the first instance, it is worth checking that the patient is actually taking her warfarin and that her INR is maintained within the therapeutic range.

The strong family history of DVT raises the possibility of an inherited thrombophilia, and various assays are used to investigate for clotting abnormalities such as Factor V Leiden, antithrombin deficiency, protein C or S deficiency, or the antiphospholipid syndrome. The coagulation cascade triggered in blood is a dynamic process, with some proteins (such as thrombin and fibrin) contributing to clot formation and others (such as antithrombin or proteins C and S) causing clot dissolution. Failure of these mechanisms leads to unwanted thrombosis and predisposes to DVT and PE.

Recurrent DVT is also linked to malignancy, and this woman should be asked closely about symptoms of cancer such a weight loss and anorexia, as well as a general systems enquiry searching for unexplained symptoms. If there are features suggestive of malignancy (symptoms, signs, or blood tests, such as a raised serum calcium), then CT scanning of the chest, abdomen, and pelvis may reveal the site.

In the meantime, she requires treatment to prevent further PEs from occurring and causing respiratory compromise. One option would be to increase her warfarin dose to achieve a higher INR. This carries a higher risk of bleeding. Another option is to arrange for an inferior vena cava filter to be fitted (under radiological guidance) to prevent leg DVTs from travelling to the lung.

4. Warfarin takes some time to reach steady state in the blood, and so common practice is to load patients with doses that are higher than what they will usually require, and then reduce the dose once the INR is in the therapeutic range—this is 2–3 for DVT and PE (in other conditions, for instance with a prosthetic heart valve, the desired INR range may be higher).

A low-molecular-weight heparin should be prescribed until the INR is in this range. It is given at 1.5 mg/kg of body weight to achieve the therapeutic goal of reducing clot size. It does this not by dissolving the clot, but by preventing it from expanding further—thrombolytic agents within blood such as plasmin actually break down the clot over time.

Warfarin is metabolized by the cytochrome P-450 enzymes in the liver. The rate of metabolism may be greatly affected by other drugs that are also metabolized this way, or which induce or impede these enzymes. For example, the antibiotic clarithromycin will slow warfarin metabolism and thus increase the anticoagulant effect (increasing the INR), whilst the over-the-counter herbal antidepressant St John's Wort will induce the P-450 enzymes, increasing metabolism of warfarin and reducing its effect on the INR. Other medications that commonly interfere with INR levels include other antibiotics, antiepileptics, and alcohol. When prescribing any medications to patients on warfarin, always check the list of interactions with warfarin (listed under 'coumarins') in Appendix 1 of the BNF.

Oral anticoagulant: Warfarin
Target INR: 2–3
Duration of treatment: 6 weeks

Date	7/9	8/9	9/9	10/9					
INR	1.0	1.4	2.2	2.8					
Dose	10 mg	10 mg	5 mg	4 mg					
Time	1800	1800	1800	1800					
Signed	DR	DR	DR	DR					
Nurse									

Drug: Enoxaparin
Instructions: Until INR >2
Signature: DR

Start: 7/9	Route: S/c								
1800	120 mg								

Further reading

Guidelines: British Thoracic Society guidelines on pulmonary embolism (http://www.brit-thoracic.org.uk/clinical-information/pulmonary-embolism/pulmonary-embolism-guidelines.aspx)

OHCM: 182, 344–345, 368, 580–581, 828

Pneumonia

This section should be used to clerk patients with acute lower respiratory tract infection—patient journeys lead from the Emergency Department to Admissions Units or General Medical Wards, or the ITU if severely unwell.

Learning challenges

- Why might three completely different antibiotic combinations be used for community acquired, hospital acquired, and ventilator-associated pneumonia?
- Which pneumonias occur in outbreaks?

History

Comment on

- Known respiratory disease; smoking
- Cough, nature of sputum—volume, colour, consistency, smell, frequency
- Chest pain, breathlessness
- Fever
- Systemic features, e.g. diarrhoea and vomiting, confusion, rashes, jaundice

Examination

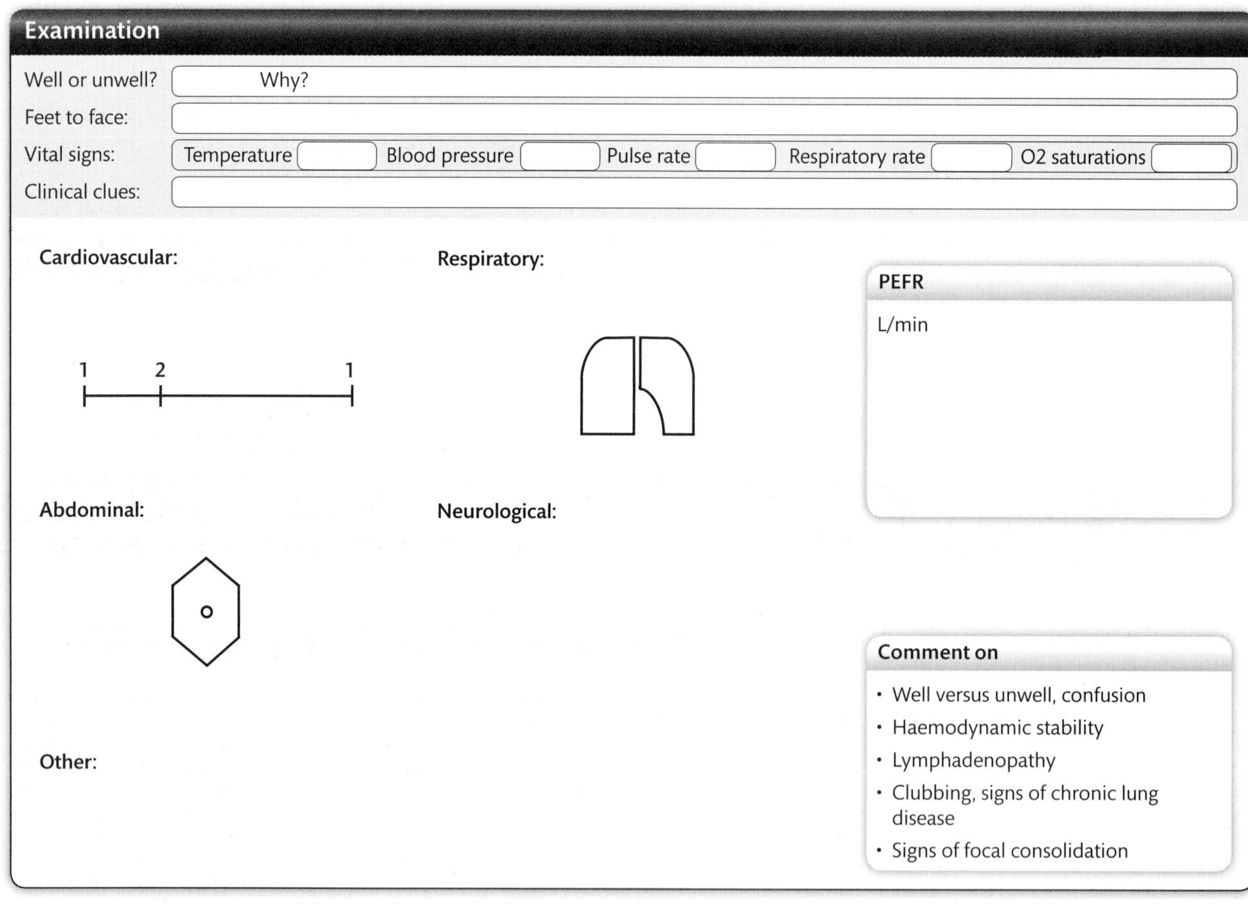

Comment on

- Well versus unwell, confusion
- Haemodynamic stability
- Lymphadenopathy
- Clubbing, signs of chronic lung disease
- Signs of focal consolidation

Chest X-ray

Comment on

- Focal consolidation versus diffuse or patchy shadowing
- Cavitation?
- Pleural effusion?

Blood tests

Comment on

- WCC and differential
- Renal impairment; hyponatraemia
- Deranged LFTs and clotting
- Lactate
- Atypical serology and viral titres

Urine

Comment on

- Legionella/pneumococcal antigen?

Arterial blood gas analysis

Comment on

- Respiratory failure?
- Acidosis?

Sputum culture

Comment on

- Organism
- Sensitivities

Blood cultures

Comment on

- Organism
- Sensitivities

Evaluation

1. Is there good evidence for lung infection? Could infection be coming from elsewhere? Do the benefits of antibiotics outweigh the risks?

2. How severe is this pneumonia? Is there evidence of systemic sepsis? What is the CURB-65 score (use SOAR scores for the over 75s)?

CURB-65 or SOAR scores for community-acquired pneumonia

CURB-65 score:	SOAR score:	For both CURB-65 and SOAR		
Confusion **U**rea >7.0 **R**R >30 **B**P <90 systolic Age >**65**	**S**ystolic BP <90 p**O**$_2$ <7.3 **A**ge >65 **R**R >30	Score	Mortality	Management
		0–1	<5%	Out-patient
		2–3	<10%	Short in-patient
		4–5	15–30%	In-patient/ITU

3. What kind of pneumonia is this? What organisms commonly cause these pneumonias? What antibiotics are appropriate?

4. How would you assess if treatment is working?

Questions

1. An 18-year-old soldier has been unwell for 5 days, initially with headache and feeling generally unwell, but now with a cough productive of a small amount of yellowish sputum. She has also had some diarrhoea and vomiting. She was otherwise fit and healthy. Examination of the chest was unremarkable, and all blood tests were within normal limits. Her chest X-ray is shown below.

(1) What does the chest X-ray show?

(2) What is the likely diagnosis and correct management of this condition?

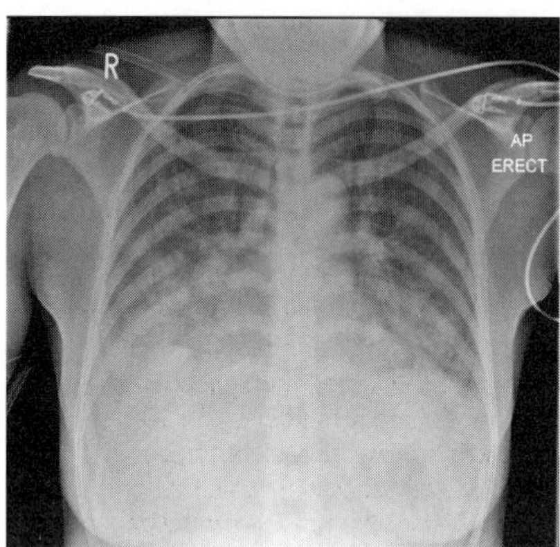

2. You are called to see an 89-year-old man on an orthopaedic ward who is recovering from right hip hemiarthroplasty, performed 6 days ago after he suffered a femoral neck fracture. He is now pyrexial (38.3°C) and confused. On examination he feels warm and well-perfused with a large-volume pulse, and has reduced breath sounds, coarse crackles and bronchial breathing throughout the left side of his chest. His heart rate is 112 bpm and his blood pressure 85/55 mmHg. His blood tests and X-ray are below.

(1) List the abnormalities and the likely causes for each.

(2) Describe the essential steps in his management.

- Sodium: 138 mmol/L
- Potassium: 3.7 mmol/L
- Creatinine: 132 µmol/L
- Urea: 11.7 mmol/L
- CRP: 112 mg/L
- Haemoglobin: 10.9 g/dL
- MCV: 85 fL
- WCC: 15.5×10^9/L
- Platelets: 199×10^9/L

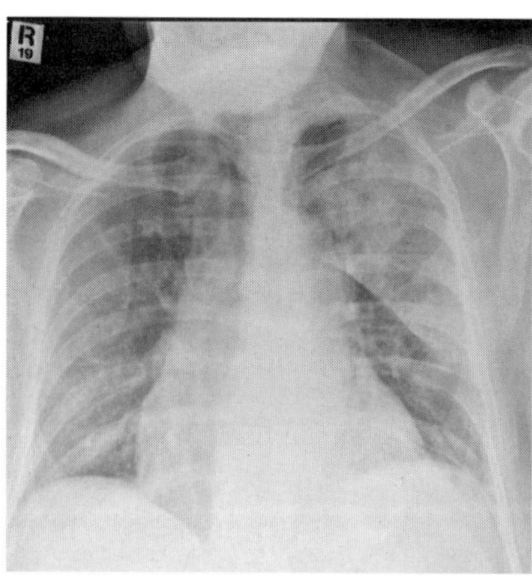

3. An 89-year-old man who has previously suffered a stroke and is fed by nasogastric tube is admitted from a nursing home with a productive cough and shortness of breath. On examination he has a heart rate of 118 bpm, blood pressure of 145/98 mmHg, a respiratory rate of 26 breaths/min, and oxygen sats of 92% on air. He has coarse crepitations and bronchial breathing at the right base. Chest X-ray confirms right lower-lobe consolidation. He has previously had various courses of antibiotics from his GP for this infection and for recurrent urinary tract infections in the past. In view of this, one of your seniors tells you to put him on 'a broad-spectrum antibiotic', and suggests ciprofloxacin. A doctor from the hospital's microbiology department overhears the conversation and suggests instead giving him intravenous benzyl penicillin and metronidazole.

(1) Why might ciprofloxacin be a good idea in this patient?

(2) What is the rationale behind the antibiotics suggested by the microbiologist?

(3) Using a sample drug chart downloaded from the Online Resource Centre, prescribe the medications suggested by the microbiology team.

Remember that you can find large-size, annotated versions of many of the X-rays and ECGs that appear in this book on the book's web site at www.oxfordtextbooks.co.uk/orc/randall/

Answers

1. The X-ray reveals:

This x-ray reveals patchy consolidation in both lungs. There is also a small right-sided effusion (the costophrenic angle cannot be seen here). The likely diagnosis her is atypical pneumonia, but similar x-ray appearances can be caused by fluid (e.g. in pulmonary haemorrhage or acute lung injury) or soft tissue shadowing (e.g. lung metastases from distant cancers).

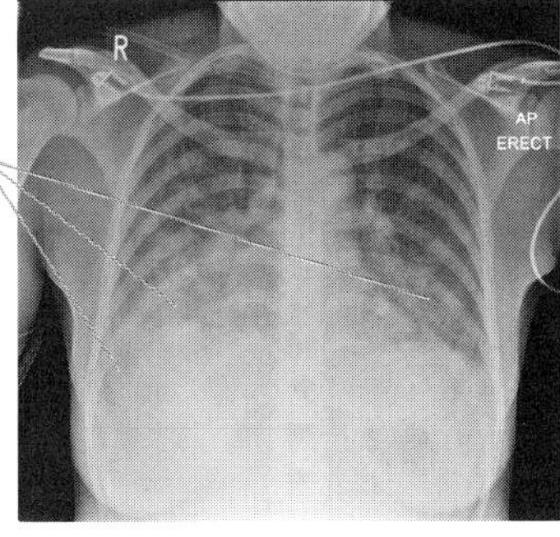

This patient has radiological evidence of pneumonia, which would of course be community acquired. However, the presentation is not classic for an ordinary lobar pneumonia, raising the possibility of an atypical pneumonia. The term 'atypical' describes:

- **History**—often present with atypical respiratory symptoms and systemic features, e.g. diarrhoea and vomiting.
- **Examination**—may present with severe respiratory distress, despite minimal clinical findings in the chest and minimal radiological changes on the chest images (the doctor 'hears nothing, sees nothing'); may also have multisystem signs.
- **Investigations**—atypical WCC and differential, hyponatraemia secondary to SIADH, deranged LFTs. Difficult to culture in routine lab media so titres of antigen and antibodies are sent.
- **Management**—may require atypical antibiotics including doxycycline, high-dose macrolides, or rifampicin.

'Typical' community-acquired pneumonia is usually caused by *Streptococcus pneumoniae*; however, atypical pathogens include *Mycoplasma*, *Chlamydia*, and *Legionella* species. *Mycoplasma* is especially associated with outbreaks in institutions and could be responsible in this woman. Appropriate treatment would include a penicillin (e.g. amoxicillin) to cover streptococcus and a macrolide (e.g. clarithromycin) to cover atypical pathogens.

2. The X-ray shows:

This x-ray shows evidence of left upper lobe consolidation - note how clearly the shadowing is defined by the oblique fissure. Right upper lobe consolidation is defined in a similar way by the horizontal fissure.

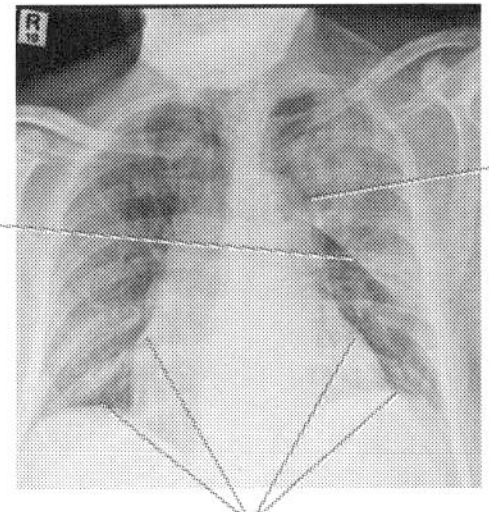

Note this air broncogram - an airway (seen here as a dark line), well defined against the more opaque surrounding lung. This is a classic feature of consolidation, caused by the lung parenchyma filling with inflammatory exudate whilst the bronchi remains relatively clear.

If there is consolidation in the lower zones, look at the heart border and diaphragm to determine where the problem lies. In lower lobe pneumonia, the heart border remains well defined but the hemi-diaphragm cannot be clearly seen. In the middle lobe (right lung) or lingula (left lung) pneumonia, the diaphragm can be seen but the heart border is lost.

His blood tests provide supportive evidence for infection (raised WCC and CRP), whilst also showing a mild anaemia (likely to be due to intraoperative blood loss) and mild renal impairment (raised urea and creatinine—very common in the context of infection, especially in the elderly).

There is enough evidence to warrant treating this man for hospital-acquired pneumonia (hospital acquired since he has been in hospital for more than 3 days). Furthermore, according to the criteria outlined in the box below, he can also be diagnosed with severe sepsis, which requires urgent treatment with antibiotics and fluids.

Systemic inflammatory response syndrome (SIRS)

Two or more of: Temperature >38°C, Heart rate >90 bpm, Respiratory rate >20 breaths/min, White cell count $>12 \times 10^9$/L

Sepsis: SIRS caused by proven infection

Severe sepsis: Sepsis accompanied by evidence of organ dysfunction, e.g. confusion or oliguria

Septic shock: Severe sepsis with hypotension (systolic blood pressure <90 mmHg) despite fluid resuscitation

SIRS is caused by the systemic effects of inflammatory mediators which are released by white blood cells in the lung, producing systemic vasodilatation and a fall in total peripheral resistance. The patient becomes tachycardic in an effort to maintain their cardiac output and blood pressure (blood pressure = cardiac output × total peripheral resistance; cardiac output = heart rate × stroke volume). This man requires quite aggressive fluid resuscitation to prevent him developing shock or worsening renal failure from inadequate renal perfusion. If he fails to improve despite adequate resuscitation then he may need transfer to intensive care for treatment with inotropic agents to maintain blood pressure and organ perfusion.

Antibiotics for hospital-acquired pneumonia need to cover the organisms causing community-acquired pneumonia, but also Gram-negative organisms such as *Klebsiella pneumoniae*. A combination of piperacillin and tazobactam is commonly used, given intravenously.

3. Using broad-spectrum antibiotics causes two problems. The first is that it predisposes to developing organisms that are resistant to multiple classes of antibiotic. The second, especially in the elderly, is that they can predispose to developing antibiotic-associated diarrhoea—especially that caused by *Clostridium difficile*. Ciprofloxacin has been particularly linked to *C. difficile* diarrhoea and most hospitals now restrict its use to only a few clinical situations.

This patient is institutionalized and has had multiple previous courses of antibiotics, so is at high risk of developing *C. difficile* infection. Therefore the antibiotic strategy should be to use antibiotics with the narrowest possible spectrum which still provide adequate cover for the likely organisms. Since the patient is also fed by nasogastric tube, he is predisposed to developing an aspiration pneumonia (which characteristically affects the right lower lobe since the right main bronchus is straighter than the left). Therefore appropriate antibiotics are benzyl penicillin (which has excellent activity against almost all streptococcal pneumonias) and metronidazole (which is active against anaerobic organisms commonly found in the bowel). They should be prescribed as below:

Drug: Benzyl penicillin
Instructions: For 5 days
Signature: DR

Start: 3/9/9	Route: IV										
0800	1.2g										
1200	1.2g										
1800	1.2g										
2200	1.2g										

Drug: Metronidazole
Instructions: For 5 day
Signature: DR

Start: 3/9/9	Route: IV										
0800	500 mg										
1200	500 mg										
2200	500 mg										

Further reading

Guidelines: British Thoracic Society guidelines for community acquired pneumonia (http://www.brit-thoracic.org.uk/clinical-information/pneumonia/pneumonia-guidelines.aspx)

OHCM: 160–169, 826

Lung cancer

This section should be used to clerk patients with presentations suggestive of lung cancer (e.g. chronic cough, haemoptysis, and weight loss) or patients with known disease. Patients may be referred up to the out-patient respiratory clinic for investigation, and then have a CT scan and bronchoscopy. Alternatively, if admitted with complications (e.g. a pleural effusion), they may be found on the Admissions Unit or Respiratory Ward.

Learning challenges

- What are the commonest types of cancer in this country, and where does lung cancer fit on that list?
- What is a paraneoplastic phenomenon, and what mechanisms may cause them?

History

Comment on

- Previous lung cancer history? (see how to take a history of malignancy p. 7)
- Cough, chest pain, haemoptysis, breathlessness
- Malaise, anorexia, weight loss
- Bony pain, personality change, neurological symptoms
- Review of symptoms

Examination

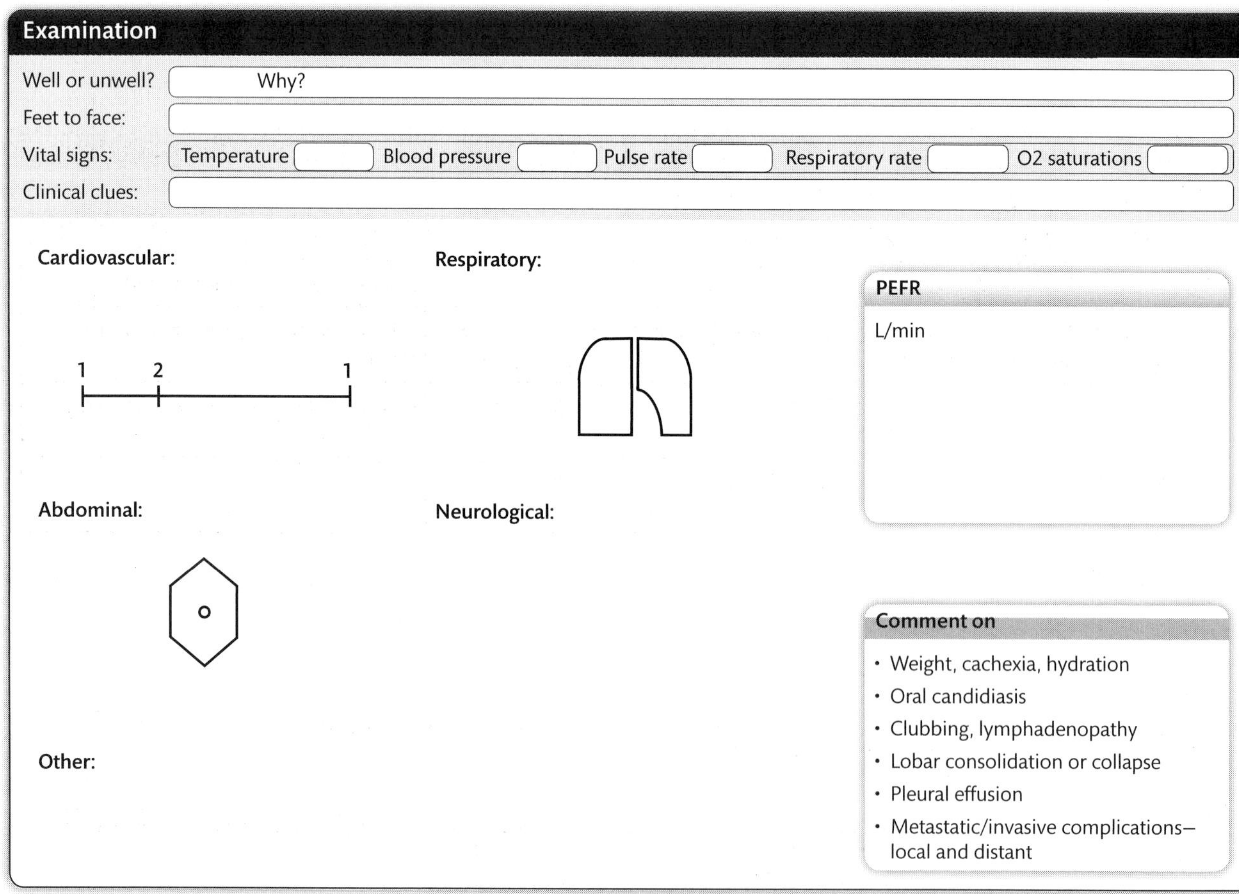

Comment on

- Weight, cachexia, hydration
- Oral candidiasis
- Clubbing, lymphadenopathy
- Lobar consolidation or collapse
- Pleural effusion
- Metastatic/invasive complications—local and distant

Chest X-ray

Comment on

- Shadows/masses
- Collapse/consolidation
- Effusion
- Rib and bony metastases/destruction

Blood tests

Comment on

- Anaemia
- Electrolyte abnormalities (Na, K, Ca)
- Deranged LFTs and clotting

CT chest, abdomen, and pelvis

Comment on

- Size and location of tumour
- Local invasion/distant spread for staging purposes

Bronchoscopy

Comment on

- Nature and location of lesion
- Bronchial obstruction

Histology

Evaluation

1. **What histological type of tumour is this? What is the staging?**

T (Tumour)	N (Nodes)	M (Metastases)
T1: Contained within lung, <3 cm across	**N0:** No nodal disease	**M0:** No evidence of distant spread
T2: 3–7 cm diameter (**2a** <5 cm, **2b** >5 cm) *or* invasion of bronchus or visceral pleura	**N1:** Disease in closest draining lymph nodes	**M1a:** Tumour in both lungs or malignant effusions
T3: >7 cm *or* invading chest wall *or* >1 tumour	**N2:** Ipsilateral mediastinal nodes	**M1b:** Distant spread, e.g. bones or liver
T4: Invasion of heart, oesophagus, vessels, diaphragm, trachea	**N3:** Contralateral mediastinal nodes or supraclavicular nodes	

- **Stage 1:** T1–T2a, N0, M0
- **Stage 2:** T1–T2b, N0–1, M0
- **Stage 3:** Any T, any N, M0
- **Stage 4:** Any T, any N, M1a or M1b

2. **Is this tumour operable? Is chemotherapy or radiotherapy indicated? What are the patient's wishes?**

3. **What symptoms are present? What can be done to alleviate these? Would the patient like to be seen by the palliative care team?**

Questions

1. A 61-year-old patient attends his GP's surgery complaining of a 2-month history of a dry cough associated with weight loss and loss of appetite. He has also noticed shooting pains down the inside of his left arm and a new hoarseness to his voice. His wife has noticed that his left eyelid has started to droop. He has no other medical problems. He has smoked 20 cigarettes per day for the whole of his adult life. On examination, the patient appeared well and was not tachypneoic. He had a notably hoarse voice. His hands exhibited bilateral clubbing. He had a left sided ptosis, with a constricted pupil and periorbital anhydrosis, but no other neurological deficits were found and examination of the chest was unremarkable.

(1) Which neurological phenomena are being described, and how might a clear understanding of neuroanatomy help piece together these disparate symptoms and signs?

(2) What is the likely unifying diagnosis?

2. A 70-year-old woman with an 80 pack-year history of cigarette smoking presents to her GP complaining of feeling weak and dizzy. She had not felt well for several months and had unexpectedly lost 7 kg in weight over this period. She had also experienced a nagging cough with occasional episodes of haemoptysis. Her GP arranged some routine blood tests (see below).

- Sodium: 124 mmol/L
- Potassium: 4.2 mmol/L
- Creatinine: 74 µmol/L
- Urea: 3.5 mmol/L
- Calcium: 3.78 mmol/L
- Haemoglobin: 9.8 g/dL
- MCV: 86 fL
- WCC: 7.6 × 10^9/L
- Platelets: 223 × 10^9/L

(1) List the abnormalities and a cause for each.

(2) List the essential further investigations and management you would arrange.

3. A 64-year-old man attends the hospital Emergency Department with a 2-day history of increasing shortness of breath. He had previously been reasonably well, but had lost 'a lot of weight' over the past month. On examination he is found to be cachetic and unwell looking, with a temperature of 39.8°C. Examination of his chest reveals decreased expansion and breath sounds throughout the whole of the left side of the chest, which is slightly dull to percussion. His chest X-ray is shown below.

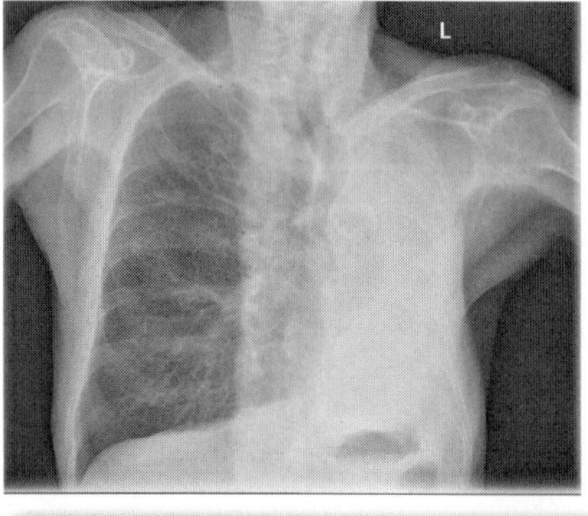

(1) What does the chest image show?

(2) List the essential investigations and management which should be arranged.

4. A 78-year-old woman with significant COPD is diagnosed with small cell cancer after CT guided biopsy (see image below). The lesion measured 8.4 cm in diameter, with invasion of the posterior thoracic wall and significant ipsilateral lymphadenopathy, as well as a likely metastasis in the liver.

(1) Using the TNM classification (see 'Evaluation' above) what is the staging of this tumour?

(2) Describe how this patient should be managed?

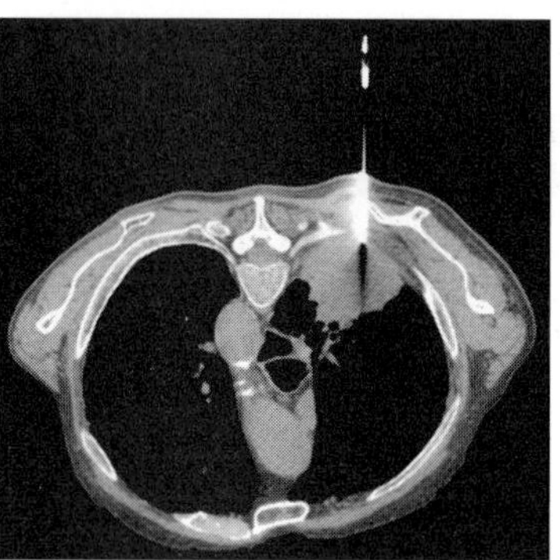

Note that for this CT-guided biopsy the patient has been positioned prone to allow for access to the tumour through the posterior chest wall. A major risk of this procedure, as well as of needle aspiration of a pleural effusion or chest drain insertion, is pneumothorax if the needle goes in too deep and punctures the lung allowing air to escape into the pleural space.

5. A 67-year-old man who had previously worked for a building demolition company presents to his GP surgery with increasing shortness of breath and persistent nagging pain on the right side of his chest. On examination he is clubbed, and has reduced breath sounds and stony dullness to percussion at the right base. After seeing his X-ray (below), his GP arranges for him to be admitted to hospital for tests.

(1) What does the chest image demonstrate?

(2) What is the best diagnostic approach to a patient with this abnormality on X-ray?

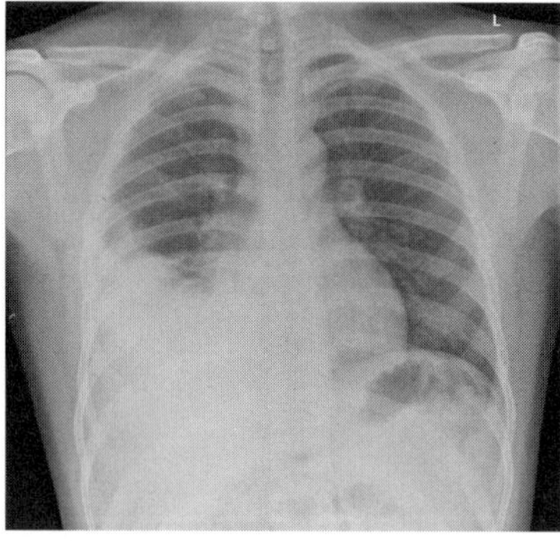

Presentation

Presented to ______ Grade ______ Date ______

Signed

Remember that you can find large-size, annotated versions of many of the X-rays and ECGs that appear in this book on the book's web site at www.oxfordtextbooks.co.uk/orc/randall/

Answers

1. Three separate groups of neurological symptoms are being described here: neuropathic arm pain (neuropathic pain is often described by patients as 'shooting'), hoarseness of voice, and loss of sympathetic innervation to the left eye (called Horner's syndrome). The single common factor to tie these deficits together is location: around the apex of the lung lie the brachial plexus (innervating the arm), the recurrent laryngeal nerve (innervating the larynx), and the upper sympathetic chain and stellate ganglion (supplying sympathetic innervation to the head).

Tumours at the apex of the lung are termed 'Pancoast tumours' if they are invasive and cause this clinical syndrome. Chronic non-productive cough with weight loss and occasional haemoptysis are symptoms of any lung cancer. This man requires a chest X-ray and review in a respiratory out-patient clinic. A tumour causing these symptoms is likely to be visible on X-ray.

2. The three abnormalities shown are hyponatraemia, hypercalcaemia, and normocytic anaemia:

- Hyponatraemia is most commonly caused by disturbances of volume status, for instance receiving too much intravenous fluid (dilutional hyponatraemia) or being dehydrated from diarrhoea or vomiting (relative excess loss of salt). If the patient's volume status is thought to be normal (to be determined clinically, by looking at the JVP, auscultating the lung bases, looking for pedal oedema, and checking for a postural blood pressure drop), then it is possible the patient has a syndrome of inappropriate antidiuretic hormone secretion (SIADH). SIADH is relatively rare, but small cell lung cancer is a recognized cause. Small cell lung cancers arise from neuroendocrine tissue and rarely secrete hormones such as ADH or ACTH.
- Hypercalcaemia is common in malignancy, sometimes caused by tumours producing a polypeptide similar to parathyroid hormone and sometimes by bony destruction from metastatic disease.
- Normocytic anaemia is most commonly associated with chronic disease, which in this patient could fit with a bronchial carcinoma.

This woman requires the following investigations:

- Chest X-ray (to establish whether a lung tumour is present). Abnormal shadows should be further investigated by CT or bronchoscopy.
- Urinary sodium level—a relatively high urinary sodium suggests SIADH as a cause for the serum hyponatraemia.
- Parathyroid hormone level (primary hyperparathyroidism remains the commonest cause of hypercalcaemia) and a whole-body bone scan to look for bony metastases.

3. This chest image reveals:

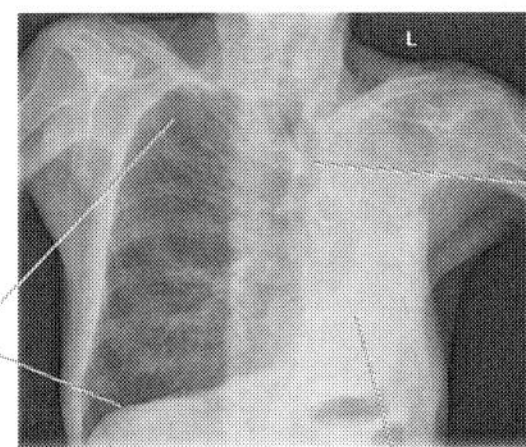

The right lung shows increased volume, decreased lung markings and a flattened hemi-diaphragm, likely due to COPD given this man's smoking history.

The key to explaining why this is a lung collapse rather than a massive effusion is the trachea. The trachea and mediastinum are pulled towards an area of collapse and pused away from a massive effusion.

The most obvious abnormality here is the 'white-out' of the left lung. The differential for a complete white-out includes collapse of the lung, massive pleural effusion, pneumonectomy (where the lung has been removed) and extensive pneumonia, only this would classically give a patchier appearance.

The primary defect here is a collapse of the left lung. Collapse occurs where a major airway becomes obstructed; distal to this obstruction the lung collapses and becomes a ready site for infection. Collapse can be seen on X-ray by a hazy translucency over the affected area, which will have decreased volume. This decreased volume causes neighbouring structures to be 'sucked in'—causing tracheal and mediastinal deviation towards the affected side, localized rib crowding, and elevation of the ipsilateral hemidiaphragm, and causing surrounding tissue to appear hyperlucent.

Airway obstruction leading to collapse may be caused by a tumour (benign or malignant), inhaled foreign body (common in children), mucous plugs, or granulomata . Some of these lesions may be amenable to reversal at bronchoscopy. In this patient, bronchoscopy revealed a bronchial carcinoma partially occluding the left main bronchus, with a thick mucous plug producing full occlusion. The mucous plug was removed by suction, and a stent was inserted to reopen the airway with resolution of the X-ray appearances of collapse.

4. This woman has stage 4 lung cancer, with her staging being T3, N2, M1b. She is clearly not a candidate for surgery, though there may be a role for chemotherapy since small cell tumours often show a dramatic initial response to chemotherapy even if they are very advanced.

She is likely to have pain where the tumour is invading her chest wall—this may be helped by local radiotherapy. As her disease progresses she may develop other physical, emotional, and spiritual needs, which can be addressed by different members of the multidisciplinary team.

All patients with lung cancer should be discussed at a multidisciplinary meeting, with respiratory physicians, cardiothoracic surgeons, radiologists, oncologists, lung cancer nurses, and the palliative care team. This allows careful discussion of the optimum management of each patient, taking into account their wishes and physical performance status.

5. This X-ray reveals:

This x-ray reveals a moderate-sized right-sided pleural effusion. Small effusions may present with only blunting of the costophrenic angle; large effusions may present with a complete 'white-out' of one lung. Note the classic 'meniscal' shape of the effusion, curving towards the chest wall.

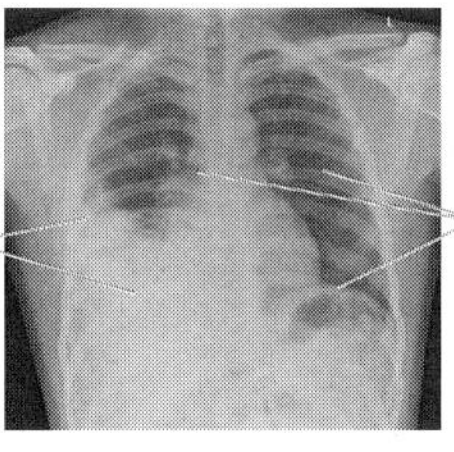

The rest of this x-ray is normal. It should be studied closely to look for evidence of what might be causing this effusion - for instance for evidence of enlarged hila (possible lung cancer or tuberculosis), upper lobe consolidation (tuberculosis), round shadows (lung cancer) or pleural plaques, often seen best against the diaphragm (which may progress to mesothelioma).

There are many causes of unilateral pleural effusions, but malignancy should always be considered. Both lung cancer and mesothelioma commonly present in this way. Essential to diagnosis of the cause of a pleural effusion is working out whether the effusion is a transudate or an exudate, with exudates suggestive of malignancy, pneumonia, or TB. This is done by performing a pleural tap and assessing various biochemical parameters, with an exudate being suggested by:

- pleural fluid protein >2.9 g/dL (29 g/L)
- pleural fluid cholesterol >45 mg/dL (1.16 mmol/L)
- pleural fluid LDH >60% of the upper limit for serum

[These criteria were determined by meta-analysis as being more specific in differentiating exudates from transudates than the previously used Light's criteria—see Heffner J, Brown L, Barbieri C (1997) 'Diagnostic value of tests that discriminate between exudative and transudative pleural effusions. Primary Study Investigators'. *Chest* **111**(4): 970–80.]

Microscopy of the fluid may also reveal malignant or inflammatory cells. If he is very symptomatic from his effusion then a drain can be inserted to improve lung volumes.

In view of this man's likely exposure to asbestos, mesothelioma is a real possibility. Mesothelioma may be suggested on chest CT scanning (which would also rule out other causes of effusion), with definitive diagnosis made by pleural biopsy, either percutaneously using a needle or at thoracoscopy. Mesothelioma carries a very poor prognosis.

Further reading

Guidelines: NICE lung cancer guidelines (http://guidance.nice.org.uk/CG24)

OHCM: 170, 184, 778

Pneumothorax

This section should be used to clerk patients with pneumothorax. Patients with pneumothoraces are commonly discharged from the Emergency Department if they are clinically stable; however, in patients with complicated or large pneumothoraces which require drainage, patient pathways lead from the Emergency Department though Admissions Units to Respiratory Wards, with possible follow-up by cardiothoracic surgeons in out-patient clinics.

Learning challenges

- What creates the negative pressure usually found in the pleural space? Why might air in the pleural space affect the mechanics of breathing?
- Cardiothoracic surgeons sometimes need to create bilateral pneumothoraces during procedures. How does the anaesthetist keep the patient alive?

History

Comment on

- Breathlessness, pleuritic pain
- Precipitating event?
- Previous pneumothoraces
- Underlying lung disease
- Connective tissue disorders

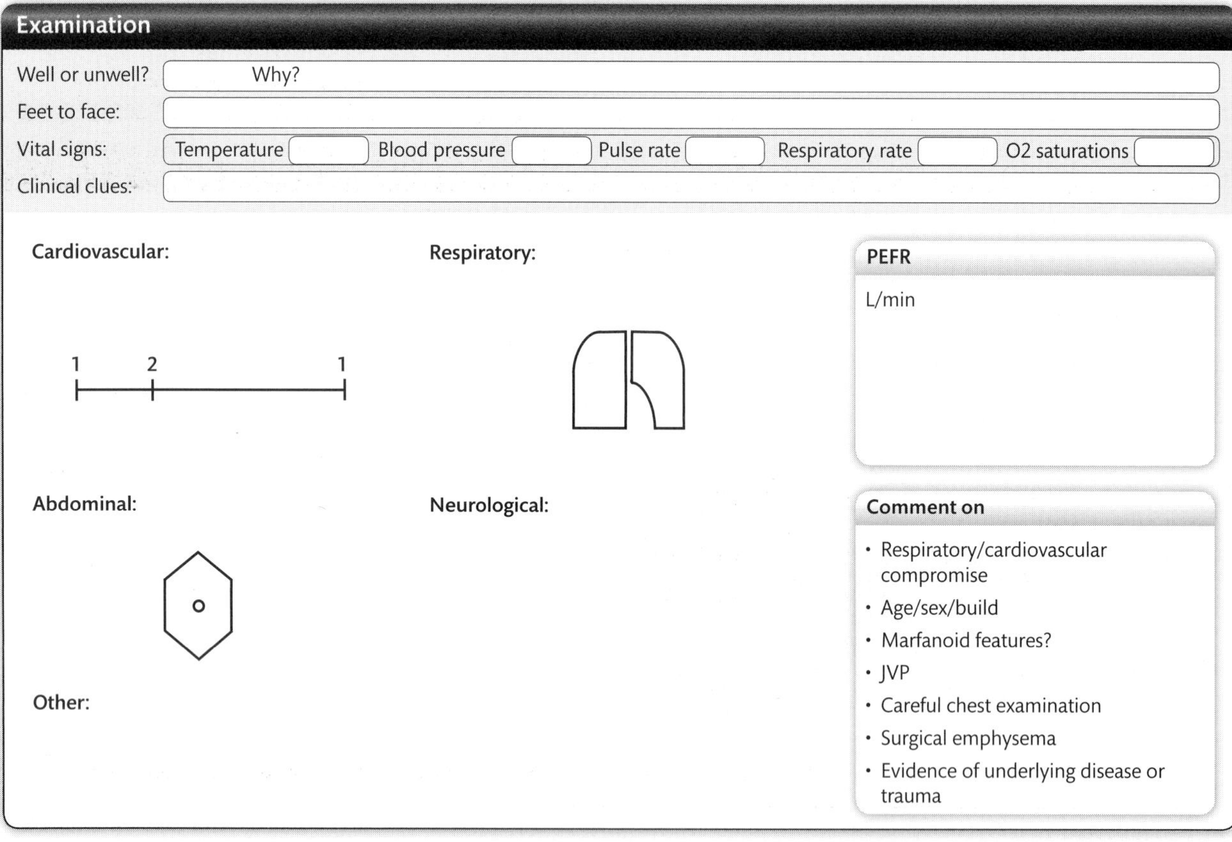

Chest X-ray

Comment on

- Large or small (>2 cm, <2 cm)?
- Localized or whole lung?
- Surgical emphysema
- Evidence of underlying disease

Arterial blood gas (if indicated by pulse oximetry)

Comment on

- Evidence of respiratory failure

CT chest (if diagnosis in doubt)

Comment on

- Size/position of pneumothorax
- Bullous lung disease?

Pleural aspiration

Comment on

- How much air aspirated?
- Repeat X-ray: resolution?

Intercostal underwater-sealed drain

Comment on

- Swinging?
- Bubbling?
- Repeat X-ray: resolution?

Evaluation

1. **How can this pneumothorax be classified?**

- **Is there any sign of a tension pneumothorax**? If so, seek help immediately.
- Primary (no underlying lung disease) or secondary (an already diseased lung)?
- Large or small (>2 cm or <2 cm)?

2. **What is the correct initial management?**

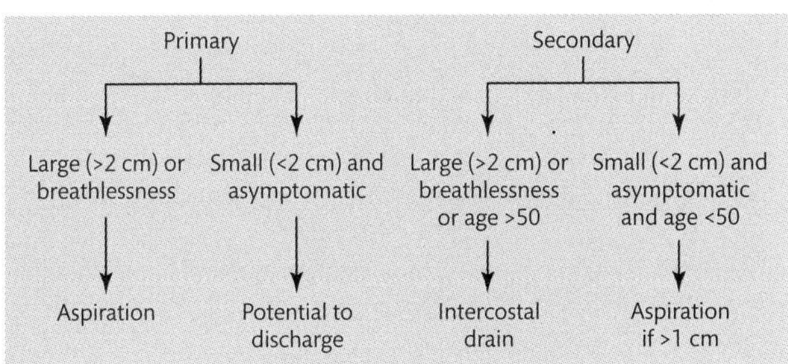

3. **Has the initial management led to resolution? What additional measures should be taken next in the case of non-resolution?**

Non-resolution:

- after aspiration—insert intercostal drain
- with intercostal drain—refer to respiratory team, apply suction

4. **Does this patient need referral to cardiothoracic surgeons (non-resolution, recurrence, complicated pneumothorax)? What surgery is potentially indicated?**

Questions

1. A 24-year-old man with presents to the Emergency Department with a history of breathlessness and left-sided pleuritic pain that began suddenly half an hour before presentation. He has no significant medical history but smokes 15 cigarettes per day. On examination he is tall and thin, with thin, tapering fingers, a high arched palate, and a back scoliosis. Further examination reveals he has a central trachea, JVP to the base of his neck, reduced chest expansion, and breath sounds on the left-hand side with a hyperresonant percussion note. Observations include respiratory rate 24 breaths/min, heart rate 105 bpm, blood pressure 112/74 mmHg, and oxygen saturations on air of 97%.

(1) Is this a tension pneumothorax?

(2) What is the likely diagnosis suggested by these findings?

(3) List your essential management steps.

2. A 68-year-old woman being investigated for chronic cough and weight loss is admitted for percutaneous CT-guided biopsy of a lesion suspected to be cancer identified on a previous CT scan of her chest. Several hours after the procedure she felt well and was keen to go home. The same evening she begins to feel short of breath and begins to panic. She calls an ambulance and is brought in to the resuscitation room in the hospital Emergency Department where the following chest X-ray is obtained.

(1) What does the chest image show when viewed online?

(2) How would you proceed?

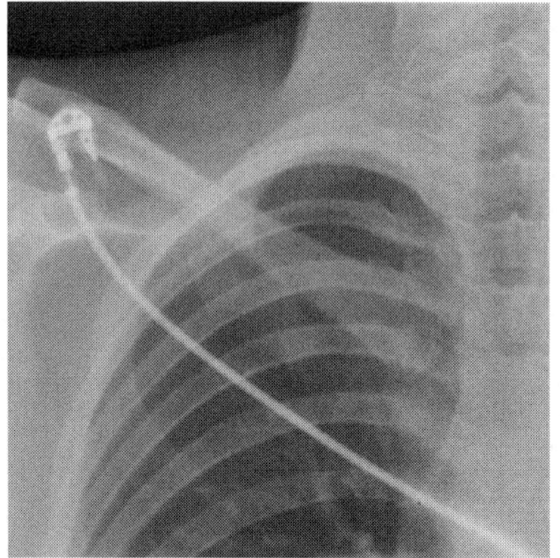

3. A 29-year-old man admitted with a large simple left-sided pneumothorax has a water-sealed chest drain inserted after aspiration of air fails to lead to resolution. He has had several previous spontaneous pneumothoraces, usually affecting the right side. In the evening you go with a senior on-call doctor to review him. On arrival he feels much improved. He is less breathless and appears comfortable in bed. Fluid in the loops of tubing in the chest drain swings up a down with each breath he takes, and when asked to cough, there is no bubbling of the drain fluid. He asks you whether you can take out the drain and let him go home.

(1) What do the chest drain findings indicate?

(2) What is the correct advice regarding his discharge?

4. A 19-year-old known asthmatic student is admitted to the ICU with an acute asthma attack. The attack is so severe that she required intubation and mechanical ventilation in the Emergency Department, with very high inflation pressures being required to maintain oxygenation. Several hours later the alarms on her monitor sound, and she is found to be newly hypoxic (saturations 90% on the ventilator). A portable chest X-ray is urgently requested, but over the next few minutes she becomes increasingly hypoxic, tachycardic (116 bpm), tachypnoeic (32 breaths/min), with a trachea deviated to the right and distended neck veins.

(1) What is the likely cause of her sudden deterioration?

(2) What emergency intervention should be performed?

Presentation

Presented to		Grade		Date	

Signed

Answers

1. The features of tension pneumothorax are those of rapidly progressive respiratory and cardiovascular impairment, with increasing breathlessness and hypoxia, cyanosis, tracheal deviation, and distension of the neck veins with elevated JVP. Tension pneumothorax is associated with trauma, underlying lung disease, or in patients being mechanically ventilated; it is rare in spontaneous pneumothorax. This patient's increased heart rate and respiratory rate are necessary to maintain oxygenation, but there are none of the sinister features suggestive of a tension pneumothorax.

This man has findings suggestive of a large uncomplicated spontaneous pneumothorax. These especially affect young men of tall, thin stature (with so-called 'Marfanoid features', as they resemble patients with Marfan syndrome), and they are associated with smoking. Simple pneumothoraces are thought to be caused by the spontaneous rupture of a small air sac (a bleb), usually at the apex of the lung, into the pleural space. The air can then expand and allow the lung to collapse, because the negative pleural pressure that usually holds the lung expanded is abolished. Pleuritic pain and breathlessness are the result.

Priorities for management of this man include putting him on high-flow oxygen (which speeds up reabsorption of the pneumothorax), and arranging a chest X-ray to confirm the diagnosis. This man's X-ray (below) revealed a large left-sided pneumothorax, with no evidence of tension and no evidence of underlying disease. An attempt should be made to aspirate the air from this; if unsuccessful then a chest drain with an underwater seal should be inserted to allow the lung to re-expand.

When looking at an x-ray showing a pnemothorax, always look at the mediastinum and trachea. Here both are relatively central though the trachea is deviated slightly to the right. In a tension pneumothorax, significant mediastinal shift will occur, preventing the heart from filling and leading to circulatory collapse.

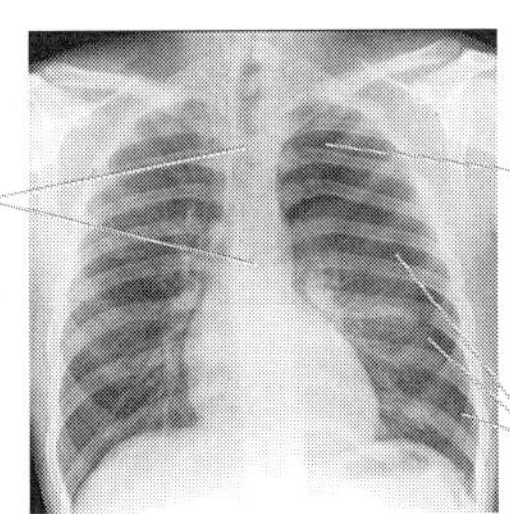

A key feature of pneumothoraces on an x-ray is that lung markings do not extend to the periphery of the lung - compare this area to the same area on the other side.

Often, as here, the edge of the lung will be clearly visible.

2. As in this case, pneumothoraces may be hard to see!

This lady has a small apical pneumothorax which would be very easily not seen - in this case, the history of the earlier biopsy prompted very careful examination of the x-ray. The lung edge is just about visible here, and there are no lung markings visible beyond this. Always look carefully at the apices on chest x-rays, along with other areas (such as behind the heart), where abnormalites may be easy to miss.

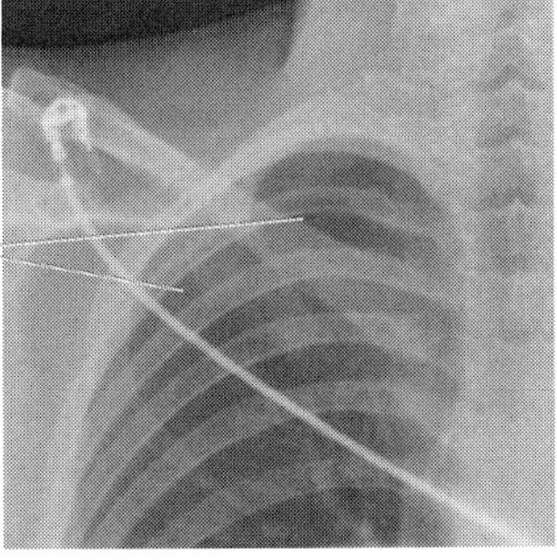

This is clearer if viewed on the Online Resource Centre.

Iatrogenic pneumothorax is a recognized complication of procedures such as lung biopsy, central venous catheter insertion, pleural fluid aspiration, or pacemaker insertion. In this case it would be impossible to aspirate this pneumothorax without the real danger of puncturing the lung again and worsening it. She should be given high-flow oxygen which leads the nitrogen in the pneumothorax air to be replaced with oxygen, which is more easily absorbed by the body. This is known to speed up resolution of pneumothoraces. The chest X-ray should be repeated in the morning. If she feels better and the X-ray has improved then she may be able to go home with strict instructions to return immediately if she becomes more short of breath or develops worsening chest pain.

3. The fact that this man is now no longer breathless implies that his pneumothorax has resolved, and the behaviour of the chest drain supports this. Assessing a chest drain involves observing whether it *swings* with normal breathing, and whether it *bubbles* when the patient coughs. A *swinging* chest drain is one that is correctly sited—the tip is in the pleural space so that the negative intrapleural pressure generated during inspiration causes fluid in the loops of tubing to swing up and down. Swinging will not happen if the tube is in the wrong place, is blocked or is kinked. Chest drains *bubble* when there is still air in the pleural space, indicating that the pneumothorax has not resolved. This may be due to a persistent air leak from the lung (forming a bronchopleural fistula). Initially, gentle suction can be applied to the drain to try to reinflate the lung, in the hope that the air leak will heal if the lung is pressed up against the chest wall. If this fails then surgical repair of the leak may be required.

In this man, the pneumothorax is likely to have resolved. He should have a repeat X-ray to confirm this. Guidelines suggest that the drain should be left in place for 24 hours after the pneumothorax has resolved. (So he should remain in hospital until the next day.) After removal of the drain the chest X-ray should be repeated again to exclude recurrence. This man has had recurrent pneumothoraces, affecting both lungs. He should be referred to a cardiothoracic surgeon for consideration of either pleurodesis or pleurectomy.

4. This patient has signs consistent with a tension pneumothorax; this is a medical emergency. Tension pneumothoraces are well-recognized complications of mechanical ventilation, particularly in patients with obstructive lung defects who require high ventilator pressures to force air in and out through narrowed airways. A 'flap' valve forms in the visceral pleura, allowing air to escape into the pleural space with each breath in, but not to escape in expiration. The mediastinum and the other lung are progressively compressed, causing breathlessness and respiratory failure and acute cardiac embarrassment, where the heart is unable to fill during diastole.

The definitive treatment for tension pneumothorax is insertion of an intercostal drain. However, to buy time, a large intravenous cannula can be inserted into the second intercostal space in the mid-clavicular line which effectively converts a tension pneumothorax into an open pneumothorax. A hiss of air escaping through the needle confirms the diagnosis. Once the chest drain has been inserted, the needle can be removed and the pneumothorax managed like a spontaneous pneumothorax. However, the tension pneumothorax may recur should the chest drain become kinked or blocked.

Further reading

Guidelines: British Thoracic Society guidelines for spontaneous pneumothorax (http://thorax.bmj.com/content/58/suppl_2/ii39.full)

OHCM: 182, 780, 824

Tuberculosis (TB)

This section should be used to clerk patients with suspected TB of any organ system. These patients may present with classic features of TB, or with other organ-specific symptoms (e.g. ascites), or simply be non-specifically unwell. Therefore patient pathways are varied, and patients may be found on any General Medical Ward or Isolation Unit.

Learning challenges

- What microbiological features of *Mycobacterium tuberculosis* have led it to be so successful (it infects one third of the world's population)?
- To what do the terms MDRTB and XDRTB refer, and why are they causing widespread fear among public health doctors?

History

Comment on

- Chronic cough, haemoptysis
- Fever, weight loss, malaise, sweats
- Systemic features
- Urinary, bowel, and meningeal symptoms, skin rashes
- Contacts with others who may be infected; recent migration/return from endemic areas (especially sub-Saharan Africa. Indian subcontinent and eastern Europe)
- Previous TB? BCG vaccination?
- Immunosuppressive agents, HIV

Examination

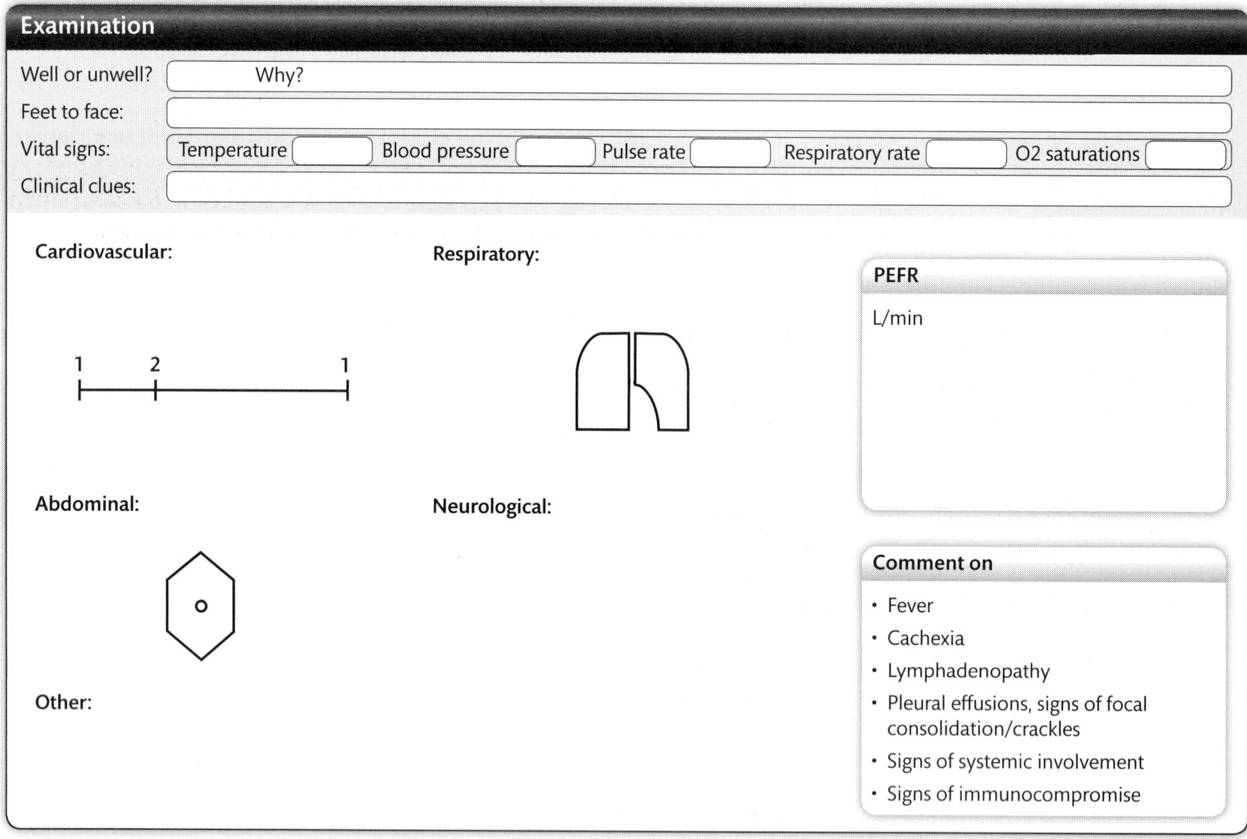

Comment on

- Fever
- Cachexia
- Lymphadenopathy
- Pleural effusions, signs of focal consolidation/crackles
- Signs of systemic involvement
- Signs of immunocompromise

Chest X-ray

Comment on

- Patchy consolidation of apices/upper zones
- Hilar lymphadenopathy, pleural effusion
- Cavitation, fibrosis, calcification, volume loss
- Miliary spread
- Evidence of previous infection/calcification

Sputum analysis, bronchoscopic washings, lymph node biopsies

Comment on

- Initial microscopy ('smear')
- Culture
- Sensitivities

Blood tests

Comment on

- HIV status
- Liver function tests

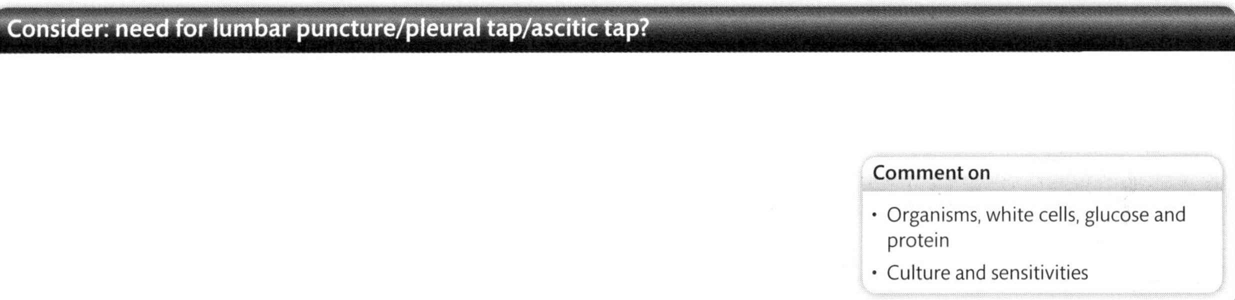

Consider: need for lumbar puncture/pleural tap/ascitic tap?

Comment on

- Organisms, white cells, glucose and protein
- Culture and sensitivities

Evaluation

1. **Is TB suspected or confirmed? Is there strong enough suspicion to warrant treatment before culture results become available?**

2. **What kind of TB presentation is this likely to be? What does this mean?**

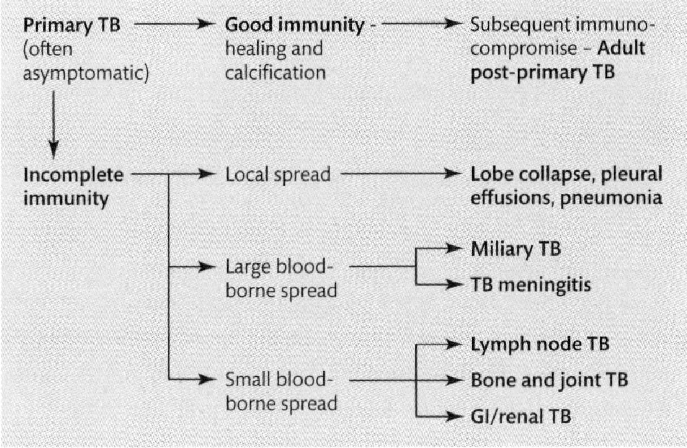

3. **What treatment is appropriate? Might adherence to treatment be an issue?**

Standard regimen	2 months: isoniazid, rifampicin, ethambutol, pyrazinamide 4 months: isoniazid, rifampicin
TB meningitis	As above but isoniazid and rifampicin alone for 10 months
Consider:	Risk factors for multidrug resistance Need for Directly Observed Treatment (DOTS)

4. **Are others at risk? Should the patient be isolated? Should contacts be tested?**

Questions

1. A 51-year-old man who grew up in rural India presents to hospital in the UK after an episode of haemoptysis. He has been feeling increasingly unwell for the past 2 months, suffering fevers and sweats. He has had a cough productive of yellowish sputum, occasionally streaked with small amounts of blood. He has also lost weight during this period. Before this all began he was fit and healthy, though a little overweight. He came to the UK 20 years ago and since then has been generally well. His blood tests show mildly raised inflammatory markers but are otherwise normal. His random capillary blood glucose is noted to be 15.6 mmol/L. His chest X-ray is shown below.

(1) What does the chest X-ray show?

(2) Describe the further management in this patient.

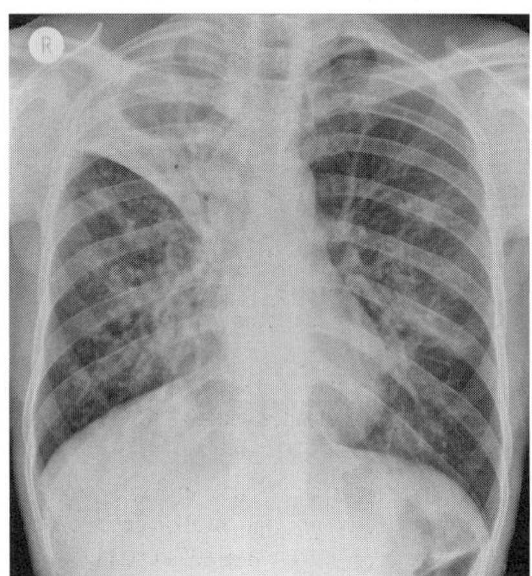

2. A 34-year-old man who has recently arrived in the country from sub-Saharan Africa is brought into hospital by ambulance after a fall. He is found to be drowsy and confused, with a GCS of 13/15. He complains of cough, headache, and neck stiffness. He is pyrexial (38.9°C) and is noted to have enlarged palpable lymph nodes in his neck. A lumbar puncture is performed, with the results of the analysis below. A chest X-ray is performed which is also shown below.

(1) What do the abnormalities of the CSF suggest?

(2) How do the radiographic appearances assist with the likely diagnosis?

(3) What is the likely unifying diagnosis?

	Results of CSF analysis	Normal values
Appearance	Clear, straw coloured	Clear, straw coloured
Protein	3.1 g/L	0.2–0.4 g/L
Glucose (serum glucose = 4.5 g/L)	2.1 g/L	60–80% plasma glucose
Cell count	143 cells/L, 78% lymphocytes	<5 white cells/L
Gram stain	No organisms seen	No organisms seen

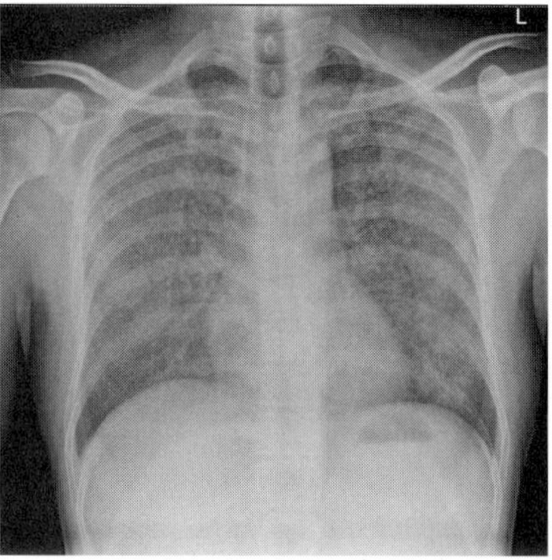

3. A 44-year-old Black-Caribbean woman is referred to hospital with a 6-week history of dry cough that began insidiously and is associated with general malaise and weakness. She has also over the previous 2 weeks developed a painful 'bruising' rash over her shins and a gritty dryness of her eyes with some misting of her vision. Examination confirms a rash over her shins, which is tender and made up of coalescing red lesions, and also confirms that both eyes are red and inflamed. Otherwise cardiovascular, respiratory, and abdominal examinations are unremarkable. Blood tests revealed a mild normocytic anaemia with slightly elevated serum calcium, but are otherwise normal. Her chest X-ray is below. She is very concerned about the possibility of TB as a cousin has contracted it.

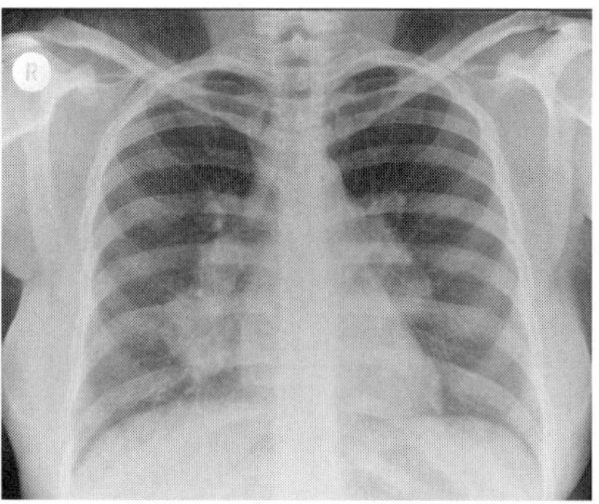

(1) What are the possible diagnoses in this patient?

(2) List three further investigations to prove the clinical diagnosis

4. A homeless man presents to hospital generally unwell with cough and fever, and is found to be 'smear positive' for TB. It transpires that he has previously been treated for TB at another hospital but that he defaulted from treatment after only 3 weeks. He tells the team that he regrets this decision and after becoming so unwell is keen now to go through with treatment.

(1) Which drugs should he be started on?

(2) How would you monitor their effectiveness?

(3) How can he be helped to adhere to the course of treatment?

Presentation

Presented to ______ Grade ______ Date ______

Signed

Answers

1. The chest image is virtually diagnostic of TB:

This x-ray shows classic changes associated with tuberculosis, including upper lobe consolidation (notice that the consolidation is limited by the horizontal fissure inferiorly), and cavitation - there is an area of lucency within the right upper lobe where infection has led to an inflammatory cavity within the lung.

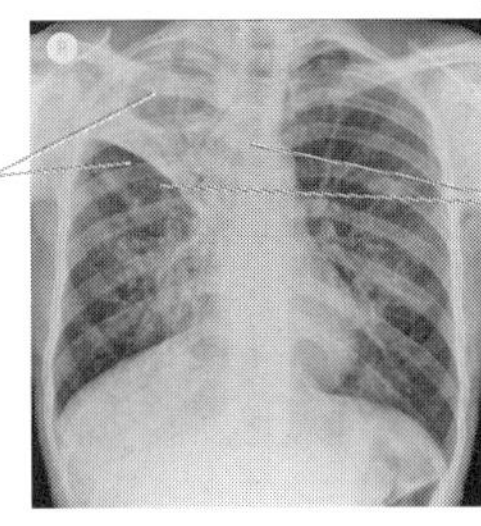

Note too that the right upper lobe is partially collapsed. The evidence for this is evidence of volume loss, 'sucking in' adjacent structures - to the trachea is deviated slightly to the right, and the horizontal fissure has been pulled superiorly.

This man's history is strongly suggestive of pulmonary TB, including the classic symptoms of fever, cough, weight loss, and a childhood in the developing world. The diagnosis of TB is further supported by a raised white cell count. A capillary blood glucose of 15.6 suggests that this man is diabetic (he was previously overweight and therefore may have developed mild type 2 diabetes but not been formally diagnosed). A fasting blood glucose level would confirm this. Diabetes causes impaired immune system function which may lead to reactivation of previously dormant TB.

Almost everyone growing up in rural areas of India and sub-Saharan Africa encounters TB as a child, where it produces a mild and often asymptomatic illness, before the body responds by enclosing the remaining bacteria within granulomas surrounded by modified macrophages (such as Langerhans' giant cells). These small granulomas may be seen on chest X-ray where they are called a Ghon focus. Subsequent immunocompromise (for instance from HIV, steroid treatment, or diabetes), can cause reactivation.

Because of his productive cough he has potentially 'open TB' (the term used for sputum production containing mycobacteria). He should be isolated in a side room, ideally one with negative pressure ventilation. Three sets of sputum should be collected on subsequent days for staining and microscopy to see if mycobacteria are detectable. These should also be cultured (even if the microscopy is negative), and any mycobacteria that grow should be tested for sensitivities. If mycobacterium TB is isolated, or if the clinical suspicion is high enough, then he should be started on anti-TB treatment. He should also receive advice and follow-up about diabetes management.

2. These CSF results are consistent with tuberculous meningitis—characteristically there is very high CSF protein, reduced CSF glucose, and raised white cells of all lineages but with lymphocytes predominant. In contrast a bacterial meningitis also produces raised protein and low glucose, but the fluid is often turbid with high numbers of neutrophils, and often with large numbers of organisms visible on microscopy.

In the context of this patient's history, the small dots seen throughout this X-ray are most likely to represent small deposits of *M. tuberculosis*, a condition known as 'miliary TB'. It occurs when TB spreads via the blood to form deposits throughout the body, especially in patients with impaired immune system function. It may be associated with TB meningitis (as in this man), where TB is thought to spread through the blood–brain barrier to infect the meninges. Deposits may also be found in lymph nodes (causing lymphadenopathy, which may suppurate), the liver and spleen (causing hepatosplenomegaly), or other sites through the body. It may present very insidiously with a pyrexia of unknown origin.

To confirm the diagnosis, CSF should be sent for culture, along with sputum samples and possibly samples from a lymph node biopsy. Any patient presenting with miliary TB should have their HIV status checked—especially someone from sub-Saharan Africa whose pre-test probability for being HIV positive is high. This man is likely to be highly infectious and should be kept in isolation. He should be started on anti-TB medication (which may cause a dramatic improvement in symptoms).

3. TB is certainly a possibility here, but the absence of fever and the presence of such prominent bilateral hilar lymphadenopathy make a diagnosis of sarcoidosis more likely. This is a multisystem disorder

The most prominent feature of this x-ray is bilateral hilar lymphadenopathy. These appearances are classically seen in sarcoidosis, but may also be seen in tuberculosis, cancers including lymphoma, lung disease caused by dusts (e.g. pneumoconiosis) and several other rare diseases.

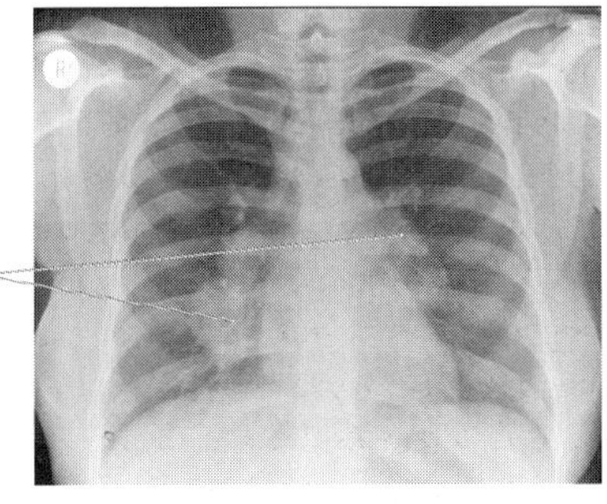

characterized by the formation of granulomas, which unlike the granulomas found in TB do not contain bacteria. It is common in people of Afro-Caribbean origin, and is more common in women than in men. The commonest finding is bilateral hilar lymphadenopathy. Pulmonary infiltration, skin lesions (such as erythema nodosum in this patient), and eye lesions (e.g. anterior uveitis, as in this patient) are common. Less commonly the heart, central nervous system, and bones and joints are affected. An anaemia of chronic disease is common, as is hypercalcaemia (since sarcoid tissue activates vitamin D in a similar way to the kidneys).

Differentiating sarcoidosis from TB is not always easy. Tests which may help to do this in this patient are:

- Serum levels of angiotensin-converting enzyme (ACE) are raised in sarcoidosis (and it is a useful screening test).
- A Heaf test (or Mantoux test) against TB antigens may exclude TB.
- Bronchoscopy with biopsy of the granulomas seen on X-ray may provide histological evidence to differentiate the two conditions.

Commonly sarcoidosis resolves spontaneously within a year or two without treatment. If there are significant symptoms or damage to organs, then the disease should be treated with steroids—usually oral prednisolone.

4. The standard treatment for TB comprises isoniazid, rifampicin, ethambutol, and pyrizinamide given for 2 months, to be followed by isoniazid and rifampicin alone for a further 4 months. These four drugs should be started in this man. However, the fact that he has received a partial course of anti-TB treatment in the past raises the possibility of drug resistance. In some centres, rapid testing for rifampicin resistance, a useful marker for multidrug resistance, can be carried out; if not, a full set of sensitivities can take up to 10 weeks to complete.

Failing to complete a course of anti-TB treatment can be disastrous both for the patient and for the wider community, since it is known to cause drug resistance. Helping this man to adhere to his treatment requires a multidisciplinary approach. Directly observed therapy short course (DOTS) may be appropriate here, where patients are allocated a TB link worker who meets them daily to observe them taking their tablets. Incentives such as free meals may help with this. Prescribing combination tablets (which limit the total number of tablets taken) is also helpful.

The patient should be warned about possible side-effects. Rifamipicin can turn secretions (e.g. sweat, urine, and tears) pink; isoniazid may cause a rash or a serious hepatitis; ethambutol can cause visual loss and colour blindness. Patients should be screened for the development of these complications (with regular blood tests, including liver function tests, in the first few weeks of treatment and afterwards less frequently). Great caution should be exercised in prescribing other medications to patients on anti-TB treatment—rifampicin induces liver enzymes, reducing plasma concentrations of certain drugs and diminishing their effect.

Further reading

Guidelines: NICE tuberculosis guidelines (http://guidance.nice.org.uk/CG33)

OHCM: 186, 398–399

Interstitial lung disease

This section should be used to clerk patients with a number of conditions, often linked to systemic diseases or caused by environmental agents, grouped together under the umbrella term 'interstitial lung diseases'. Hospital admission occurs when shortness of breath becomes severe, and patient pathways lead from the Emergency Department through the Admissions Unit to the Respiratory Ward. These patients are also all seen in out-patient clinics.

Learning challenges

- What does the term 'fibrosis' mean? Which other organs may be affected by this process?
- How does the body adapt to chronic hypoxia?

History

Comment on

- Shortness of breath, cough, wheeze, sputum
- Known environmental precipitants
- Multisystem diseases, careful systemic enquiry
- Occupational history, pets, travel
- Medication history

Examination

Well or unwell? Why?

Feet to face:

Vital signs: Temperature Blood pressure Pulse rate Respiratory rate O2 saturations

Clinical clues:

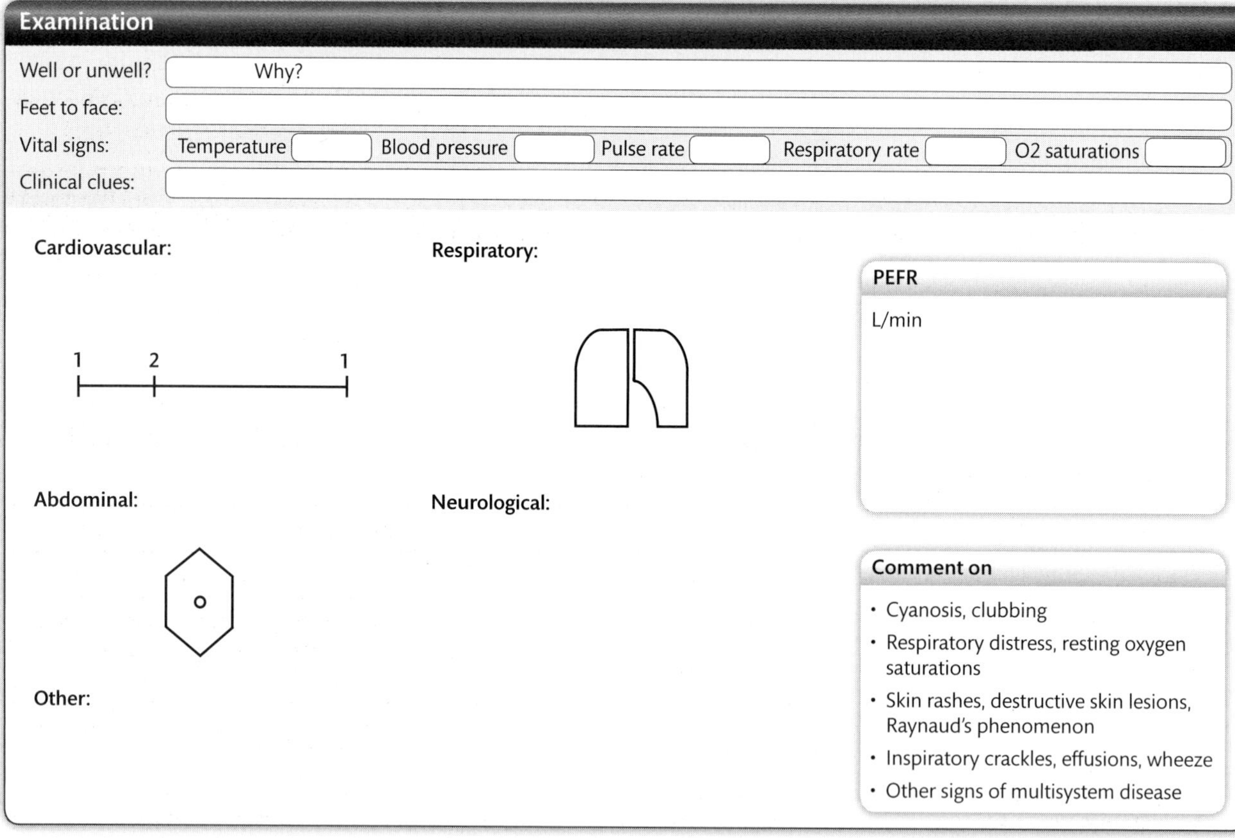

Comment on

- Cyanosis, clubbing
- Respiratory distress, resting oxygen saturations
- Skin rashes, destructive skin lesions, Raynaud's phenomenon
- Inspiratory crackles, effusions, wheeze
- Other signs of multisystem disease

Chest X-ray

Comment on

- Shadowing: reticular (streaky) or nodular (small dots)
- Localized (zonal–apical, mid or lower zones), or diffuse involvement
- Loss of volume with mediastinal/diaphragm displacement
- Enlarged hila

High resolution chest CT scan

Comment on

- Fibrosis
- Granulomas

Blood tests

Comment on

- Inflammatory markers, white cell differential
- Specific tests: ANCA, rheumatoid factor, anti-GBM, ESR, immunoglobulin (especially IgE), Aspergillus antibody, serum ACE

Spirometry

Comment on

- Restrictive lung defect

Arterial blood gas

Comment on

- Respiratory failure – usually type I

ECG/echocardiogram

Comment on

- Cor pulmonale

Evaluation

1. What is the likely diagnosis? What is the evidence to support this?

Class of disease	Example	Diagnostic features
Granulomatous lung disease	Sarcoidosis	Granulomas on chest X-ray, serum ACE
Connective tissue diseases and vasculitides	Rheumatoid disease, systemic lupus, systemic sclerosis, Wegener's granulomatosis, Churg–Strauss	Arthritis, Raynaud's phenomenon, vasculitic rashes, renal disease, rheumatoid factor, ANCA, ANA
Pulmonary eosinophilia	Allergic bronchopulmonary aspergillosis	Wheeze, fever, raised IgE, *Aspergillus* antibody
Idiopathic pulmonary fibrosis		Diffuse fibrosis, respiratory failure
Extrinsic allergic alveolitis	Farmer's lung, pigeon-fancier's lung	Diffuse fibrosis, antigen exposure
Occupational lung disease	Pneumoconiosis, asbestosis	Diffuse fibrosis, occupational exposure

2. What treatment is available?

3. Are there clear risk factors that can be avoided? If the cause is occupational, is the patient eligible for compensation?

4. Is the patient a candidate for home oxygen/lung transplantation?

Questions

1. A 59-year-old woman presents to hospital with worsening shortness of breath and left-sided chest pain. The breathlessness has been developing slowly for many months and is now severe, leaving her short of breath on minimal exertion. The chest pain, which is pleuritic in nature, had come on over the previous day leading the Emergency Department doctor to suspect a pulmonary embolism. On systemic enquiry, the patient also said she had noticed rashes which tended to occur on sunny days, on skin exposed to the sun. She did not have any other medical conditions and was not on any regular medication. On examination the patient is hypoxic (saturations of 92% on room air) with fine end-inspiratory crackles heard through both lung fields. Her chest X-ray is shown below.

(1) What are the abnormalities shown?

(2) Describe your further investigations.

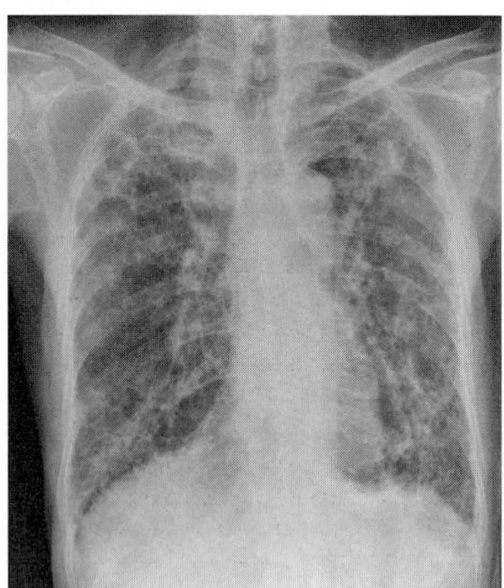

2. A 54-year-old farmer is referred to respiratory out-patients by his doctor with a disease the doctor believes might be farmer's lung (extrinsic alveolitis). He has noticed for several years that he becomes short of breath and wheezy whilst working in his barn, especially when he has been involved in work that produces dust, for example tossing hay or pouring grain into sacks. Chest examination is unremarkable, and the chest X-ray is reported as normal. Blood tests are all normal except for a raised serum IgE level. Spirometry revealed FVC 4.4 L (predicted FVC based on height is 4.9 L), with an FEV1 of 2.7 L. However, the FEV1 improved to 3.4 L after 5 mg of nebulized salbutamol was given.

From the given information, explain the likelihood of the doctor's diagnosis being correct.

3. A 49-year-old woman presents with haemoptysis, on the background of a worsening, dry cough that had been troubling her for 2 weeks. She feels generally unwell and has left-sided pleuritic chest pain. On further questioning she reports that over the past few years she has had a sore, persistently runny nose, with ulcers inside the nostrils which sometimes bleed. A chest X-ray is performed which is shown below.

(1) List the most likely cause for her symptoms and a possible differential diagnosis.

(2) List five investigations that would confirm this diagnosis.

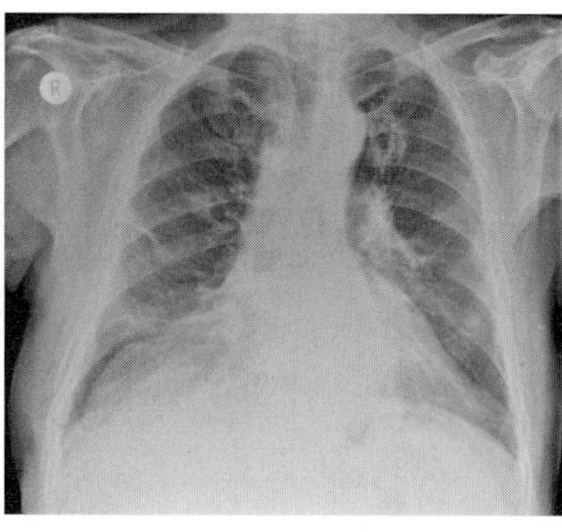

4. A 59-year-old woman with known idiopathic pulmonary fibrosis is seen in a medical polyclinic complaining of progressive breathlessness that is having a significant effect on her quality of life. She was diagnosed with idiopathic pulmonary fibrosis 2 years ago, and takes azathioprine daily. She has a medical history including systemic sclerosis and autoimmune hepatitis. She is noticed to have clubbing of the fingernails and has peripheral and central cyanosis. Arterial blood gas analysis reveals significant type I respiratory failure, with a pO2 of 7.2. Her chest X-ray is shown below.

Describe the management options available to improve her symptoms.

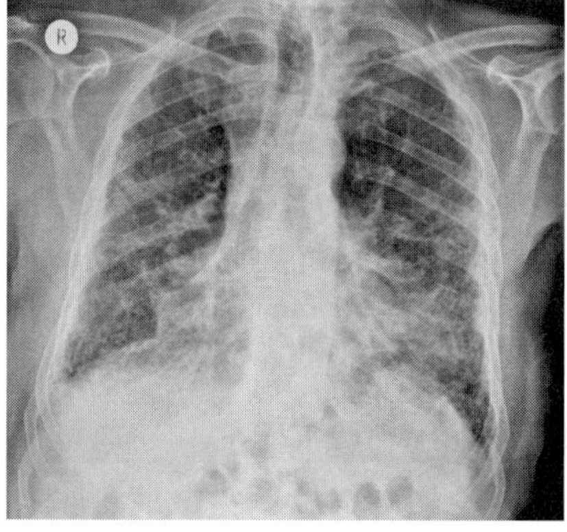

5. A 48-year-old man with a previous history of pulmonary TB presents to hospital worried about recurrence or reactivation. He has been completely well ever since completing TB treatment 5 years earlier, but today coughed up a small amount of fresh, red blood. His chest X-ray is shown below.

(1) How would you confirm or refute his concerns?

(2) What is the arrowed lesion likely to represent?

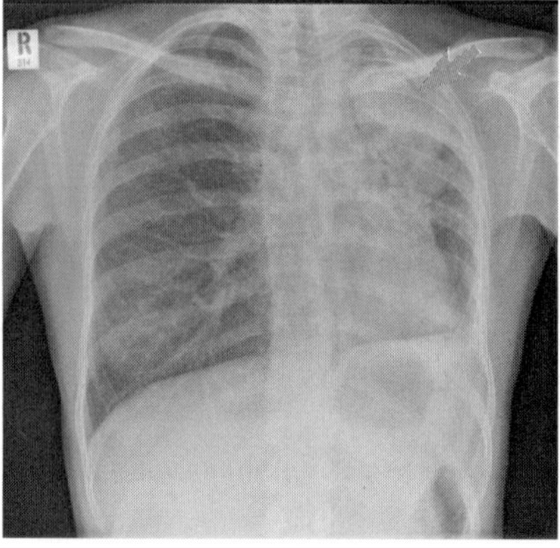

Answers

1. This woman's chest X-ray reveals:

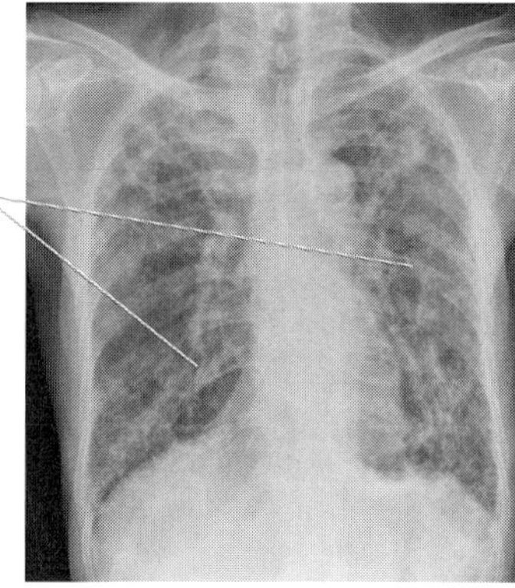

This x-ray shows bilateral interstitial shadowing (slightly worse on the left), consistent with pulonary fibrosis. The shadowing of pulmonary fibrosis can be described on x-ray as reticular ('net-like' or streaky), or nodular (with multiple small opacities), or commonly as reticulonodular where both appearances are seen.

Pulmonary fibrosis causes hypoxia relative to the amount of lung affected, and classically produces fine, fixed crackles (i.e. they don't change with position or coughing) heard just before the end of inspiration.

There are many causes of pulmonary fibrosis, and a correct approach to patients begins with a good history and examination, which rules out certain causes (for instance, iatrogenic (drug) causes in this lady) and makes other diagnoses more likely. This patient suffers with photosensitivity rashes which are often caused by systemic lupus erythematosus (SLE), a known cause of pulmonary fibrosis, which can also cause pleuritic chest pain and pleural effusions. Patients with SLE may be positive for antinuclear antigen (ANA) or antidouble-stranded DNA (anti-dsDNA) antibodies. Other immunological tests worth performing in this patient include ANCA (for vasculitic conditions) and rheumatoid factor (for rheumatoid arthritis). Sometimes no obvious cause is found for pulmonary fibrosis, in which case it is termed 'idiopathic pulmonary fibrosis'. However, the other symptoms complained of by this lady suggest that her fibrosis is likely to be caused by a multisystemic disease.

2. Farmer's lung is the most common type of extrinsic allergic alveolitis (EAA). In this condition, inhalation of spores from the *Micropolyspora* species of fungus (which are often found in damp hay) leads to an inflammatory reaction in the lungs including granuloma formation and eventually pulmonary fibrosis. Initial exposure to the antigen produces an acute hypersensitivity response with fever, shortness of breath, malaise and cough several hours after exposure. This resolves after removal of the environmental agent. With on-going exposures the patient develops chronic fibrosis, usually in the upper zones. Other forms of EAA include pigeon fancier's lung (bird antigens), maltworker's lung (fungal antigen in beer production), and humidifier fever (bacteria or fungi from air conditioning units).

There are several features of this presentation that make EAA unlikely. EAA rarely produces wheezing, and the breathlessness experienced by this man comes on earlier than expected after antigen exposure were this to be EAA. Examination and X-ray are normal (no evidence of granuloma formation or fibrosis), and the serum IgE is raised (although this may occur in some forms of EAA). Also the pattern of respiratory deficit is obstructive rather than restrictive (FEV1 is only 61% of FVC, whilst the FVC is near normal), with significant reversibility after a nebulized bronchodilator. This all suggests that a more likely diagnosis is occupational asthma, perhaps triggered by wheat dust.

3. This chest X-ray reveals:

One key feature of this cheat radiograph is fibrosis - seen here as streaky shadowing predominantly affecting the lower zones. These appearances are known as recticular shadowing.

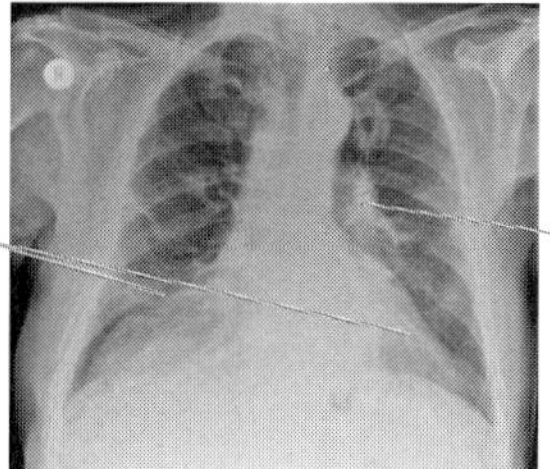

The hila are key places to look in assessing a chest radiograph, and here there is a prominent opacity near to the left hilum. In this case its shape and position make it most likely to be a vascular shadow caused by the pulmonary arteries.

In view of the history, the following tests may all help characterize this patient's disease:

- High-resolution CT chest—to confirm fibrosis and look for other disease processes
- Serum ACE—sarcoidosis may cause pulmonary infiltration
- ANCA—to identify a systemic vasculitis
- ANA/rheumatoid factor—to identify autoimmune causes of fibrosis
- Serum inflammatory markers and ESR—to suggest whether an infective or inflammatory process could underlie this presentation

This lady had a positive ANCA (indicative of a vasculitic condition), and the chest CT scan demonstrated multiple small granulomas with some pulmonary infiltrates. In view of her history of nasal ulceration the most likely diagnosis is Wegener's granulomatosis. This is characterized by a triad of upper respiratory tract ulcerative granulomas, lower respiratory tract granulomas with fibrosis and haemorrhage, and glomerulonephritis (which often occurs after the respiratory tract pathologies). It responds well to immunosuppressive therapy such as cyclophosphamide.

4. The X-ray reveals advanced, extensive fibrosis producing a 'honeycomb lung' appearance. Idiopathic pulmonary fibrosis (previously known as cryptogenic fibrosing alveolitis) is an autoimmune condition related to other autoimmune diseases such as SLE and autoimmune hepatitis. It classically affects the lower zones but may go on to cause diffuse pulmonary fibrosis. This patient is severely affected—clinically symptomatic and chronically hypoxic.

No single drug treatment has been shown to influence the poor prognosis of this condition. Despite recent trials of newer, novel therapies, the main stay of treatment remains palliation. This lady may benefit from home oxygen, especially ambulatory oxygen to increase her range of activity. High-dose steroids may also help with breathlessness but the risks of long-term high steroid doses must be balanced against possible benefit to the patient. Younger patients may be considered for lung transplant, but without such radical intervention prognosis remains limited to a few years.

5. The fact that this man is otherwise completely asymptomatic suggests that the haemoptysis he has experienced is probably not caused by a recurrence of TB. Absence of fever, night sweats, constitutional symptoms and weight loss also make TB recurrence unlikely.

His chest X-ray reveals:

The arrowed structure in this patient's left upper lobe is an aspergilloma - a ball of fungus which forma in a pre-existant lung cavity (for instance, caused by tuberculosis). Note the 'halo' of air surrounding the aspergilloma.

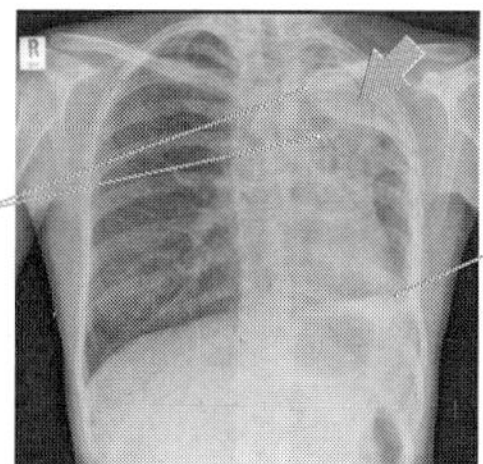

Did you notice that this patient also seems to have a left-sided pleural effusion? This may represent pleural thickening after his previous TB. An ultrasound-guided pleural aspiration or CT-scanning of the chest may help determine the significance of this abnormality.

This is characteristic of an aspergilloma—a ball of fungus (normally found in the environment) which can form within pre-existing lung cavities where immune cells can't penetrate. (*Aspergillus* can also grow on the walls of airways producing a chronic eosinophilic pneumonia, or even invasive disease in immunocompromised individuals.)

Aspergillomas are commonly harmless and asymptomatic, existing within unaware patients for many years. They are often impossible to treat (because of poor penetrance of antifungal agents into the lung cavity), which is rarely a problem since they cause few problems. If haemoptysis or other symptoms become problematic, lobectomy of the affected lung lobe may be required.

Further reading

Guidelines: British Thoracic Society guidelines on interstitial lung disease (http://www.brit-thoracic.org.uk/clinical-information/interstitial-lung-disease-(dpld)/interstitial-lung-disease-(dpld)-guideline.aspx)

OHCM: 186–192

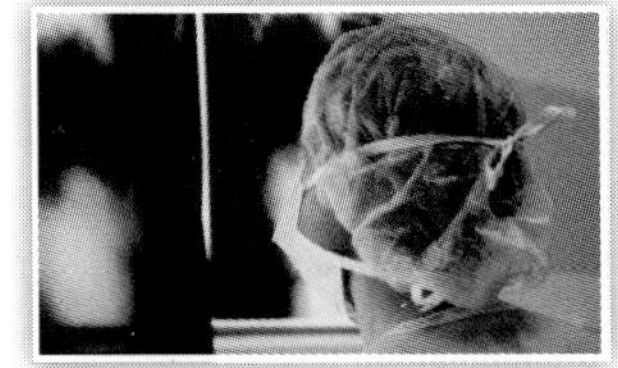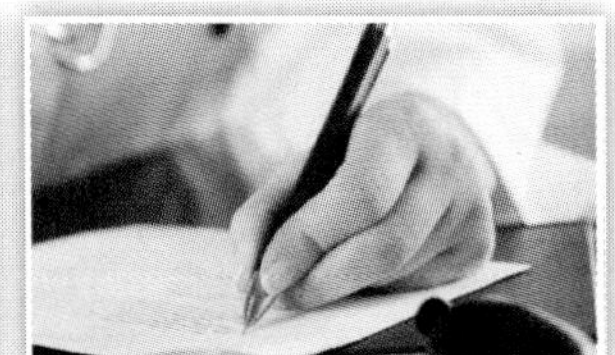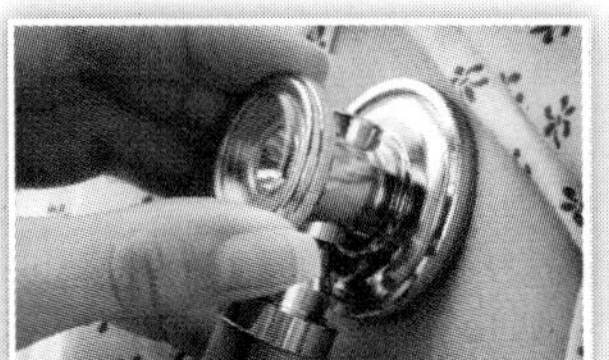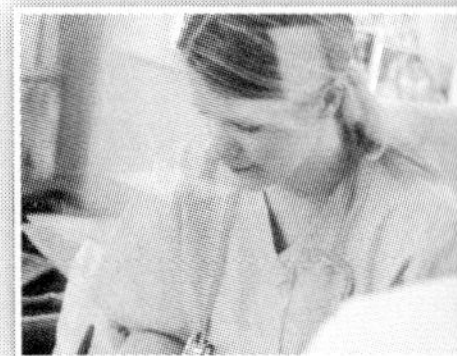

Unit 3
Gastroenterology

Key learning outcomes in gastroenterology include:

- Being able to take a comprehensive gastrointestinal (GI) history including patients presenting with dysphagia, upper and lower GI bleeding, a change in bowel habit, and weight loss.
- Recognizing 'red flag' symptoms for GI cancers.
- Being able to take a history from a patient with jaundice, to include a comprehensive alcohol history and other major risk factors for chronic liver disease.
- Recognizing the clinical signs of acute, decompensated liver disease.
- Understanding and applying objective scoring systems to estimate the severity of a GI haemorrhage.
- Appreciating the benefits and risks of upper and lower GI endoscopy.
- Understanding the presentations and management strategies for inflammatory bowel disease

Tips for learning gastroenterology on the wards:

- Clerk a patient presenting with an acute upper GI bleed; follow their patient journey from admission to endoscopy, and discharge.
- Attend the cancer multidisciplinary team meetings to discover how patients with GI cancers present, are investigated, and managed.
- Attend sessions of endoscopic retrograde cholangiopancreatography (ERCP) and magnetic resonance cholangiopancreatography (MRCP).
- Attend community clinics for patients with inflammatory bowel disease; you should be familiar with the members of the expert multidisciplinary team.
- Clerk a patient with ascites; recognize the investigations necessary to identify the aetiology of the ascites and the therapeutic interventions used to reduce the ascitic volume.
- Appreciate and understand the common screening tests used to identify the aetiology of a patient's liver disease, including blood tests, viral hepatitis screening, and radiological investigations.

History

There are numerous GI and hepatobiliary symptoms. They may be divided into:

(1) upper GI symptoms

(2) lower GI symptoms

(3) hepatobiliary symptoms

(4) red flag symptoms suggestive of malignancy.

1. Upper GI symptoms

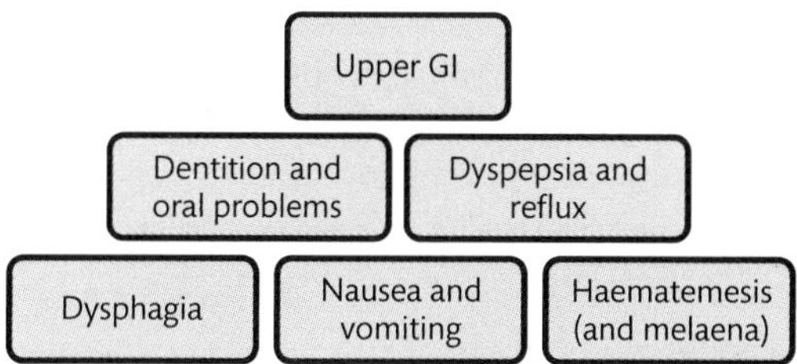

Dysphagia: Difficulty in swallowing. Your history needs to include level (back of the throat to the base of the neck, upper, mid, and lower chest), duration, rate of progression, what consistency of food/fluids the patient can manage, GI and systemic features. Think also about nutrition—is the patient able to eat and drink adequately?

One of the key aims of a dysphagia history is to suggest whether the dysphagia is more likely to be **anatomical** (caused by malignant of benign strictures) or **neuromuscular** (caused by abnormal nerve or muscle function):

Anatomical dysphagia—usually occurs within the thorax or upper abdomen	Neuromuscular dysphagia—usually occurs above the base of the neck
Progressive	Intermittent (at least initially)
Worse for solids than liquids	Worse for liquids than solids
Feeling that food 'gets stuck' (define the level at which this occurs)	Pronounced coughing and spluttering; classically nasal regurgitation
Associated features of GORD (benign stricture) or systemic features (malignancy)	Associated speech problems or other neurological phenomena

Dyspepsia and 'heartburn': Upper abdominal pain is common, and can be caused by a number of conditions including gastro-oesophageal reflux disease (GORD), peptic ulcer disease, gastritis, biliary colic, pancreatitis, basal pneumonias, and ischaemic heart disease. Even a thorough history bearing all of these differentials in mind may still not be enough to make the correct diagnosis—it is known that patients' descriptions of dyspeptic symptoms correlate poorly with the underlying pathological process.

If worrying causes of pain (which require urgent endoscopy) and non-GI causes of pain are excluded the epigastric pain may be divided into **reflux-type dyspepsia** and **non-reflux-type dyspepsia**. Reflux-type pain is worse on lying down, may be felt in the chest (retrosternally), and may be accompanied by a bitter, acidic taste in the mouth or regurgitation of partially digested food.

Nausea and vomiting: There are numerous GI and extra-intestinal causes of nausea and vomiting. As ever it is important to keep an open mind and consider all the possible causes. One should define the onset, duration, and frequency of vomiting, exacerbating and relieving factors, relationship to eating and drinking, volume and content of vomitus, i.e. altered or unaltered food, and the presence of blood (haematemesis; see below).

Haematemesis: The vomiting of blood. It is important to define onset, duration, number of episodes, volume(s), and content—fresh blood, clots, altered blood, coffee grounds (blood mixed into fluid like vomitus).

2. Lower abdominal symptoms

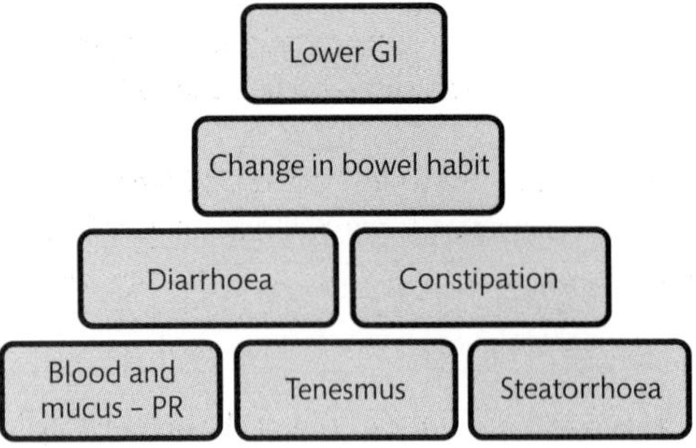

The principal symptoms of lower abdominal disorders are related to a **change in bowel habit**, i.e. diarrhoea and constipation. Once this change has been established, the patient needs to be asked when and what their normal bowel habit was before the change started. Progression and associated GI and systemic features also need to be established.

Diarrhoea: Common causes include:

- Infection, e.g. viral gastroenteritis (short duration of symptoms, other contacts affected, associated vomiting)
- Infection by *Clostridium difficile* (previous antibiotic use, recent hospital admission, or resident of care home)
- Inflammation, e.g. inflammatory bowel disease (frequent stool containing blood and mucous)
- Cancer—the commonest symptom of colonic carcinoma is a 'change in bowel habit' towards looser stool
- Overflow—in the presence of constipation (for instance in those using opiate analgesia)
- Bleeding—some patients may describe upper or lower GI bleeding (either fresh blood or melaena), as diarrhoea
- Others—medications (e.g. antibiotics), hyperthyroidism

Always ask patients:

- To define their 'normal bowel habit'—when and what was it.
- The duration and progression of symptoms—getting better, getting worse, or staying the same?
- The frequency and quantity of stool—how often are they passing stool? how much?
- Consistency and colour—loose, watery, clear, black, brown, green, pale
- Associated blood or mucous.
- Associated symptoms—abdominal pain? fevers? extra-abdominal symptoms of inflammatory bowel disease or malignancy?

Constipation: Absolute constipation means failure to pass stool or flatus. This is a sinister symptom and suggests bowel obstruction. Non-obstructive constipation is very common, especially in the elderly, and may be associated with severe abdominal pain. Common causes include:

- Drugs—opiates, anticholinergics, iron
- Large bowel malignancy
- Poor oral intake or inadequate dietary fibre
- Diverticular disease
- Rectal/anal disease—fissures and haemorrhoid
- Metabolic causes—hypocalcaemia, diabetes mellitus, and hypothyroidism
- Spinal cord compression

3. Hepatobiliary symptoms

The principal symptom of hepatobiliary disease is jaundice which may be associated with fever, nausea and vomiting, pruritus, and upper abdominal pain. A full systemic review may also be required.

Jaundice: The diagnosis of jaundice will often be apparent immediately on looking at a patient. Jaundice is a sign of acute hepatic dysfunction and may be associated with acute fulminant liver failure. This is manifest by jaundice, signs of encephalopathy including asterixis, confusion, a depressed level of conscious, and hepatic fetor.

It is worth considering the mechanisms of jaundice:

- Haemolysis (**pre-hepatic** jaundice)—this rarely produces severe jaundice, but ask about haemolytic anaemias (e.g. sickle-cell), drugs, mechanical valves, and infective symptoms.
- Intrinsic liver disease [intra-hepatic **(hepatic)** jaundice]—possibly accompanied by a dull right upper quadrant ache. Ask about risk factors for liver disease.
- Bile duct obstruction (post-hepatic **'obstructive'** jaundice)—often accompanied by colicky right upper quadrant pain, dark urine, and pale stools.

Asking about risk factors for intrinsic liver disease includes:

- A full medical history—especially previous liver disease or autoimmune diseases
- An alcohol history—what do they drink? how regularly? how much? do they binge?
- An illegal drug history—including previous use. Most importantly, have they ever injected drugs intravenously?
- A sexual history—how many sexual partners in the past 3 months? what activities? do they use condoms?
- A travel history—where have they been? any risky behaviours (see above) whilst there?
- Others—tattoos, blood transfusions

4. Red flag symptoms

Weight changes: A forensic approach is needed! Most people know their 'fighting weight', i.e. the weight they normally are; ask when they were last that weight, and then weigh them directly in the ward, clinic, or surgery. You now know that they have lost/gained that amount of weight in a given time. By measuring their height, you can then work out their body mass index (BMI).

Cancer symptoms: Since almost all symptoms in gastroenterology can be caused by malignancies, always keep the question 'could this be cancer' at the back of your mind—and ask about constitutional symptoms which may indicate malignant disease:

'Red flag' features suggestive of malignancy

- Rapid weight loss
- Anorexia
- General malaise
- Relatively short duration of symptoms (e.g. 'a 2-month history of...')
- Progressively worsening symptoms
- Symptoms of metastasis—bony pain, jaundice, cough, neurological symptoms

Examination

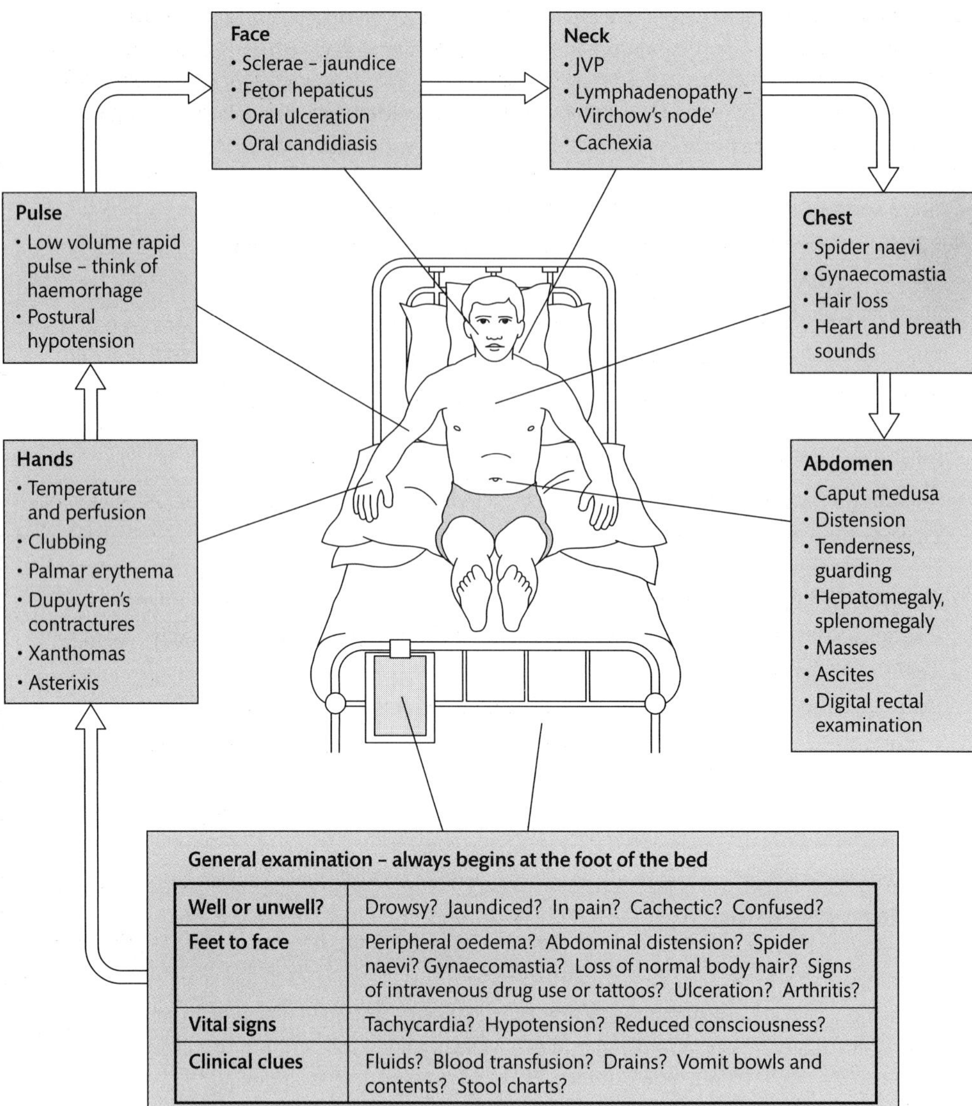

General examination – always begins at the foot of the bed

Well or unwell?	Drowsy? Jaundiced? In pain? Cachectic? Confused?
Feet to face	Peripheral oedema? Abdominal distension? Spider naevi? Gynaecomastia? Loss of normal body hair? Signs of intravenous drug use or tattoos? Ulceration? Arthritis?
Vital signs	Tachycardia? Hypotension? Reduced consciousness?
Clinical clues	Fluids? Blood transfusion? Drains? Vomit bowls and contents? Stool charts?

Assessing a patient with liver disease

Patients with liver dysfunction present with a wide spectrum of symptoms. They may be asymptomatic and the dysfunction may be found incidentally on blood testing or they may present with one of the complications of liver disease such as jaundice, ascites, or variceal bleeding. A lot can be deduced from physical examination about the likely level of liver functioning using the stepwise approach below.

Is there evidence of an acute decompensation of liver function?

- Encephalopathy? Asterixis, personality change, confusion, stupor, or coma.
- Jaundice?
- Ascites? Flank dullness, shifting dullness. Fluid thrill indicates tense ascites. Generalized tenderness may indicate spontaneous bacterial peritonitis
- GI bleeding? Haematemesis, melaena, haemodynamic instability

Is there evidence of chronic liver disease?

- Clubbing, Dupuytren's contracture, palmar erythema, leuconychia, spider naevi, male hair loss, gynaecomastia, testicular atrophy

Is there hepatomegaly? What does it feel like?

- A **smoothly enlarged** liver may indicate fatty liver (of any cause) or acute hepatitis, when the liver may be tender to palpate
- An **irregularly enlarged** liver may contain metastases or primary cancer
- A **pulsatile** liver may be caused by right sided heart failure. Cirrhotic livers are normal sized or small

Are there signs of portal hypertension?

- These include **ascites**, **splenomegaly**, and **distended abdominal wall veins**, often radiating from the umbilicus in a pattern known as '**caput medusa**'

Signs of GI bleeding

Acute bleeding	Chronic bleeding
Haematemesis and melaena Tachycardia, tachypnoea, hypotension Postural drop in blood pressure Pallor	Pallor Koilonychia Angular stomatitis Glossitis

Beware of:

- Younger patients who maintain their blood pressure for a long period before suddenly decompensating (they are often well but tachycardic).
- Patients on beta-blockers who do not become tachycardic despite substantial fluid loss.
- Patients with signs of active bleeding (ongoing haematemesis/melaena /fresh rectal bleeding, haemodynamic instability) require urgent endoscopy to 'turn off the tap' as well as fluid resuscitation.

Investigations

Upper GI endoscopy

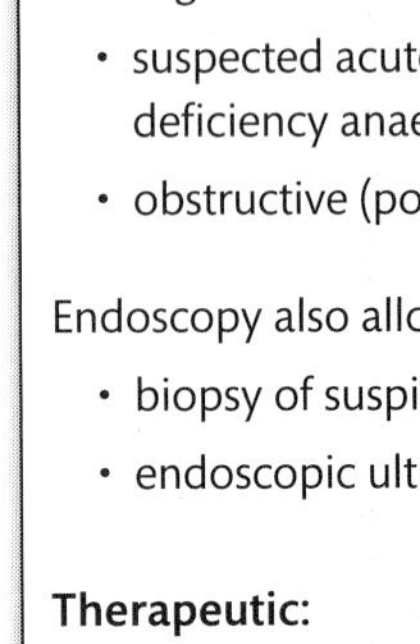

Common indications for upper GI endoscopy include the following.

Diagnostic:

Investigation of

- suspected acute upper GI bleeding, iron deficiency anaemia, dysphagia, dyspepsia
- obstructive (post-hepatic) jaundice (ERCP)

Endoscopy also allows:

- biopsy of suspicious lesions
- endoscopic ultrasound

Therapeutic:

- Haemostasis of oesophageal varices through injection of sclerosant or banding of oesophagogastric varices.
- Haemostasis of bleeding ulcers and other lesions with a variety of methods including injection of sclerosant and laser photocoagulation.
- Insertion of expanding stents (e.g. to relieve dysphagia or biliary obstruction).
- Allowing release of gallstones by sphincterotomy (cutting the sphincter of Oddi at ERCP).

The diagram above shows the possibilities of different types of endoscopy:

- **Oesophagogastroduodenoscopy (OGD)** allows good visualization of the oesophagus, stomach, and early duodenum, and allows biopsy of lesions or therapeutic intervention (e.g. banding of varices)
- **Endoscopic retrograde cholangiopancreatography (ERCP):** insertion of a side-viewing endoscope into the second part of the duodenum allows a small cannula to be inserted into the ampulla of Vater. Contrast can then be injected allowing X-ray visualization of the pancreatic duct and biliary tree. The ampulla can be cut (sphincterotomy) to allow the passage of gallstones, or biliary stents can be inserted.
- Visualizing the small bowel: **capsule endoscopy** involves ingestion of a pill containing a camera whilst wearing a belt containing radio receivers that pick up images recorded by the camera. **Double-balloon enteroscopy** uses a modified endoscope with overlying sheath and two balloons via a push-pull technique to allow conventional endoscopy, including biopsy taking or stent insertion, of the whole bowel.

Lower GI endoscopy

- Proctoscopy, commonly performed in surgical out-patient clinics, gives good visualization of the anal canal and distal rectum and allows banding of haemorrhoids.
- Rigid sigmoidoscopy can also be carried out in clinic and allows visualization of the rectum and distal sigmoid colon.
- Flexible sigmoidoscopy is performed in the endoscopy suite and allows visualization of the descending colon.
- Colonoscopy is a major endoscopic procedure allowing visualization of the whole colon and terminal ileum.

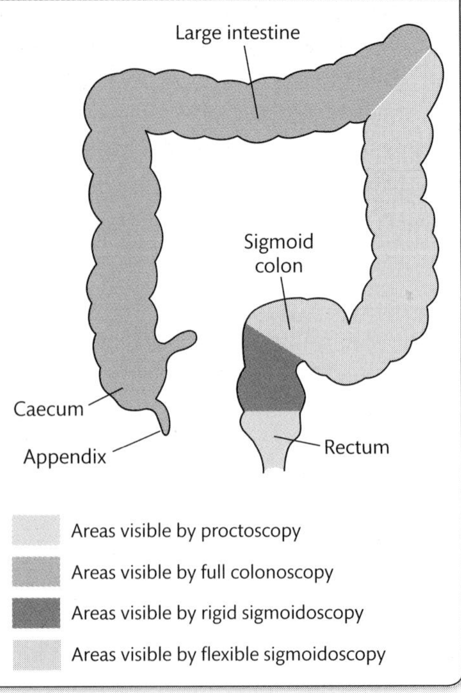

Interpreting the liver function tests (LFTs)

- **Bilirubin:** This is a breakdown product of haemoglobin, which is conjugated in the liver and then excreted in bile. Raised bilirubin produces jaundice, which may be detectable clinically from levels of 35 μmol/L. An isolated rise in bilirubin without abnormalities in other LFTs may indicate **haemolysis (pre-hepatic jaundice)**.
- **ALT and AST:** These are the **transaminases**. They are usually maintained within hepatocytes, but their plasma concentration increases with hepatocyte death. They particularly increase with hepatic injury, e.g. caused by viral infection, toxins (like paracetamol). or acute ischaemia.
- **ALP and GGT:** These are normally located on the epithelial surfaces of bile canaliculi, and rise significantly in bile duct obstruction or alcohol excess. The ALP may also rise in disorders of bone, e.g. Paget's disease.
- **Albumin and INR:** These reflect the liver's synthetic function. Low albumin or high INR in the context of liver disease may indicate significant disease, for instance, the presence of **cirrhosis**.

Markers of good nutrition

Poor nutrition caused by inadequate diet is common in the elderly, alcoholics, the homeless, and throughout the developing world. Poor nutrition may also be caused by diseases affecting the small intestine (such as coeliac disease or Crohn's disease), by pancreatic insufficiency, or by any medical condition causing the patient to be made 'nil by mouth' for a prolonged period. Gastroenterologists have an important role in ensuring good nutrition for such patients. Markers of nutrition and malabsorption include:

- **Low albumin:** In the absence of severe liver disease (e.g. cirrhosis) or renal disease (e.g. the nephrotic syndrome), serum albumin is a good marker of a patient's overall nutritional status. Low albumin in elderly patients may indicate self-neglect or an inability to prepare food for themselves.
- **Vitamin B_{12} and folate deficiency:** These are absorbed by the small intestine and have important roles in cell synthesis. Malabsorption is common in diseases of the small bowel, and a particularly profound vitamin B_{12} deficiency is caused by autoimmune destruction of gastric parietal cells with subsequent lack of intrinsic factor secretion which is needed for vitamin B_{12} absorption. Deficiency of both folate and vitamin B_{12} can lead to a macrocytic anaemia; however, in the presence of iron deficiency (see below), microcytosis and macrocytosis may cancel each other out to produce a normal MCV.
- **Electrolyte abnormalities:** Prolonged starvation (>5 days) can lead to serious depletion of electrolytes including magnesium, phosphate, calcium, and potassium. If feeding is commenced before these have been replaced then a sudden increase in cellular metabolism can lead serum levels of these electrolytes to plummet, which in severe cases can lead to multiorgan failure (the 'refeeding syndrome'). In patients at risk of refeeding syndrome, levels of these electrolytes should be monitored regularly once feeding had recommenced with intravenous replacement being given as required.
- **Iron deficiency:** This is very rarely due to poor nutrition. By far the commonest cause of iron deficiency is chronic blood loss, with gynaecological causes most common in younger women and GI blood loss most common in the elderly. Iron deficiency causes a microcytic anaemia, which can be confirmed as iron deficient by low ferritin and raised total iron-binding capacity (TIBC). Signs include koilonychias, angular stomatitis, glossitis, and brittle hair.

Interventions

Antiemetics

Numerous different antiemetic drugs exist, each of which may be particularly effective for nausea and vomiting of different causes:

- Histamine antagonists (such as cyclizine) are often used as first-line antiemetics in general use.
- Dopamine antagonists (such as metoclopramide or domperidone) stimulate gastric emptying and are also often used as a first line.
- Serotonin antagonists (such as ondansetron) are often used as second-line antiemetics, or first-line in situations (such as chemotherapy) where powerful antiemetic action is needed.
- Steroids (such as dexamethasone) may have an important antiemetic role in palliative care, where they may also be useful in reducing distress and stimulating appetite.

Drugs in inflammatory bowel disease

Patients with acute exacerbations of inflammatory bowel disease may be acutely unwell. Management has two phases: establishing remission (where steroids are used because of their potent anti-inflammatory effects), and maintaining remission (where steroids are avoided because of their long-term side-effects). Mainstays of treatment for inflammatory bowel disease are the 5-aminosalicylate drugs such as mesalazine. These drugs are nephrotoxic, but this problem is avoided by formulations which prevent their absorption in the small intestine, for instance by using an enteric coating that only breaks down in the large bowel.

Laxatives and enemas

Laxatives are useful for preventing and treating constipation. There are two broad categories: bulk and osmotic laxatives which produce soft, well-formed stool, and stimulant laxatives which cause colonic stimulation.

Osmotic and bulk-forming laxatives	Stimulant laxatives
Lactulose Isphagula husk Bran Sodium docusate	Senna Bisacodyl Glycerine suppositories

Enemas such as the phosphate enema are effective in distal constipation (when hard stool is felt on digital examination of the rectum), and consist of hypertonic solutions introduced rectally which soften stool and irritate the rectum, producing (often forceful) defecation.

The laxative lactulose is also indicated in hepatic encephalopathy, where cognitive function is affected by nitrogenous waste products which are not 'filtered' and metabolized by the liver in advanced liver disease. Here lactulose speeds passage of stool through the gut. The aim should be to induce several soft bowel openings every day.

Common gastroenterology medications

Class	Examples	Mechanism	Indications	Contraindications	Side-effects	Special notes
Histamine H_1 antagonists						
Dopamine D_2 antagonists						
Serotonin antagonists						
Antifungals						
Antacids						
Proton pump inhibitors						
Histamine H_2 inhibitors						
Vasopressin analogues						
Secondary bile salts						
Colestyramine						
Antispasmodics						
Aminosalicylates						
Steroids	Oral: IV:					
Steroid-sparing anti-inflammatory drugs						
Anti-TNFα drugs						
Osmotic and bulk-forming laxatives						
Stimulant laxatives						
Enemas						
Antidiarrhoea medicine						
Iron						
Vitamins						

Upper gastrointestinal bleeding

This section should be used to clerk patients admitted as an emergency with an acute upper GI bleed, or admitted with symptomatic anaemia as a result of chronic bleeding. Patient pathways lead from the Emergency Department through the Medical Admissions Unit to Gastroenterology, via the Endoscopy Unit at some point.

Learning challenges

- What might lead to you suspect that a patient is bleeding from oesophageal varices, and how might this influence management?
- What Nobel prize-winning discovery by Barrie Marshall and J. Robin Warren in the 1980s has had a profound impact on the management of upper GI disease?

History

Comment on

- Haematemesis—volume, character (frank blood, clots, altered blood), number of episodes
- Melaena—number of episodes, fresh blood passed rectally
- Epigastric pain, dyspepsia, reflux symptoms
- Previous stomach or liver disease
- NSAIDs, warfarin, aspirin, and other antiplatelet drugs
- Alcohol use

Examination

Well or unwell? Why?

Feet to face:

Vital signs: Temperature Blood pressure Pulse rate Respiratory rate O2 saturations

Clinical clues:

Cardiovascular:

1 2 1

Respiratory:

Weight/kg

Height/m

BMI (kg/m^2)

Abdominal:

Neurological:

Other:

Comment on

- Signs of hypovolaemia and shock—perfusion, BP, HR
- Pallor, signs of iron deficiency
- Signs of chronic liver disease
- Encephalopathy
- Digital rectal examination: melaena

Blood tests

Comment on

- Haemoglobin, MCV
- U&Es—high urea:creatinine ratio?
- Cross-match—how many units?
- Clotting, INR, platelets
- LFTs, albumin
- Repeat haemoglobin (if transfused)

Chest X-ray

Comment on

- Aspiration? Perforation?

Endoscopy

Comment on

- Macroscopic appearances
- Evidence of active/recent bleeding
- Interventions carried out
- Rapid urease test

Histology

Evaluation

1. **How severe is this patient's haemorrhage (ATLS grading below)? What resuscitation do they need?**

Class I haemorrhage	Class II haemorrhage	Class III haemorrhage	Class IV haemorrhage
<15% blood volume	15–30% blood volume	30–40% blood volume	>40% blood volume
No change in observations	Tachycardia	Tachycardia with hypotension (shock)	Profound hypotension
No signs/symptoms	Cool skin, slight behavioural changes	Drowsy, cool, capillary refill >2 seconds	Moribund
No resuscitation needed	IV fluids, e.g. saline, required	Blood transfusion needed	Aggressive fluids and blood needed

2. **Does the patient need urgent endoscopy (if there is ongoing active bleeding)? What is found? Is endoscopic intervention possible?**

3. **What is the patient's chance of further complications (Rockall score, below)?**

Rockall risk scoring system attempts to identify patients at risk of adverse outcome followng acute upper gastrointestinal bleeding.

	Score 0	Score 1	Score 2	Score 3
Age	<60	60-79	>79	
Shock	None	Tachycardia (>100)	Hypotension (<100 systolic)	
Comorbidity			Cardiac or other major disease	Liver or renal failure, cancer
Diagnosis	Mallory-Weiss, nothing seen	All others	Malignancy	
Endoscopic findings	Nothing seen	All others	Active/recent bleeding, spurting vessel	

Score <3 = Low risk, aim for early discharge. **Score >8** = High risk of death/rebleeding

4. **What follow up is indicated?**

Questions

1. A 55-year-old woman with severe rheumatoid arthritis presents to hospital feeling dizzy and faint. She reports having passed black stool for the previous 2 days. On examination she appears pale and somewhat drowsy, with cool, pale peripheries. Her heart rate is 115 bpm with a blood pressure of 105/78 mmHg (and a postural drop of 25 mmHg on sitting upright). She has a soft, non-tender abdomen and an empty rectum on digital examination. Blood tests reveal: Hb 7.9 g/L, MCV 81 fL, urea 18.7 mmol/L, and creatinine 116 μmol/L. She is carrying a list of her regular medications in her handbag, shown below:

Co-codamol 30/500: Take two tablets four times per day
Methotrexate 10 mg: Take one tablet once per week
Naproxen 500 mg: Take one tablet twice per day with food

(1) List the differential diagnosis for this patient's presentation.
(2) What is the significance of the urea:creatinine ratio in this case?
(3) Describe the essential steps in her management.

2. A 62-year-old man is brought in to the Emergency Department by ambulance vomiting copious amounts of fresh blood. He is an alcoholic, who is well known to the hospital, and is known to have cirrhosis and oesophageal varices. On arrival the haematemesis has slowed, though he is drowsy and mumbling incoherently. His hands and feet are cold with a capillary refill time of 4 seconds. His pulse is 126 bpm, of poor volume, and difficult to palpate; his BP is 84/48 mmHg. He is pale and chronically unwell looking, with jaundice, Dupuytren's contracture, palmar erythema, and multiple spider naevi. His hands flap gently when he is asked to hold them in front of him with extended wrists. Abdominal examination reveals a tense, distended abdomen with shifting dullness. His blood tests are shown below:

Sodium: 132 mmol/L	Haemoglobin: 6.1 g/dL
Potassium: 4.8 mmol/L	MCV: 107.5 fL
Urea: 8.9 mmol/L	WCC: 10.7 × 10^9/L
Creatinine: 89 μmol/L	Platelets: 64 × 10^9/L
Bilirubin: 43 μmol/L	INR: 3.2
ALT: 68 IU/L	ALP: 168 IU/L
Albumin: 23 g/L	

(1) List the abnormalities shown in his routine blood tests with an explanation for each; what is the unifying diagnosis in this case?
(2) List the immediate, essential management steps you would take before he is sent for urgent upper GI endoscopy.

3. A 59-year-old woman is admitted to hospital after vomiting twice. She describes the vomitus as being about half to a full pint of brownish, watery fluid. There are no fresh blood or clots in it. The triage nurse says that the patient's blouse was covered in 'coffee grounds'. The patient tells the doctor that she has had upper abdominal pains for the past few years, which seem to get better with antacids that she takes from time to time. She had no other medical history. On arrival in the Emergency Department her heart rate was 95 bpm and her blood pressure 114/68 mmHg. Her haemoglobin was 10.7 g/dL, and remained well overnight on the Medical Admissions Unit. Upper GI endoscopy the following morning revealed a 3 cm ulcer in the first part of the duodenum, but with no evidence of active or recent bleeding, no blood, and no obvious vessels seen. A biopsy of the gastric antrum was taken for urease testing; however, unfortunately due to confusion in the endoscopy unit the sample was lost. She is now back of the ward and is keen to go home.

(1) Is it safe to let her go home?—Explain your reasoning.
(2) Name a non-invasive test that you could arrange to replace the lost urease test.
(3) What further therapeutic intervention(s), if any, might you arrange.

4. A 24-year-old man is brought to the Emergency Department by his friends from a party. He had been drinking heavily and had then begun to vomit. After dry retching for several minutes, he vomited about a cupful of fresh blood. On examination, all basic observations were within normal ranges. His haemoglobin is 14.5 g/dL. You discuss the patient with the on-call endoscopist who tells you to admit him to the observation ward and discharge him as soon as he is sober, but adds as an afterthought, 'but make sure he hasn't got any surgical emphysema'.

(1) What is the likely underlying cause for the bleeding?
(2) What is surgical emphysema and why is the endoscopist concerned about it in this case?

5. A 78-year-old woman is admitted to a gastroenterology ward following a significant upper GI bleed. Upper GI endoscopy reveals a 3 × 2 cm ulcer on the lesser curve of the stomach. The bleeding had stopped by the time of the endoscopy, though the area was nonetheless injected with alcohol to induce vasoconstriction. She received two units of blood on admission and but had not needed any further transfusions since. She had been progressing well but 4 days after admission, on the morning proposed for discharge, she passed a large amount of black tarry stool. Her initial observations on the ward show HR 110 bpm regular, BP 105/78 mmHg, temperature 37.2°C, RR 18 breaths/min, oxygen sats 97% on air. Blood tests revealed a drop in haemoglobin from 10.5 g/dL (2 days before) to 7.2 g/dL. She was transfused two units before a repeat endoscopy, where the stomach was found to be full of fresh and altered blood, with active bleeding from the site of the earlier identified ulcer. After the endoscopy a repeat FBC found that despite two units of blood, her haemoglobin was 7.6 g/L.

(1) What does the repeat Hb, post-endoscopy, signify?
(2) List the essential steps in this patient's further management.

Presentation

Presented to ______ Grade ______ Date ______

Signed

Answers

1. This patient has had a significant upper GI bleed, with melaena, hypovolaemia, and a drop in haemoglobin. A normal MCV implies that the bleeding is acute (if she had been bleeding slowly over time then iron deficiency would have developed). The differential diagnosis here includes all causes of upper GI bleeding, for instance oesophageal and gastric varices, peptic ulcers, gastritis, and upper GI malignancies. However, the most likely cause here is gastric erosions secondary to the use of the NSAID naproxen (especially since the patient was not taking a prophylactic medication such as a proton pump inhibitor to protect the stomach).

This woman has a high urea:creatinine ratio. This is a pattern commonly seen in upper GI bleeds because blood is digested in the intestine and then all the protein it contains is absorbed into the circulation, rather like taking a large high-protein meal. A raised urea can be a useful indication that a patient has suffered a GI bleed. High urea:creatinine ratios are also seen in pre-renal renal failure.

The first step in this woman's management is fluid resuscitation. The presence of a tachycardia and postural blood pressure drop suggests compensated hypovolaemia (the blood pressure only falls once raised heart rate and peripheral vasoconstriction are unable to maintain a normal level). The best fluid to use in resuscitation of this lady is cross-matched blood; however, saline or colloid solutions can also be used. There is also evidence for use of an intravenous proton pump inhibitor (such as omeprazole) in the management of upper GI bleeds. Once stable she should have an endoscopy to determine the cause of the bleeding and determine definitive management. The NSAID should be stopped.

2. The abnormalities shown here are characteristic of advanced alcoholic liver disease. This has caused:

- Derangement of LFTs (essentially markers of liver damage)
- Derangement of the synthetic function of the liver (low albumin and a high INR)
- Secondary splenomegaly (producing low platelets)
- Macrocytosis (caused both by the direct effect of alcohol on bone marrow and by chronic liver disease)
- Variceal bleeding with a low haemoglobin and raised urea:creatinine ratio
- Slight hyponatraemia, commonly seen in advanced liver disease

Once again, good fluid resuscitation is key: this man is in hypovolaemic shock. He should be urgently cross-matched for between six and ten units of blood, and in the meantime boluses of fluid given to maintain his blood pressure adequately to achieve cerebral perfusion. The drug terlipressin is licensed for use in upper GI bleeding of known variceal origin (not in other upper GI bleeding), and works by reducing splanchnic blood flow and raising the blood pressure. Once the patient has been resuscitated then urgent endoscopy is required to stop the bleeding. Oesophageal varices can have elastic bands placed around them or can be injected with sclerosant. Since the patient is drowsy and is still actively vomiting blood, the hospital's anaesthetic team should be called to consider intubating the patient to protect his airway whilst the endoscopy is performed, to prevent aspiration.

3. This woman has had a small GI bleed from a duodenal ulcer which does not contain any large vessels. Her Rockall score is 2, indicating that she is at low risk of rebleeding and can safely be sent home.

By far the commonest cause of duodenal ulcers is the bacterium *Helicobacter pylori*, accounting of 90% of duodenal ulcers (and 50% of stomach ulcers). The rapid urease test, carried out immediately on biopsy specimens of duodenal or stomach mucosa, is the best way for diagnosing infection. However, for this woman an alternative would be breath testing (where the patient drinks radiocarbon-labelled urea and the breath is tested for radiolabelled CO_2), or blood or stool antigen tests (different tests are available in different hospitals, and no test is 100% accurate).

If she tests positive for *H. pylori* then she should be discharged with 'triple therapy' aimed to eradicate it. This consists of an antacid drug (e.g. Lansoprazole) along with two antibiotics (e.g. amoxicillin and clarithromycin). After completing a 2-week course, she could be retested using one of the non-invasive methods described above, or a repeat endoscopy could be carried out to ensure that the ulcer has healed.

4. The most likely cause for bleeding in this man is a Mallory–Weiss tear—a small lesion in the lining of the oesophagus caused by vigorous retching. These tears may produce significant bleeding, but heal up well without intervention, and so if the diagnosis can be made confidently on clinical grounds, endoscopy is not necessary.

Surgical emphysema describes air trapped in subcutaneous tissue, which may produce a 'crackly' feeling on palpation of the patient's skin. In this case, the registrar is concerned that the patient's prolonged retching may have caused him to rupture his oesophagus (called Boorhaave's syndrome after the Dutch admiral said to have suffered it after a bout of prolonged vomiting). Air can escape from the oesophagus into the mediastinum and the subcutaneous tissues around the neck. It causes a severe inflammation of the mediastinum and may require urgent oesophageal stent insertion to cover the hole, or even intervention by cardiothoracic surgeons.

5. Each unit of blood transfused to a patient should raise the Hb by approximately 1 g/dL. The fact that this woman's Hb has not risen significantly despite two units of blood implies that she is continuing to bleed from the ulcer. A consideration whenever large amounts of blood are transfused (and this woman has had four units in one day), is to correct any associated clotting abnormalities. In most western hospitals, units of packed red cells (rather than of whole blood) are transfused in order to minimize transfusion reactions generated by, for example, white cells. What this means is that when large volumes are transfused, accompanying transfusions of fresh frozen plasma (containing clotting factors) and platelets, should also be given.

This woman will die unless the bleeding in her stomach can be stopped, and failed endoscopic therapy is an indication for surgical treatment. The hospital's upper GI or general surgeons should be contacted immediately and asked to review the patient. Often a limited operation to remove the wedge of stomach containing the ulcer can be performed, though more radical surgery (such as a partial gastrectomy) may be required. In the meantime, the key consideration is resuscitation. Two large-bore intravenous cannulae should be inserted, and a urinary catheter put in to monitor urine output. Fluid should be given (ideally in the form of blood) to maintain a urine output of 0.5 mL/kg/hour.

Further reading

Guidelines: Scottish Intercollegiate Guidelines Network guidelines on management of acute upper and lower intestinal haemorrhage (http://www.sign.ac.uk/guidelines/fulltext/105/index.html)

OHCM: 240–243, 252–257, 830–831

Gastric and oesophageal cancer

This section should be used to clerk patients being investigated either as an in-patient or out-patient for upper GI cancer. They may be found on the Gastroenterology Ward or in the Endoscopy Unit, or being discussed at upper GI cancer multidisciplinary team meetings.

Learning challenges

- How does the histological finding of Barrett's oesophagus fit within the pathological process of tumour development?
- Why are survival rates from gastric cancer much higher in Japan than in the rest of the developed world? Why has a Japanese approach to screening not been adopted elsewhere?

History

Comment on

- Dysphagia—level, consistency of food/fluids that get stuck; regurgitation
- Dyspepsia pain and reflux symptoms
- Early satiety
- Malaise, anorexia, weight loss
- Symptoms of local and distant metastases, e.g. bony pain or jaundice

Examination

Well or unwell? Why?

Feet to face:

Vital signs: Temperature | Blood pressure | Pulse rate | Respiratory rate | O2 saturations

Clinical clues:

Cardiovascular:

1 2 1

Respiratory:

Weight/kg

Height/m

BMI (kg/m²)

Abdominal:

Neurological:

Other:

Comment on

- Cachexia and dehydration
- Lymphadenopathy—Virchow's node
- Signs of aspiration
- Abdominal masses—epigastric
- Hepatomegaly

Blood tests

Comment on

- Anaemia (microcytic)
- LFTs and clotting
- Calcium—hypercalcaemia of malignancy

Endoscopy

Comment on

- Macroscopic appearance
- Evidence of bleeding

Histology

Comment on

- Tumour type
- Differentiation
- Neurovascular invasion

CT chest/abdomen

Comment on

- Local invasion
- Lymph node enlargement
- Distant metastases

Endoscopic ultrasound

Comment on

- Extent of local spread
- Lymphadenopathy

Evaluation

1. What histological type of tumour is this? What is the staging?

T (Tumour)	N (Nodes)	M (Metastases)
T1: Submucosal	**N0:** No nodes involved	**M0:** No evidence of distant spread
T2: Muscular invasion	**N1:** *Oesophageal:* any nodes involved. *Gastric:* <6 nodes involved	**M1:** Evidence of distant spread
T3: Breached serosal surface	**N2:** *Gastric:* 7–15 nodes involved	
T4: Invasion of other organs	**N3:** *Gastric:* >15 nodes	

2. **Is surgical resection possible? Could chemotherapy or radiotherapy improve survival or symptoms?**

3. **How can the patient be supported nutritionally if the cancer is preventing eating?**

4. **Which other professionals should be involved in helping to care for this patient?**

Questions

1. A 49-year-old man had attended his GP surgery 10 years before complaining of intermittent upper abdominal pain; the pain often settled with food or with an antacid preparation. On each occasional he had been otherwise well, had suffered with no other medical conditions, and had not taken any other medications. His weight had been stable and he had had no other upper or lower abdominal symptoms, including dysphagia. Examination had been normal, and the doctor had prescribed a proton pump inhibitor (PPI), which the patient found very helpful; he stopped the PPI within a few months as the symptoms resolved.

He now returns, complaining of similar worsening upper abdominal pain but also of weight loss of almost 10 kg during the previous 2 months. The doctor referred him urgently for endoscopy, where an ulcerating tumour of the gastric fundus was found. Subsequent tests revealed liver metastases making the tumour inoperable. The patient was upset that he had not been referred for endoscopy 10 years ago.

(1) If you were the doctor what might you have done differently in this case?

2. A 64-year-old woman presents to her family doctor with a 6-week history of worsening dysphagia, which was initially to solids, such as bread and butter, but in the last 2 weeks has included custard, and now tea and water. During this period she has lost more than 5 kg in weight. She had no significant medical history other than some heartburn, which she has had for 'years'. An urgent endoscopy is arranged that reveals a thickened, irregular stricture in the lower third of the oesophagus, surrounded by streaks of red mucosa running up into the oesophagus from the stomach. The histology report is shown below.

> **Histology report:** Four 2 mm × 1 mm sections of reddish tissue from the distal oesophagus. Three showed evidence of moderately differentiated adenocarcinoma with invasion through the lamina propria into the muscularis mucosa. The fourth section shows evidence of severely dysplastic columnar epithelium.

(1) What is the cause of her dysphagia?

(2) List the generic and specific stages of her further management.

3. A previously fit and well 34-year-old man presents to his family doctor with an insidious, 2-month history of 'difficulty swallowing'. He finds liquids especially difficult, causing him to cough and splutter, 'like I'm choking'. He gets a feeling low down behind his sternum that the food and drink 'isn't getting through', sometimes accompanied by severe 'squeezing' chest pain. He sometimes regurgitates undigested food into his mouth. In view of his age and symptoms, a barium swallow rather than an endoscopy is arranged.

(1) What does the barium study show?

(2) What is the most likely underlying cause?

(3) What are the management options?

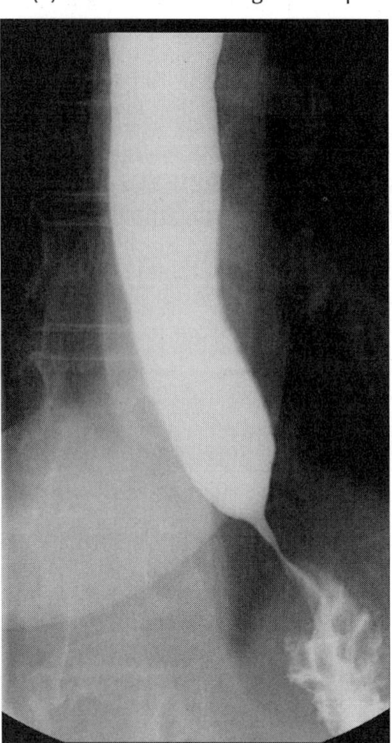

4. A 64-year-old woman is being investigated in hospital after being found to have a haemoglobin of 6.4 g/dL, MCV 61 fL, after presenting to her doctor complaining of feeling tired all the time. Upper GI endoscopy reveals a 3 × 2 cm gastric ulcer on the greater curvature; the ulcer has rolled edges and there is evidence of bleeding at the base. Histology confirms a moderately differentiated adenocarcinoma. She has been transfused and now feels much better.

How might you discuss the endoscopy findings with the patient, including the management options? Write out the generic and specific issues you would cover.

5. A 68-year-old man with a known inoperable tumour of the gastric fundus is admitted to hospital because he is rapidly deteriorating, and becoming increasingly symptomatic. He is in severe pain from bony metastases which is not controlled by the regular tramadol he was prescribed. He has suffered worsening dysphagia and has hardly eaten anything in the past week. He feels very nauseated and has been vomiting and retching regularly. On examination the patient is extremely cachectic and dehydrated. He has marked oral candidiasis and dry mucous membranes. He is clinically anaemic. Digital rectal examination reveals hard stool per rectum. He confides in you his despair at his condition, and that he wishes he were dead. He asks if there is anything you can do to 'send him off to sleep'.

(1) What is your duty as the 'doctor' in this case?

(2) List five palliative interventions to help him.

(3) What would you do if he refuses further intervention?

Presentation

Presented to ______ Grade ______ Date ______

Signed

Remember that you can find large-size, annotated versions of many of the X-rays and ECGs that appear in this book on the book's web site at www.oxfordtextbooks.co.uk/orc/randall/

Answers

1. Dyspepsia is extremely common, and symptoms fit poorly with the underlying pathology. Guidelines from the National Institute of Health and Clinical Excellence (NICE) suggest that endoscopy is not indicated for diagnosis unless 'alarm features' exist, including chronic GI bleeding, dysphagia, unexplained weight loss, an epigastric mass, or iron deficiency anaemia. Endoscopy is also indicated for unexplained and persistent dyspepsia in patients aged over 55. Otherwise, after offending drugs have been stopped, a trial of a PPI can be prescribed. Testing for *Helicobacter pylori* can also be carried out, though at the moment there is inadequate evidence of the value of this. *H. pylori* is the major cause of duodenal ulcers, and also causes gastritis, gastric ulcers, and upper GI malignancies, including gastric cancer. If *H. pylori* is detected, it can be eradicated with a short course of 'triple therapy', consisting of two antibiotics and a PPI (e.g. amoxycillin, metronidazole, and lansoprazole).

According to the NICE guidelines, the doctor's management of this patient was entirely appropriate. He could have referred for *H. pylori* testing, though the evidence for doing so is equivocal. In the UK patients with gastric cancer often present in the later stages of their disease, but because of its relatively low incidence in the UK a screening programme is not warranted. Japan has a much higher incidence of gastric cancer than the UK and has a well-developed screening programme that does pick up a number of early gastric cancers, which can be resected with a good prognosis. Outside of the Japanese system, early detection of gastric cancer depends on doctors looking carefully for the 'alarm features' listed above and referring promptly for endoscopy if they are present.

2. This patient's history of heartburn is likely to have been caused by acid reflux, leading to metaplasia, dysplasia, and finally neoplasia in her lower oesophagus. She has oesophageal cancer; the next step is to work out the staging. She will require endoscopic ultrasound to determine how deeply the cancer has invaded her oesophageal wall and whether local lymph nodes are affected. A CT scan of the chest and abdomen will reveal the presence of other lymphadenopathy or metastasis. She can then be considered for surgery if it has not spread, or otherwise for palliative interventions.

The two major histological types of oesophageal cancer are squamous cell carcinoma and adenocarcinoma. Squamous cell carcinomas arise from the normal squamous lining of the oesophagus and tend to affect the middle third of the oesophagus. They are associated with tobacco and alcohol use and dietary factors. Adenocarcinomas arise from dysplastic oesophageal mucosa that has become columnar (like stomach mucosa), in response to persistent acid reflux. This altered mucosa is known as 'Barrett's oesophagus', and is an example of metaplasia. Barrett's oesophagus is a pre-malignant condition which requires regular surveillance with 6-monthly endoscopies.

3. The barium swallow demonstrates:

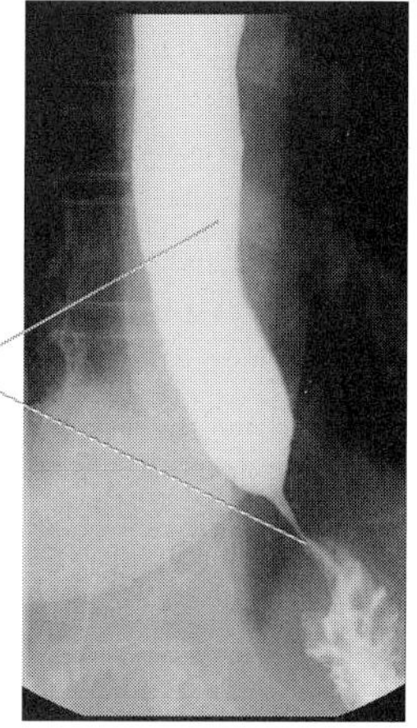

This x-ray reveals a grossly dilated oesophagus which is completely full of barium contrast. This tapers distally, where the lumen of the distal oesophagus is extremely narrow (though some contrast has reached the stomach). The smooth mucosal edges here contrast with the irregular 'apple-core' appearance caused by an oesophageal carcinoma.

These findings are classical of **achalasia**, a condition where the lower oesophageal sphincter fails to relax, associated with loss of peristalsis in the lower oesophagus. The patient presents with a classical history of achalasia, with **long-standing dysphagia** to both solids and liquids associated with **chest pain** where the oesophagus forcefully contracts to squeeze food through, and **regurgitation of undigested food** trapped in the oesophagus. This history is quite different from the classic history given by a patient with oesophageal cancer who complains of rapidly progressive dysphagia to solids and then liquids.

Treatment is initially by balloon dilatation, performed endoscopically under radiological guidance. If this is unsuccessful then surgical debulking of the muscular sphincter may be required. At endoscopy, biopsies should be taken for histology in case a cancer underlies the tight sphincter.

4. Breaking bad news is difficult, especially to someone who may have no inkling of what you are about to tell them. The points below offer some structure to help with this task:

- Prepare the environment—go to a side room off the ward, ensure you are free from distractions or interruptions, and turn off your bleep.
- Ask the patient to tell their story from the beginning, describing the symptoms they have had and what tests have been done.
- Explain that the test results are now back, and simply and briefly what they show. Try to be brief and sympathetic. Include the word 'cancer'.
- Allow pauses and emotional reactions. Don't be frightened of tears, and don't argue too hard if the patient denies what you say. Allow time for things to sink in.
- Answer any initial questions they may have, and encourage them to write down other questions they think of to ask you later.
- Ensure that they have someone to talk to. Think about family, friends, or religious leaders. Ask if they would like to have a nurse sit with them for a while, or if they would like to speak to the hospital chaplain.
- Go back later once the news has sunk in and ask if there is anything else they want to ask.

Spend time watching more experienced doctors break bad news. Talk to them about how they learned to do it. If you have bad experiences or if breaking bad news brings up difficult memories from your own life, try to talk about this with someone.

5. Physician-assisted suicide remains illegal in the UK, but suicide is almost certainly not what this man actually wants. What he wants is good quality palliative care.

Almost all hospitals have a palliative care team who can come and see patients on the wards. They have the experience and time to address issues faced by patients and find solutions to help make patients more comfortable. This man will need powerful opiate analgesia and a regular antiemetic to make him feel more comfortable. Intravenous fluids (and possibly a blood transfusion) will correct his dehydration and make him feel better. The issue of his dysphagia will need to be addressed—perhaps by an expanding metal stent to lie across the gastro-oesophageal junction and maintain patency. An enema and laxatives will relieve his constipation and antifungal treatments and good mouth care will remove the candidiasis. He may also need antidepressant therapy and psychological support.

The palliative care team also provide a valuable link to the community. This man may need daily carers at home, or visits from cancer support nurses. He may want to discuss going into a hospice if he is unable to cope at home. His family may need support, whether financial, emotional, or through respite care. There are often excellent care networks set up to help care for patients with terminal cancer, fully addressing their physical, mental, emotional, and spiritual needs. These networks provide hope for patients facing an appalling prognosis and allow them to die in as much comfort and dignity as is humanly possible.

If he is competent to make the decision to refuse further intervention his wishes must be respected and he should be palliated as much as he will allow.

Further reading

Guidelines: British Society of Gastroenterology guidelines for the management of gastric and oesophageal cancer (http://www.bsg.org.uk/clinical-guidelines/gastroduodenal/guidelines-for-the-management-of-oesophageal-and-gastric-cancer.html)

OHCM: 240, 244, 256, 621

Acute hepatitis

This section should be used to clerk patients with an acute hepatic illness. These patient may be admitted to the Medical Admissions Unit or Gastroenterology Ward, or may be managed in primary care and gastroenterology out-patient clinics.

Learning challenges

- What different patterns of derangement of LFTs are associated with pre-hepatic, intrahepatic and post-hepatic jaundice?
- What are the indications for liver transplant in acute liver failure?

History

Comment on

- Duration of symptoms—when did this all start?
- Jaundice and associated symptoms (e.g. change in stool and urine colour, pruritus)
- Abdominal pain—location and character
- Established liver disease/problems, e.g. gallstones, viral hepatitis
- Contacts with similar symptoms or signs
- Recent foreign travel
- Risk factors for blood borne viruses—IVDU, blood transfusions, migration from endemic areas, e.g. Southeast Asia
- Medications history, including illicit drugs
- Alcohol (and other possible toxins)
- Family history—gallstones, autoimmune liver disease
- Systemic features—other systems involved

Examination

Well or unwell? Why?

Feet to face:

Vital signs: Temperature Blood pressure Pulse rate Respiratory rate O2 saturations

Clinical clues:

Cardiovascular:

1 2 1

Respiratory:

Weight/kg

Height/m

BMI (kg/m^2)

Abdominal:

Neurological:

Other:

Comment on

- Jaundice
- Signs of chronic liver disease (see Introduction)
- Signs of encephalopathy—asterixis, confusion, decreased level of consciousness, seizures, hepatic fetor
- Hepatomegaly, ascites

Blood tests

Comment on

- FBC and U&Es
- LFTs—hepatitic versus obstructive
- Clotting profile
- Viral markers—HAV, HBV, HCV, HEV
- Paracetamol level (if overdose suspected)
- Other relevant parts of 'liver database'

Liver ultrasound

Comment on

- Diameter of common bile duct
- Presence of stones
- Flow in portal vein

Evaluation

1. Is the patient acutely unwell from any of the complications of liver failure (below)? What supportive treatment is required?

Complication	Evidence
Encephalopathy	Grade I: Impaired mental state—agitation, euphoria, anxiety
	Grade II: Disorientation, personality change, asterixis
	Grade III: Somnolence or stupor, marked asterixis
	Grade IV: Coma, seizures
Coagulopathy	High INR, risk of bleeding
Bleeding	Haematemesis or melaena, falling haemoglobin
Infection	Pyrexia, raised inflammatory markers, abdominal tenderness
Cerebral oedema	Progressively worsening cognitive function, drowsiness, coma, fixed dilated pupils
Renal failure	Rising creatinine and urea, low urine output

2. Is there any evidence of previous liver disease?

3. Are signs, symptoms, and test results more suggestive of a pre-, intra-, or post-hepatic cause? What is the likely cause?

4. What specific management is indicated?

Questions

1 A 23-year-old fashion student is admitted to hospital after presenting to the Emergency Department with a 2-week history of worsening jaundice. He has not experienced any abdominal pain or changes in his urine or faeces; however, he has felt generally unwell, tired and lethargic.

(1) List 10 possible causes of his jaundice.

(2) With this list in mind, list 10 further questions you would wish to ask him to help with the diagnosis.

(3) List the steps you might take in approaching some of the more sensitive questions.

2. A 21-year-old student is brought to hospital by ambulance at 02:00. Her flatmate had found her at home with a suicide note. She was drowsy but rousable, and said that she had taken a total of 32 paracetamol tablets at around 20:00 the previous evening. She suffers with epilepsy and takes carbamazepine regularly. She admitted to drinking a bottle of wine at the same time as taking the overdose. On examination she was drowsy and confused but her vital signs were all normal, and examination was otherwise unremarkable. Selected blood results are shown below, along with a graph to guide treatment for paracetamol overdose.

(1) What do the blood results and paracetamol levels indicate?

(2) List the important steps in her management

Bilirubin: 11 μmol/L	INR: 1.1
ALP: 113 IU/L	Haemoglobin: 14.6 g/dL
ALT: 38 IU/L	Urea: 3.5 mmol/L
Albumin: 42 g/L	Creatinine: 81 mmol/L
Paracetamol level: 90 mg/L	

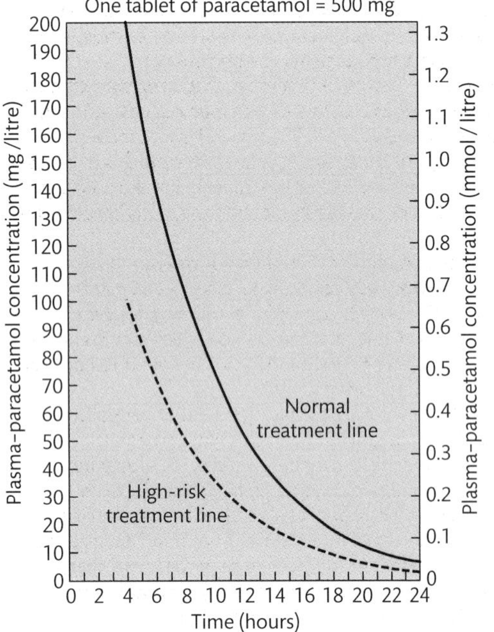

3. A homeless man with a long history of alcohol abuse is admitted to hospital acutely unwell after a long alcohol binge. He is drowsy but fully rousable, confused, and unsteady on his feet. He is unable to give any further clear history. He shows you a box of tablets that include thiamine and spironolactone and says he is taking both 'occasionally'. On examination he is mildly icteric, confused, and has a coarsened flap of his hands when asked to hold them outstretched in full dorsiflexion. He has a number of spider naevi across his chest where there is very little hair growing. Examination of the abdomen reveals moderate ascites and a tender, mildly enlarged liver. The rectum is empty on digital examination. His blood tests are shown below.

Sodium: 124 mmol/L	Haemoglobin: 10.2 g/dL
Potassium: 5.5 mmol/L	MCV: 114 fL
Creatinine: 105 μmol/L	WCC: 16.1 × 10^9/L
Urea: 6.8 mmol/L	Platelets: 67 × 10^9/L
Bilirubin: 86 μmol/L	INR: 2.7
ALP: 1198 IU/L	
ALT: 471 IU/L	
Albumin: 18 g/L	

(1) What is the likely diagnosis?

(2) What are the abnormalities shown? How do they support your diagnosis?

3 Gastroenterology

Answers

1. This patient has presented with acute jaundice; in a young man the differential will include:

(1) Viral hepatitis—HAV, HBV, HCV, HEV
(2) HIV
(3) Other infectious causes—EBV, CMV, toxoplasmosis, *Legionella*, brucellosis, malaria, leptospirosis
(4) Alcohol excess
(5) Illicit drug taking
(6) Medications including overdose (accidental or intentional)
(7) Less common causes will include congenital disease (Wilson's disease, haemochromatosis), Budd-Chiari syndrome, and malignancy (lymphoma or leukaemia, secondary cancer such as testicular cancer in a young man)

You will thus need to ask questions about

- Alcohol—what is their favourite drink? Do they drink it every day? How much? Do they binge drink? How regularly? Do they drink any other drinks?
- Sex—How many sexual partners have they had in the last 6 months? Which sex (gender) were they? What sort of sexual activity have they been involved in—vaginal, oral, anal, or other forms. During these activities do they always use a condom?
- Intravenous drug use—Have they ever injected themselves with drugs? Where did they get their needles from—were they sterile? Did they ever share needles?
- Tattoos, blood transfusions overseas, tribal markings—any of these procedures, especially if done in a potentially unsafe place (e.g. unregistered tattoo parlour) carry the risk of transmission of hepatitis B and C viruses, as well as HIV.
- Foreign travel—All of the hepatitis viruses are more common in the developing world than in the developed world, especially if whilst there the person was involved in risky behaviour, for instance eating seafood or salad (hepatitis A), or unprotected sex, injection of drugs, or blood transfusions (hepatitis B and C).
- Medications—Several commonly used drugs can cause an acute hepatitis, including several antibiotics, anti-TB treatments and antiepileptics. Ask also about over-the-counter medications or traditional remedies, which may contain a variety of biologically active ingredients.
- Overdose—how has their mood been? Have they ever felt low enough to want to take their life? Have they taken an overdose of paracetamol, or any other medication?
- Close contacts—is anyone else they know/live with acutely ill or jaundiced?

Many of the questions you will need to ask are of a very personal nature, which may make both the patient and you as the doctor or medical student feel very uncomfortable. There are a number of simple steps to apply in such situations:

- As with all patient interactions, but especially ones of a sensitive nature, one should guarantee as **safe, private, and supportive an environment as possible.** The patient may not want accompanying relatives or friends to be present, and may ask for the information not to be recorded. If this information impacts on possible healthcare and interactions with other colleagues, some explanations should be offered around how the information will be used; you should not make promises that you are unable to keep.
- When you come to ask them, be direct and introduce the change in questioning (**signposting**), e.g. 'I'm afraid I need to ask you some personal questions now which are important in helping us to make a diagnosis'.
- **Reassure** the patient that what they tell you is in confidence and will be shared only with other members of the direct clinical team.
- Then try to discuss the issues in a relaxed, adult, non-judgemental manner; do not make assumptions and do not use euphemisms, e.g. ask 'did you use a condom' rather than 'did you practice safe sex'. Try to guide the patient by asking open questions and listening to the full answer. This avoids having to choose expressions or statements that they may not understand or wish to hear.

2. Don't be deceived—liver biochemistry is usually normal for up to 24 hours after ingestion of a significant paracetamol overdose. Hepatic and renal damage is caused by a toxic metabolite of paracetamol which is only produced when the normal pathway for paracetamol metabolism is saturated:

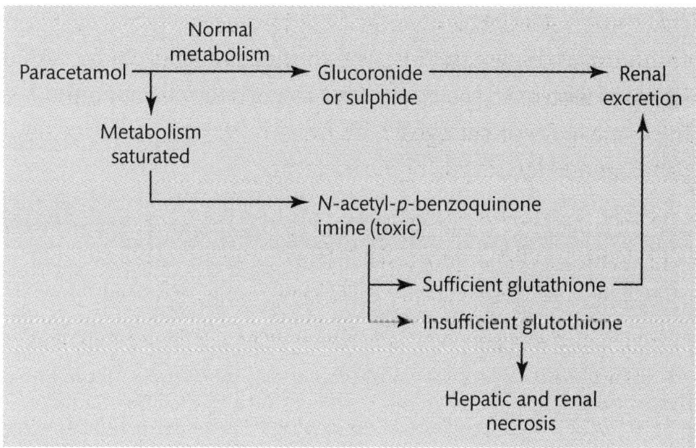

Toxicity is increased in patients who have induced liver enzymes (for instance caused by drugs such as rifampicin or carbamazepine), or in patients with reduced glutathione stores (e.g. long-term alcohol abusers). The specific antidote, *N*-acetylcysteine, acts to replenish stores of glutathione, but is effective only if given early in an overdose (efficacy decreases greatly if started more than 8 hours after the overdose is taken).

Serum paracetamol levels are only relevant at between 4 and 24 hours after the overdose. In this patient, the paracetamol level is below the 'normal' treatment line at 6 hours after the overdose is taken. However, since the patient is regularly taking an enzyme-inducing drug (carbamazepine), the lower ('high risk') treatment line should be used, and the patient should receive intravenous *N*-acetylcysteine.

This patient requires admission for an intravenous infusion of *N*-acetylcysteine and for regular monitoring. She should be monitored clinically for signs of acute liver damage (level of consciousness, evidence of bleeding, presence of right upper quadrant tenderness, encephalopathy) and have her liver biochemistry, clotting, and renal function checked regularly. Severe cases of paracetamol overdose (through a high dose taken or more commonly delay in seeking help) can cause fulminant hepatic failure requiring a liver transplant. If this patient remains well then she should not be discharged from hospital until she had been reviewed by a member of the psychiatry liaison team.

3. This patient has clinical and biochemical evidence of chronic liver disease—probably due to alcohol consumption. His acute deterioration could be down to decompensation of chronic liver disease, perhaps caused by an infection, or alcoholic hepatitis. More uncommonly an obstructive cause may be responsible.

Common sources of sepsis should be ruled out by examination and investigation. Investigations should include blood cultures, urinalysis and MSU, chest X-ray, and ascitic fluid analysis (if spontaneous bacterial peritonitis (SBP) is suspected). A liver ultrasound is of primary importance here to rule out bile duct obstruction. If there is no sign of obstruction or infection then acute alcoholic hepatitis becomes the most likely cause.

Excessive alcohol consumption (e.g. after a binge) can cause acute damage to hepatocytes, producing an alcoholic hepatitis. This presents as in this case with signs of liver failure, a tender and enlarged liver, and raised inflammatory markers. This man has grade II encephalopathy. If need be the diagnosis can be confirmed by liver biopsy (once clotting is normalized).

Supportive treatment includes managing his encephalopathy with laxatives (lactulose) and possibly a phosphate enema, to empty his bowel of nitrogen-containing material. He should be given intravenous vitamin K to bring down his INR and reduce the chances of bleeding. All alcoholics should receive intravenous vitamin supplementation (most are malnourished), and also sedation to prevent delirium tremens (to be given as required rather than regularly in this man, since he is already drowsy). Spironolactone should be withheld because of his raised potassium.

Definitive treatment for alcoholic hepatitis may include steroids—these should be started only after senior review.

Further reading

Guidelines: American Association for the Study of Liver Diseases acute liver failure guidelines (http://www.aasld.org/practiceguidelines/Documents/Practice%20Guidelines/Acuteliverfailurepg.pdf)

OHCM: 250, 258, 268, 282, 406–407, 856–857

Chronic liver disease

This section should be used for clerking patients presenting with a decompensation of chronic liver disease, for instance through infection or worsening fluid overload. Patient journeys lead from the Emergency Department through the Medical Admissions Unit to the Gastroenterology Ward.

Learning challenges

- How does nitrogenous waste from the bowel contribute both to confusion and fluid retention in patients with chronic liver disease?
- What problems are caused by portal hypertension?

History

Comment on

- Jaundice and itching
- Abdominal swelling/distension
- Haematemesis and melaena
- Risk factors including alcohol intake, risks for chronic viral hepatitis (HBV and HCV)
- Other medical conditions—especially autoimmune disease

Examination

Well or unwell? Why?

Feet to face:

Vital signs: Temperature | Blood pressure | Pulse rate | Respiratory rate | O2 saturations

Clinical clues:

Cardiovascular:

1 2 1

Respiratory:

Weight/kg

Height/m

BMI (kg/m^2)

Abdominal:

Neurological:

Other:

Comment on

- Signs of chronic liver disease
- Signs of acute and chronic encephalopathy—confusion, reduced level of consciousness and liver flap (acute), chronic cognitive impairment, constructional dyspraxia, VIth nerve palsies (chronic)
- Ascites and abdominal tenderness
- Hepatosplenomegaly
- Peripheral oedema
- Digital rectal examination: melaena?

Blood tests

Comment on

- FBC—looking for macrocytosis; WCC and differential
- Clotting and platelets
- U&Es
- Liver biochemistry
- Alpha-fetoprotein
- Relevant parts of the 'liver database'

Abdominal ultrasound

Comment on

- Cirrhosis
- Splenomegaly
- Ascites

Ascitic fluid analysis

Comment on

- White cells, organisms
- Albumin

Daily weight (to assess fluid loss–target is approximately 1 kg/24 hours)

Urinary sodium

Upper GI endoscopy

Comment on

- Varices - suitable for intervention?
- Gastritis

Stool chart (to exclude melaena, and ensure no constipation)

Evaluation

1. What are the acute medical problems faced by this patient and how should they be managed?

Ascites	Spironolactone, possibly paracentesis
Encephalopathy	Laxatives and enemas
Coagulopathy	Vitamin K, fresh frozen plasma, or platelets if bleeding
Renal failure	Meticulous fluid management
Infection	Antibiotics to cover spontaneous bacterial peritonitis

2. What is this patient's prognosis (use the Child-Pugh score below)?

	1 point	2 points	3 points
Bilirubin	<34	34–50	>50
Albumin	>35	28–35	<28
INR	<1.7	1.71–2.2	>2.2
Ascites	None	Mild	Severe
Encephalopathy	None	Grade I–II	Grade III–IV

Score 5–6: Grade A, 2-year survival 85%; **Score 7–9:** Grade B, 2-year survival 57%; **Score 10+:** Grade C, 2-year survival 35%.

Child Pugh score reference

- Child CG, Turcotte JG. Surgery and portal hypertension. In: *The liver and portal hypertension.* Edited by CG Child. Philadelphia: Saunders 1964:50–64.
- Pugh RN, Murray-Lyon IM, Dawson JL, Pietroni MC, Williams R (1973). "Transection of the oesophagus for bleeding oesophageal varices". *The British Journal of Surgery* **60**(8): 646–9.

3. What can be done long-term to control symptoms? Is the patient a candidate for liver transplant?

Questions

1. A 61-year-old woman with known chronic hepatitis C infection and cirrhosis is brought to hospital by ambulance having been discovered by her daughter drowsy and confused. She complains of worsening abdominal swelling over the previous few weeks.

On examination she is chronically unwell looking and is mildly icteric, with numerous scattered spider naevi. Asterixis is present. She has tense ascites with shifting dullness and an obvious fluid thrill. 20 ml of ascitic fluid is removed by needle aspiration; the fluid appears straw coloured but slightly cloudy. Serum electrolytes and markers of renal function are within normal ranges. The CRP is 21 mg/L and the WCC 15.6 × 10^9/L. The results of ascitic fluid analysis are below:

Appearance: slightly cloudy
Protein: 0.8 g/dL
Neutrophils: 346/mm^3, no organisms seen
Culture: pending

(1) Describe how you would manage this patient's ascites.

(2) How would you monitor the effectiveness of the treatment given?

2. You see a patient on the Medical Admissions Unit with the medical registrar. The patient, a 43-year-old merchant banker has been admitted with acute decompensation of alcoholic liver disease. He has been started on diuretics and antibiotics. After examining him, the other doctor feels that he has grade I encephalopathy and is at risk of alcohol withdrawal. He asks you to write up laxatives to manage the encephalopathy, a reducing regime of chlordiazepoxide to prevent alcohol withdrawal ('with something written up as-required as well—just in case'), and 'vitamin prophylaxis'.

Using the BNF and/or local guidelines please prescribe the necessary regime on a sample drug chart downloaded from the Online Resource Centre.

3. A 58-year-old man is referred urgently to the gastroenterology out-patient clinic with a 2-month long history of tiredness, malaise, and significant weight loss of approximately 10 kg. . There are no localizing symptoms, though physical examination reveals a mildly tender mass in the right upper quadrant, which is confirmed on ultrasound examination as arising within the liver. LFTs are as follows: bilirubin 14 µmol/L, ALP 112 IU/L, ALT 89 IU/L, albumin 39 g/L. 'Liver screen' blood tests revealed a positive hepatitis C antibody and a significantly raised alpha-fetoprotein. A contrast enhanced abdominal CT scan is arranged (shown below).

(1) What is the radiological abnormality shown?

(2) What is the likely diagnosis?

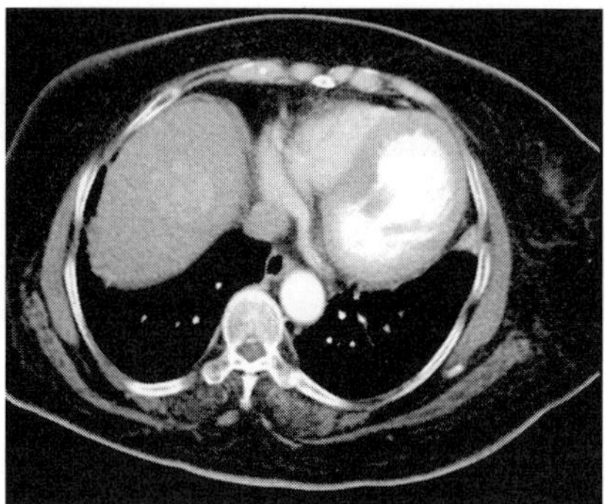

4. A 29-year-old woman of Indian origin is referred to the gastroenterology out-patient clinic after routine screening blood tests carried out at the ante-natal clinic revealed she is hepatitis B surface antigen positive. She has subsequently suffered a miscarriage. Her further blood tests are below.

(1) What do the investigation results signify?

(2) List three investigations to guide the further management.

Bilirubin: 12 µmol/L	Hepatitis B 's' antigen: POSITIVE
ALP: 123 IU/L	Hepatitis B 'e' antigen: POSITIVE
ALT: 98 IU/L	Hepatitis B anti-'e': NEGATIVE
AST: 104 IU/L	Hepatitis B DNA: 350,000 copies/mL
Albumin: 42 g/L	Full blood count normal
	Renal function normal

Remember that you can find large-size, annotated versions of many of the X-rays and ECGs that appear in this book on the book's web site at www.oxfordtextbooks.co.uk/orc/randall/

Answers

1. Cloudy ascitic fluid with a high neutrophil count (>250/mm^3) indicates spontaneous bacterial peritonitis (SBP), in this case in the context of decompensated hepatitis C liver disease. Her CRP is not as significantly raised as might be expected by her WCC and acute illness; this is due to poor synthetic function in the liver as a result of chronic liver disease. Ascitic fluid—especially with a low protein content—is a rich medium for developing bacterial infection. It often presents with a marked functional decline in a patient who is known to have advanced liver disease. The mainstay of treatment for SBP is intravenous antibiotics (according to hospital policy, often a broad-spectrum penicillin or third-generation cephalosporin), followed by life-long prophylaxis with oral antibiotics (e.g. ciprofloxacin).

Tense ascites requires urgent drainage if it is compromising respiration (by restricting the movement of the diaphragm). However, such drainage (by paracentesis, using an ascitic drain over a period of several hours) carries a significant risk of developing hypovolaemic renal failure, and intravenous human albumin solution should be given to prevent this. If there is no respiratory compromise, ascites can be treated medically. Firstly, patients are told to restrict their salt and fluid intake—to take no added salt with foods, and to drink no more that 1.5 L of water per day. The aldosterone antagonist spironolactone can also be used. This should not be given in the presence of hyperkalaemia (because it is a potassium-sparing diuretic which raises serum potassium), and serum potassium and renal function should be monitored regularly.

The effectiveness of treatment can be monitored by daily weights (aim for weight loss of 0.5–1 kg/day) and urinary sodium analysis. A high sodium:potassium ratio in the urine implies negative sodium balance and successful fluid removal from the body.

2. The in-patient management of withdrawing alcoholics can be extremely challenging—once they begin to withdraw from their alcohol excess, they often become acutely confused, agitated, and aggressive, and can suffer serious medical problems such as psychosis ('delirium tremens') and fits. Signs of alcohol withdrawal include agitation, sweating, and tremor. Chlordiazepoxide is most commonly used to control and prevent this, in a reducing regime over several days. Additional doses should be written up as-required in case of acute agitation. Since alcoholics are often malnourished, high-dose intravenous vitamins [particularly vitamin B_1 (thiamine)] are given to help prevent the development of Wernicke's encephalopathy. This man is also suffering mild hepatic encephalopathy, caused by the direct effect of products of protein breakdown on the brain (usually these would be metabolized by healthy liver tissue). Lactulose is proven to reduce symptoms by speeding up bowel transit. Accompanied by a low-protein diet, lactulose significantly improves hepatic encephalopathy. Appropriate medications for this man would include:

Drug: Chlordiazepoxide		Instructions: If alert				Signature: DR					
Start: 13/10/9	Route: O	30mg	20mg	15mg	10mg	10mg					
0800	30mg						X	X	X	X	X
1200	30mg					X	X	X	X	X	X
1800	30mg						X	X	X	X	X
2200	30mg					X	X	X	X	X	X
Drug: Pabrinex		**Instructions:**				**Signature: DR**					
Start: 13/10/9	Route: IV										
0800	I+II										
1200											
1800	I+II										
2200											

Drug: Lactulose		Instructions:				Signature: DR					
Start: 13/10/9	Route: O										
0800	15ml										
1200	15ml										
1800	15ml										
2200	15ml										

Drug: Chlordiazepoxide		Date	Time	Nurse
Dose: 20mg	Start: 13/10			
Route: O	Frequency: prn			
Indication: Agitation	Signature: DR			

3. There is a large mass in the left lobe of the liver which enhances with intravenous contrast.

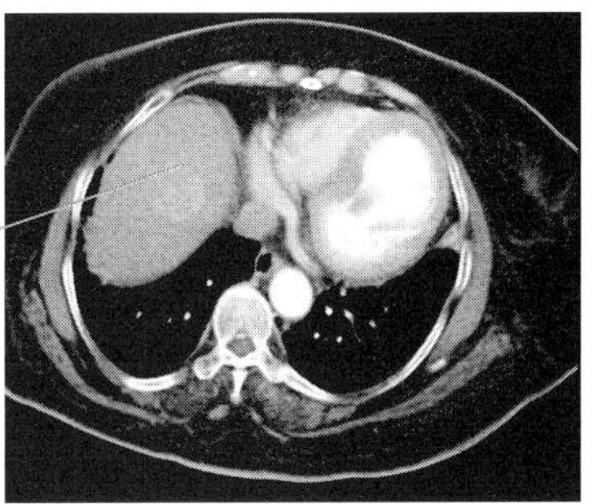

The major abnormality here is a lesion within the liver which appears hyperdense (brighter than the surrounding tissue), because the cells are metabolocally active and have taken up intravenous contrast. Note correspondingly how bright the chambers of the heart and descending aorta look; they contain blood with high concentrations of intravenous contrast.

A multiphase CT scan helps to differentiate different types of soft tissue lesions within the liver. An initial pre-contrast scan is performed, after which an intravenous contrast is given. Around 30 seconds later an arterial phase scan is performed, followed by a portal venous scan around 90 seconds post-contrast and a delayed phase scan 5–10 minutes later. Classically hepatocellular carcinomas show increased uptake in the arterial phase, which then 'washes out' by the portal venous phase.

In the developed world, the commonest kind of liver tumours seen are metastases from colon, breast, lung, or other tumours. However, worldwide, primary liver cancer or primary hepatocellular carcinoma (HCC) are common, and are is especially likely in this man since he has chronic HCV infection and a raised serum alpha-fetoprotein level, a tumour marker associated with hepatocellular carcinoma. These cancers carry a very poor prognosis. This man needs early referral to a hepatobiliary surgeon since surgical resection offers the only hope of cure.

4. Adults infected by hepatitis B often develop an acute hepatitis with raised 's' and 'e' antigens, but then clear the virus completely, developing anti-'s' antibody—the sign of immunity. Children infected by hepatitis B rarely become acutely unwell, but may often become chronically infected (with persistently raised 's' antigen). They may simply be carriers of hepatitis B ('s'-antigen positive, 'e'-antigen negative), or they may develop a chronic hepatitis (both 's'- and 'e'-antigen positive).

This woman has a chronic 'active' hepatitis, i.e. ongoing viral replication, evidenced by the 's'- and 'e'-antigen positivity; she also has viral DNA present in her blood and has raised transaminases indicating ongoing liver damage. She is at high risk of developing cirrhosis or hepatocellular carcinoma. She requires:

- alpha-fetoprotein levels (which if raised suggest HCC may be developing)
- formal ultrasound imaging of her liver
- a liver biopsy (performed under ultrasound guidance).

If there is evidence of fibrosis or active inflammation then she should be treated with a prolonged course of medication aimed at eradicating the virus, with antiviral agents and pegylated interferon. The success rate of treatment is around 40%.

Further reading

Guidelines: British Society of Gastroenterology guidelines on managing ascites in cirrhosis (http://www.bsg.org.uk/images/stories/docs/clinical/guidelines/liver/ascites_cirrhosis.pdf)

OHCM: 254, 260–271, 282, 406

Inflammatory bowel disease

This section should be used for clerking patients presenting with inflammatory bowel disease (IBD). Patients with IBD are managed in the community but may require hospital admission for exacerbations of their disease. Pathways lead from the Emergency Department to the Gastroenterology Ward, though patients with known or suspected IBD may also be encountered in the Endoscopy Unit.

Learning challenges

- How and why is ulcerative colitis linked to colorectal cancer?
- How is a capsule endoscopy carried out, and why is it especially useful in the investigation of IBD?

History

Comment on

- Diarrhoea—define normal bowel habit, change, duration, present frequency of defecation, stool consistency, offensive smell, features of steatorrhoea, blood and mucous passed rectally
- Abdominal pain—localizing or diffuse
- Weight change—'fighting weight', present weight (get them weighed), duration of change
- Other upper and lower GI symptoms including oral and perianal disease
- Systemic symptoms
- Extraintestinal manifestations

Examination

Well or unwell? Why?

Feet to face:

Vital signs: Temperature Blood pressure Pulse rate Respiratory rate O2 saturations

Clinical clues:

Cardiovascular:

1 2 1

Respiratory:

Weight/kg

Height/m

BMI (kg/m²)

Abdominal:

Neurological:

Other:

Comment on

- BMI [weight in kg/(height in m)²]
- Dentition, mouth ulcers, angular stomatitis, signs of anaemia
- Abdominal tenderness—localized versus diffuse, signs of peritonism
- Abdominal masses, fistuale, scars
- Rectum: anal fistulae
- Extraintestinal manifestations—uveitis, erythema nodosum, pyoderma gangrenosum, arthritis

Blood tests

Comment on

- Anaemia
- Signs of malabsorption—raised MCV, B12, folate and ferritin, calcium and magnesium, trace elements
- Inflammatory markers—WCC and differential, ESR, CRP

Abdominal and chest X-ray

Comment on

- Obstruction—loops of dilated small bowel
- Perforation—air under diaphragm
- Toxic dilatation (>6 cm)
- 'Featureless bowel'—with thickened walls lacking the normal indurations of normal mucosa

Stool cultures

Stool chart

Comment on

- Number/day
- Presence of blood/mucus

Sigmoidoscopy or colonoscopy

Comment on

- Macroscopic appearance
- Histology

Barium studies/CT/capsule endoscopy

Comment on

- Extent of disease

Evaluation

1. **Is there evidence of impending surgical disaster (e.g. toxic megacolon or intestinal obstruction)?**

2. **Is the flare-up improving with steroids? If not, should more powerful drugs be considered (e.g. ciclosporin)? Does the patient need to be seen by a surgeon?**

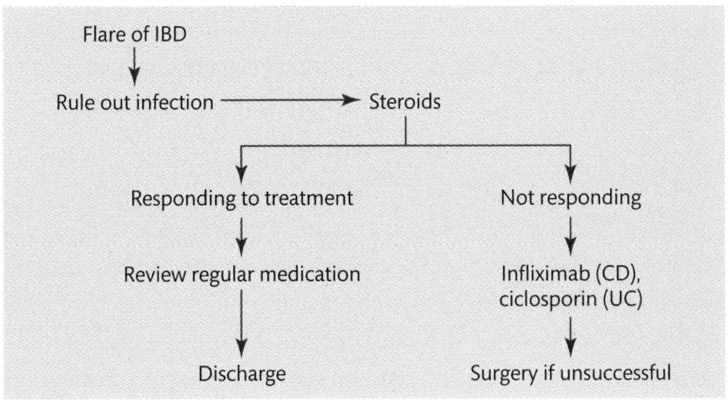

Flare of IBD
↓
Rule out infection → Steroids
↓ Responding to treatment → Review regular medication → Discharge
↓ Not responding → Infliximab (CD), ciclosporin (UC) → Surgery if unsuccessful

3. **How can remission be maintained?**

4. **Is there evidence of malabsorption? How can the patient be supported nutritionally?**

5. **Can a suitable level of remission be maintained medically? Would surgery improve quality of life?**

Questions

1. A 21-year-old man is referred to hospital by his GP complaining of a 3-week history of opening his bowels up to five times per day. The stool he passes is pale coloured, greasy (often leaving oily droplets floating on top on the water in the toilet), and is hard to flush away. There is no associated blood or mucous per rectum. He has also suffered bouts of mild to moderate, cramping central abdominal pain which comes and goes in waves. He feels he has lost weight recently as his clothes are feeling loose but he is unable to quantify this exactly. Physical examination is unremarkable.

(1) List five further questions to ask this patient regarding his presentation.

(2) List five possible differential diagnoses.

(3) List five investigations to prove the likeliest one.

2. A 45-year-old man with known ulcerative colitis presents to his local hospital with a 1-week history of passing bloody stool up to 15 times per day. He usually takes mesalazine and azathioprine to control his disease, but had stopped taking them 2 weeks earlier because he felt his symptoms were well controlled and he disliked taking regular medications.

On examination he appears unwell, has a temperature of 37.8°C, HR 110 bpm, and BP 120/76 mmHg. His abdomen is soft but diffusely tender and there is both blood and mucus in his rectum on digital examination. His CRP is 190 mg/L and ESR 75 mm in the first hour. Stool is sent for culture and an abdominal X-ray is ordered (shown below).

(1) What are the abnormalities shown?

(2) Describe your immediate and subsequent management.

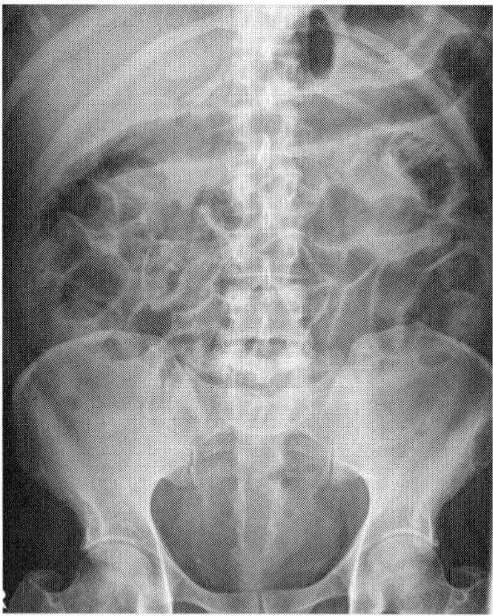

3. A 19-year-old woman presents to her GP feeling generally weak and tired. On further questioning she tells the GP that she has also had intermittent diarrhoea and generalized abdominal pain which is present on most days. The GP makes an initial diagnosis of irritable bowel syndrome and the patient is reassured and told to return in 3 months if symptoms continued.

Six weeks later she returns with no resolution of her symptoms. A routine set of blood tests is organized and the results are shown below. Referral to the local gastroenterology out-patient clinic is followed by an upper GI endoscopy. The jejunal biopsy results confirm, 'villous atrophy'.

Renal function normal	Hb: 9.2 g/dL
Liver function normal	MCV: 97.1 fL
CRP: 5 mg/L	ESR: 14 mm/hour
Tissue transglutaminase raised	

(1) Given the history and investigation results what is the likely diagnosis?

(2) Describe the further management including the lifestyle modifications you would recommend.

4. A previously fit and well 36-year-old Caucasian man, with no previous history of bowel problems, presents to the local hospital with a short history of lower abdominal pain and frequent, bloody diarrhoea. He is admitted under the gastroenterology team and the following day a colonoscopy is arranged. The endoscopy and histology reports are shown below.

Endoscopy report
The entire colon was visualized, with intubation through the ileo-caecal valve into the terminal ileum. The mucosa of the whole colon was reddened and inflamed, with contact bleeding throughout. There were areas throughout the colon of severe ulceration with islands of preserved oedematous mucosa. The rectum and anal canal are not affected but there is significant disease extending into the terminal ileum. Six biopsies taken throughout length of colon.

Histology report
Macroscopic appearance: six small sections of red mucosal tissue.
Microscopic appearance: all specimens reveal evidence of acute inflammation along with evidence of chronic inflammatory exudates. Crypt abscesses are seen along with goblet cell depletion. The inflammation appears to be confined to the mucosa. No granulomas or malignant cells are seen.

Given the above reports, what is the likely diagnosis?

5. A 31-year-old woman is admitted to hospital with severe abdominal pain and bloody diarrhoea. Subsequent endoscopy and histology confirm a new diagnosis of Crohn's disease. The disease affects predominantly her terminal ileum and ascending colon. Her symptoms respond well to a course of steroids and mesalazine, and after 5-days she is clinically ready for discharge. The registrar decides to switch her to azathioprine and to continue mesalazine. The patient asks you to explain how these two drugs work and why she needs to be monitored regularly in clinic now that her symptoms have settled.

List the essential information you would provide regarding her acute and chronic management, including the modes of actions and side-effects of her new medications.

Presentation

Presented to | Grade | Date

Signed

Answers

1. If a diagnosis of IBD is suspected, then other relevant questions to ask the patient include:
    - Has he had any symptoms of mouth disease, or anal disease?
    - Has he had any symptoms, such as rashes, skin changes, or joint pains?
    - Does he have a family history of IBD?
    - Has he travelled abroad recently? (consider tropical sprue or *Giardia* infection.)
    - Are his symptoms related to what he eats? (consider coeliac disease)

This man is describing colicky abdominal pain, steatorrhoea, and weight loss. These may be associated with Crohn's disease of the small bowel, but may be the result of any small bowel enteropathy that leads to malabsorption. Steatorrhoea describes loose stools that are pale, bulky, fatty, oily, and difficult to flush away. They are the result of malabsorption of fat in the small intestine. As well as Crohn's, other conditions that need to be excluded include **coeliac disease**, **infections**, including tropical sprue, giardiasis, and Whipple's disease, **infiltration of the small bowel**, including systemic sclerosis and lymphoma, and **bacterial overgrowth**.

Blood tests for coeliac disease should be requested since this is the main differential diagnosis. Upper and lower GI endoscopy may reveal evidence of mucosal inflammation, and allow histology to produce a firm diagnosis. If these are normal, then CT scanning may reveal bowel wall thickening and surrounding mesenteric stranding characteristic of Crohn's; however, CT appearances can be hard to interpret and have low diagnostic accuracy. Capsule endoscopy (where the patient swallows a pill containing a camera) is rapidly becoming the method of choice for searching for small intestine pathology in the presence of normal upper and lower conventional endoscopy.

2. This man is quite unwell, with symptoms and signs of an acute colitis. The abdominal X-ray shows:

The transverse colon here displays some classic features of acute colitis. The overall appearance is described as looking like a lead pipe - the mucosa is featureless and straight, there is a loss of haustrations and the bowel wall is thickened due to oedema.

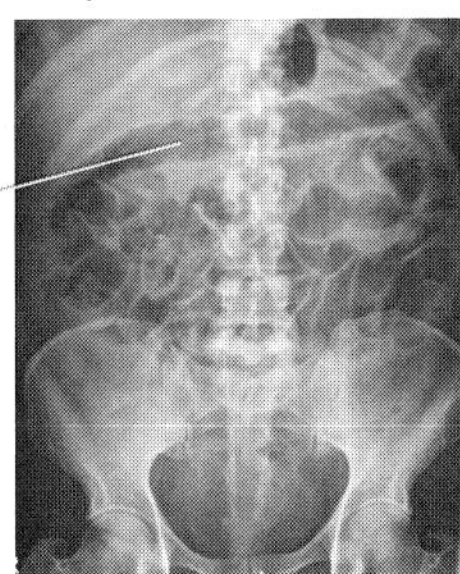

When reviewing an abdominal x-ray of a patient with acute colitis, measure the maximum diameter of the colon. Any dilatation over 5.5 cm should prompt urgent surgical review. A total colectomy is often required to prevent colonic perforation and subsequent peritonitis.

This man needs urgent treatment to avoid developing serious complications. Since he has known ulcerative colitis (and has been non-compliant with maintenance medications), steroids should be started before stool cultures are completed. He should be given an intravenous steroid (hydrocortisone) four times per day, and oral mesalazine should be restarted. He should also be given antibiotic prophylaxis (with oral metronidazole) until stool cultures are found to be negative. An erect chest X-ray should be ordered to look for air under the diaphragm, to exclude intestinal perforation. A surgical opinion should be sought to consider a partial or total colectomy. This man will require daily review, with review of his stool chart, abdominal X-ray, blood tests, and clinical examination of his abdomen. If he fails to respond to steroids then intravenous ciclosporin should be used. Failure to respond to this warrants surgery. Patients with more than eight stools per day or raised CRP > 45 mg/L after 72 hours will probably require surgical intervention.

3. This patient's symptoms may produced by IBD, but this should only be diagnosed if other more serious causes for abdominal pain and diarrhoea can be confidently excluded. In this case, raised tissue transglutaminase is a specific marker for coeliac disease, and endoscopy confirmed the classic pattern of villous atrophy in the jejunum associated with this condition.

Coeliac disease may present non-specifically with the symptoms of malabsorption and anaemia, possibly accompanied by abdominal pain and diarrhoea/steatorrhoea. A macrocytic anaemia may be seen, as a result of folate deficiency. Coeliac disease is caused by a hypersensitivity reaction to gluten, a protein found in wheat and other cereals. Inflammation in the small bowel (worse proximally than distally) leads to a loss of villi and decreased surface area for absorption of nutrients.

There is no treatment, but eating a gluten-free diet (avoiding wheat, barley, and rye), leads to resolution of symptoms. Gluten-free foods may be expensive and can be prescribed by doctors to help patients to cope with the costs.

4. Differentiating between Crohn's disease and ulcerative colitis can be difficult, and in up to 10% of cases no firm diagnosis can be made. The table below lists features distinguishing between the two conditions. The patient described in the question is likely to have severe ulcerating colitis.

Crohn's disease	Ulcerative colitis
Affects the entire GI tract, especially the terminal ileum, ascending colon, and anus. Produces areas of severe inflammation with 'skip lesions' of normal bowel in between	Affects the colon, typically sparing the rectum and working proximally from there with continuous ulceration. Severe cases can cause a 'backwash ileitis'
Produces 'cobblestone' mucosa with deep fissures, ulcers, and abscesses	Produces red, oedematous mucosa which bleeds easily
Microscopically, inflammation extends through all layers of the bowel wall. There are granulomas and possibly deep abscesses	Microscopically, inflammation is limited superficially. There are chronic inflammatory exudates with overgrowth of lymphoid tissue
Can erode into other tissues producing anal fistulae, discharging sinuses or visceral fistulae	Disease is limited to the colon and does not erode into other organs
Both diseases are associated with extra-intestinal manifestations, including an inflammatory arthritis, eyes problems including uveitis, skin problems such as pyoderma gangrenosum and erythema nodosum, liver disease including sclerosing cholangitis, and an association with deep vein thrombosis	

5. **Azathioprine** is a steroid-sparing agent that helps maintain remission in IBD that has been achieved using steroids. It avoids the side-effects of long-term steroid use such as weight gain, osteoporosis, hypertension, and diabetes. However, it can cause bone marrow suppression and so it is necessary to monitor the patient's full blood count.

Mesalazine is a 5-aminosalicylate drug. These are absorbed in the small bowel and can be toxic to the kidneys, so preparations are given (in ulcerative colitis or Crohn's disease affecting the colon) that only break down in the large bowel—either triggered by time after ingestion or by changes in pH. They suppress inflammation locally.

Patients with IBD should be cared for by a specialist multidisciplinary team, including specialist nurses, physicians and surgeons, dieticians, and others. Disease control is judged by how symptomatic the patient is, and a range of medications can be used to maintain remission. Explaining treatments to patients is essential to help improve compliance with medications. Patients with Crohn's disease (in particular) and ulcerative colitis should be encouraged to stop smoking.

Further reading

Guidelines: British Society of Gastroenterology guidelines for the management of inflammatory bowel disease (http://www.bsg.org.uk/clinical-guidelines/ibd/guidelines-for-the-management-of-inflammatory-bowel-disease-in-adults.html)

OHCM: 246, 272–277, 280–281

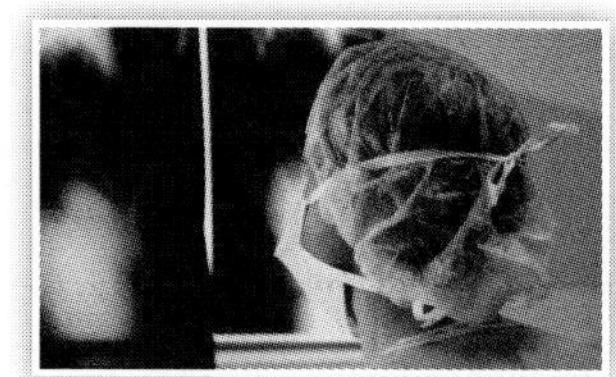
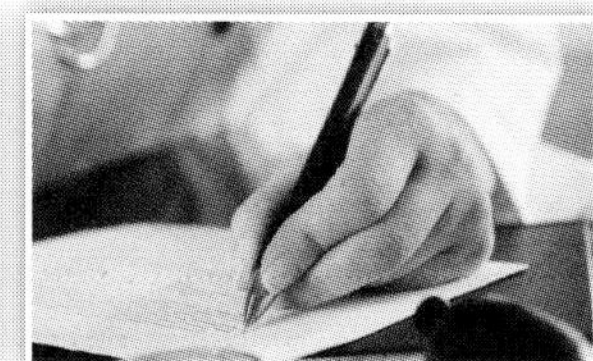
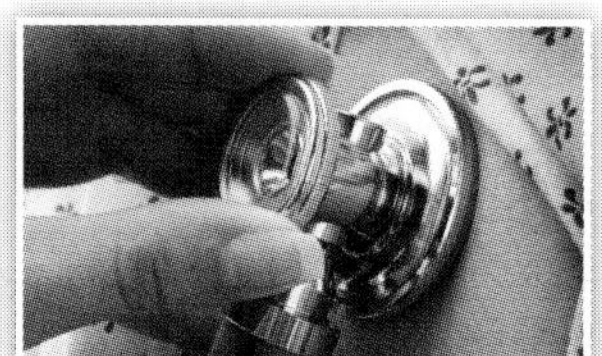
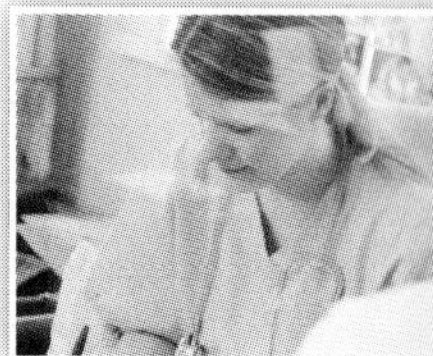

Unit 4
Renal medicine

Key learning outcomes in renal medicine include:

- Knowing and understanding the common causes of pre-renal, intrarenal, and post-renal (obstructive) kidney failure.
- Being able to take a focused history from a patient presenting with renal disease.
- Being able to examine a patient to determine whether they are hypovolaemic, euvolaemic, or fluid overloaded.
- Understanding the difference between hypertension and fluid overload, and between hypotension and hypovolaemia.
- Knowing how to interpret electrolyte, urea, creatinine, and eGFR results.
- Understanding the principles of systemic sepsis using the example of urinary sepsis.
- Recognizing the life-threatening complications of acute kidney injury.
- Understanding the indications for, and principles of, haemofiltration and haemodialysis.

Tips for learning renal medicine on the wards:

- Try to work out the likeliest causes of electrolyte, urea, and creatinine derangement in the unwell patients that you see.
- Attend rounds in high-dependency areas such as the ITU or HDU. Try to map out patients' urea and creatinine levels in response to fluid resuscitation. From their fluid balance chart, calculate fluid input and outputs. What other losses might you need to consider?
- Follow patients with multiorgan failure to ITU; what features of their condition might require them to have haemofiltration?
- Visit the local dialysis unit. Talk to patients about their experiences of dialysis or being on a transplant list, and talk to doctors and nurses about the science behind dialysis.

History

At presentation to healthcare professionals, renal patients are often asymptomatic, or have vague, non-specific symptoms of ill-health. The medical history is therefore particularly important in elucidating the likeliest cause(s) and risk factors for their renal disease. In this section, learn how to ask the relevant questions about:

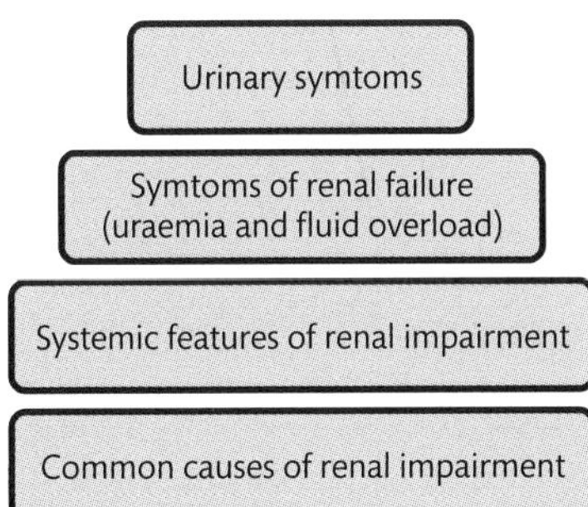

1. Urinary symptoms

Sometimes referred to as lower urinary tract symptoms or LUTS, ask carefully about the nature of the symptoms the patient describes, suggesting either a diagnosis of 'irritant LUTS' (commonly caused by urinary tract infection) or 'obstructive LUTS' (commonly caused by bladder outflow tract obstruction):

Irritant LUTS	Obstructive LUTS
Dysuria (pain on passing urine) Increased **frequency** of micturition **Nocturia** (needing to wake in the night to pass urine) **Haematuria** **Urgency** (sudden strong desire to micturate) **Incontinence** (especially in the elderly)	**Frequency** (with small volumes of urine passed) **Nocturia** **Hesitancy** (reduced ability to initiate micturition) **Straining** to initiate micturition **Poor stream** **Terminal dribbling** (inability to stop urinating) **Acute retention**

Irritant LUTS may be accompanied by symptoms of systemic response to infection—for instance **fevers**, **sweats**, **rigors**, or **vomiting**. There may be suprapubic pain in cystitis or loin pain if the infection has ascended to the kidney (pyelonephritis). **Key investigations** include urine dipstick, inflammatory markers, and urine microscopy, culture, and sensitivities.

Obstructive LUTS suggests outflow obstruction to the bladder, with the most common cause being prostate disease in men. Reduced appetite, weight loss, and the presence of bony pain may suggest a diagnosis of prostate cancer, though benign prostatic enlargement is just as common. **Key investigations** include urine dipstick, cultures, radiological imaging (primarily ultrasound scanning) of the renal tract (including ureters and bladder), and in men, prostatic investigation including digital rectal examination, PSA, and prostate biopsy (if appropriate)

2. Symptoms of renal failure (uraemia and fluid overload)

These are often vague and not specific to renal disease. They may be divided into:

- **Symptoms of uraemia:** Malaise, anorexia, insomnia, itching, nausea and vomiting, drowsiness, confusion, restlessness, paresthesia from polyneuropathy, intractable hiccups
- **Symptoms of fluid overload and dysregulation:** Ankle/leg/genital/abdominal swelling from oedema and ascites, breathlessness from pulmonary oedema and pleural effusions, nocturia and incontinence from a reduced ability to concentrate urine

3. Systemic features of renal failure

- **Symptoms of anaemia:** Breathlessness, reduced exercise tolerance, dizziness
- **Symptoms of bone disease:** Joint aches and bony pain, paraesthesia and tetany from hypocalcaemia

4. Common causes of renal failure

<table>
<tr><th>Pre-renal</th><th>Renal</th><th>Obstructive</th></tr>
<tr><td>Hypotension or intravascular depletion, i.e. poor renal perfusion
Renal artery stenosis, particularly coupled to use of an ACE inhibitor or angiotensin-2 receptor antagonist</td><td>• Acute tubular necrosis secondary to significant hypovolaemia or hypotension.
• Glomerulonephritis—causes include:
Infections, e.g. streptococcal, malaria, meningitis
IgA nephropathy
Malignancy—lung, breast, myeloma
Systemic vasculitides—SLE
Systemic sclerosis
• Acute and chronic pyelonephritis (reflux nephropathy)
• Metabolic—diabetic renal disease; nephrocalcinosis (any cause of chronic hypercalcaemia)
• Tubulo-interstitial nephritis (TIN)—acute (antibiotic and NSAIDs) and chronic (sickle cell disease, NSAIDs)
• Congenital disease—polycystic kidney disease
• Renal carcinoma
• 'Myeloma kidney'—there are five causes of renal failure associated with myeloma and it is therefore common in undergraduate examinations! The causes are tubular obstruction by the light chains, increased infections and dehydration, nephrocalcinosis, glomerulonephritis, and amyloidosis
• Infiltrative—amyloidosis</td><td>Stones—renal and bladder
Benign and malignant tumours
Strictures
Foreign bodies
Extrinsic compression, e.g. retroperitoneal fibrosis</td></tr>
<tr><td>Ask about:
Acute illness
Vascular disease
ACE inhibitors</td><td>Ask about:
Any systemic disease
Diabetes, hypertension, other vascular risk factors
Medications—antibiotics, NSAIDS, reno-active drugs
Family history
Previous UTIs</td><td>Ask about:
Abdominal pain
Haematuria
LUTS
Weight loss, general health</td></tr>
</table>

Examination

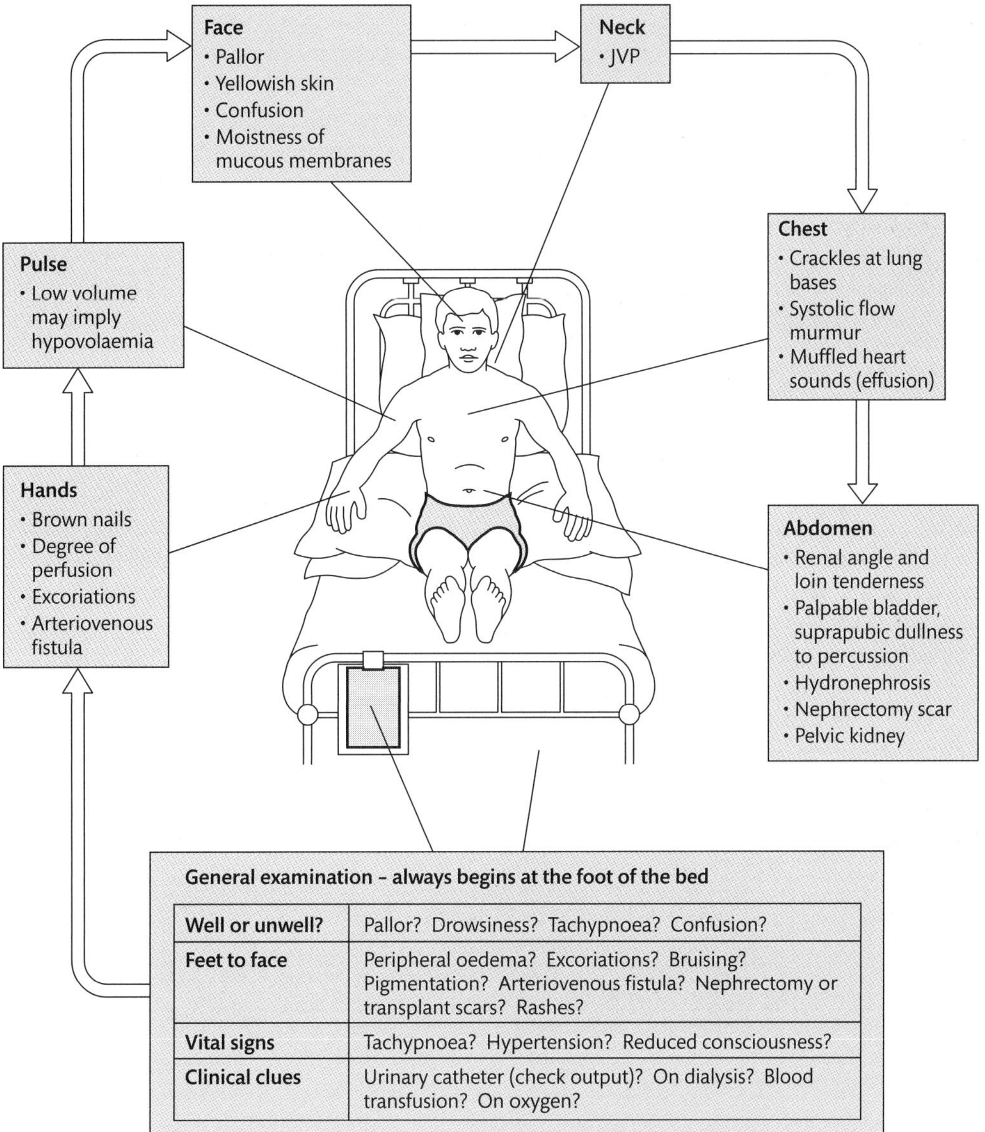

General examination – always begins at the foot of the bed

Well or unwell?	Pallor? Drowsiness? Tachypnoea? Confusion?
Feet to face	Peripheral oedema? Excoriations? Bruising? Pigmentation? Arteriovenous fistula? Nephrectomy or transplant scars? Rashes?
Vital signs	Tachypnoea? Hypertension? Reduced consciousness?
Clinical clues	Urinary catheter (check output)? On dialysis? Blood transfusion? On oxygen?

Estimating a patient's fluid status

This can be very clinically challenging! Patients who are seriously ill and grossly oedematous may also commonly be intravascularly fluid depleted. Thus the aim of therapy is to 'revascularize' some of the fluid, so improving their renal perfusion pressure and in turn their renal function. With poor perfusion pressure (as with intravascular depletion) the addition of diuretics to improve urine output may paradoxically make things worse.

Essential clinical clues suggesting a diagnosis of either dehydration or fluid overload include:

Signs of dehydration	Signs of overload
Cool peripheries Hypotension (if severe), postural hypotension Capillary refill time >2 seconds Reduced skin turgor Sunken eyes Dry mucous membranes Axillary dryness Reduced urine output (<0.5 ml/kg/hour)	Peripheral, genital, sacral, and abdominal wall oedema and ascites (not always reliable) Raised JVP Third heart sound Systolic flow murmur Crackles at lung bases Urine output may be normal or reduced

Because fluid status in the very sick patient is often (1) difficult and (2) essential to determine, invasive monitoring is commonly required. Initially a urinary catheter should be inserted to allow hourly monitoring of urine output. A close record of all fluid input and output (including oral fluids and other fluid output '**insensible losses**', e.g. vomiting, stomas, or drains) should be kept. The aim of fluid resuscitation should be to maintain a systolic blood pressure >100 mmHg, HR <100 bpm, and urine output >0.5 ml/kg/hour.

Placement of a central venous catheter into a central vein such as the internal jugular vein (usually performed under ultrasound guidance), allows objective measurement of the **central venous pressure** (**CVP**)—effectively, the pressure in the right atrium. Patients with CVP lines *in situ* should be managed in a high-dependency area, for instance the ICU.

- **Normal CVP** is 5–10 cmH_2O
- **Low CVP** indicates dehydration—boluses of fluid should be given until the CVP is maintained in the normal range.
- **High CVP** indicates fluid overload—if the patient is symptomatic (e.g. in pulmonary oedema) then treatment with nitrates and diuretics may be indicated.

Signs of renal replacement therapy

- **Dialysis:** If this is required acutely (for instance, in acute kidney injury or in chronic kidney disease where there was inadequate time to prepare an AV fistula), dialysis is usually preformed using a **central venous catheter** inserted into the internal jugular vein. If a patient with chronic kidney disease has been adequately prepared for starting dialysis then they will usually have an AV fistula created by anastomosing an artery and vein in the forearm, usually several months before starting dialysis. This is felt as a thickened, rubbery, pulsatile subcutaneous tube on the palmar surface of the forearm.
- **Transplant:** Donor kidneys are transplanted into the pelvis and anastomosed to the iliac vessels. They are felt as a mass with an overlying scar, usually in the right iliac fossa. The need for long-term immunosuppression may lead to the development of skin cancers or pre-malignant growths.

Investigations

Urea, creatinine, and the eGFR

Urea and **creatinine**, both products of protein breakdown, are excreted by the kidney and therefore rise in renal failure. Levels of both are also dependent on the level of protein catabolism in the body, thus levels of urea will rise after a high-protein meal. Creatinine is a reflection of muscle mass within the body, thus normal levels of creatinine will be much higher in a young man with large muscle bulk than in a frail, elderly woman.

The **GFR** (glomerular filtration rate, measured in mL/minute) is the amount of fluid filtered by the glomeruli in the kidneys. It is the most accurate measurement of renal function. Since it is very difficult to calculate directly, an estimated GFR or '**eGFR**' is usually used. This is calculated using the patient's serum creatinine level, weight, and sex. Renal function in patients with chronic kidney disease can be monitored by eGFR.

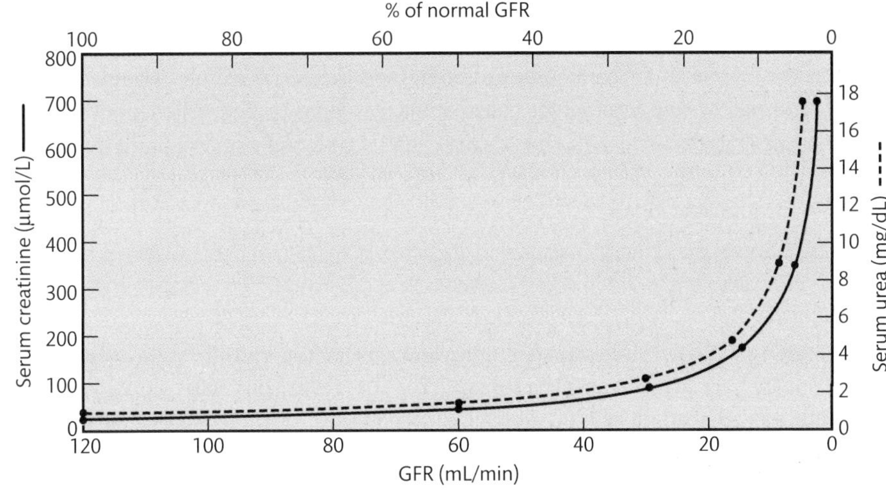

The importance of using the eGFR in calculations of renal function is shown by the graph above. Almost 50% of renal function (measured by eGFR) can be lost before the serum urea and creatinine rise above normal levels. Therefore relying only on urea and creatinine levels prevents early intervention to slow the decline in renal function.

Many hospital laboratories calculate eGFR and list it as part of the blood results they release.

Analysis of urine

Urine dipstick analysis

This is a widely available, useful, and cheap test of the urine. Key components include:

- **Nitrites** and **leucocytes**—especially if both are present; these are highly suggestive of a urinary tract infection. Nitrites are derived from nitrates, catalysed by enzymes produced by certain bacteria, e.g. *E. coli*. The absence of nitrites does not exclude bacterial infection, just the absence of these nitrate-converting organisms. In the absence of any other features of infection, leucocytes indicate inflammatory conditions, e.g. renal stones. This is known as **sterile pyuria**.
- **Protein (proteinuria)** in the urine may also be seen in infection but is a significant feature of kidney disease affecting the glomeruli. If positive on dipstick testing it should be quantified either by 24-hour protein collection or by measuring the protein:creatinine ratio in the urine. **Microalbuminuria** is also assessed and quantified in diabetic patients to monitor the development of diabetic nephropathy.
- **Blood (haematuria)** is most commonly caused by infection, stones, or urinary tract malignancy. False positives are commonly caused by menstruation in women. Haematuria requires follow-up. In acute kidney injury, haematuria may indicate glomerulonephritis.
- **Glucose (glycosuria)** is present in the urine once tubular reabsorption mechanisms are saturated—usually once the serum glucose level is significantly raised. All such patients should have diabetes mellitus excluded.
- **Ketones** are found in the urine of normal non-diabetics in significant dehydration or fasting. High levels of ketones are found in type 1 diabetics in acute diabetic ketoacidosis and require urgent attention.

Other urinary testing should include **urinary culture and sensitivities** looking for the causative organism of a urinary tract infection, and **microscopy**. This may reveal: **pus cells** (supportive evidence for infection), **malignant cells** (in urological malignancies), or **casts** of collecting ducts in the kidney: **red cell casts** indicate intrinsic renal damage, e.g. glomerulonephritis, **white cell casts** may indicate pyelonephritis, and **granular casts** are caused by proteinuria of any cause.

Distinguishing between acute kidney injury and chronic kidney disease

Patients being admitted to hospital often have abnormal renal function (low eGFR or raised urea or creatinine). An important question to ask is whether this is **acute kidney injury**, **chronic kidney disease**, or **acute-on-chronic kidney disease**. This may be obvious, for instance if previous blood results from the patient are available showing normal or abnormal values from months or years previously. As with most parameters we measure in medicine, trends are often more important than absolute numbers. Has this been a slow insidious deterioration or is this a catastrophic acute event?

If no previous results are available then the following tests may all be useful in suggesting whether kidney disease is acute or chronic. The tests listed may obviously be deranged for other reasons in the seriously ill patient, and these are only a guide.

	Acute kidney injury	Chronic kidney disease
Hb and MCV	Normal	Normocytic anaemia
Sodium	Normal	Low
Potassium	HIgh	High end of normal range or lower limit of high range
Bicarbonate	Normal	Low
pH	Normal or low	Low
Albumin	Normal	Low
Calcium	Normal	Low
Phosphate	Normal	High
Renal ultrasound	Normal size kidneys (or enlarged if obstructed)	Shrunken kidneys (or enlarged if obstructed or polycystic)

Tests for glomerulonephritis

This section is complex—only a basic understanding is required at undergraduate level. Kidney failure may be pre-renal (caused by inadequate renal blood flow), intrarenal, or post-renal (caused by obstruction for urinary flow). The intrarenal causes are often complex and a fuller list of causes is provided earlier, in the 'History' section of this unit introduction. A major group of causes of intrarenal kidney failure is **glomerulonephritis**—immune-driven damage to the glomeruli which may present with kidney failure or the nephrotic syndrome. If a glomerulonephritis is suspected, it can only be confirmed by microscopy after **renal biopsy**, when a specific histological diagnosis can be made (for instance, crescentic or minimal-change glomerulonephritis). The following tests are performed to help elicit the specific cause—in each case these are tests for complex, multisystem diseases that often involve the kidney.

Complement protein (C3 and C4)	Associated with immune complex deposition and glomerulonephritis of any cause
Antinuclear antibody (ANA), antidouble-stranded DNA and antiextractable nuclear antigen (ENA)	Markers of systemic lupus erythematosus (SLE)
Antineutrophil cytoplasmic antibodies (ANCA)	Vasculitic conditions such as Wegener's granulomatosis (cANCA) or polyarteritis nodosa (pANCA)
Antiglomerular basement membrane (anti-GBM) antibody	Goodpasture's syndrome—associated with renal dysfunction and pulmonary haemorrhage
Cryoglobulins	Raised in cryoglobulinaemia
Antistreptolysin-O titre	Post-streptococcal nephritis
Hepatitis B and C, and HIV serology	Can cause cryoglobulinaemia or immune complex deposition

Interventions

Drugs causing or worsening kidney failure

Pre-renal kidney failure is caused by poor renal perfusion–this is usually as a result of **dehydration** (causing **hypovolaemia**) or **hypotension**. Drugs often to blame in pre-renal kidney failure include:

- **Diuretics**, e.g. furosemide–these may cause significant dehydration and hypovolaemia and are commonly prescribed in the elderly for heart failure.
- Any **anti-hypertensive medications**–e.g. beta-blockers or calcium-channel blockers, in overdose. This is especially the case if a patient on antihypertensives becomes unwell, for instance develops sepsis. Patients being admitted with sepsis should usually have the antihypertensives withheld whilst they are acutely unwell.
- **ACE inhibitors**, as well as potentiating hypotension along with other antihypertensives, they may also cause dramatic worsening of renal function in patients with bilateral renal artery stenosis.

Intrarenal kidney failure can be caused by several mechanisms including chronic and acute tubulo-interstitial nephritis, acute tubular necrosis, or glomerulonephritis. Culprit drugs include:

- **Antibiotics**, particularly aminoglycosides (e.g. gentamicin) and penicillins.
- **NSAIDs**
- **Heavy metals**, e.g. gold which can be used to treat rheumatoid arthritis

Post-renal kidney failure caused by drugs is very rare, but some drugs may cause retroperitoneal fibrosis and others may contribute to stone formation: both processes that can lead to ureteric obstruction.

Prescribing in kidney failure

Most drugs are excreted, eventually, by the kidneys. Poor renal function may reduce clearance of these drugs, leading to increased (possibly toxic) concentrations in the blood. This is a particular problem with drugs (such as gentamicin, digoxin, or phenytoin) which have narrow therapeutic windows, with toxic effects occurring at levels only slightly above therapeutic levels. Kidney failure may also have other complex effects on drug levels, for instance the kidneys have a role in direct catabolism of insulin, meaning that diabetics who develop significant kidney failure require less insulin than previously. Strategies for prescribing safely in kidney failure include:

- Consulting formularies, e.g. Appendix 3 of the BNF which deals with kidney failure
- Only prescribing drugs which are absolutely necessary
- Monitoring drug levels where possible, e.g. gentamicin
- Reducing doses
- Monitoring for toxic side-effects

Common medications in renal medicine and affecting the kidney

Class	Examples	Mechanism	Indications	Contraindications	Side-effects	Special notes
Loop diuretics						
Thiazide diuretics						
Potassium-sparing diuretics						
ACE inhibitors and Angiotensin-2 receptor antagonists						
Beta-blockers						
Calcium-channel antagonists						
Statins						
Vitamin D						
Calcium supplementation						
Erythropoietin						
Sodium bicarbonate						
Aminoglycosides						
Trimethoprim						
Penicillins						
NSAIDs						
Gold preparations						

Acute kidney injury

This section should be used to clerk patients with acute kidney injury, developing in previously well patients who suffer an acute renal insult or in patients with known renal disease (acute-on-chronic disease). It may complicate the admission of patients on any ward, medical, surgical, or obstetric, with patients with severe disease possibly being managed on the ICU or dialysis units.

Learning challenges

- What is acute tubular necrosis, what is the natural course of this process, and why does this justify intensive care treatment even for extremely severe renal failure?
- What processes actually lead to death in acute kidney injury?

History

Comment on

- Irritant lower urinary tract symptoms
- Obstructive lower urinary tract symptoms
- Systemic features of uraemia
- PMHx—known vascular disease, systemic vasculitides, hypertension, diabetes mellitus
- Medications—NSAIDS, reno-active medications, e.g. ACE inhibitors or diuretics
- SHx—smoking, occupation, e.g. worker in the dye industry (bladder TCC)

Examination

Well or unwell? Why?

Feet to face:

Vital signs: Temperature | Blood pressure | Pulse rate | Respiratory rate | O2 saturations

Clinical clues:

Cardiovascular:

1 2 1

Respiratory:

Abdominal:

Neurological:

Other:

Comment on

- Vital signs—BP (hyper- and hypotension), HR, CBG, temperature, oxygen sats and RR, GCS
- Fluid status: (1) signs of fluid overload—pulmonary oedema, peripheral oedema, ascites, raised JVP; (2) signs of fluid depletion/hypovolaemia—hypotension including postural hypotension, dry mucous membranes
- Signs of uraemia
- Signs of chronic renal impairment and renal replacement therapy
- Abdomen—scars secondary to renal or bladder operations, indwelling catheter (urethral or suprapubic), renal masses

Fluid balance

Comment on

- Urine output (mL/hour), other fluid losses
- Fluid intake: IV and oral

Urine analysis (if passing urine)

Comment on

- Urinary protein:creatinine ratio
- Red cell casts (intrinsic renal damage), bacteria, white cells

Blood tests

Comment on

- Urea and creatinine
- Potassium—hyperkalaemia
- Evidence of infection
- 'Renal screen' including CBG, albumin, ESR, vasculitic screen

Ultrasound kidneys/ureters/bladder

Comment on

- Size of kidneys
- Evidence of obstruction

Arterial blood gas

Comment on

- Metabolic acidosis

Chest X-ray

Comment on

- Presence of fluid overload

ECG

Comment on

- Evidence of hyperkalaemia

Renal biopsy: undertaken principally in renal centres (i.e. not on general wards)

Evaluation

1. In the context of rising urea and creatinine, is there evidence of any of the following emergency complications developing? Are they being managed appropriately?

Complication	Assessment	Initial management
Hyperkalaemia	Serum K^+, peaked T waves on ECG	Calcium gluconate, insulin, salbutamol, ion-exchange resins
Pulmonary oedema	Basal crepitations, fluid overload on chest X-ray	Careful fluid balance, cautious diuretics
Acidosis	Arterial blood gas—reduced pH, low pCO_2 and HCO_3^-	Ensuring good renal perfusion
Uraemia	Serum urea, drowsiness	Ensuring good renal perfusion
Sepsis	Pyrexia, raised CRP and WCC	Antibiotics—but beware toxicity

2. Is this likely to be due to pre-renal causes, intrinsic renal disease, or post-renal causes?

3. How much fluid does the patient need (= total fluid output + 500 ml for insensible losses over a 24-h period)?

4. Are the above complications improving with standard initial management? If not, would the patient benefit from haemofiltration or dialysis on the intensive care unit?

5. Review the patient's drug chart. Do any of the patient's current medications worsen renal failure? Should doses be reduced of any others that are renally excreted?

Questions

1. A 78-year-old man is recovering 6 days after a right hemiarthroplasty following a fractured neck of femur. Two days earlier the patient had been drowsy and pyrexial on the morning ward round and had been prescribed intravenous antibiotics for a suspected urinary tract infection. His routine blood tests this morning reveal Na^+ 139 mmol/L, K^+ 5.2 mmol/L, urea 21.4 mmol/L, creatinine 215 μmol/L, all of which had been within normal ranges on admission. His observation chart is shown below. His fluid chart is unavailable. His current medications include bendroflumethiazide 2.5 mg od, amlodipine 5 mg od, tamsulosin 400 μg od, gentamicin 300 mg od, and diclofenac 50 mg tds. On examination he is drowsy, with basic observations including temperature 37.2°C, HR 120 bpm regular, BP 130/87 mmHg. Physical examination is otherwise unremarkable, other than some tenderness and dullness to percussion over the suprapubic region. His surgical wound appears clean.

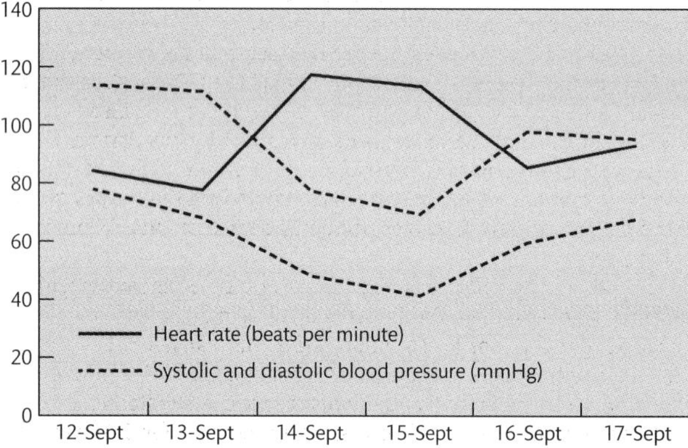

(1) List five possible causes of renal impairment in this case, and divide them according to whether they are pre-renal, intrarenal, or post-renal.

(2) List five important steps in the management of this patient.

2. A 64-year-old woman is admitted to hospital following a fall and subsequent 'long lie' on the floor. She was unable to get up after having tripped over her cat, and so lay on her left side for over 12 hours, before being found by her daughter the next day. On admission she is clinically septic. She is vasodilated and hot to the touch, her temperature is 39.8°C and HR 120 bpm regular, blood pressure 89/56 mmHg. She is clinically dehydrated.

Routine blood tests reveal

- FBC: Hb 12.9 g/dL, MCV 88 fL, WCC 15.9 × 10^9/L (neutrophils 12.6 × 10^9/L), platelets 222 × 10^9/L
- U&Es: Na^+ 154 mmol/L, K^+ 5.3 mmol/L, urea 28.3 mmol/L, creatinine 431 μmol/L
- CBG: 5.9 mmol/L
- CK: 21,087 IU/L

She is started on intravenous antibiotics and is given several litres of fluids to normalize her blood pressure. An indwelling catheter is sited and she is admitted to the acute care of the elderly ward.

The next morning the biochemist rings to tell you that her repeat serum potassium is 7.2 mmol/L (normal 3.5–5). You ask for an ECG which is shown below.

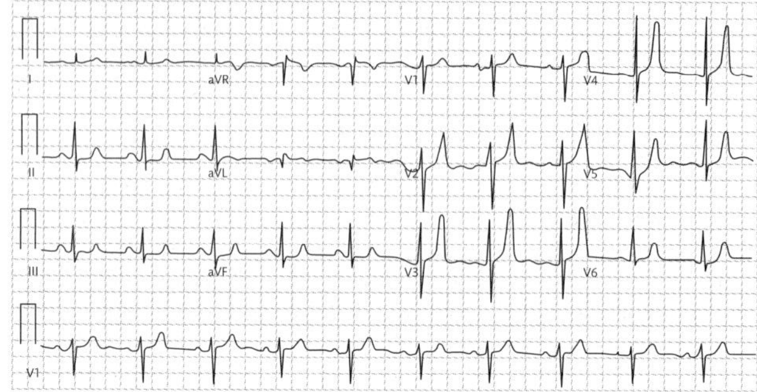

(1) What are the contributing causes to her acute kidney injury?

(2) What does the ECG show?

(3) List five essential management steps.

3. A 45-year-old man is admitted to hospital after complaining to his GP of a 2-week history of increasing swelling of his lower limbs. Initially the swelling just affected his ankles, but now affects both lower limbs and his genitalia as well.

On examination he is relatively well looking but short of breath at rest. Pulse 100 bpm regular, BP 140/79 mmHg, temperature 37.0°C, oxygen sats 96% on room air. On examination of his cardiovascular system his JVP is raised to the angle of the jaw, auscultation of the heart is unremarkable, and there is marked pitting oedema of the lower limbs, genitalia, lower anterior abdominal wall, and sacral pad.

Initial investigations revealed heavy proteinuria (4+) on urine dipstick analysis, urea 12.5 mmol/L, creatinine 134 μmol/L, total blood cholesterol 7.8 mmol/L, and a serum albumin of 12 g/L.

(1) What syndrome has this man developed?

(2) What are the common causes of this syndrome in a man of this age?

(3) List five further investigations to confirm the diagnosis and the underlying cause.

Presentation

Presented to ______ Grade ______ Date ______

Signed

Answers

1. In clinical practice it is common for patients to present with a number of factors contributing to the development of acute kidney injury. The patient's management should consider and address all of these factors. They should receive careful monitoring to ensure their renal function improves and serious complications do not develop.

Pre-renal causes	Intrarenal causes	Post-renal causes
The observations chart reveals a period of **prolonged hypotension**, which will have led to hypoperfusion of the kidneys. This will have been caused by systemic vasodilatation (as a result of sepsis), the patient's antihypertensive medications (which should have been stopped), and **dehydration**, caused by reduced oral intake (as a result of being drowsy) and increased losses (sweat)	Both **gentamicin** and **diclofenac** (a non-steroidal anti-inflammatory drug) are directly nephrotoxic. Another potential intrarenal cause of this man's kidney injury is **acute tubular necrosis**. This is a destruction of the kidney tubules brought about by prolonged hypotension (there are also other causes, including several commonly used drugs). If it develops it can take several weeks to resolve even in the presence of adequate blood pressure	Clinically this man has developed **urinary retention**, evidenced by the suprapubic tenderness and dullness to percussion. Bladder outflow tract obstruction is more likely in this man as he is already on tamsulosin (used in benign prostatic hypertrophy) and he has undergone hip surgery (which is a recognized cause of urinary retention)

Key management priorities include:

- Catheterization—to relieve urinary obstruction and allow monitoring of urine output
- Stopping antihypertensive medications
- Stop diclofenac—find an alternative analgesic if required. Check gentamicin levels and reduce or omit doses if levels are high
- Adequate intravenous fluid resuscitation to maintain a systolic BP >100 mmHg and a urine output of >0.5 ml/kg/hour
- Hourly monitoring of urine output and basic observations, daily monitoring of U&Es

2. This patient's acute kidney injury is due to (1) prolonged poor renal perfusion, secondary to systemic hypotension caused by sepsis, (2) the resultant **acute tubular necrosis**, and (3) renal tubular obstruction as a result of the **rhabdomyolysis**. The 'long lie' on the floor has caused a crush injury to her muscles, resulting in the release of myoglobins. These collect in the tubules and cause an obstructive nephropathy. Intravenous fluid resuscitation is normally enough to 'unblock' the tubules, but severe cases may require renal replacement therapy.

This ECG displays features of hyperkalaemia:

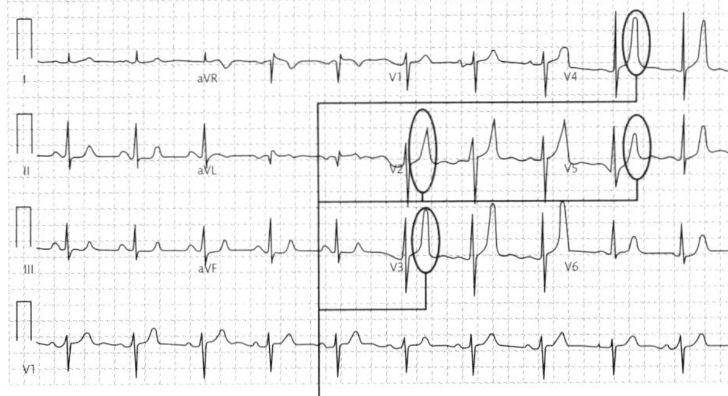

Note the tall 'peaked' T waves seen here in the anterior leads. This is an early sign of hyperkalaemia on the ECG.

Other sinister, late signs on ECG (which precede a life-threatening arrhythmia) include prolongation of the PR interval, flattening of the P waves, broad QRS complexes and eventually a 'sine wave' appearance with loss of constituent parts of the normal ECG.

Hyperkalaemia is a potentially life-threatening complication of acute kidney injury. It causes life-threatening ventricular dysrhythmias such as ventricular fibrillation and asystole. Calcium gluconate should be given immediately to stabilize the heart and decrease the likelihood of a dysrhythmia. The next priority is to decrease potassium concentrations. Both **intravenous insulin** (which must be given with 50% dextrose to prevent hypoglycaemia) and **nebulized salbutamol** have the effect of causing potassium to enter cells from the bloodstream, thus reducing serum concentrations but not total body potassium. Ion exchange resins (e.g. **calcium resonium**) work in the gut to remove excess potassium from the body; however, their action is slow and they can only be used to prevent further hyperkalaemia rather than treat it if it already exists. The effects of insulin and other medications are short lived, and administration may need to be repeated several times before safe potassium levels are maintained. 'Resistant' hyperkalaemia is one of the indications for acute dialysis therapy. Others include severe metabolic acidosis, fluid overload, acute renal impairment associated with poorly resolving diabetic ketoacidosis, and acute drug overdose, e.g. severe salicylate overdose.

3. This patient has developed the **nephrotic syndrome**. This is defined by the triad of **hypoalbuminaemia**, **heavy proteinuria** (3–5 g in 24 hours), and **gross peripheral oedema**. It is associated with a high serum cholesterol, and carries a high risk of venous thromboembolism, e.g. renal vein thrombosis.

The nephrotic syndrome is caused by disease of the glomerulus, the part of each nephron that initially filters blood. Damage to these makes them very leaky, so large amounts of protein are passed into the urine. Low plasma osmotic pressure (caused by low plasma protein concentrations) leads to oedema, intravascular fluid depletion, and fluid retention. Renal clearance of urea and creatinine, as well as of potassium, may be preserved, though a degree of renal failure is often also seen.

The nephrotic syndrome is often caused by a glomerulonephritis, which can be described histologically on renal biopsy. A range of blood tests can look for common causes, for instance SLE (ANA and antidouble-stranded DNA), vasculitis (ANCA), immune complexes (C3), hepatitis B and C viruses, group A *Streptococcus* (antistreptolysin-O titre) or Goodpasture's syndrome (antiglomerular basement membrane antibody) . Other common causes of the nephrotic syndrome include diabetes and drugs, such as those containing heavy metals, e.g. gold therapy in rheumatoid arthritis.

This man needs fluid restriction (e.g. 1 L of drinking water per day, or water equivalent to the previous day's urine output + 500 mL) and a high-protein diet. Diuretics can be helpful in trying to cause excretion of additional fluid. Protein loss should be quantified—either by 24-hour protein concentration or by urine protein:creatinine ratio. A kidney biopsy is likely to be needed to determine the precise diagnosis so that definitive treatment can be initiated.

Further reading

Guidelines: The Renal Association acute kidney injury guidelines (http://www.renal.org/clinical/GuidelinesSection/AcuteKidneyInjury.aspx)

OHCM: 294–299, 303, 306–307, 644, 682, 688, 848

Chronic kidney disease

This section should be used to evaluate patients with chronic impairment of kidney function. These patients, like patients with any chronic disease, are managed in the community, only being admitted to hospital acutely with exacerbations or complications. They may be found on the Renal Ward, in the nephrology out-patient clinic, or in large numbers on dialysis units.

Learning challenges

- List as many functions of the kidney as you can. Does this help you to understand the problems caused in chronic kidney disease?
- What ethical issues surround organ donation from living donors? What are heart-beating and non-heart-beating cadaveric organ donors, and how are organs harvested from them?

History

Comment on

- Symptoms of renal tract disease, haematuria, dysuria, symptoms of outflow tract obstruction
- Symptoms of fluid overload, oliguria/anuria.
- Known renal disease or impairment
- Significant previous medical conditions—diabetes mellitus, hypertension, IHD, systemic vasculitides (SLE, systemic sclerosis, Wegener's granulomatosis)
- Drug history—NSAIDs, antibiotics, diuretics, ACE inhibitors and angiotensin-2 receptor blockers, gold therapy
- Family history of renal disease

Examination

Well or unwell? Why?

Feet to face:

Vital signs: Temperature Blood pressure Pulse rate Respiratory rate O2 saturations

Clinical clues:

Cardiovascular:

1 2 1

Respiratory:

Abdominal:

o

Neurological:

Other:

Comment on

- Signs of chronic renal impairment and uraemia
- Pallor
- Stigmata of renal replacement therapy—AV fistula, scars from insertion of venous access, peritoneal dialysis catheter, transplanted pelvic kidney
- Fluid status
- Blood pressure and glycaemic control

Urine dipstick

Comment on

- Proteinuria
- Haematuria

Urine analysis

Comment on

- Urinary protein:creatinine ratio
- Presence of red cell casts, inflammatory cells, bacteria

Renal ultrasound

Comment on

- Size of kidneys
- Evidence of obstruction
- Changes in renal architecture

Blood tests

Comment on

- Estimated glomerular filtration rate (eGFR)
- Urea, creatinine, potassium
- Haemoglobin
- Calcium, alkaline phosphatase, parathyroid hormone
- Specific tests for causes of chronic kidney disease

Renal biopsy

Echocardiogram

Comment on

- Pericardial effusion

Evaluation

1. **What stage of chronic kidney disease does this patient have?**

   Source: Clinical Practice Guidelines for Chronic Kidney Disease: Evaluation, Classification, and Stratification. National Kidney Foundation Disease Outcomes Quality Initiative, 2002. Available from http://www.kidney.org/professionals/KDOQI/guidelines_ckd/toc.htm

Stage 1	Normal eGFR (>90 mL/min/1.73 m^2) but evidence of renal damage on urine dipstick/ultrasound/blood tests
Stage 2	eGFR slightly reduced (60–89 mL/min/1.73 m^2) with evidence of renal damage
Stage 3	Moderately reduced eGFR (30–59 mL/min/1.73 m^2)—consider nephrology referral
Stage 4	Significantly reduced eGFR (15–29 mL/min/1.73 m^2)-prepare for renal replacement therapy
Stage 5	Established renal failure. Renal replacement therapy

2. **Why does this patient have renal failure? Is the cause treatable and can progression be slowed?**

3. **Is there evidence of renal bone disease or anaemia? How could these complications be managed?**

4. **What can be done to reduce this patient's long term cardiovascular risk?**

5. **Would this patient be suitable for renal replacement therapy? Do they understand what it entails, and would they be keen to start this?**

Questions

1. A 29-year-old woman moves to a new area and registers with a GP. Routine urine dipstick analysis reveals 'Protein +++', and follow-up blood testing shows urea 9.4 mmol/L and creatinine 147 μmol/L, which is calculated to give an eGFR of 39 mL/min/1.73 m². She has no medical history and feels herself to be in excellent health. Her mother had suffered from 'kidney disease' but died of a 'heart attack' aged 58, and her maternal grandfather also died in early middle age.

On examination she looks slightly plethoric but is otherwise well looking. Her blood pressure is 156/90 mmHg, HR 88 bpm regular, and her aural temperature and capillary blood glucose are within normal limits. Abdominal examination reveals bilateral ballotable masses in the left and right flank. Her doctor arranges an abdominal ultrasound scan to investigate these abnormalities, and images from this are shown below:

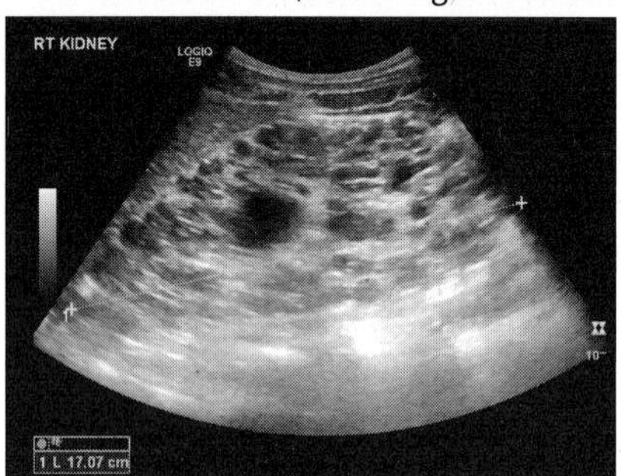

(1) What do these images reveal, and how does this explain the abnormalities found on examination?

(2) What is the prognosis of this condition, and how should this lady be managed?

2. A 54-year-old patient previously known to have stage 3 diabetic kidney disease attends her family doctor complaining of feeling lethargic and generally unwell over the preceding 2 months. She was last seen 10 months ago in the community renal clinic. Her investigations from the polyclinic and today's results are shown below:

	Polyclinic	Today
eGFR	30 mL/min/1.73 m²	18 mL/min/1.73 m²
Hb, MCV	9.1 g/dL, 88 fL	7.8 g/dL, 84 fL
HbA1c	8.5%	9.8%
Albumin	31 g/L	25 g/L

She reports no acute medical problems and that she is compliant with her medications, which include metformin 1 g tds, ramipril 10 mg od, atenolol 100 mg od, aspirin 75 mg od, and simvastatin 40 mg od.

You are the medical student reviewing the patient with the GP

(1) List five members of the multidisciplinary team you may involve in this case

(2) Why might this woman be feeling so unwell?

3. A 61-year-old man who is on long-term renal dialysis is reviewed by the local nephrologist. He complains of 'a few aches and pains' in his arms, legs, and spine. There is no clinical evidence of arthritis or fracture. Blood tests to investigate for renal bone disease are shown below:

- Corrected calcium: 2.10 mmol/L (2.2–2.6)
- ALP: 156 IU/L (70–110)
- Phosphate: 5.1 mmol/L (2.5–4)
- Parathyroid hormone: 80 pg/mL (10–55)

(1) What do the biochemical abnormalities signify?

(2) Describe your further management of this patient.

4. A 76-year-old woman has a history of chronic kidney disease (baseline urea 15.4 mmol/L, creatinine 148 μmol/L, eGFR 32 mL/min/1.73 m² as checked 2 weeks before by her GP). Last year she suffered a myocardial infarction which has left her with significant heart failure. She is admitted to hospital after becoming drowsy and confused with evidence of systemic sepsis. Her urine dipstick is positive for protein, nitrites, and leucocytes. Blood tests reveal raised inflammatory markers (WCC 16.3 × 10⁹/L, CRP 231 mg/L), with decreased renal function (urea 22.5 mmol/L, creatinine 251 μmol/L, eGFR 17 mL/min/1.73 m²). Her potassium is 5.3 mmol/L and her blood pH is 7.28. She appears clinically dehydrated. Her regular medications are shown below:

Ramipril 5 mg od	
Metformin 850 mg tds	
'Humalog 30' insulin 36 units bd	
Simvastatin 40 mg od	
Aspirin 75 mg od	
Spironolactone 25 mg	

(1) Describe what you would do in the short and long term for each of her medications shown in the above table.

(2) You are asked to prescribe a stat dose of gentamicin and a course of low-molecular-weight heparin; using a BNF write out these prescriptions.

Remember that you can find large-size, annotated versions of many of the X-rays and ECGs that appear in this book on the book's web site at www.oxfordtextbooks.co.uk/orc/randall/

Answers

1. The renal ultrasound shows multiple large cysts in both kidneys, consistent with a diagnosis of polycystic kidney disease, a common inherited kidney disease where the renal parenchyma is replaced by large fluid-filled cysts, leading eventually to destruction of the remaining kidney tissue with loss of function. On the ultrasound opposite, her kidney measures over 17 cm in length—normal kidney size is 10–13 cm, with almost all causes of chronic kidney disease (except polycystic kidney disease) producing shrunken kidneys. The gross enlargement of her kidneys can be seen on the coronal CT scan shown below.

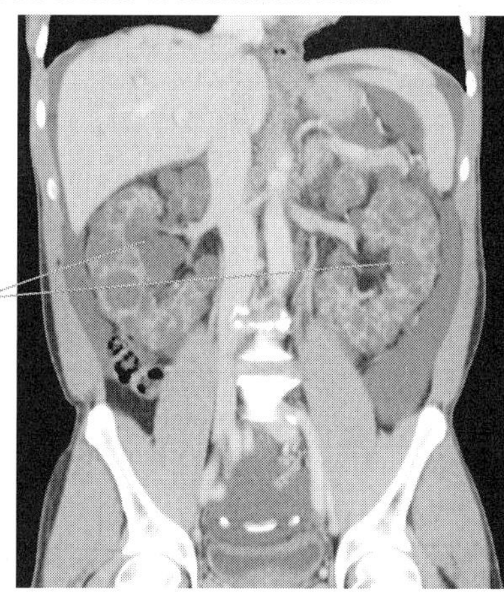

Coronal CT from the same patient, showing markedly enlarged kidneys bilaterally containing multiple large cysts. As the disease progresses there is increasing destruction of normal renal tissue with an accompanying fall in eGFR.

Adult polycystic kidney disease is caused by an autosomal dominant genetic defect. Presentation may be with hypertension, worsening kidney failure, loin discomfort caused by enlarging kidneys, or acute loin pain where there is haemorrhage into or infection of a cyst.

This woman already has stage 3 chronic kidney disease. Little can be done to halt the progression of the disease, which may progress rapidly to chronic kidney disease (below a GFR of 50 mL/min, GFR can fall by 5 mL/min/year). Controlling this woman's hypertension will be of primary importance, generally using an ACE inhibitor. She needs referral to a hospital nephrologist to monitor her disease and arrange a smooth transition to renal replacement therapy when this becomes necessary.

2. The key referral here is to nephrology out-patients. This woman has severe advanced renal failure (now stage 4 chronic kidney disease) and is likely to require renal replacement therapy (dialysis or transplant) within a few months or years. Patients at this stage do better when referred early to a nephrologist so that the transition to renal replacement therapy can be well planned and not done as an emergency. She should:

- Have her blood pressure control reviewed—controlling blood pressure is one of the surest ways to slow the progression of chronic kidney disease.
- Be considered for erythropoietin treatment—anaemia is likely to be one of the main reasons why she us feeling so unwell.
- Receive genetic testing to determine her HLA compatibility: being put on the transplant list offers real hope for patients otherwise facing a lifetime of dialysis.

Other referrals that should be made include:

Endocrinology out-patient review	Even at this woman's stage of kidney impairment, progression can be slowed by achieving good control of diabetes (this will also help control other diabetic complications). Since she is fully compliant with her oral medications and her high HbA1c indicates poor glycaemic control she may need to commence regular insulin
Appointment with a dialysis nurse	Starting dialysis has huge lifestyle implications, usually requiring three 4 to 6-hour-long sessions at hospital every week. Having the chance to talk about this with a dialysis nurse helps the patient understand the implications for them
Retinal screening	Development of significant renal disease in diabetes is strongly suggestive of the development of other diabetic complications. Diabetic retinopathy is highly treatable with laser surgery

3. This man has secondary hyperparathyroidism. A crucial step in the metabolism of vitamin D is carried out in the kidney, resulting in low levels of vitamin D in patients with chronic kidney disease, which in turn produces hypocalcaemia. The body responds by increasing production of parathyroid hormone—a process known as secondary hyperparathyroidism (secondary to low calcium). One of the effects of parathyroid hormone is to raise serum calcium by reabsorbing bone—a good serum marker of this is alkaline phosphatase (which also rises in liver disease). The situation is worsened by retention of phosphate which should be excreted by normally functioning kidneys. This can produce several clinical presentations including osteomalacia, osteoporosis, and osteosclerosis, which are grouped together under the label of 'renal osteodystrophy'. Radiological findings may include fractures (e.g. vertebral crush fractures in osteoporosis), evidence of bone erosion (e.g. a 'pepperpot skull'), or alternating bands of sclerotic and porotic bone in the vertebrae—'rugger-jersey spine'. Management of renal bone disease centres on:

- restriction of dietary phosphate
- oral calcium and vitamin D supplementation.

4. This woman has acute-on-chronic kidney disease—acute worsening of already impaired renal function. Prescribing is very important since some drugs will worsen kidney failure, others will accumulate owing to decreased excretion and therefore cause toxic effects.

Ramipril 5 mg od	Ramipril is an excellent drug for slowing the development of renal impairment. However, in the presence of acute sepsis it should be omitted for a few days since it will contribute to hypotension and under-perfusion of the kidneys
Metformin 850 mg tds	Metformin should be omitted since it worsens lactic acidosis
'Humalog 30' insulin 36 units bd	Insulin requirement rises in infection owing to the production of steroids by the adrenal glands. The dose should also be increased as metformin will be withheld
Simvastatin 40 mg od	Simvastatin can safely be continued unless there is any evidence of rhabdomyolysis (e.g. a raised serum creatinine kinase)
Aspirin 75 mg od	Aspirin can safely be continued
Spironolactone 25 mg	Spironolactone should be stopped. It is a potassium-sparing diuretic and will worsen hyperkalaemia and dehydration

- The normal prophylactic dose or low-molecular-weight heparin is 40 mg which is reduced to 20 mg in renal impairment.
- Gentamicin is nephrotoxic, and also accumulates rapidly in renal impairment. Instead of giving the normal dose of 5 mg/kg, a reduced dose of 2.5 mg/kg should be given with daily monitoring of levels to exclude accumulation. Doses should be withheld if the levels are high.

Further reading

Surviving Sepsis Campaign: International guidelines for management of severe sepsis and septic shock: http://www.survivingsepsis.org/About_the_Campaign/Documents/Final%2008%20SSC%20Guidelines.pdf

OHCM: 306–314, 558–559, 682–684, 690, 698

Urinary tract infection

This section should be used to clerk patients sufficiently unwell from urinary tract infection (UTI) to warrant admission to hospital. Patient pathways lead to the Admissions Unit, General Medical Ward or Care of the Elderly Ward, or if very severe to the ICU.

Learning challenges

- What is the 'surviving sepsis' campaign and what does their suggested early sepsis care bundle consist of?
- What is the significance of extended spectrum beta-lactamase (ESBL)-producing organisms for antibiotic prescription?

History

Comment on

- Dysuria, frequency, haematuria, urinary incontinence (especially in the elderly)
- Pain—urethral, suprapubic, or loin/lumbar
- Fever and rigors
- Nausea and vomiting
- Previous/recurrent UTIs (especially in men)

Examination

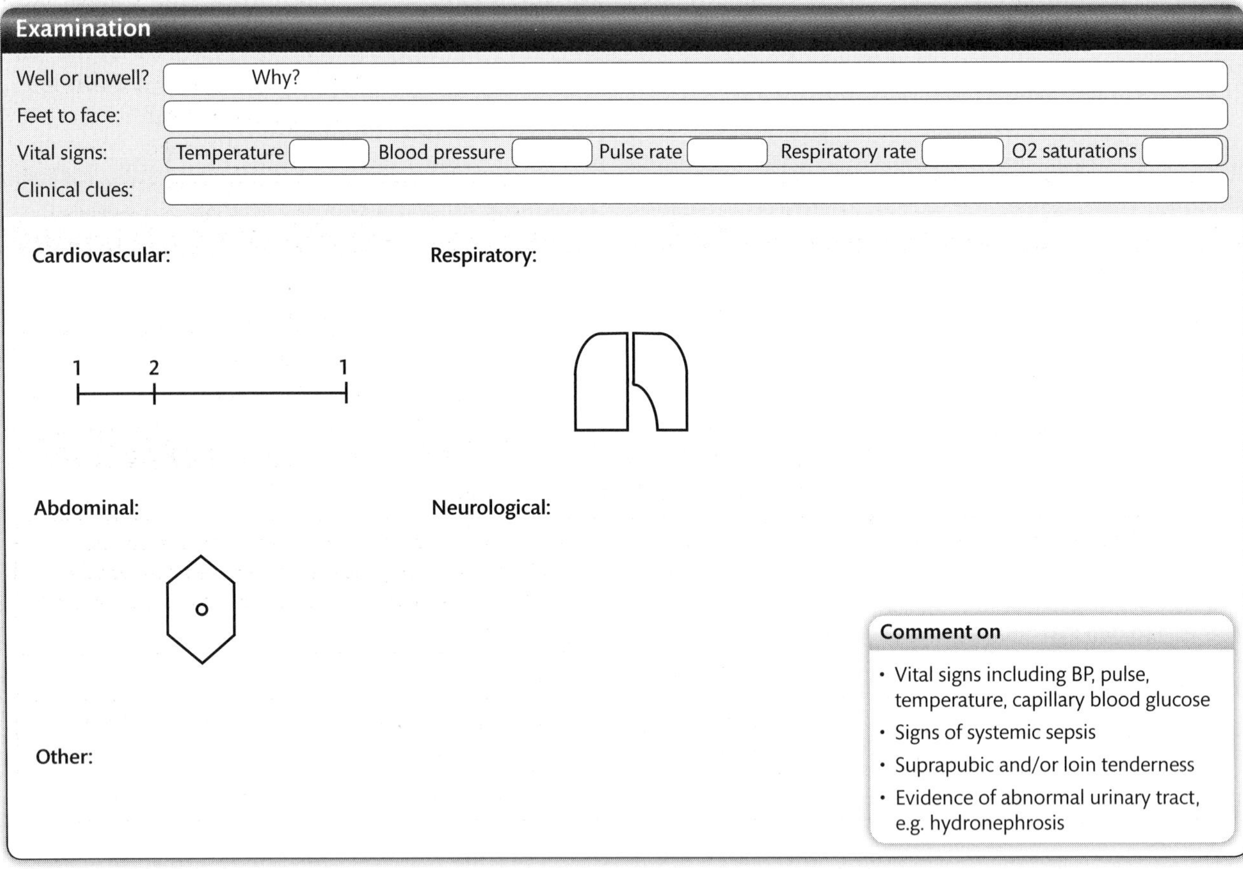

Comment on

- Vital signs including BP, pulse, temperature, capillary blood glucose
- Signs of systemic sepsis
- Suprapubic and/or loin tenderness
- Evidence of abnormal urinary tract, e.g. hydronephrosis

Urine dipstick

Comment on

- Leucocytes
- Nitrites (positive when bacteria convert nitrates to nitrites—absence does not exclude bacteriuria)
- Blood
- Protein

Blood tests (in patients being considered for admission)

Comment on

- FBC—WCC and differential
- CRP
- U&Es, CBG

Urine analysis

Comment on

- Pus cells
- Culture
- Antibiotic sensitivities

Blood cultures

Ultrasound kidney/ureters/bladder (in complicated or recurrent sepsis)

Comment on

- Structural abnormalities
- Abscesses or collections

Post-voiding bladder scan (where incomplete voiding and retention is considered)

Comment on

- Residual volume

Evaluation

1. **Is there evidence of sepsis or septic shock? How should the patient be resuscitated?**

Systemic inflammatory response syndrome (SIRS)	The body's response to a variety of attacks, including infection, trauma, burns or sterile inflammatory conditions. SIRS is diagnosed by two or more of: temperature <36 or >38°C, heart rate >90 bpm, respiratory rate >20 breaths/min, white cell count >12 or <4 × 10^9/L
Sepsis	SIRS caused by proven infection
Severe sepsis	Sepsis leading to organ dysfunction—for example, drowsiness or agitation (brain dysfunction) or oliguria (renal dysfunction).
Septic shock	Severe sepsis with a systolic blood pressure <90 mmHg despite fluid resuscitation

2. **What is the evidence for urinary tract infection?**

3. **What antibiotics are appropriate empirically? How should they be amended once the patient improves clinically? For how long should the patient be treated?**

4. **Are there any factors predisposing to urinary tract infection that can be addressed?**

Questions

1. A 24-year-old woman presents to the Emergency Department with a 2-day history of urinary frequency, dysuria, and haematuria. She has vomited several times today and has not been able to keep down any food or drink. Her baseline observations are: temperature 38.9°C, heart rate 108 bpm, blood pressure 105/78 mmHg, respiratory rate 18 breaths/min, oxygen saturations 98% on room air. She looks unwell but is fully alert and conscious. On examination of her abdomen she has marked suprapubic tenderness and is very tender in the left loin. Urine dipstick is positive for nitrites and leucocytes.

(1) What is the likely diagnosis?

(2) List the key investigations.

(3) List the key steps in managing this patient.

2. An 87-year-old man is referred to hospital from a nursing home by his GP. He is bed-bound and has advanced dementia and very limited verbal communication. He has been drowsy and pyrexial over the previous few days, which has not improved despite a course of oral trimethoprim. He is too drowsy to give a history. On examination he has a temperature of 38.5°C, heart rate of 113 bpm, and a blood pressure of 74/44 mmHg. His chest is clear and his abdomen is soft but there is some tenderness and dullness to percussion suprapubically. A catheter is inserted which rapidly drains 1.5 L of urine. Dipstick analysis is positive for leucocytes only. His blood tests, all of which had been normal when checked routinely by the GP 2 weeks earlier, are shown below.

Sodium: 154 mmol/L	Haemoglobin: 10.5 g/dL
Potassium: 5.9 mmol/L	MCV: 85 fL
Urea: 20.7 mmol/L	White cells: 18.5 × 10^9/L
Creatinine: 356 μmol/L	Platelets: 478× 10^9/L
CRP: 215 mg/L	

(1) List the essential steps in his management.

(2) What special considerations would you need to make in this case?

3. A 92-year-old man is admitted to hospital after being found drowsy and confused at home by his daughter. He has a long-term urinary catheter because of benign prostatic hypertrophy and has had several previous urinary tract infections which presented in a similar way. He has a slight temperature and mildly raised inflammatory markers, with no possible source of infection except his urine. He is known to be allergic to penicillin and has significant chronic kidney disease caused by diabetes (with a creatinine of 350 μmol/L). He is started on a course of oral trimethoprim and plans are made for an early discharge. However, after 3 days of antibiotics he has made no clinical improvement, remaining pyrexial, with rising inflammatory markers. His urine microbiology result is shown below:

Red cells: None seen			
Pus cells: ++			
Significant growth of *Escherichia coli*			
Amoxicillin	R	Ciprofloxacin	S
Co-amoxiclav	S	Nitrofurantoin	S
Cefalexin	S	Gentamicin	S
Trimethoprim	R	Piperacillin/tazobactam	S

(1) Given the results of this urine sample, what change in the management would you instigate now?

(2) Please prescribe any change in the management on a sample drug chart downloaded from the Online Resource Centre.

Answers

1. Clinically this woman has the classic features of pyelonephritis—an ascending urinary tract infection, affecting the kidney. Patients can be very unwell, with severe pain, vomiting, significant dehydration, and renal impairment. The management plan shown below would :

- treat the cause,
- treat the symptoms, and
- confirm the microbiological cause.

Interventions	Investigations
Intravenous antibiotics—following the hospital's antibiotics policy, though a penicillin (e.g. co-amoxiclav) or aminoglycoside (e.g. gentamicin) would commonly be used in this situation	**Routine blood tests**—to support the diagnosis of infection (raised CRP and white cell count). Renal function can be deranged in sepsis and should be checked, and deranged blood glucose may reflect underlying diabetes which is unmasked during infection
Intravenous fluids—to maintain hydration whilst the patient is vomiting, and counteract the hypovolaemia associated with sepsis	**Blood culture**—to rule out bacteraemia which would require longer courses of intravenous antibiotics. Organisms grown and sensitivities guide antibiotic treatment
Paracetamol—to reduce pyrexia and reduce pain (although if the patient is vomiting this may need to be given per rectum or even intravenously). Stronger **analgesia** including opiates may often be required	**Urine culture**—to confirm the bacterial diagnosis and to allow antibiotics to be selected according to sensitivities
Intravenous antiemetic such as cyclizine or metoclopramide, to reduce nausea and vomiting	**Renal tract ultrasound**—to identify the presence of stones, anatomical abnormalities, or abscess formation complicating infection

2. This man is extremely unwell, with septic shock (pyrexia, hypotension, and tachycardia), and has acute kidney injury. He is bed-bound and has advanced dementia. His prognosis is poor and this should be explained to relatives. He is very unlikely to survive a 'cardiac arrest' and management should not be escalated beyond intravenous antibiotics, fluids, and antipyretics. This needs senior agreement and support from an early phase of his admission and should be recorded clearly in his notes. He should be nursed on a pressure-relieving mattress on an appropriate elderly care ward.

Treatment of this man will be based around fluid resuscitation and intravenous antibiotics. His renal impairment is due to a combination of urinary retention (obstructive kidney failure) and systemic hypotension and dehydration (pre-renal kidney failure). Having relieved the obstruction, it is important to give intravenous fluids to attempt to achieve a systolic blood pressure of >100 mm Hg and a urine output ≥0.5 mL/kg/hour. Intravenous antibiotics are essential for this man; however, they must be given cautiously in view of his kidney failure. Drugs such as gentamicin should be given in reduced doses, adjusted based on the estimated glomerular filtration rate (for instance, gentamicin is given at 2.5 mg/kg/day rather than the usual dose in sepsis of 5 mg/kg/day). Speak to a hospital pharmacist or look in Appendix 3 (renal impairment) of the BNF.

3. Common urinary pathogens such as *Escherichia coli*, *Proteus mirabilis*, *Enterococcus faecalis*, and *Staphylococcus saprophyticus* are increasingly resistant to first and second-line antibiotics. Problems of resistance are compounded in this the patient as he is allergic to penicillin. The antibiotics this organism (*E. coli*) is sensitive to are:

Co-amoxiclav and piperacillin/tazobactam	These combination antibiotics contain penicillin and are therefore contraindicated due to allergy, particularly if the allergic reaction was of a true anaphylactic type with hypotension and airway compromise
Cefalexin	Up to 10% of those truly allergic to penicillin are also allergic to the cefalosporins. Cefalosporins are also associated with a high risk of developing antibiotic-associated diarrhoea (due to *Clostridium difficile* infection), and are therefore generally avoided, especially in the elderly
Ciprofloxacin	This is one of the antibiotics most associated with *Clostridium difficile* diarrhoea
Nitrofurantoin	This antibiotic is bacteriostatic (slows bacterial growth), rather than bacteriocidal (killing bacteria). However, its limited use in the recent past means it is becoming increasingly useful in the treatment of uncomplicated UTI
Gentamicin	This is likely to be the appropriate choice in this patient; however, it should be used with caution, in reduced renal doses, and with close monitoring of levels. Renal function should be monitored in view of its nephrotoxicity

Gentamicin is probably the best choice of antibiotic here (though antibiotic policies vary between hospitals and if in doubt it is best to speak to a microbiologist). Gentamicin is commonly given once daily, with trough levels being taken just before the third dose. Subsequent doses are then increased or decreased accordingly. The way this is written on the chart is shown below:

Drug: *Gentamicin*		**Instructions:** *Levels after 3rd dose*			**Signature:** *BW*						
Start: *10/9*	**Route:** *IV*	*10/9*	*11/9*	*12/9*	*13/9*	*14/9*	*15/9*	*16/9*	*17/9*	*18/9*	*19/9*
0800	*150mg*			↑							
				levels							

Further reading

Surviving Sepsis Campaign: International guidelines for management of severe sepsis and septic shock: http://www.survivingsepsis.org/About_the_Campaign/Documents/Final%2008%20SSC%20Guidelines.pdf

Gentamicin dosing: www.nuh.nhs.uk/nch/antibiotics/A-Z/gentobeseimpkg.asp

OHCM: 292, 640-641, 647

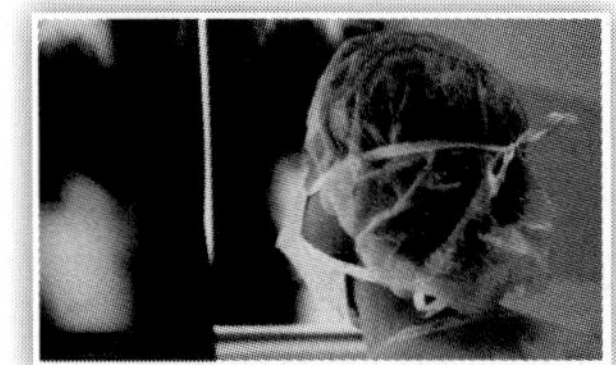 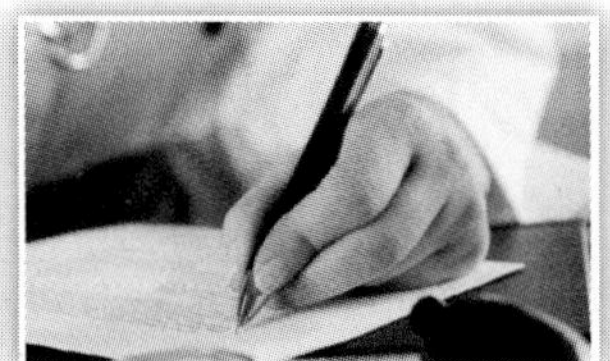 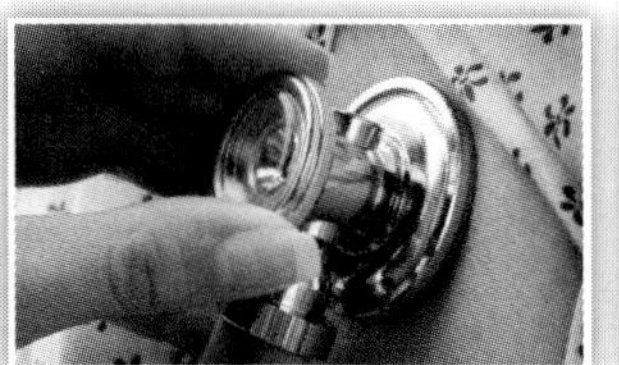 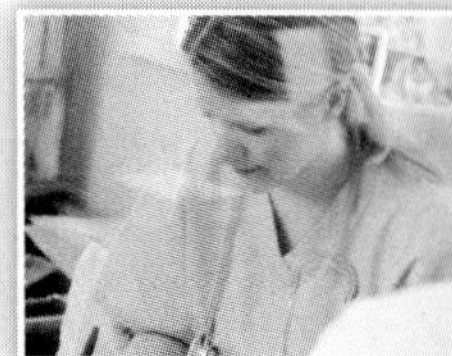

Unit 5
Endocrinology

Key learning outcomes in endocrinology include:

- Being able to take a history from a patient presenting with a new diagnosis of diabetes mellitus.
- Being able to take history from a patient with chronic complications of diabetes mellitus.
- Being able to perform a focused examination screening for common complications of diabetes mellitus—including macro- and microvascular disease and neurological complications.
- Understanding the mechanism of hyperosmolality and ketoacidosis in hyperglycaemic emergencies, and the principles of their management.
- Knowing about the different forms of insulin therapy and oral hypoglycaemic agents.
- Being able to recognize the clinical features of hyper- and hypothyroidism, and to examine both for the patient's thyroid state but also for a goitre.
- Recognizing the clinical features of Cushing's syndrome and Addison's disease, and knowing how to begin investigating the cause of such presentations.

Tips for learning endocrinology on the wards:

- Try to clerk (or observe a clerking of) a patient being admitted with diabetic ketoacidosis. Try to understand the significance of the arterial blood gas results and the key blood test results.
- On ward rounds when your team are seeing a diabetic patient, look through the nursing notes to find out what the patient's capillary blood glucose readings have been. Look at their drug chart to see what medication they are on.
- Observe the nursing staff looking after a diabetic patient on an insulin sliding scale
- Attend an endocrinology out-patient clinic and ask to clerk patients before your seniors see them, so that you can present to them your findings and clinical impressions.
- Look out for signs of Cushing's syndrome in patients on long-term steroids. See if they have been prescribed protection against gastric erosion or osteoporosis.

History

Hormones exert effects on all organs and systems within the body. Classical syndromes, symptoms, and biochemical abnormalities may be present, but endocrine disorders often produce a wide range of symptoms, many of which may be vague and non-specific, for instance malaise and lethargy.

Since endocrine disease may affect all organ systems, asking a wide range of questions in a 'review of systems' may be appropriate:

General symptoms:
- Tiredness and malaise
- Changes in weight
- Hot and cold intolerance
- Anorexia
- Sweating
- Changed voice

Neurological symptoms:
- Tremor
- Poverty of movement
- Syncope
- Restlessness
- Insomnia

Psychiatric symptoms:
- Low mood
- Irritability
- Psychosis

Neck:
- Goitre
- Other lumps and bumps

Eyes:
- Sore bulging eyes
- Visual disturbances

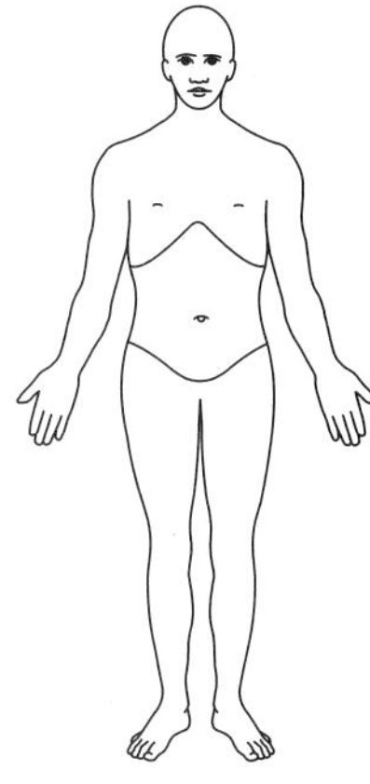

Cardiovascular:
- Palpitations
- Ischaemic heart disease

Changes in appearance:
- Rashes
- Dry skin
- Brittle hair
- Changed pigmentation
- Coarsened facial features
- Facial puffiness
- Central obesity
- Striae
- Bruising

Sex and reproduction:
- Subfertility
- Reduced libido
- Menorrhagia or oligomenorrhoea

Gastrointestinal:
- Diarrhoea
- Constipation
- Vomiting
- Abdominal pain

Also ask about:
- Symptoms of hyperglycaemia (below)
- Autoimmune disease
- Cardiovascular disease and risk factors

Musculoskeletal:
- Myalgia
- Arthralgia
- Limb weakness
- Fractures

Symptoms of hyperglycaemia

Developing symptoms of hyperglycaemia are often the presenting feature of diabetes mellitus. Since early diagnosis of diabetes is critical in reducing the incidence of both diabetic emergencies and long-term diabetic complications, recognizing these symptoms is critical.

The **symptoms of hyperglycaemia** are a classical triad of:
- thirst (polydipsia)
- polyuria
- weight loss

Other features include:
- visual blurring
- increased infections, e.g. candidiasis and cellulitis

The first two of the classical triad of symptoms (thirst and polyuria) are caused by high levels of glucose in blood, producing an osmotic diuresis and fluid dysregulation. Weight loss is caused by an inability of the body to use the high levels of circulating glucose to produce energy, leading to catabolism of energy stores of fat and protein. This has been described as 'starvation in the midst of plenty', where the body is unable to make use of high levels of circulating glucose because of insulin deficiency or insensitivity. As well as helping in the diagnosis of diabetes, asking patients known to have diabetes about the presence of these symptoms can give a clue to how well their diabetes is controlled.

Assessing control of diabetes and compliance with medication

A young person diagnosed with diabetes will face a lifetime of diet restrictions, injections, and blood sugar monitoring. This may produce a combination of fear, resentment, and embarrassment which may combine to produce poor adherence with prescribed insulin.

Assessment of diabetic control includes the following aspects of history, examination, and investigations:

- Reported adherence to medications
- Symptoms of hyperglycaemia
- Number and frequency of serious complications, e.g. ketoacidosis or hypoglycaemia
- Problems with injecting—local symptoms at injection sites
- Diary of capillary blood glucose measurements at different times of the day
- Ability to adjust insulin doses according to capillary blood glucose measurements
- Examination of injection sites for local complications, e.g. lipohypertrophy
- Objective evaluation of glycaemic control—glycosylated haemoglobin (HbA1c)

Proceed gently and non-judgementally: the aim is to encourage the patient to understand their condition and take responsibility for managing it.

Prevention of longer-term complications

At any review of a diabetic patient, questions should be asked about:

- Macrovascular complications—cardiac disease, stroke, or peripheral vascular disease
- Microvascular complications—focusing on the development of retinal disease or neuropathy
- Neurological complications—sensory neuropathy (often a 'glove and stocking' sensory loss), amyotrophy, autonomic neuropathy, stroke disease, mononeuritis multiplex
- Eyes—ask about complications including retinopathy, cataracts, and glaucoma. These may present as visual loss or blurring
- Feet—reduced sensation in the feet or ulceration
- Cardiovascular risk: hypertension, smoking, hyperlipidaemia,
- Diet—does the patient understand which foods are appropriate and which are best avoided in diabetes? Have they ever seen a dietician?
- Exercise—does the patient take regular exercise? How could this be built into their daily routine?

Examination

This page considers two crucial aspects in the examination of the diabetic patient—examination of the legs and of the fundi. On the facing page are four classic endocrine presentations—hyper- and hypothyroid, Addison's disease, and Cushing's disease.

Examination of the lower limbs

Observation

- Proximal muscle wasting may complicate diabetic neuropathies (amyotrophy)
- Ulceration: **neuropathic ulcers** are painless and occur over pressure areas, e.g. the balls of the feet; **vascular (ischaemic) ulcers** are painful and affect mainly the heels and toes, possibly with evidence of gangrene (dry or wet) or deep infection with sinus formation
- Ischaemic legs feel cool to touch and are pale or dusky in colour, becoming red when hung over the edge of the bed
- Neuropathic feet have a 'clawed', high-arched appearance, but are pink, warm, and well-perfused

Neurological assessment

- Tone and power are often normal in diabetic neuropathy
- Reflexes are often absent, especially the ankle jerk
- There is glove-and-stocking sensory loss (a distal sensory neuropathy)—often the first modalities to be lost are vibration sense and joint position sense

Vascular assessment

- Are the feet pink and warm? If pale, do they become red when hung from the bed?
- Aortic, femoral, popliteal, posterior tibial, and dorsalis pedis pulses should all be palpated
- If absent an attempt should be made to detect them using a Doppler probe
- Using the Doppler probe the ankle:brachial pressure index (ABPI) should be calculated

Fundoscopy

Looking into the back of the eye with an ophthalmoscope should be practised in a darkened room. The patient's pupils should be dilated, using a pupillary dilator such as tropicamide (patients should be told they must not drive for the rest of the day after having their pupils dilated). Tell the patient to focus on a point on the wall behind you and warn them that you will be coming in very close to their face.

First locate the optic disc and inspect it: then follow vessels out to the periphery of each eye quadrant. Finally, tell the patient to look at the light, then inspect the macula. Diabetic maculopathy (any disease affecting the macula) requires urgent ophthalmological assessment.

Background retinopathy:

- dots—microaneurysms
- blots—small blood leaks
- hard exudates—protein-rich fluid leaks

Pre-proliferative retinopathy: cotton-wool spots

Proliferative retinopathy: new vessel formation

Maculopathy—classically a 'macular star'

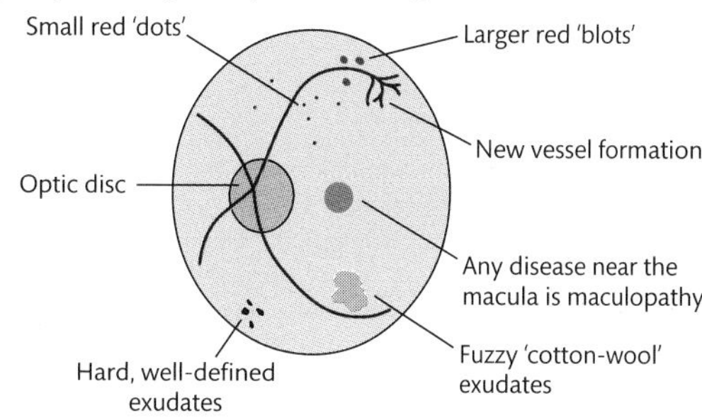

Thyroid signs

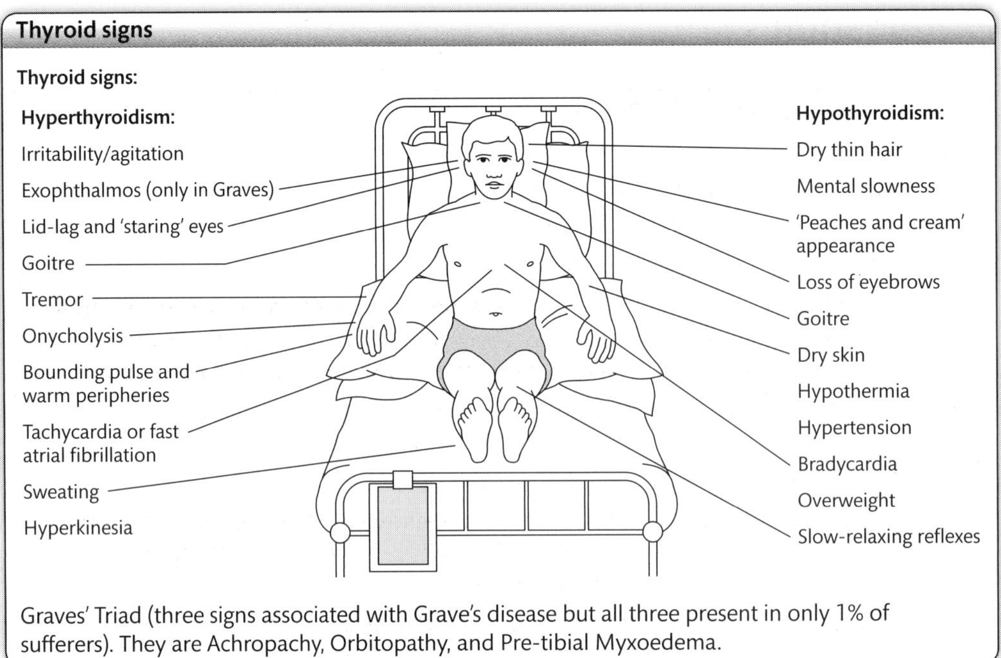

Graves' Triad (three signs associated with Grave's disease but all three present in only 1% of sufferers). They are Achropachy, Orbitopathy, and Pre-tibial Myxoedema.

Signs of disorders of the steroid axis

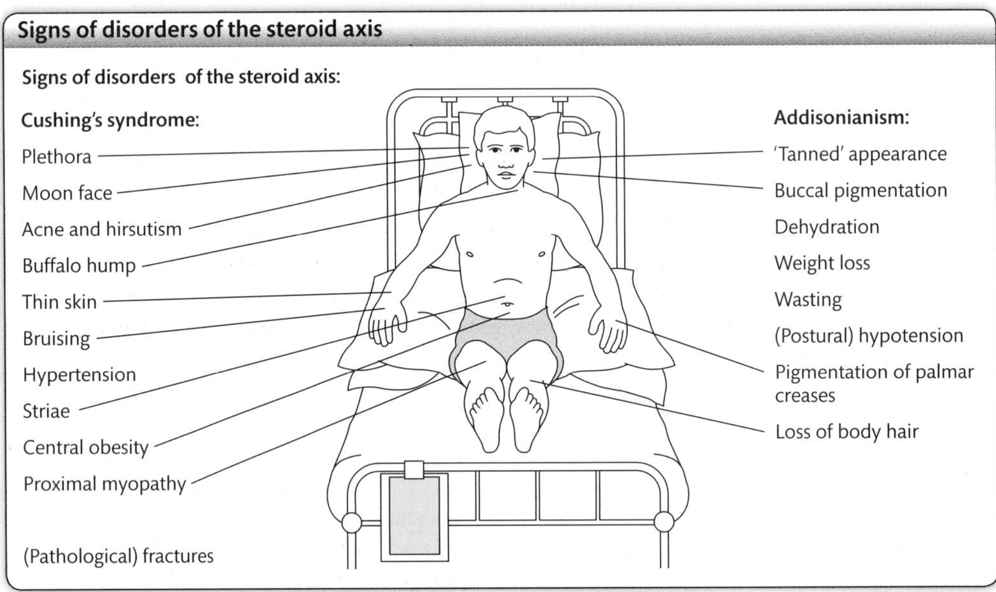

Investigations

Confirming the diagnosis of diabetes mellitus

Diabetes is diagnosed by:

- a random plasma glucose level of ≥11 mmol/L,
- a fasting glucose level of ≥7.0 mmol/L, or
- a positive oral glucose tolerance test (OGTT)

An OGTT is performed in patients with borderline random or fasting glucose levels, or in patients where there is a strong suspicion of diabetes despite normal random and fasting glucose levels. In this the patient fasts overnight, has a glucose measurement before eating and then a repeat level 2 hours after eating 200 mg of glucose. Diabetes is diagnosed if:

- the initial (fasting) blood glucose level is >7 mmol/L, or
- the blood glucose level after eating is ≥11 mmol/L

The World Health Organization also recognizes two 'pre-diabetic' conditions, impaired fasting glucose (IFG) and impaired glucose tolerance (IGT), which are associated with increased cardiovascular risk and developing frank diabetes mellitus

- WHO criteria for IFG fasting blood glucose of 6.1–6.9 mmol/L
- WHO criteria for IGT = 7.0–10.9 mmol/L 2 hours after an OGTT

Investigations used in monitoring the diabetic patient

- **HbA1c** (glycosylated haemoglobin) is a measure of the patient's glycaemic control over the previous 3 months. It can be used to assess the effectiveness of treatment, and the level of adherence to what has been prescribed. Guidelines from the support and research group Diabetes UK suggest a target of HbA1c < 6.5% to indicate good control of diabetes, with a target of HbA1c < 7.5% in those particularly at risk of hypoglycaemia (see http://www.diabetes.org.uk).
- **Renal function** should be assessed in all diabetic patients, both by measuring their urea and creatinine (and calculating the estimated glomerular filtration rate, eGFR) but also by **urine dipstick analysis**. Microalbuminuria is a specific marker of renal damage and is linked with increased long-term cardiovascular risk.
- A patient's **lipid profile** is also important, since lipid abnormalities and diabetes often co-exist, raising further the patient's risk of cardiovascular death.

The acutely unwell diabetic patient

The three common diabetic emergencies are: hypoglycaemia, diabetic ketoacidosis (DKA, affecting type 1 diabetics), and hyperosmolar hyperglycaemic state (HHS, affecting type 2 diabetics). Key investigations include:

- **Capillary blood glucose (CBG)** and a '**lab glucose**' measurement.
- **Arterial blood gas analysis** in hyperglycaemic patients.
- **Urine dipstick**—the presence of ketones in the urine can confirm that the acidosis is secondary to the presence of ketone bodies (in DKA); it is also important to exclude urosepsis as a possible precipitant of DKA or HHS.
- **Urea, creatinine, and sodium**—hyperglycaemic patients (especially those with HHS) can become extremely dehydrated and hyperosmolar, shown by a raised serum sodium, urea, and creatinine.
- **White cell count and CRP**—often DKA or HHS are precipitated by infection, which must be treated at the same time as fluids and insulin are administered.

The essence of hormonal regulation and testing

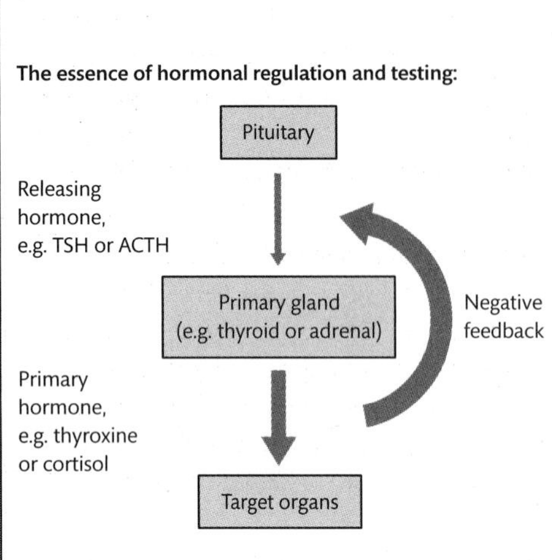

Many hormones in the body are secreted in response to the presence of another, controlling hormone—for instance, cortisol is secreted by the adrenal glands when they are stimulated by adrenocorticotrophic hormone (ACTH) from the anterior pituitary gland. In turn the secretion of pituitary hormones is under positive control by releasing or stimulating hormones secreted from the hypothalamus.

Patients may present with disease caused by excess or lack of the main (primary) hormone—for instance, with hyperthyroidism (excess T_3 and T_4), Addison's disease (cortisol deficiency), or hypercalcaemia caused by hyperparathyroidism (PTH excess). These abnormalities could be caused by disease of the primary gland (e.g. the adrenal gland) or by problems higher up (e.g. in the hypothalamus or pituitary).

Questions for determining the level at which the problem lies include the following.

1. Are the abnormal levels of the primary hormone explained by abnormal levels of releasing hormones?

This determines whether there is a problem with the primary gland or with the gland secreting the releasing hormone. For example, in Cushing's syndrome excess cortisol is *explained* by excess ACTH—implying that the problem is with ACTH production in the pituitary (or more rarely, with corticotrophin releasing hormone production from the hypothalamus). Excess cortisol is *not explained* by a low ACTH (the negative feedback has suppressed ACTH, showing the pituitary function is normal)—implying that the problem lies with cortisol production by the adrenals.

2. Are other hormones affected?

Sometimes the same gland secretes different hormones. Co-existing abnormalities of several hormonal systems suggest where the primary disease lies. For instance: abnormalities of thyroid hormones, cortisol, sex hormone, growth hormone, and prolactin levels imply pituitary disease while abnormalities of corticosteroids, mineralocorticoids, and sex steroids imply adrenal disease.

3. Can low levels of primary hormone by stimulated by administering the releasing hormone?

The short and long Synacthen tests use a synthetic ACTH to stimulate the adrenal glands, and are used in the diagnosis of low cortisol levels. If cortisol levels *rise* after Synacthen is given then the adrenals are functioning well. If cortisol levels *do not rise* after Synacthen then there is primary adrenal insufficiency—true Addison's disease.

4. Can high levels of primary hormone be suppressed by stimulating negative feedback mechanisms?

The dexamethasone suppression test is used in the diagnosis of unregulated cortisol production (Cushing's syndrome), especially in identifying true cases of steroid disease from patients who may appear Cushingoid for other reasons (e.g. obesity or alcoholism). The synthetic steroid dexamethasone is given. Subsequent *non-suppression* of cortisol levels implies excess cortisol secretion (confirms Cushing's syndrome).

Interventions

Trying to maintain normoglycaemia

The risk of developing long-term complications in diabetes is closely related to the patient's glycaemic control. Type 1 diabetes is characterized by pancreatic (islet cell) failure and a deficiency of insulin. Thus all type 1 diabetics require insulin replacement. The primary abnormality in type 2 diabetes is insulin resistance (though insulin deficiency may develop as the disease progresses), and so oral hypoglycaemic agents are the mainstay of therapy.

The therapeutic steps below should be used in all diabetic patients, **although step 3 is not applicable to patients with type 1 diabetes**.

- **Step 1: Lifestyle.** Blood sugars can be much more easily controlled in diabetics who are of an appropriate weight than in those who are obese—indeed, after significant weight loss some type 2 diabetics who had previously required insulin to achieve good glycaemic control may be able to revert to using only oral agents. The two primary lifestyle strategies for reducing weight are diet control and exercise. One strategy for encouraging patients to take more exercise is by suggesting that they get off the bus one or two stops early and walk the rest of the way to work. All major cardiovascular risks such as smoking, hypertension, and hyperlipidaemia should be addressed.
- **Step 2: Diet.** In normal individuals, insulin levels rise dramatically after eating and control blood glucose levels very tightly. Diabetic patients are unable to produce such good control (either by injectable insulin or by residual pancreatic insulin production in type 2 diabetics), so efforts are made to minimize the degree of glycaemic load placed on the body. Advice is for regular, small meals and snacks (rather than irregular feasts), and primarily eating foods that release energy slowly, such as complex carbohydrates that require prolonged digestion. Sweet foods contribute to poor diabetic control because all the energy they contain is absorbed rapidly after ingestion.
- **Step 3: Oral hypoglycaemics.** The two most commonly used classes are the sulphonylureas (such as gliclazide, which stimulate pancreatic production of insulin) and the biguanides (such as metformin, which increase peripheral sensitivity to insulin). These can be started in type 2 diabetics who are unable to achieve adequate glycaemic control with diet alone. Biguanides are often preferred to sulphonylureas, partly because they do not cause weight gain and partly because they do not cause hypoglycaemia. You should be aware of the other classes of oral hypoglycaemics including meglitinides, thiazolidinediones, and the new glucagon-like peptide-1 analogues.
- **Step 4: Insulin.** Modern insulins are generally produced synthetically using recombinant DNA technology. They can be short-acting, long-acting, or come in formulations containing a mixture of the two. Standard insulin regimes include the 'basal-bolus' regime where a long-acting insulin is injected at night and short-acting insulin injected (usually three times) during the day. Alternatively a simpler regime uses a combination insulin preparation (a mixture of short- and long-acting insulins) injected twice daily. Basal-bolus regimes generally achieve better glycaemic control, but require high levels of motivation from the patient, so twice-daily regimes may be preferred for less adherent patients.

Hypoglycaemia is a potentially life-threatening acute complication of diabetes. It should be treated as soon as it is discovered using oral glucose (e.g. sugary drinks or sweets) if the patient is conscious, or if the patient is too drowsy or cannot swallow, by buccal or intravenous glucose preparations—for instance 50 ml of 50% dextrose. A cause for the hypoglycaemia should always be sought and any obvious precipitant treated or removed.

Common medications in endocrinology

Class	Examples	Mechanism	Indications	Contraindications	Side-effects	Special notes
Short-acting insulins						
Long-acting insulins						
Combination insulins						
Oral/buccal glucose preparations						
IV glucose preparations						
Sulphonylureas						
Biguanides						
Meglitinides						
Thiazolidinediones						
α-Glucosidase inhibitors						
Glucagon-like-peptide-1 analogues						
Thyroid hormones						
Antithyroid drugs						
Synthetic corticosteroids						
Synthetic mineralocorticoids						

Hyperglycaemic emergencies

This section should be used to clerk patients presenting with diabetic ketoacidosis (DKA) or hyperosmolar hyperglycaemic state (HHS; formerly referred to as hyperosmolar non-ketotic state or HONK). Patient pathways often begin in the resuscitation room of the Emergency Department, where the patient may be extremely unwell and almost comatose, and then lead either to the ICU or medical admissions units.

Learning challenges

- Why do most type 2 diabetics, despite being extremely hyperglycaemic, not become ketotic?
- How should diabetics be told to adjust their insulin during infections, and why?

History (see generic history of long-term conditions)

Comment on

- Previous diabetic history
- Previous DKA/HHS
- Weight loss/polyuria/thirst
- Adherence to treatment
- Evidence of infection or other systemic illness
- Duration and character of present episode
- Possible underlying causes, e.g. sepsis, systemic illness, poor adherence

Examination

Well or unwell? Why?

Feet to face:

Vital signs: Temperature Blood pressure Pulse rate Respiratory rate O2 saturations

Clinical clues:

Cardiovascular:

1 2 1

Respiratory:

Weight/BMI:

CBG:

Abdominal:

Neurological:

Other:

Comment on

- Capillary blood glucose; BP, HR, temperature, oxygen sats
- Level of consciousness
- Kussmaul respiration
- Ketotic breath
- Fluid status
- Evidence of infection—chest, skin, urine, others, e.g. meningitis

Urine dipstick

Comment on

- Glucose
- Ketones
- Evidence of infection

Arterial blood gas

Comment on

- Metabolic acidosis—marked depression of pH and bicarbonate
- Respiratory alkalosis (attempted compensation)

Blood tests

Comment on

- Evidence of infection (WCC and differential, CRP)
- Renal function—potassium, urea:creatinine ratio
- Serum osmolality
- Lab blood glucose

Microbiology

Comment on

- Blood cultures
- Urinary cultures (MSU)

Chest X-ray

Comment on

- Evidence of infection

ECG

Comment on

- Signs of IHD, LVH (hypertension), arrhythmia, e.g. AF

Evaluation

1. **Is this a hyperglycaemic emergency? If so, treat!**

2. **Is the patient responding? How should management be changed?**

Parameter to measure	Intended response	Action if not responding
Capillary blood glucose	Should fall, but beware hypoglycaemia	If high, continue high-dose insulin. Slow insulin once <12 mmol/L
pH	Should rise to normal range	Consider ITU for haemofiltration
Potassium	Should remain >3.5 mmol/L	Replace in IV fluids
Urinary ketones	Should be removed completely	Continue high-dose insulin until completely removed
Urine output	Should be high (>1 ml/kg/hour)	Ensure aggressive fluid resuscitation

3. **What is likely to have caused this emergency?**

4. **Once the patient has recovered, what issues need to be addressed to prevent this from recurring?**

Questions

1. A 19-year-old man is brought by ambulance to the resuscitation room of his local Emergency Department. He is feeling generally unwell and is noticed to be confused and 'hyperventilating' in the ambulance. According to his girlfriend, who accompanies him, he has not had any previous medical problems, but for the past 2 weeks has been feeling generally 'under the weather', with weight loss, intense thirst, and passing large amounts of urine. For the past 2 days he has been feeling very unwell and increasingly short of breath. On examination he appears flushed and unwell, and has a very dry mouth. His respiratory rate is 32 breaths/min but chest examination is unremarkable. His capillary blood glucose is 35.6 mmol/L. Arterial blood gas analysis reveals:

pH: 7.01	HCO_3^-: 13 mmol/L
pCO_2: 2.11 kPa	pO_2: 45.6 kPa
Base excess: −17.8 mmol/L	Lactate: 6.3 mmol/L

(1) What are the abnormalities shown on this patient's arterial blood gas analysis?

(2) The patient has two large-bore cannulae in place. Please write up the initial fluids, insulin infusion, and sliding scale on a downloaded chart from the Online Resource Centre.

2. Ten hours later you are asked to go back and review the patient in Question 1. He was reviewed during the previous day and you have been told that he is making good progress and can probably be switched to oral fluids and subcutaneous insulin injections. He was reviewed 4 hours before when his capillary blood glucose was 12.3 mmol/L and his pH had risen to 7.32. In response his insulin infusion had been reduced to 3 units/hour. Since admission he has received a total of 3.5 L of normal saline and is currently receiving a further litre, being given over 8 hours and which has 20 mmol of KCl added. You go to see the patient and find him fully alert and conscious, still feeling unwell and thirsty but better than before. You perform a range of investigations, the results of which are below.

(1) What changes would you make to this patient's current management?

Arterial blood gas:	Potassium: 3.1 mmol/L
• pH: 7.28	Urea: 8.4 mmol/L
• pCO_2: 3.44 kPa	Creatinine: 111 µmol/L
• pO_2: 12.6 kPa	Glucose: 15.1 mmol/L
• HCO_3^-: 17 mmol/L	Urine output: 35, 32, and
• Base excess: −4.3 mmol/L	38 ml/L in past 3 hours

3. A 56-year-old woman is admitted to the Emergency Department in a coma. She was found at home by family members slumped in a chair. She is known to have COPD, and is receiving a course of prednisolone and co-amoxiclav from her GP for a chest infection. On arrival she has a GCS of 8 (E1, V2, M5) and is markedly dehydrated. CVS, respiratory, abdominal, and neurological examinations are unremarkable. Her urinalysis shows glucose ++++ but nothing else of note. Her CBG reading is > 48 mmol/L. Her blood test results are shown below.

Sodium: 160 mmol/L	Haemoglobin: 16.0 g/dL
Potassium: 4.7 mmol/L	White cells: 12.3×10^9/L
Urea: 21.0 mmol/L	Platelets: 465×10^9/L
Creatinine: 144 mmol/L	Glucose: 64.9 mmol/L

(1) Using the formula **osmolality = 2(Na⁺ + K⁺) + urea + glucose**, calculate her serum osmolality (normal serum osmolality = 285–295 mOsmol/L).

(2) What do the U&Es imply about her renal function?

(3) List five interventions you would employ in this case.

4. There is sudden commotion on the ward during the morning round. A patient with known type 2 diabetes is noticed to be slumped in her chair and not responding to verbal or tactile stimuli. She is moved onto her bed and a set of observations are performed, all of which are within normal ranges except for her CBG which is found to be 1.2 mmol/L.

(1) Describe your initial management.

After giving emergency treatment, you review the patient's drug chart. She is taking a combined short-acting/long-acting insulin preparation twice daily, 30 units in the morning and 24 units in the evening. You check with the nursing staff who assure you that she is taking all her medications and that she has a good appetite for her meals. Her capillary blood glucose chart is shown below.

(2) How could her insulin regime be altered to reduce the likelihood of this complication arising again?

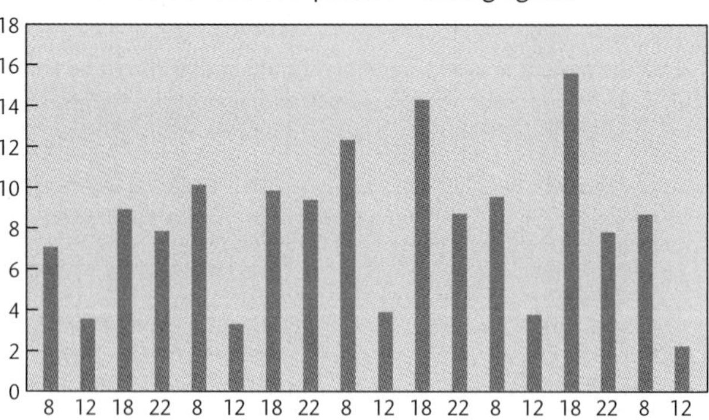

Presentation

Presented to ____ Grade ____ Date ____

Signed

Answers

1. This man's arterial blood gas analysis shows a severe metabolic acidosis. Follow the process in the introduction to Unit 2 whenever you are faced with the results of an arterial blood gas analysis:

> **1. Is this primarily an acidosis or an alkalosis?** Because the pH is low (<7.35), this is a primary acidosis.
>
> **2. Is the pH explained by the pCO_2?** Acidosis is caused by a high pCO_2, but in this man the pCO_2 is low. So this is NOT a primary respiratory acidosis, meaning instead it is a primary metabolic acidosis–proved by the LOW bicarbonate and negative base excess.
>
> **3. Is there any compensation?** Since the primary problem here is metabolic, any compensation will be provided by the respiratory system. Here, the pCO_2 is low, showing that the patient is hyperventilating to blow off CO_2 and raise the pH to compensate.
>
> **4. Is there respiratory failure?** The pO_2 here is elevated, because the patient has been put on high-flow oxygen (because he is tachypnoeic–it is not really needed). There is no evidence of respiratory failure.

The metabolic acidosis here is partly as a result of excess of serum ketones (ketones are acidic), and partly as a result of lactic acid produced by tissues with inadequate blood supply. Lactate levels rise in any shock or hypovolaemia (caused here by dehydration), since tissues are underperfused and switch from aerobic to anaerobic respiration. Normally production of ketones is suppressed by circulating insulin, but in its absence they are produced (by the breakdown of fat), and this leads to the acidosis. His apparent hyperventilation is in fact his attempt to blow off his CO_2. This is known as Kussmaul's respiration.

Initial treatment of hyperglycaemic emergencies is based on fluid resuscitation and insulin. Fluid resuscitation should be aggressive, as patients with DKA are extremely dehydrated. Typically 6–7 L of saline are given over the first 24 hours. A litre is given as quickly as possible (stat), followed by one over 30 minutes, 1 hour, 2 hours, and then 4 hours. All fluids should be titrated against the patient's clinical response, monitored by their urine output (target 0.5–1 ml/kg/hour), BP (target systolic pressure >100 mmHg), and HR (<100 bpm). Potassium should be added to each litre (of fluid) after the stat litre. As a guide if K^+ > 5.5 mmol/L no K^+ should be added; if K^+ is 3.5–5.5 mmol/L add 20 mmol/L of KCl; if K^+ < 3.5 mmol/L add 40 mmol/L of KCl. Insulin in DKA is given according to a 'sliding scale' at an infusion rate titrated to blood glucose measurements every 30 minutes.

Date	Time	Infusion fluid	Volume	Added drug	Infusion rate	Signature
27/10	21.00	Normal saline	1 L	-	Stat	DR
27/10	21.00	Normal saline	1 L	20 mmol KCl	30 min	DR
27/10	21.00	Normal saline	50 mL	Soluble insulin 50 units	According to sliding scale (see below)	DR

Capillary blood glucose	Infusion rate
0–3.9 mmol/L	0.5 ml/hour
4–6.9 mmol/L	1 ml/hour
7–10.9 mmol/L	2 ml/hour
11–14.9 mmol/L	3 ml/hour
15–19.9 mmol/L	4 ml/hour
>20 mmol/L	6 ml/hour

2. Close monitoring of patients with DKA is necessary. In this case, the patient's blood glucose level has actually risen again, and his plasma pH has worsened. 'Yo-yoing' of blood sugars is a common problem in managing patients with DKA, as insulin infusion rates are cut in accordance with the sliding scale. Alternatively, in other patients hypoglycaemia can develop. It is essential that capillary blood glucose levels be checked by nursing staff every 30 minutes and the insulin rate adjusted accordingly. The insulin infusion should be increased again in accordance with the sliding scale. 5% dextrose (glucose) can be given to prevent hypoglycaemia.

There are also problems with this patient's fluid resuscitation. His raised urea and creatinine (and desire to drink) suggest he remains somewhat dehydrated, and his urine output is at the lower end of normal (estimating the weight of a healthy young man as 70 kg).. Patients in DKA are thought to have a fluid deficit of around 5 L, and fluid replacement should be aggressive, aiming to produce a good diuresis. This patient would benefit from faster fluids (say two bags of normal saline over 2 hours each), with appropriate added potassium.

This man has presented with DKA on the background of a 2-week history of the symptoms of hyperglycaemia. Many type 1 diabetics present like this. Once his pH, blood glucose, renal function, and electrolytes are all normal he can be converted onto injectable (subcutaneous) insulin and oral fluids, and after education about diabetes and its management can be discharged home with out-patient follow-up.

3. This woman has an extremely high serum osmolality of 415.8 mOsmol/kg which will be contributing, alongside the direct effect of hyperglycaemia, to her coma. Hyperosmolar hyperglycaemic state presents more insidiously than DKA, and though patients do not become acidotic they are often more profoundly dehydrated than patients with DKA.

The high urea:creatinine ratio here suggests that her renal failure is pre-renal in origin. Here her urea has risen three times above normal, but her creatinine is less than 1.5 times above the normal range.

It is likely that this woman has had undiagnosed type 2 diabetes for several years. This acute problem is likely to have been caused by both infection and the prescription of steroids, both of which raise blood glucose levels:

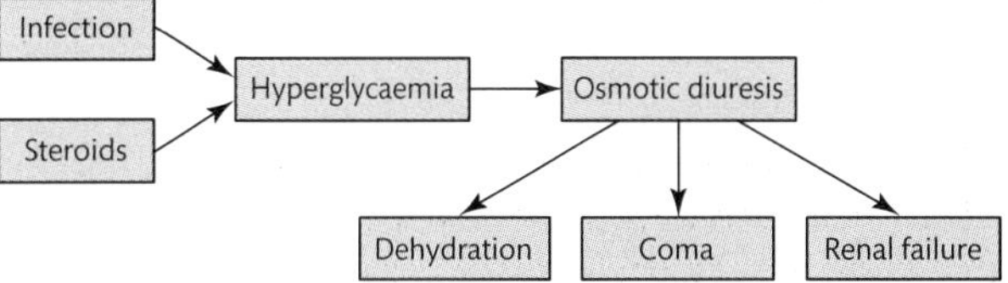

Type 2 diabetics have enough circulating insulin to suppress the production of ketones, so they do not become ketotic or acidotic. The management of hyperosmolar hyperglycaemic state and DKA are similar, though more caution may be required in giving fluids and insulin more slowly to prevent the complications of cerebral oedema and fluid overload to which older patients are more prone. BOTH require prophylactic heparin to reduce the risk of venous thromboembolism whilst their blood is so hyperosmolar and therefore hypercoagulable.

4. The treatment for hypoglycaemia is, unsurprisingly, glucose! If the patient is fully conscious she can be given sugary drinks or biscuits to eat; if unconscious, as in this case, then intravenous 50% dextrose (or more rarely intramuscular glucagon) can be given–once the patient is more alert she can then be given some longer-acting carbohydrates, such as jam and toast, to eat. If the patient has been made nil by mouth, intravenous dextrose should be used. The cause of the hypoglycaemia should be sought and treated.

Hypoglycaemia in diabetics occurs due to reduced food intake or high doses of insulin (or oral hypoglycaemic agents such as gliclazide). Hypoglycaemia can be a real problem for patients as well as being potentially very dangerous. Attempts should be made to establish the patterns of hypoglycaemia and the likely causes, adapting diet and insulin regime to produce better glycaemic control without recurrent hypoglycaemia.

This woman seems to have reasonable control of her blood sugars, but to be prone to hypoglycaemia mid-morning. One way to solve this problem may be to reduce her morning dose of insulin to, say, 26 units. An alternative (given a reasonable degree of variation between days) might be to start a qds 'basal-bolus' insulin regime with a long-acting insulin at night and smaller doses of short-acting insulin three times during the day with meals. Well-motivated patients may be competent to recognize hypoglycaemia and measure their blood glucose levels regularly, making day-to-day adjustments in their doses. Patients unable to do this should be prescribed insulin doses that err on the side of caution–achieving less good glycaemic control but avoiding hypoglycaemia.

Further reading

Guidelines: Joint British Diabetes Societies Inpatient Care Group guidelines on managing DKA in adults (http://www.library.nhs.uk/Diabetes/ViewResource.aspx?resID=345687)

OHCM: 206, 590, 842–844

The diabetic review

This section should be used in general practice, diabetic out-patient clinics, or with diabetic patients on the wards to assess how they are coping with managing their disease and to identify any developing complications.

Learning challenges

- Apart from diabetes, what other medical problems are associated with obesity?
- Why is diabetes such a problem for society at large? How does it lead to disability?

History

Comment on

- Monitoring including hyper- and hypoglycaemic episodes
- Glycaemic diary—glycaemic control at home
- Diet and exercise in normal lifestyle
- Adherence to medications
- If on insulin—Insulin injection technique
- Macro- and microvascular complications—IHD, stroke, and PVD; kidney and eyesight problems
- Neurological: **symptoms of autonomic dysfunction** (dizziness, falls, loss of consciousness); **peripheral sensory changes**—numbness, paraesthesiae, burns, trauma to peripheries; symptoms suggestive of **mononeuritis (multiplex)**—multiple peripheral nerve lesions
- Feet—sensory problems (ask also about hands), symptoms of vascular insufficiency, ulcers

Examination

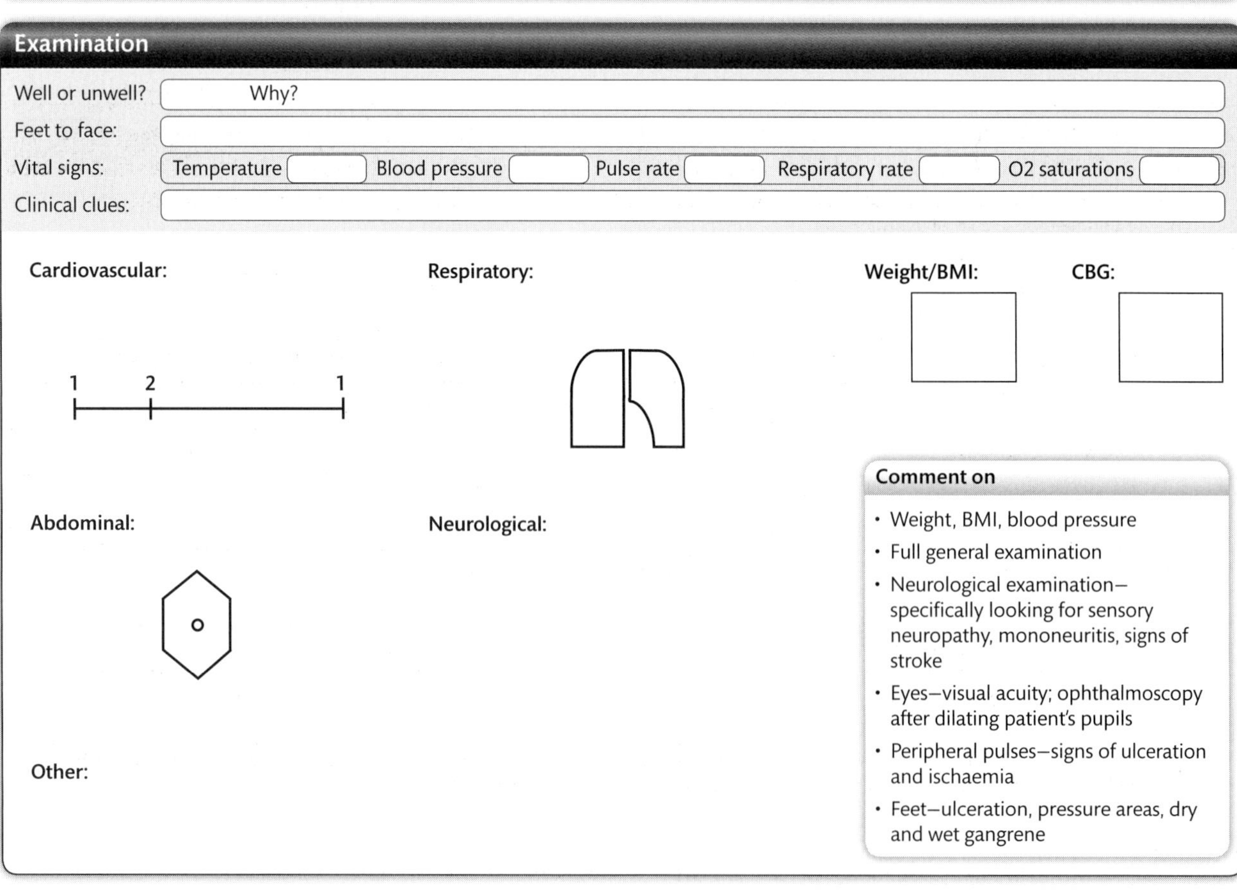

Comment on

- Weight, BMI, blood pressure
- Full general examination
- Neurological examination—specifically looking for sensory neuropathy, mononeuritis, signs of stroke
- Eyes—visual acuity; ophthalmoscopy after dilating patient's pupils
- Peripheral pulses—signs of ulceration and ischaemia
- Feet—ulceration, pressure areas, dry and wet gangrene

Blood tests

Comment on

- HbA1c
- Fasting lipid profile (cholesterol and triglycerides)
- Renal function

Fundoscopy or retinal screening (see above)

Comment on

- Diabetic retinopathy
- Cataracts

Ankle/brachial pressure index

Urine dipstick

Comment on

- Protein
- Urine for microalbuminuria estimation

Evaluation

1. **What does the patient understand about their disease? Do they understand the need for good diabetic control to reduce the chance of developing complications?**

2. **How good is this patient's glycaemic control? Are changes in their medications indicated?**

3. **How well is this patient's long-term cardiovascular risk being managed? What interventions could improve their prognosis?**

	Target	Lifestyle interventions	Medications
Blood pressure	< 130/80	Weight loss	ACE inhibitor, calcium-channel blocker, others
Lipids	Total cholesterol <4 mmol/L, LDL cholesterol <2 mmol/L	Diet, exercise	Statin, fibrate
Glycaemic control	HbA1c < 6.5%	Diet, exercise, compliance with medication	Insulin, oral hypoglycaemic drugs
Smoking	Complete cessation	Counselling	Nicotine patches

Consider the need for **aspirin** prophylaxis, and medication such as **orlistat** or even **bariatric surgery** to aid weight loss.

4. **Are complications such as retinopathy, neuropathy, nephropathy, or peripheral vascular disease developing? How can these be managed? Should the patient be referred to an ophthalmologist, nephrologist, podiatrist, or vascular surgeon?**

Questions

1. A 28-year-old man with type 1 diabetes, diagnosed 10 years ago, is reviewed on a general diabetes and endocrine ward after being discharged from the ITU where he was being managed for severe DKA. Over the previous 2 years he had been admitted to hospital five times with DKA, this being his second admission to ITU. He admits that adherence to his basal-bolus insulin regime is sporadic. He is currently homeless and lodging with a friend, and admits to regular alcohol binges. He has a HbA1c of 11.6%, an eGFR of 41 mL/min with 2+ proteinuria on urine dipstick analysis and has evidence of background retinopathy on fundoscopy. He says he wants to 'sort his life out', and asks for your help in doing so, but says he hates injecting himself all the time.

(1) Make a list of the issues that have arisen in this case. For each of these issues describe the appropriate interventions that could help this patient gain control of his diabetes and life.

2. A 26-year-old woman is referred to the diabetes out-patient clinic after undergoing investigation for infertility. Fasting blood tests had revealed a glucose of 8.9 mmol/L and total cholesterol of 7.1 mmol/L, with LDL of 4.9 mmol/L. She is generally well, but has struggled with her weight since her teenage years and also complains of excessive hair growth on her upper lip and chin, as well as suffering from long-standing acne. She works as a receptionist. On examination she is obese, with a BMI of 34 kg/m^2. Her blood pressure is 155/94 mmHg. An abdominal ultrasound organized as part of her fertility investigations revealed multiple small cysts in both ovaries, and also detected changes in the architecture of the liver consistent with fatty infiltration. Her LFTs were normal except for a mildly raised ALT.

(1) List the conditions she has developed. What is the collective name for this group of disorders?

(2) What lifestyle and therapeutic interventions would you recommend?

3. A 72-year-old woman who has suffered with type 2 diabetes for many years presents to hospital with an ulcer she recently noticed on the sole of her left foot. She also complains that the left ankle has been becoming progressively swollen and red for the previous 3 months. On examination she appears well, with no signs of systemic upset. Both feet appear deformed, with unusually high arches and clawed toes. Light touch, sensation, and joint position sense are decreased in a 'stocking' distribution bilaterally. On the left-hand side the ankle joint is generally swollen and red, but not unduly hot to touch and is non-tender. There is a 3 cm × 2 cm punched out, well-demarcated ulcer on the plantar aspect overlying the first and second metatarsophalangeal joints. There are no acute changes to the surrounding skin and the ulcer base is covered with yellowish odourless slough. Serum inflammatory markers are not significantly raised (WCC 9.9 × 10^9/L, CRP 14 mg/L). The ankle:brachial pressure index is 0.8. A lateral X-ray of the ankle is shown below.

(1) What is the clinical and radiological diagnosis?

(2) Describe the further management of this patient.

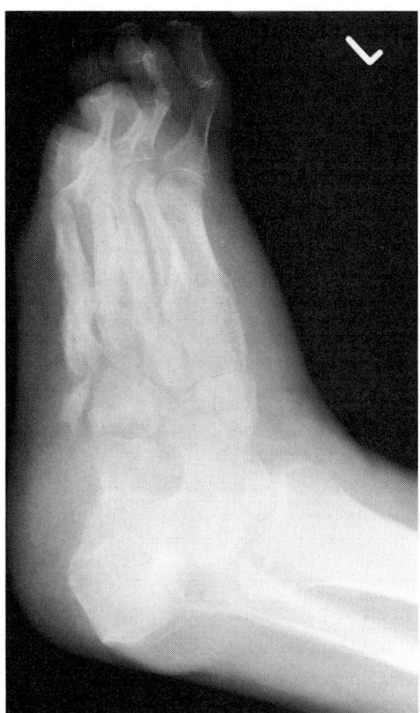

Remember that you can find large-size, annotated versions of many of the X-rays and ECGs that appear in this book on the book's web site at www.oxfordtextbooks.co.uk/orc/randall/

Answers

1. This patient is clearly not coping with his diabetes, suffering regular hyperglycaemic emergencies and already showing evidence of microvascular complications, i.e. retinopathy and nephropathy. This is a complex case with many clinical and social challenges. By listing all the issues, in the form of a problem list, patients, carers, and members of the clinical team can identify strategies to help get the patient's diabetes and life back under control. As well as the regular members of the clinical staff, social services and a psychologist may be of help in this case.

Poor adherence to medications and lifestyle advice	Explaining the nature of diabetes and the need for close glycaemic control. Giving the patient the information necessary to take ownership of their diabetes
Early retinopathy	Regular retinal screening
Early nephropathy	Good control of blood pressure. ACE inhibitors are of proven benefit in slowing the progression of diabetic kidney disease
Homelessness	Referral to the homeless persons' unit at the local council. They should be able to arrange hostel accommodation for this man, especially if the request is supported by a doctor's letter explaining why adequate housing is important for medical reasons
Alcohol addiction	Alcohol in moderation is safe in diabetes, and guideline daily intakes are the same as for the normal population. However, binges of alcohol predispose to hypoglycaemia, especially if drinking alcohol replaces eating food, and is also likely to worsen adherence to medications. This man should be reviewed by a substance misuse counsellor whilst he is motivated to change. They should be able to arrange community support in abstaining from alcohol
Needle phobia	Basal-bolus regimes of insulin, where a long-acting insulin is injected at night and three boluses of rapid-acting insulin are injected with meals, achieves good glycaemic control by adequately mirroring physiological insulin secretion. However, in this man it may be better to offer a twice-daily regime (where a mixture of rapid- and longer-acting insulin is injected twice daily). Although glycaemic control may be poorer on this regime, if adherence is improved then it will be better overall for the patient

2. This woman has developed:
    - Diabetes (since she has a fasting blood glucose level of >7.0 mmol/L)
    - Hypertension (for this to be treated the blood pressure should be sustained at >160/90 mmHg)
    - Hypercholesterolaemia (with the more dangerous LDL cholesterol especially raised)
    - Polycystic ovarian syndrome (multiple cysts on both ovaries, often associated with subfertility and hirsutism)
    - Non-alcoholic fatty liver disease

The '**metabolic syndrome**' is a term used to describe individuals who suffer from a range of conditions which together predispose to the development of cardiovascular disease. Various diagnostic criteria have been suggested, including combinations of impaired glucose tolerance or diabetes, obesity, raised cholesterol or triglycerides (or low HDLs), hypertension, and microalbuminuria (a sign of early kidney damage). The term is controversial, with few doubting that these conditions do cluster together but some doubting the usefulness of an umbrella term.

Other conditions associated with the metabolic syndrome (and displayed by this patient) include **fatty liver** and **polycystic ovarian syndrome**. Fatty liver describes a process where hepatocytes contain large amounts of fat, and can progress to **steatohepatitis** if there is inflammation present. It is frequently caused by alcohol, but non-alcoholic steatohepatitis (NASH) is associated with the metabolic syndrome. Both may progress to cirrhosis.

Polycystic ovarian syndrome is a poorly understood syndrome causing symptoms of androgen overactivity (such as male-pattern hair growth, baldness, acne, and increased muscle mass), along with menstrual irregularity and reduced fertility. The ovaries often contain large numbers of fluid-filled cysts. The cause of the syndrome is unclear, but there are strong associations with obesity, diabetes, and altered lipid metabolism.

This woman has a relatively high risk of developing premature cardiovascular disease. She would benefit from lifestyle advice regarding her diet and exercise; losing weight may significantly improve each of her present conditions. She may be a candidate for weight loss interventions including orlistat or bariatric surgery. A statin, antihypertensive (e.g. an ACE inhibitor), and aspirin may also be prescribed as primary prophylaxis. Oestrogen supplementation (in the form of the oral contraceptive pill) will reduce ovarian production of androgen and reduce masculinizing symptoms. Metformin can be a particularly useful drug in polycystic ovarian syndrome producing improvements in glycaemic control alongside weight loss, and improving cardiovascular risk.

3. The first problem with this woman's foot is a diabetic foot ulcer. These are a common problem and may be responsible for multiple clinic reviews and hospital admissions for the diabetic patient. The two main aetiological groups are **ischaemic ulcers**, where tissue damage cannot be repaired due to inadequate blood flow, and **neuropathic ulcers**, more likely in this patient. Neuropathic feet have a characteristic appearance with a high arch and clawed toes—this leads to pressure areas developing in ill-fitting footwear causing pressure necrosis and damage. A lack of sensation from sensory neuropathy means developing damage is not detected until ulceration has occurred.

Her second foot problem, another common feature of diabetic neuropathy, is **Charcot's joint** (neuropathic osteoarthropathy). This is caused by microtrauma leading to small fractures in the joints. Because of loss of pain sensation protective rest is not instituted so further damage occurs. Joints are red and swollen, with reduced movement but no pain. X-ray, as in this case, may show considerable bony destruction.

Management of diabetic ulcers depends on the aetiology. Sterilized dressings may be used, along with cleaning (and possible debridement) of the wound. Systemic antibiotics should be used only if there is evidence of infection (for instance, a surrounding cellulitis)—not in this case. Rest is an important part of management, to allow healing to occur.

Ischaemic ulcers may require surgical or other therapeutic interventions to improve oxygenation of tissues (for instance bypass surgery or intravascular stenting). Neuropathic ulcers improve with careful management to ensure pressure is avoided on the damaged tissue; this may include specially designed footwear. This patient has good peripheral circulation (shown by a relatively normal ankle:brachial pressure index) and so management should be focused on pressure relief and optimizing diabetic control. Without due care and rest, diabetic ulcers can prove difficult to heal; up to 50% of lower limb amputations are carried out on diabetic patients, but with adherence to diet, medications, and lifestyle changes, careful monitoring, and surveillance for complications, preventative measures may stop this potentially serious set of events occurring.

Further reading

Guidelines: NICE guidelines on managing type 2 diabetes (http://guidance.nice.org.uk/CG66)

OHCM: 198–206, 590

Thyroid disease

Patients with thyroid disease may present acutely with hyper- or hypothyroidism, and are managed on specialist endocrine units. More commonly they present with other unrelated problems, but the following questions can be used to assess their thyroid status and their level of disease control.

Learning challenges

- What is the physiological function of thyroid hormones and how does this explain features of their excess/deficiency?
- How might you approach a patient who complains of being 'tired all the time'?

History

Comment on

- Main presenting problems
- Heat/cold intolerance
- Changes in weight
- Bowels
- Other autoimmune disease
- Local symptoms—neck swelling, dysphagia, hoarseness

Examination

Well or unwell? Why?

Feet to face:

Vital signs: Temperature Blood pressure Pulse rate Respiratory rate O2 saturations

Clinical clues:

Cardiovascular:

1 2 1

Respiratory:

Weight/BMI:

CBG:

Abdominal:

Neurological:

Other:

Comment on

- General examination—hot and sweaty versus cool peripheries; proximal weakness
- Heart rate, (tachy- versus bradycardia) temperature
- Behaviour—slow and sleepy versus agitated and anxious
- Fine tremor of fingers
- Quality of skin and hair
- Acropachy, pre-tibial myxoedema
- Eye signs—lid lag versus others
- Examination of goitre
- Reflexes

Blood tests

Comment on

- T_3, T_4 and TSH
- Thyroid antibodies (seen in autoimmune thyroid disease)
- Electrolytes, calcium (calcium regulated by calcitonin and parathyroid hormone)
- Blood glucose
- Pituitary hormones (if indicated)

ECG

Comment on

- Fast AF, SVT, bradycardia

Thyroid ultrasound

Fine needle aspiration (FNA)

Thyroid cytology or biopsy

Evaluation

1. What is the patient's clinical thyroid status—hyperthyroid, hypothyroid, or euthyroid?

2. Comparing TSH and T_4 levels, is the primary problem likely to lie in the pituitary or in the thyroid? What is the likely cause?

	TSH high	TSH low
T_4 high	Very rare—pituitary TSH-secreting tumour	Primary thyroid disease—commonest causes including Graves' disease, toxic multinodular goitre or solitary toxic nodule
T_4 low	Primary thyroid disease—commonly autoimmune (atrophic) thyroiditis or Hashimoto's thyroiditis, or after thyroid surgery.	Pituitary disease—look for signs that other pituitary hormones are deficient

3. Is there a goitre? Is this large enough to be causing any compressive or cosmetic symptoms? Are there any features of malignancy?

4. What treatment can be used to restore this patient's thyroid status to normal?

5. Are there any eye complications which warrant specialist management (Graves' disease)?

Questions

1. A 24-year-old student complains to her doctor of feeling anxious. She also complains of having a tremor, of feeling hot all the time, and suffering loose bowels and palpitations. On examination she is thin, with warm well-perfused peripheries and a fine resting tremor of her outstretched hands. Her heart rate at rest is 125 bpm and there is a systolic murmur. She has evidence of proptosis but no other eye signs and no obvious goitre. Her thyroid function test results are shown below.

(1) What is the likely underlying diagnosis?

(2) Describe the generic and specific management steps in this case.

T_4: 186 mmol/L
TSH: 0.02 mU/L
Thyroid-stimulating globulin: Positive
Antithyroid globulin: Positive

2. A 60-year-old woman presents to her GP with several neck lumps. She first noticed them 6 months ago but 'was too busy to do anything about them'. She is now very concerned as they are increasing in size and she is worried that she may have cancer. She also reports than the lumps have been causing her some difficulties in swallowing, and that she has taken to wearing scarves to cover them up. She has not had any difficulty in breathing and is otherwise well. On examination she appears clinically euthyroid. There are multiple lumps visible inferior and lateral to the thyroid cartilage. They are smooth and firm on palpation and move superiorly on swallowing. It is impossible to palpate below the swelling and there is some dullness to percussion over the manubrium. She has normal levels of T_4 with slightly suppressed TSH.

(1) What is the likely diagnosis suggested by the history and examination findings?

(2) How would you investigate the 'lumps' to reassure the patient that this is not a malignant condition?

3. A 56-year-old woman presents to her general practitioner with a 6–8 month history of 'feeling tired all the time' and 'lacking the energy to leave the house'. She feels generally run down and miserable, which has been worse since being made redundant 3 months previously. On examination she is overweight and has an 'expressionless' face. She is speaking in a flat monotone. Her skin appears thick and she has dry, brittle hair. There is a modest diffuse goitre which rises with swallowing and with a lower border that is easily palpable above the sternum. Her ankles are swollen, though they do not pit when compressed.

(1) What is the differential diagnosis in this case?

(2) List five further investigations to prove the underlying cause of her symptoms.

4. A 42-year-old housewife is recovering in hospital 2 days after a total thyroidectomy, carried out for a large toxic multinodular goitre On the consultant ward round she reports feeling well, and that the pain from the wound is well controlled. All basic observations are within normal ranges. However, she complains of a hoarse voice which is new since the operation. She has been started on 75 μg of thyroxine once daily. Her blood tests are below.

(1) What are the differential causes of her hoarseness of voice?

(2) List the abnormalities of the blood results below, then likely causes and their treatments.

Sodium: 140 mmol/L	Haemoglobin: 10.5 g/dL
Potassium: 4.5 mmol/L	MCV: 84 fL
Urea: 4.3 mmol/L	White cells: 10.2×10^9/L
Creatinine: 87 μmol/L	Platelets: 213×10^9/L
Corrected calcium: 2.11 mmol/L	T_4: 44 mmol/L
TSH: 11 mU/L	

5. A middle-aged man presents to his GP concerned by a painful swelling in his neck. He has noticed the swelling over the past 2 weeks, just inferolateral to his 'Adam's apple', and for the previous day he has experienced pain when he touches it. He is otherwise well and does not complain of any symptoms suggestive of thyroid dysfunction. On examination he appears euthyroid. A smooth, tender mass in felt in the thyroid gland on the right-hand side, which measures about 1 cm across. There is no evidence of oesophageal or tracheal compression and there is no surrounding lymphadenopathy.

(1) Are there any sinister features to concern you regarding this presentation?

(2) Which two investigations are crucial to perform to assist with the further management?

Presentation

Presented to ______ Grade ______ Date ______

Signed

Answers

1. This woman displays classic signs and symptoms of thyrotoxicosis (**hyperthyroidism**); the diagnosis of primary hyperthyroidism (i.e. arising from the thyroid gland) is confirmed biochemically by the elevated T_4 level and suppressed TSH levels. The positive antibodies suggest that this is autoimmune in nature so the most likely unifying diagnosis is **Graves' disease**: Over 99% of hyperthyroidism is caused by intrinsic thyroid disease (hardly any is of pituitary origin), and of these Graves' disease is the commonest single cause. Graves' disease is an example of type V hypersensitivity where disease is caused by the blocking or stimulating effect of autoantibodies—in the case of Graves' disease, antibodies bind to and stimulate the TSH receptor on thyroid cells causing oversecretion of T_3 and T_4.

A range of treatments are available, with the least invasive that can achieve adequate control being preferred. **Carbimazole** (or **propylthiouracil**) are used to suppress thyroid hormone synthesis, but because T_4 has a half-life of 7 days in the blood, effects may not be seen for 2 weeks. In the meantime propranolol can be used to control tachycardia and tremor (but is contraindicated in asthma). Two strategies can be used with carbimazole—either the dose is titrated carefully to achieve good control of T_4 levels, or high doses are used to suppress all endogenous thyroxine production, with thyroxine supplementation being given—the '**block-and-replace**' strategy.

If carbimazole fails to control symptoms then treatments to destroy thyroid tissue may be required. **Radioactive iodine** (**^{131}I**) is used for this purpose, but is contraindicated in pregnancy and where there is Graves' eye disease. The alternative is thyroid surgery, which whilst being successful does carry small but significant risks.

Graves' disease also produces retro-orbital inflammation and mucopolysaccharide deposition, leading to proptosis and possibly optic nerve compression. Graves' eye disease (**orbitopathy**) can lead to loss of sight and patients should be referred to an ophthalmologist for review and potentially for medical management, surgery, or radiotherapy to reduce swelling behind the eyes. Treating the hyperthyroidism does not improve eye disease.

2. This woman has a multinodular goitre, which can be confirmed using ultrasound should this be required but is readily apparent clinically. Multinodular goitres can become extremely large, causing cosmetic issues. Most patients with this condition are euthyroid but single active nodules within the goitre can render the patient thyrotoxic (this patient has compensated hyperthyroidism, with a normal T_4 and suppressed TSH). There is little potential for malignancy. Multinodular goitre is the commonest cause of compressive symptoms in the neck. CT or MRI imaging can confirm the extent of compression, and should include the thoracic inlet and upper chest since these tumours often extend retrosternally.

Given the presence of dysphagia and the fact that this goitre continues to enlarge, surgical resection is likely to be necessary. Total thyroidectomy is the commonest operation, though a subtotal thyroidectomy can be performed if the swelling is largely unilateral. Lifelong thyroxine replacement will be needed if the whole gland is removed.

3. Patients complaining of tiredness in the absence of other localizing symptoms can be a real diagnostic dilemma. This woman has some features to suggest a possible diagnosis of hypothyroidism, but equally well could be depressed, anaemic, vitamin D deficient, or suffer from systemic lupus erythematosus, chronic kidney disease, diabetes mellitus, or a whole range of other diseases. A few initial tests such as measuring full blood count, renal function, liver function, and thyroid function can help to differentiate these non-specific presentations and diagnose common problems; if these are all normal then after assessing for clinical depression, a period of watching and waiting may be indicated to see whether symptoms improve or whether additional problems become evident. This lady's thyroid function tests are below:

> T_4: 3.1 mmol/L (4.5–11 mmol/L)
> TSH: 7.8 mU/L (0.5–5.0 mU/L)

The high TSH confirms primary hypothyroid disease and a low-normal T_4 is in keeping with this. Thyroid antibodies may suggest a possible diagnosis—the two most likely are **atrophic** (**autoimmune**) **hypothyroidism**, where autoantibodies lead to the destruction of the thyroid gland, or **Hashimoto's thyroiditis** where **thyroid peroxidase** (**TPO**) **antibodies** lead to tissue destruction and regeneration, causing goitre formation. Both conditions require treatment with thyroxine replacement, which is essential to improve symptoms and reduce cardiovascular risk. Patients with hypothyroidism have an increased cardiovascular risk compared with the normal population.

4. This woman is likely to have a hoarse voice because of recurrent laryngeal nerve injury: The recurrent laryngeal nerve supplies the vocal cords, and lies in close association to the thyroid gland in the neck. Thyroidectomy may lead to damage of the nerve, which may vary from temporary palsy and hoarseness to more permanent damage. Less commonly there may be bilateral nerve injury which leads to paralysis of both vocal cords and airway obstruction, requiring emergency tracheostomy. Most commonly hoarseness in the post-operative period is due to difficult or traumatic intubation.

This patient displays several of the common complications of major thyroid surgery. These need to be discussed with the patient when obtaining consent and are important to be aware of in the post-operative period.

- **Bleeding:** This woman's mild normocytic anaemia is likely to have been due to intraoperative blood loss. The thyroid is very vascular and blood loss is common in such procedures. Post-operatively, significant bleeding may cause a compressive haematoma around the upper airway. If this occurs it is imperative that the pressure be released as soon as possible by immediate removal of the sutures.
- **Hypocalcaemia:** Calcium metabolism is regulated in the body by parathyroid hormone, produced in the parathyroid glands which can be very hard to dissect out during thyroid surgery. Usually hypocalcaemia is transient, but if all parathyroid tissue has been accidentally removed or destroyed, lifelong supplementation with calcium may be necessary.
- **Hypothyroidism:** This is to be expected in total thyroidectomy, and to be anticipated in subtotal thyroidectomy. This patient may require an increase in her thyroxine dose to maintain her TSH within physiological levels.

5. The majority of isolated thyroid lumps are '**simple cysts**' with no malignant potential. However, a proportion will prove to be malignant. Differentiating them on clinical grounds can be very difficult. This man's presentation has some sinister features suggestive of malignancy including: (1) the short history (i.e. rapid onset of symptoms) and (2) presence of pain. These are indications for rapid referral and investigation.

Thyroid function tests should be performed but are unlikely to differentiate the causes. The two most useful investigations are **thyroid ultrasound** which, in the hands of an experienced operator, can give very useful information on the possibility of malignancy. **Fine needle aspiration** (**FNA**) (which can be carried out in the clinic) may sometimes be diagnostic, but more commonly raises or lowers the index of suspicion for thyroid cancer. If results of both tests indicate a moderate or high probability of cancer then surgical resection is carried out with perioperative histology confirming or refuting the diagnosis, and guiding further management.

Most thyroid cancers, if caught early, carry an excellent prognosis if fully resected. The commonest are **follicular** and **papillary** carcinomas. Poorly differentiated anaplastic tumours are rare, affecting older people, but are very aggressive and rapidly fatal.

Further reading

Guidelines: British Thyroid Association guidelines on the use of thyroid function tests (http://www.british-thyroid-association.org/info-for-patients/Docs/TFT_guideline_final_version_July_2006.pdf)

OHCM: 208–212, 215, 593, 602, 844

Disorders of steroid axis

This section should be used to clerk patients suffering with diseases of the steroid axis—Cushing's syndrome (or disease) or Addison's disease. These patients may rarely be encountered outside specialist endocrine units, so this section can also be used to review patients taking prolonged courses of steroids for any reason.

Learning challenges

- What is the difference between Cushing's syndrome, Cushing's disease and pseudo-Cushing's syndrome?
- What is the physiological role of cortisol and how does this help explain some of the features of Cushing's syndrome?

History

Comment on

- Tiredness and constitutional symptoms
- Changes in weight
- Changes in appearance (does the patient have any old photos?)
- Skin changes—pigmentation, bruising, thin skin
- Dizziness or syncope
- Amenorrhoea, lack of libido

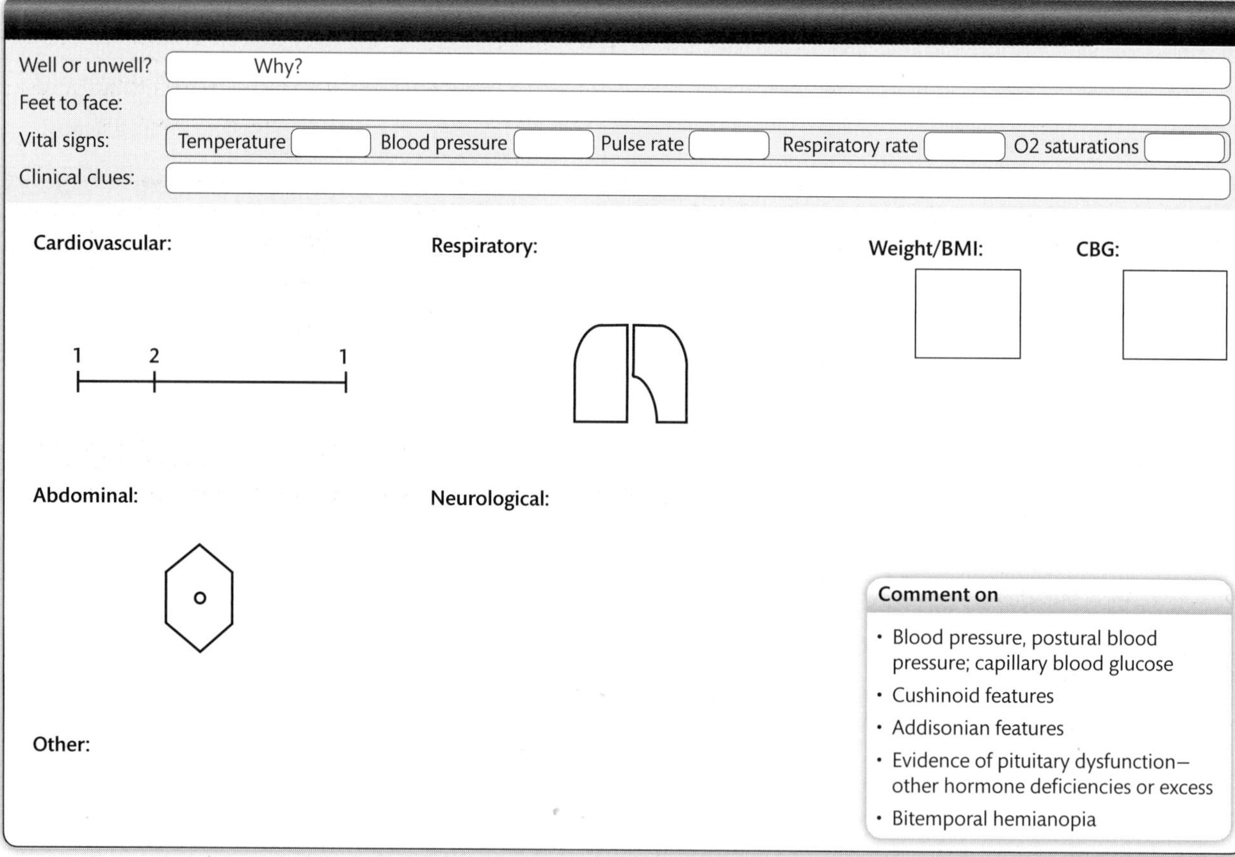

Comment on

- Blood pressure, postural blood pressure; capillary blood glucose
- Cushinoid features
- Addisonian features
- Evidence of pituitary dysfunction—other hormone deficiencies or excess
- Bitemporal hemianopia

Blood tests

Comment on

- Electrolytes
- Glucose
- 9.00 a.m. cortisol
- Thyroid function tests
- Pituitary hormones
- Adrenal antibodies

Confirmatory tests

Comment on

- Dexamethasone suppression test (Cushing's)
- ACTH Synacthen stimulation tests (hypoadrenalism)

Chest X-ray

Comment on

- Evidence of TB (commonest cause of Addison's disease worldwide)
- Evidence of bronchial carcinoma (possible source of ectopic ACTH secretion)

Abdominal X-ray

Comment on

- Evidence of adrenal calcification

Pituitary MRI

Comment on

- Evidence of adenoma (cause of Cushing's disease)

Adrenal MRI/CT

Comment on

- Evidence of adenoma/carcinoma
- Diffuse hyperplasia

Evaluation

1. **What evidence is there to suggest Cushing's syndrome or hypoadrenalism? Is there any evidence of an Addisonian crisis requiring urgent steroid and fluid support?**

2. **Is this clinical suspicion supported by a positive suppression/stimulation test?**

3. **What is the likely cause?**

- Cushing's syndrome
  - High ACTH
    - Pituitary adenoma
    - Ectopic source of ACTH e.g. lung tumour
  - Low ACTH
    - Adrenal adenoma or cancer
- Hypoadrenalism
  - High ACTH
    - Autoimmune adrenalitis or adrenal TB
  - Low ACTH
    - Hypopituitarism or adrenal suppression by exogenous steroid

4. **How can the patient be managed?**

Cushing's: surgery to treat cause, control symptoms with metyrapone

Hypoadrenalism: steroid supplementation, patient advice, steroid card

Questions

1. A 56-year-old man is referred to the local hospital by his doctor for investigations. Over the past month he has been feeling generally unwell and has been gaining weight around his abdomen (though he feels that his arms and legs are now thinner than before). He also has 'stretch marks' on the skin of his abdomen. His son who is away at university, felt that his father's face had changed shape when he returned from his term away, becoming much rounder and with a darker complexion than before, and the patient also complains of troublesome acne. He has never smoked cigarettes and has no other complications. Physical examination provides evidence for all of the patient's complaints, as well as revealing thinning skin, with several large bruises, and weakness of the proximal limb muscles. His blood pressure is 162/96 mmHg, and his random capillary blood glucose measures 8.6 mmol/L. The patient is given 1 mg of dexamethasone which he is told to take at 23:00 that night before going to bed, and then to return for a blood test at 09:00 the following morning. This reveals a blood cortisol level of 143 nmol/L (normal <100 nmol/L).

(1) Explain the significance of this result?

(2) Describe the further investigations to confirm the likely diagnosis.

2. A 43-year-old woman is brought to the hospital Emergency Department after collapsing on the train on the way to work. She says she stood up to get off the train and felt very dizzy and then lost consciousness, fully recovering a few moments later. She has felt dizzy, especially on standing up, several times over the previous few weeks, during which time she has also been feeling very tired. She has lost weight over this period and her periods have stopped. Her previous medical history includes vitiligo, and she does not take any medications. On examination she appears tanned (apart from some hypopigmented patches on her arms which she explains are caused by vitiligo), though she has not spent any time in the sun for many months. Areas of pigmentation are also noted on the buccal mucosa inside her mouth and in the creases on her palms. Her blood pressure is 102/74 mmHg lying down, falling to 78/66 mmHg after standing up for 2 minutes. Otherwise physical examination is unremarkable. Her chest X-ray is unremarkable.

(1) List the differential diagnosis for someone with a history of collapse and postural hypotension.

(2) What is the likely diagnosis in this case?

(3) Describe the further investigations to prove this diagnosis.

3. An 84-year-old man is diagnosed with giant cell arteritis after presenting acutely with a severe headache and scalp tenderness. He is started on prednisolone 80 mg od, which he is told will slowly be reduced, depending on his response, over the next 12 months or so. Two years later he remains on 7 mg od.

(1) What are the risks of being on high doses of steroids for a prolonged period of time?

(2) What steps should be taken to manage specific risks?

(3) Describe how you would try to stop his steroids if he were clinically well.

4. A 39-year-old man is seen in the endocrinology out-patient clinic after his GP diagnosed Addison's disease on the basis of reduced serum cortisol after stimulation with synthetic ACTH (Synacthen). He also complained of a headache that had been present for over a month, and of a problem with his vision which he described as 'tunnel vision': when he looked straight ahead he could no longer see things on either side of himself. Examination is relatively normal except he has marked bitemporal hemianopia. By the time he was seen in the out-patient clinic the result of the ACTH assay ordered by the patient's family doctor had become available: it was at 54 ng/L (normal range 100–500 mg/L). The endocrinologist orders several more blood tests, the results of which are shown below.

T_4: 62 mmol/L (normal 70–140 mmol/L)
TSH: 0.3 mU/L (normal 0.5–5 mU/L)
LH: 0.12 U/L (normal 2–14 U/L)
FSH: 0.32 U/L (normal 1–12 U/L)
Testosterone: 84 ng/dL (normal 300–1000 ng/dL)
Prolactin: 1081 ng/mL (normal <15 ng/mL)

(1) Given these results what is the likely diagnosis?

(2) Describe the principles of further management of this patient.

5 Endocrinology

Presentation

Presented to | Grade | Date

Signed

Answers

1. This patient's symptoms and clinical signs are suggestive of Cushing's syndrome. However, Cushing's syndrome remains relatively rare and many patients presenting like this will prove simply to have obesity with accompanying diabetes and hypertension. Tests are needed to confirm the diagnosis of Cushing's.

The simplest test is simply a **random serum cortisol**. However, since levels fluctuate diurnally and between individuals this is highly unreliable. A **9 a.m. cortisol** (the time when, apart from illness or other stresses, cortisol levels should be at their peak), can serve to rule out Cushing's if it is very low, but cannot confirm the diagnosis. The **overnight dexamethasone (suppression) test** undergone by this patient is much more suggestive of Cushing's syndrome if (as here) the morning cortisol level is high. However, for full confirmation of the diagnosis the patient should undergo a **low-dose dexamethasone suppression test**, where a total of eight 0.5 mg doses of dexamethasone are given a 6-hourly intervals, with cortisol levels being measured before and after the course.

To begin investigating the cause of the Cushing's syndrome, he should have a 9 a.m. ACTH level measured. If this is low then it suggests that there is a primary problem with the adrenal glands—they are over-secreting cortisol independently of ACTH control. Benign adenomas or adenocarcinoma of the adrenal gland are the commonest causes, which may be visualized on abdominal CT or MRI. If, however, the 9 a.m. plasma ACTH levels are high, then the adrenal glands are 'behaving normally', i.e. secreting high levels of cortisol in response to high levels of ACTH. The ACTH may be coming from a pituitary adenoma, in which case the diagnosis is **Cushing's disease**. This may be visualized on a pituitary MRI scan. Alternatively the ACTH could be coming from an ectopic source such as a bronchial carcinoma. Chest X-ray, CT scan of the chest, and bronchoscopy may confirm this diagnosis. Rarely there is no obvious source of ACTH secretion found in the chest or the pituitary. Invasive investigations such as angiography with venous blood sampling from different areas of the body may reveal local variations in venous ACTH levels which may suggest where the source of secretion is, for instance (rarely) ovarian or GI cancers.

2. Postural hypotension (where the systolic blood pressure falls by >20 mmHg after standing for 2 minutes) is caused either by the inability of the body to cause sufficient vasoconstriction to increase blood pressure on standing or by hypovolaemia:

Causes of a decreased ability to vasoconstrict	Causes of hypovolaemia
Failure of autonomic nervous system, e.g. autonomic neuropathy in diabetes Drugs that cause peripheral vasodilatation, e.g. alpha-adrenoceptor antagonists Vasodilatation caused by sepsis	Haemorrhage GI fluid losses, e.g. diarrhoea and vomiting Diuretics Other renal losses, including in Addison's

In this patient there is no evidence of infection or systemic disease, and she is not on any regular medications. She has a history of vitiligo, which is associated with an increased incidence of autoimmune disease. The presence of widespread pigmentation (which can be caused by high ACTH levels), alongside evidence of fluid depletion and a history of feeling generally unwell, points to a possible diagnosis of **Addison's disease.** Addison's disease describes destruction of both adrenal glands; the two commonest causes are TB and autoimmune disease.

The diagnosis can be confirmed by the **short Synacthen test**, where an ACTH analogue is given and cortisol levels are measured just before and 30 minutes after its administration. If the cortisol fails to rise it suggests that the adrenal glands are not working (Addison's disease). If the pre-administration level of plasma cortisol is low but is seen to rise 30 minutes later, then the patient has secondary adrenal failure, e.g. loss of pituitary or hypothalamic stimulation. If Addison's disease is confirmed, the patient will require lifelong steroid replacement with hydrocortisone, as well as possible mineralocorticoid and sex steroid supplementation.

3. Long-term steroid therapy may lead to Cushing's syndrome (steroid excess) or adrenal suppression (inadequate steroids).

Cushing's syndrome has several major sequelae, including:

Complication	Monitoring/treatment
Hypertension and diabetes	Regular review of blood pressure and blood glucose, treat appropriately
Peptic ulceration	Consider prophylaxis with a proton pump inhibitor if the patient is high risk
Osteoporosis	Prescribe a bisphosphonate
Infection	Aggressive antibiotics if evidence of infection. Consider TB reactivation if any evidence of this
Weight gain	Lifestyle advice
Depression or psychosis	Monitor for signs

Adrenal suppression: Being on steroids (more than 5–7.5 mg/day) for any significant length of time suppresses the hypothalamic–pituitary–adrenal (HPA) axis, so that if the patient's steroid dose is reduced, or withdrawn too rapidly, the HPA axis is unable to 'recover' and the patient can suffer acute hypoadrenalism.

It can be extremely difficult to wean patients off long-term steroids; the process takes many months and must be tailored to the patient's clinical response. The dose should be reduced by 5 mg every few weeks until it reaches a total dose of 10 mg/day; thereafter the dose should be reduced by1 mg/week. For these reasons **steroid-sparing agents** are utilized wherever possible in long-term inflammatory conditions, e.g. azathioprine in ulcerative colitis. Short courses of steroids (such as the 5 days of prednisolone commonly used for exacerbations of asthma) do not produce adrenal suppression.

4. The commonest cause of pituitary disease is pituitary adenoma, 'functional' (secreting hormones) or non-functional. They can produce three groups of symptoms:

- **Local, compressive symptoms**—including headache, bitemporal hemianopia (compression of the optic chiasm), or hydrocephalus (compression of the ventricles).
- **Secretory symptoms**—caused by uncontrolled secretion of pituitary hormones. The three commonest hormones are ACTH (Cushing's disease), growth hormone (acromegaly), and prolactin causing hyperprolactinaemia and galactorrhoea.
- **Deficiency symptoms**—destruction of the pituitary by a large adenoma leads to a deficiency of pituitary hormones. Panhypopituitarism is a loss of all pituitary hormones including TSH (hypothyroidism), ACTH (hypoadrenalism), GH (growth hormone deficiency), LH, and FSH (disorder of sexual function). A large adenoma will interfere with the pituitary stalk, removing the negative inhibition from above. This leads to hyperprolactinaemia.

This man has evidence of compressive symptoms and panhypopituitarism, making the most likely diagnosis a non-functioning pituitary adenoma. This should be confirmed by pituitary MRI. Pituitary tumours may be amenable to surgical resection (by an 'up the nose' trans-sphenoidal approach).

Once resected the patient will require hormone replacement therapy, including hydrocortisone (started first to avoid adrenal crises), thyroxine, and sex hormones (oestrogen and testosterone).

Further reading

Guidelines: The Endocrine Society guidelines on investigating Cushing's syndrome (http://www.endo-society.org/guidelines/Current-Clinical-Practice-Guidelines.cfm)

OHCM: 216–221, 224–229, 593, 846

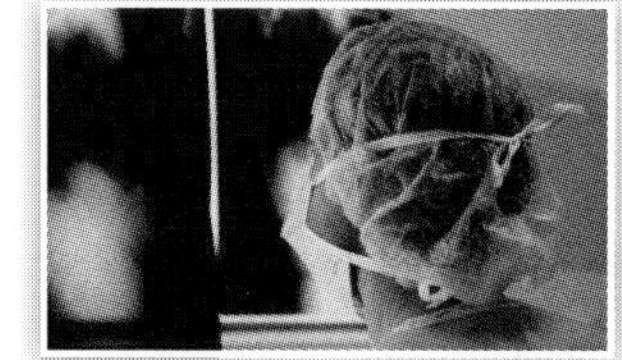
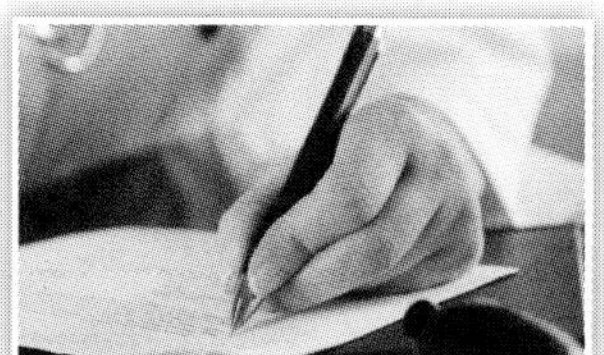
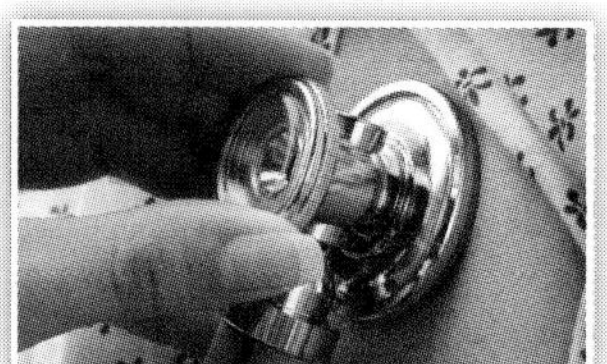
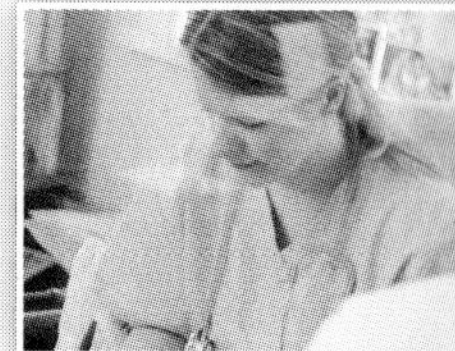

Unit 6
Neurology

Key learning outcomes in neurology include:

- Being able to take a focused history of the major neurological symptoms including headache, altered level of consciousness, weakness, and speech and language problems.
- Being able to explain the differences between upper and lower motor neuron signs and to determine the likely site of a neurological lesion based on clinical signs elicited at examination.
- Understanding the causes of stroke and how to investigate patients presenting with transient ischaemic attacks (TIAs).
- Being aware of the common causes of an acute confusional state (delirium) and of the differences between this and dementia.
- Understanding the indications for CT and MRI scan of the brain and lumbar puncture.

Tips for learning neurology on the wards:

- Clerk patients presenting with severe headache, loss of consciousness, stroke, and acute confusion in the acute clinical areas.
- Clerk patients presenting with fits, falls, and funny turns, concentrating on eliciting a clear history to suggest the likely aetiology of the episode.
- Practice assessing the level of consciousness and applying the Glasgow Coma Scale in patients who are drowsy.
- Visit the hospital's stroke unit to practice neurological examinations.
- Attend the hospital's rapid access TIA clinic to assess patients with possible cerebrovascular disease.
- Observe a lumbar puncture being performed and try to understand the significance of the results of CSF analysis.

History

The nervous system is responsible not just for directing and coordinating the body, but also for more abstract functions such as volition, personality, reasoning, and conscious thought. In some conditions such as dementia or epilepsy, gaining a history from the patient may be impossible and collateral history (from family, friends, or carers) will be essential.

Neurological patients present with a vast range of symptoms. A typical neurological history therefore will focus in detail on the presenting complaint, but will also include a brief assessment of all areas of neurological function to include or exclude other key differential diagnoses. For instance, in a patient presenting with seizures, it is not only important to take a comprehensive 'seizures' history, but also to ask screening questions about **headache** (are there features suggestive of raised intracranial pressure?), **limb weakness** or numbness (a focal brain lesion could be causing the seizures), and **mood** and **behaviour** (could these be pseudo-seizures caused by emotional disturbance?).

One approach to patients with neurological disease, following a 'top-down' approach, asks:

1. Is there global neurological dysfunction?
2. Are there localizing symptoms?
3. What is the likely cause?

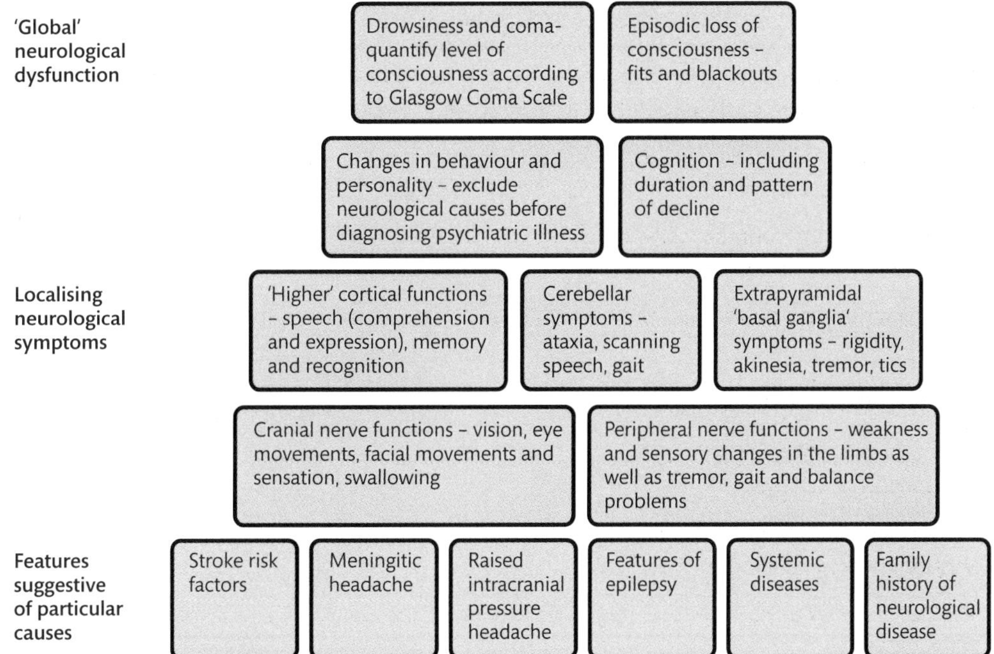

Neurological symptoms are often hard to describe—for instance patients may use the term 'numbness' to describe weakness, sensory loss, paraesthesia, or even pain. Precise definition is very important—what exactly is being described? Where is it? For how long has it been a problem? Does it come and go? Have they had it before?

The commonest causes of neurological disease in the western world are:

- Stroke—thus a vascular risk assessment should be made.
- Demyelination (often first presents in the 20–40-year-old age group).
- Space-occupying lesions including intracranial haemorrhage, benign tumours, and primary and secondary malignant tumours.

The time course of the history is also important in confirming the likely aetiology:

Time course of onset/development of symptoms	Possible aetiologies
Minutes	Vascular events, e.g. stroke Seizure-like activity
Hours	Inflammatory and infectious processes
Days and weeks	Demyelination Tumours
Months and years	Degenerative diseases

Weakness and altered sensation

A basic working knowledge of motor and sensory pathways in the central nervous system, and of the anatomy of peripheral nerves, is crucial in suggesting a location for lesions causing motor and sensory symptoms.

Localized symptoms in one particular area of the body may be caused by damage to a **peripheral nerve** (1) if the symptoms fit with one dermatome or myotome. A classic example is carpal tunnel syndrome caused by median nerve entrapment, or footdrop caused by injury to the common peroneal nerve. Alternatively a lesion may correspond to a **spinal root** myotome or dermatome, suggesting a radiculopathy (2).

Unilateral symptoms, e.g. symptoms affecting the left side of the face and the left arm or leg, suggest a lesion of the central nervous system (3), either the spine or brain. Causes include vascular events (stroke), compression by a space-occupying lesion, localized epileptic activity, or localized demyelination (for instance in multiple sclerosis).

Symmetrical symptoms affecting the lower limbs, e.g. hemiplegia, suggest disease of the spinal cord (4). There may be a sensory level (e.g. at the T12 dermatome) and bowel and bladder dysfunction.

Sensory and motor pathways

Pain and temperature sensation crosses the midline at the level it enters the spinal cord.
Light touch sensation and motor control both travel ipsilaterally in the spinal cord, crossing the midline in the brainstem.

Four reasons for neurological symptoms in the legs

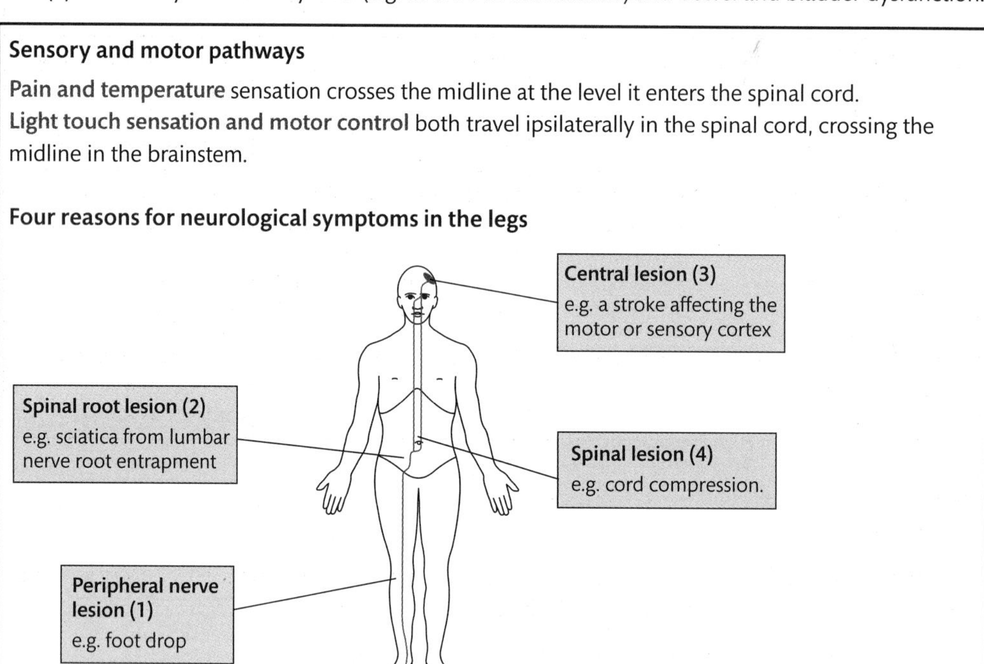

Funny turns—fits, faints, and TIAs

Patients often describe having a 'funny turn' or 'blackout', which are imprecise terms used to describe a large range of different phenomena. A good general history should be taken, including asking in detail about prior epilepsy, strokes, or cardiac disease. In particular, has the patient ever had any similar episodes previously? The history of the presenting episode should then be structured carefully to ask about **precipitating factors**, symptoms **preceding** the episode, the patient's behaviour **during** the episode, and how the patient felt **afterwards**. Getting a collateral history from an onlooker is essential. This information helps to decide whether an event is likely to be an epileptic seizure, a TIA, or cardiovascular syncope.

	Seizures	TIA	Cardiovascular syncope
Precipitant	Often none, but consider trauma and alcohol or drug withdrawal. Adherence to medication should be discussed with known epileptics	None	Straining, micturition, defecation, emotional stress, heat, standing up, exercise
Preceding symptoms	Sometimes none, sometimes a focal neurological 'aura', e.g. an unusual smell or jerking in one limb	None	Lightheadedness, feeling flushed, nausea, pallor, ringing in the ears, a feeling of a 'lump in the throat'
Symptoms during episode	Jerking of all limbs, eye rolling, foaming at the mouth. May become cyanosed during prolonged seizure. Usually a loss of consciousness	Focal neurological deficits, e.g. loss of vision in one eye, loss of power on one side, inability to speak, facial droop. Usually preserved consciousness	Loss of consciousness. Extreme pallor, hard to palpate pulses. Snorting or grunting, occasionally twitching of limbs
Symptoms after episode had resolved	Post-ictal drowsiness and deep sleep	Rapid recovery of function	Rapid return of colour to face and normal consciousness

Headache

Everyone experiences headaches, and the vast majority are completely harmless. Worrying symptoms suggesting the need for urgent investigation include:

- 'Thunderclap' acute onset—suggests subarachnoid haemorrhage
- Scalp tenderness with a unilateral headache—suggests temporal (giant cell) arteritis
- Photophobia, neck pain and stiffness, rash—suggests meningitis
- Early morning headache, worse on lying or straining—suggests raised intracranial pressure

Other headaches to consider include cluster headaches, migraine, stress headaches, benign intracranial hypertension, and sagittal vein thrombosis.

Examination

Global neurological dysfunction and coma

A distinction is made in neurology between 'focal' neurological signs, usually caused by pathological processes in specific areas in the brain, and globally decreased function which may be caused by systemic pathologies that exert direct effects on the whole central nervous system.

Levels of global neurological dysfunction

GCS	AVPU: alert, voice, pain, unresponsive	Level of functioning	Behaviour
15	**A**lert	Normal	Normal level of functioning, normal behaviour
15	**A**lert	Subtle alteration in consciousness	May be confused, irritable, or apathetic—subtle changes in consciousness or functioning with a normal GCS. May be a sign of delirium in the elderly
13–14	Responds to **V**oice	Drowsy	Fully rousable and answering appropriately but falls asleep again when not stimulated
8–12	Responds to **P**ain	Stuporous	Hard to rouse, does not answer appropriately
<8	**U**nresponsive	Comatose	Impossible to rouse. Patients with a GCS <8 are unable to protect their airway—they are at risk of aspiration and should be intubated and managed in a high dependency area unless a decision has be made that invasive treatments are inappropriate.

Common causes of global neurological dysfunction include trauma, raised intracranial pressure, toxins, alcohol, hypoxia, hyper- and hypoglycaemia, hepatic encephalopathy, and inadequate cerebral perfusion—generally **systemic** processes which if severe lead to brain malfunction. Patients with global impairment should be monitored with 'neuro obs'—regular checks of basic observations, GCS, and measurement of pupil diameter.

Upper and lower motor neuron signs

Examination of the peripheral nervous system in a patient complaining of weakness will objectify the level of impairment and also indicate which muscles are affected. Objective limb weakness is conventionally described as either an upper motor or lower motor neuron pattern:

	Upper motor neuron pattern	Lower motor neuron pattern
Bulk	Normal but will get disuse atrophy after months to years	Wasting sometimes associated with fasciculation
Tone	Increased—'spastic' and very stiff, associated with clonus (> three beats)	Reduced—hypotonic and floppy
Power	Reduced	Reduced
Reflexes	Increased—'spastic', with upgoing (extensor) plantars	Decreased or absent. Downgoing (flexor) plantars
Causes	Brain and spinal cord problems, e.g. stroke	Peripheral nerve problems, e.g. Guillain-Barré

MRC grading of muscle power (0–5)
0: no movement
1: flicker is perceptible in the muscle
2: movement only if gravity eliminated
3: can move limb against gravity
4: can move against gravity and some resistance exerted by examiner
5: normal power

Disorders of gait, balance, and movement

Problems with walking may be caused by a range of things, including physical deformity, painful joints, or muscle weakness. However, problems with walking, balance, and fine movement may also be caused by disease of the basal ganglia (which initiate movements), or the cerebellum (which coordinates movements and maintains gait). The two most common presentations—Parkinsonism and cerebellar dysfunction—are described below. These often present with difficulty moving despite normal power in the limbs and no signs of injury.

Parkinsonism	Cerebellar ataxia (using the mnemonic DANISH)
• **Akinesia or bradykinesia** (slow movements which are difficult to initiate) • **Resting tremor** • **Rigidity** (stiffness of limbs), may be: lead-pipe rigidity (increased tone on manipulating joints which is consistent through the whole range of movement) or cogwheel rigidity (intermittent jerky rigidity on manipulating the wrists) • **Serpentine stare** (caused by a paucity of facial expressions) • **Shuffling gait** with difficulty turning	• **D**ysdiadochokinesia (the inability to perform rapid alternating movements, e.g. turning one hand over and over whilst clapping) • **A**taxic gait (staggering as if drunk, using a broad base to avoid falling) • **N**ystagmus (saw-tooth side-to-side movements of the eyes) • **I**ntention tremor and past-pointing (very jerky attempts to perform simple motor tasks such as touching the nose with a finger) • **S**taccato, scanning speech (slow and slurred) • **H**ypotonia and hyporeflexia on the ipsilateral side to the lesion

Signs of cerebral dysfunction

Different parts of the cerebral cortex are involved in different levels of functioning, and lesions involving areas of higher function may produce functional deficits that are not as immediately obvious as those caused by a lesion in, say, the primary motor cortex. The following are all signs that localize lesions to different areas of the brain.

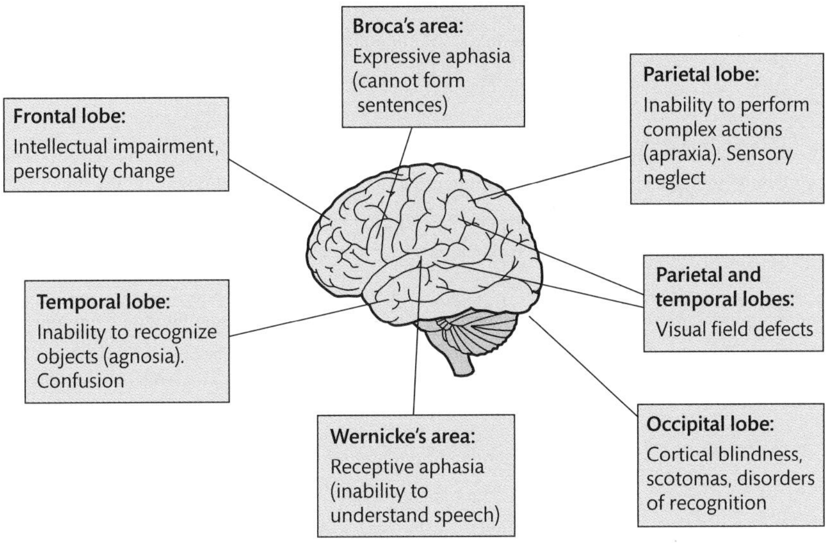

Investigations

Imaging of the brain–CT and MRI scanning

CT and MRI scans are complex radiological investigations and need review and interpretation by a radiologist. However, it is worthwhile becoming familiar with the basic appearance of the brain and skull and being able to recognize obvious abnormalities. We have set out a schema for reviewing a CT head scan below (this is a normal scan):

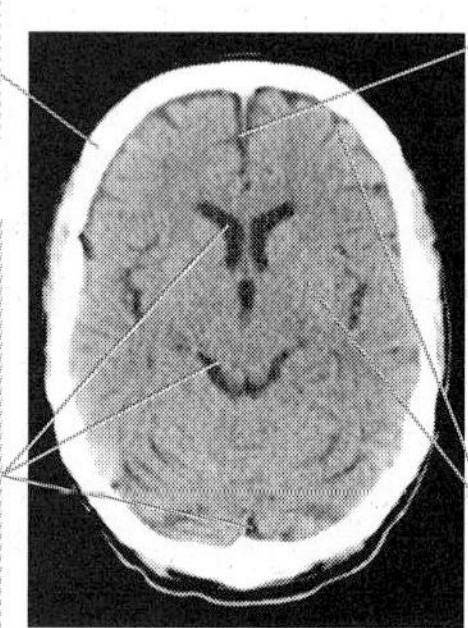

Other than the amount of radiation involved in a CT scan, the main drawback is in imaging soft tissue–for instance, plaques of demyelination will rarely be seen on CT, and so for imaging of soft tissue lesions MRI is preferred despite being slower and more expensive. MRI scanning is becoming increasingly utilized in acute stroke disease. CT with the addition of intravenous contrast is particularly used in the investigation of space-occupying lesions such as tumours or abscesses.

Electroencephalography (EEG)

Sixteen electrodes are attached to the scalp and electrical activity is monitored. A specific locus of epileptic activity is sometimes identified, though the test is often negative when the patient is not having a seizure. At specialist centres EEG is coupled with video recording for investigation of complex abnormalities of consciousness.

Investigation of TIA or stroke

Transient ischaemic attacks (TIAs) are sometimes referred to as the harbingers of stroke, since they are often followed by a full stroke with symptoms which do not resolve. Because of this, patients suffering a TIA are risk-assessed, and then investigated rapidly either as in-patients or out-patients according to their risk scoring.

The beautifully simple **ABCD**^{2} risk score of Rothwell and colleagues (Johnston SC *et al.* (2007) *Lancet* **369**(9558), 283–92) is now utilized to assess patients presenting with a TIA.

- **A**ge ≥60 years = 1
- **B**lood pressure: ≥140 mmHg or diastolic ≥90 mm = 1
- **C**linical features: focal weakness = 2; speech impairment without focal weakness = 1
- **D**uration of symptoms: ≥60 min = 2; 10–59 min = 1
- **D**iabetes (at presentation) = 1

Risk: Low = 0–3, Moderate = 4–5, High = 6 and 7; patients with scores > 5 should be admitted and investigated.

Remember that you can find large-size, annotated versions of many of the X-rays and ECGs that appear in this book on the book's web site at www.oxfordtextbooks.co.uk/orc/randall/

Patients presenting with symptoms of stroke or TIA need a full cardiovascular risk assessment. Investigations should include:

- **Bloods-**including FBC, U&Es, glucose, ESR, lipids
- **Radiology**—chest X-ray and CT head scan
- **ECG**: Looking for signs of: (1) old ischaemic heart disease including left bundle branch block, left axis deviation, and poor anterior R-wave progression; (2) left ventricular hypertrophy (according to voltage criteria); (3) left atrial hypertrophy (widened P waves, called *P-mitrale*); but perhaps most importantly of all (4) atrial fibrillation (AF). AF is one of the biggest single risk factors for developing stroke, because thrombi form in the non-contracting atria and are then 'thrown off' into the cerebral circulation. Depending on the patient's risk of developing further strokes and the nature of the abnormality detected, aspirin or warfarin thromboprophylaxis may be instituted.
- **Echocardiogram**: Various abnormalities of heart structure and function predispose to intracardiac thrombus formation. These include chamber hypertrophy, valvular lesions, and chamber wall hypokinesis following myocardial infarction. Patients with proven intracardiac thrombus, or those at risk of developing it, should be started on warfarin or aspirin as above.
- **Doppler ultrasound scanning** of the carotid arteries: Significant stenosis of the common or internal carotid arteries is strongly linked to developing stroke after a TIA. If the patient has greater than 70% stenosis then they should be considered for carotid endarterectomy where atheroma is removed from the carotid artery wall.

Analysis of cerebrospinal fluid (CSF)

Lumbar puncture is an invasive procedure where a spinal needle is inserted into the subarachnoid space in the lumbar spine under local anaesthetic and CSF is removed for analysis. This should always undertaken below the level of L1 since this is where the spinal cord ends. The commonest complication is a severe headache (reduced by bed rest, analgesia, and fluid replacement), but rare complications include nerve damage and meningitis. It should not be performed if there is raised intracranial pressure since suddenly relieving CSF pressure in the spinal cord can cause brainstem herniation through the foramen magnum ('coning'), leading to death.

Diagnoses that can be made or confirmed by lumbar puncture include:

- Subarachnoid haemorrhage—if there is a large amount of blood or xanthochromia (a haemoglobin breakdown product).
- Meningitis—if white cells or organisms are seen. (TB meningitis is suggested by large numbers of lymphocytes and very high protein levels.)
- Viral encephalitis—rapid polymerase chain reaction (PCR) testing is used to look especially for herpes simplex encephalitis.
- Demyelinating disease—isolated high protein, in oligoclonal bands, is strongly suggestive of demyelinating disease such as multiple sclerosis or Guillain-Barré syndrome.

Interventions

Cerebrovascular disease

Patients with cerebrovascular disease require a full assessment of their modifiable cardiovascular risk factors. Once the diagnosis has been confirmed, antiplatelet therapy should be initiated, commonly consisting of aspirin, clopidogrel and slow-release dipyridamole. The seven crucial steps for combating vascular disease remain:

1. Smoking cessation—many hospitals have counsellors to help patients with this
2. Diet
3. Exercise to promote weight loss, better blood pressure and glycaemic control
4. Blood pressure control—treat in line with standard hypertension protocols
5. Glycaemic control—test for diabetes and treat to control the HbA1c at <6.5% if possible
6. Aspirin to prevent clot formation in the event of plaque rupture
7. Statin, to control lipid levels as well as to stabilize atheromatous plaques and reduce inflammation

Epilepsy

Caution is exercised in prescribing antiepileptic medications—they should be reserved only for patients suffering regular seizures that are affecting the quality of life. These medications are never started after a 'first fit', partly because of their side-effects but also because a significant proportion of patients will suffer only one fit in their life and should not be labelled 'epileptic'.

There are various classes of antiepileptic drugs, which may act to block ion channels and stabilize neuronal membranes (e.g. phenytoin) or to increase inhibitory transmission in the central nervous system (e.g. sodium valproate). Many of these medications have complex interactions and side-effects and are therefore common in undergraduate assessments. The rule of thumb to follow in epilepsy is 'the fewest drugs, at the lowest doses'

The following points should always be borne in mind when seeing a patient on an anticonvulsant:

- **Therapeutic range:** Both phenytoin and carbamazepine cause toxicity at concentrations only slightly above those necessary to produce an anticonvulsant effect. Their plasma concentrations should be monitored every few months.
- **Cardiac effects:** Any drugs that interfere with sodium channels (again, phenytoin and carbamazepine in particular) cause changes in cardiac conduction predisposing to arrhythmia. In particular the QT interval on ECG may be prolonged, which can lead to ventricular tachycardia.
- **Liver metabolism:** Both phenytoin and carbamazepine induce the cytochrome P-450 enzymes in the liver and may therefore reduce the plasma levels of other drugs.
- **Pregnancy:** Most anticonvulsants are potentially teratogenic; however, the risk to the fetus of fits with subsequent cyanosis is considered greater and so generally pregnant women are encouraged to take lamotrigine (believed to be the safest drug) during pregnancy.

Common medications in neurology

Class	Examples	Mechanism	Indications	Contraindications	Side-effects	Special notes
Antiplatelet drugs						
Thrombolytics						
5-HMG-CoA-reductase inhibitors						
Sodium channel stabilizers						
GABA transaminase inhibitors						
GABA agonists						
Benzodiazepines						
Barbiturates						
Levodopa						
Dopa-decarboxylase inhibitor						
Dopamine agonists						

Stroke and transient ischaemic attacks (TIAs)

This section should be used to clerk patients with acute strokes. The management philosophy of stroke has changed a lot over the past 10 years, with the emphasis on early intervention to achieve reperfusion. Patient pathways often now begin at a centralized, regional hyperacute stroke unit (HASU), where they may be thrombolysed, and then lead to smaller stroke units for rehabilitation and physiotherapy.

Learning challenges

- Why is getting a CT scan of the brain as early as possible crucial in managing patients with strokes, when changes associated with infarction show up better later on?
- What can be done to prevent a patient who has suffered a TIA from going on to suffer a stroke?

History

Comment on

- Time when symptoms began
- Visual loss
- Speech and language loss (including comprehension)
- Confusion or drowsiness
- Facial weakness or sensory changes
- Limb weakness—mono-, hemi-, paraparesis (spinal)
- Limb sensory changes—numbness/paraesthesiae
- Vascular risk factors—previous stroke, hypertension, IHD, PVD, DM, smoking and alcohol excess, hyperlipidaemia, family history of premature vascular-related death
- Other specific stroke risks, including atrial fibrillation, clotting disorders, use of anticoagulants, and antiplatelet therapies
- Dominant hand ('which hand do they write with?'—useful for localizing lesions)

Examination

Well or unwell? Why?

Feet to face:

Vital signs: Temperature | Blood pressure | Pulse rate | Respiratory rate | O2 saturations

Clinical clues:

Cardiovascular:

1 2 1

Respiratory:

GCS [ ]E [ ]V [ ]M

Abdominal:

Neurological:

Other:

Comment on

- GCS, blood pressure, HR, CBG, oxygen sats, temperature
- Signs of vascular risk—tar staining of fingers, xanthelasma
- Cardiovascular: pulse—rate and regularity; cardiac murmurs
- Vascular tree—central and peripheral pulses, aortic aneurysm, bruits
- Eyes—hemianopia, visual neglect, eye movements and pupillary responses
- Speech and language—dysphasia (receptive and/or expressive) versus dysarthria
- Cerebellar signs, posterior fossa signs, e.g. vertigo, nystagmus
- Swallowing assessment
- Limbs—motor/sensory assessment

CT head (prove the diagnosis, exclude the differentials)

Comment on

- Evidence of infarction
- Evidence of intracranial haemorrhage
- Evidence of other pathologies, e.g. space-occupying lesion

Blood tests

Comment on

- FBC, clotting screen
- Random glucose and lipids
- ESR/CRP—evidence of vasculitis

ECG

Comment on

- Atrial fibrillation; voltage criteria of LVH; signs of IHD, e.g. LAD, LBBB

Chest X-ray

Comment on

- Cardiomegaly, left atrial enlargement

Carotid Doppler

(only for patients with (1) anterior circulation strokes and (2) eligible or willing to have secondary investigations and intervention, i.e. carotid angiography and endarterectomy)

Comment on

- Degree of carotid stenosis

Echocardiogram

Comment on

- Dilated chambers
- Valvular disease

Evaluation

1. Is there evidence of stroke? Which stroke syndrome is suggested?

Syndrome	Features
Total anterior circulation stroke (TACS)	All three of: (1) higher cortical dysfunction (e.g. aphasia), (2) homonymous hemianopia, (3) motor and sensory deficits in face/arm/leg
Partial anterior circulation stroke (PACS)	Two of the three features of TACS
Posterior circulation stroke (POCS)	Altered consciousness, dysarthria, nystagmus, vertigo, cranial nerve abnormalities, bilateral motor/sensory disturbance
Lacunar stroke (LACS)	Small strokes, e.g. purely motor. Often there is evidence of small earlier strokes

2. If the symptoms wore off within 24 hours (a TIA), what is the risk of developing a full stroke (ABCD^2 score)? **See p. 184**

- **A**ge ≥60 years = 1
- **B**lood pressure: ≥140 mmHg or diastolic ≥90 mm = 1
- **C**linical features: focal weakness = 2; speech impairment without focal weakness = 1
- **D**uration of symptoms: ≥60 min = 2; 10–59 min = 1
- **D**iabetes (at presentation) = 1

Risk: Low = 0–3, Moderate = 4–5, High = 6 and 7; patients with scores > 5 should be admitted and investigated.

3. Is there haemorrhage on CT? How long since the symptoms came on? Is this patient suitable for thrombolysis, aspirin or dipyridamole?

4. What is the likely cause? What interventions can reduce the risk of future events?

5. Is this patient safe to swallow? How can nutrition and other areas of rehabilitation be addressed in the longer term?

Questions

1. A 54-year-old right-handed man presents to the Emergency Department with sudden-onset of loss of power in his right arm and problems with his speech. The episode started whilst he was sitting at his desk at work about an hour ago. He remained fully conscious throughout and the symptoms resolved completely within 10 minutes. He has no significant previous medical history, but is a 'social smoker', having a 20 pack-year history.

On physical examination, the patient is alert and well with a GCS of 15. His pulse is regular at 64 bpm and his blood pressure is 165/93 mmHg. Examination is otherwise remarkable, with no neurological deficit.

Routine blood tests including FBC, U&Es, and CBG are normal, as is a CT scan of the head. His ECG confirms normal sinus rhythm.

(1) Calculate his $ABCD^2$ score

(2) Describe your further management of this patient.

2. A 64-year-old left-handed man presents to the Emergency Department with a dense left-sided hemiparesis and facial droop that came on suddenly an hour earlier whilst at work. His past medical history includes hypertension and diabetes, and he is clinically obese. Two years before he had suffered a stroke that he left him with stiffness on his right-hand side. His medications include amlodipine 10 mg od, bendroflumethiazide 2.5 mg od, aspirin 75 mg od, enalapril 20 mg bd, and gliclazide 80 mg bd. He is a non-smoker.

On examination he is fully alert. He is able to speak but his speech is slurred and difficult to understand. His blood pressure is 184/92 mm Hg, pulse 86 bpm, regular. Neurological assessment confirms a flaccid left-sided paralysis, with hypotonia, areflexia, and power 0–1/5 in all muscle groups of the upper and lower left limbs. There is a left-sided facial palsy with drooling of saliva from the corner of his mouth. He has a spastic paraparesis on the right-hand side, but his wife reports that this has been the case ever since his stroke 2 years before. Cardiovascular examination including cardiac auscultation and assessment of the pulses is notable only for a right-sided carotid bruit. An urgent CT is performed which is shown below.

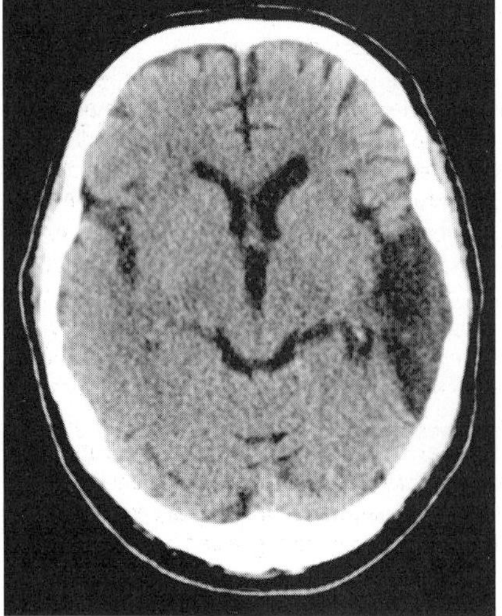

(1) What is the major abnormality demonstrated on this scan?

(2) What is the most important negative finding on this scan?

(3) List the essential steps in your further management of this patient.

3. A 63-year-old right-handed man is brought to the Emergency Department by ambulance. His wife had noticed he became 'suddenly vague' whilst sitting watching television, he was unable to speak, and she noticed his right arm was 'lying by his side'. The paramedics describe both his right upper and lower limb being flaccid and weak, and say that he couldn't answer any of their questions. A CT head scan confirms the diagnosis of an acute left-hemisphere infarct.

Over the next week his upper limb weakness improves considerably, though there is still some residual weakness in the lower limb, which is noted after a few days to be stiffer than at first, with exaggerated reflexes (that were initially absent) and an extensor plantar reflex (which previously was equivocal). Although he seems to be fully alert and able to follow instructions, he shows great difficulty in trying to speak and despite obviously trying hard, can only say the words 'hi', 'yes', and 'no' in response to questions.

(1) What is the arterial distribution of this stroke?

(2) Which particular areas of the brain have been affected?

(3) Which particular members of the multidisciplinary team would you involve in this man's on-going rehabilitation?

4. A 72-year-old right-handed woman is admitted to hospital after developing a left-sided hemiparesis and dysarthria. Her swallow is assessed by the admitting doctor who finds that she coughs and splutters when given sips of water to drink. The nursing staff are instructed that she is to be kept nil by mouth and intravenous fluids are prescribed. A CT head scan shows an area of early infarction in the right internal capsule. She is managed with aspirin and dipyridamole and transferred to the hospital's acute stroke unit. Over the next 10 days she is seen by physiotherapists and speech therapists, and finally by an occupational therapist. She improves somewhat and is able to walk with a frame, but she is still unsafe when she swallows and after a few days began to be fed by nasogastric tube.

(1) How would you manage this patient's long term nutrition if her swallow doesn't improve?

(2) What steps should be taken to get this patient home?

Remember that you can find large-size, annotated versions of many of the X-rays and ECGs that appear in this book on the book's web site at www.oxfordtextbooks.co.uk/orc/randall/

Blood tests

Comment on

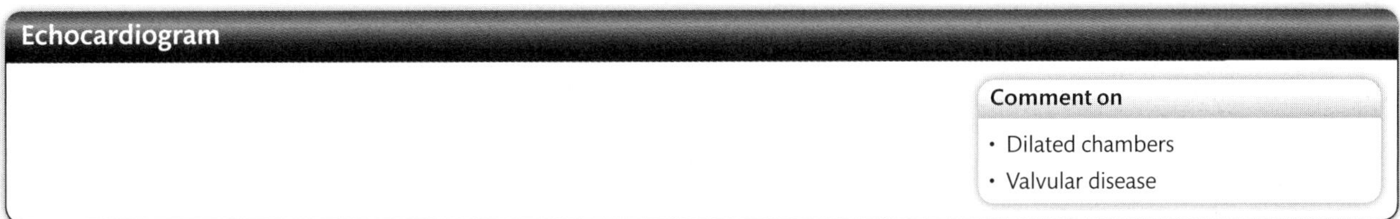

6 Neurology

Answers

1. This man has had a transient ischaemic attack (TIA). His ABCD^2 score is 3 and therefore he does not require admission but requires 'urgent' referral to the hospital TIA clinic. He should also have his modifiable risk factors addressed—secondary prophylaxis to prevent further stroke/TIAs should be started as soon as a CT head scan has excluded haemorrhagic disease or other differential diagnoses; with immediate management including the following:

- Antiplatelet therapy—aspirin (or clopidogrel)
- Statin—simvastatin or similar is started independent of lipid status in stroke disease
- Education to address smoking, weight loss, diet, appropriate exercise, and moderation of alcohol intake

At a TIA clinic efforts are made to discover what led to this TIA. The two commonest causes of ischaemic stroke are carotid artery stenosis (detected by Doppler ultrasound of the carotid arteries), and atrial fibrillation:

- In appropriate patients with anterior circulation stroke/TIA disease a Doppler scan of the carotids should be arranged. If the scan reveals a stenosis on the 'symptomatic side' of greater than 70% patients should be referred for carotid endarterectomy. Whilst endarterectomy significantly reduces the chance of having a further event, it carries significant risk (mortality 3%, risk of suffering a perioperative stroke 3%) and so patients need to be carefully selected and fully involved in the management decisions. Patients should also be started on aspirin and a statin, along with having any underlying diabetes and hypertension well controlled.
- Warfarin therapy is advised for patients with: (1) echocardiogram-proven thrombus within the heart or areas of myocardial hypokinesia (predisposing to mural thrombus formation), or (2) atrial fibrillation.

2. This man has clinical evidence of acute stroke. His CT shows:

The most clinically relevent feature of this CT scan is that there is no sign of intracerebral haemorrhage - this would show up as a bright white smudge within the brain parenchyma, and would directly affect management since treatment reduces the coagulability of the blood (for instance aspirin or thrombolysis) would be contraindicated. Approximately 15% of strokes are haemorrhagic. Acute ischaemic strokes may cause no acute CT changes (as here), or may cause cerebral oedema.

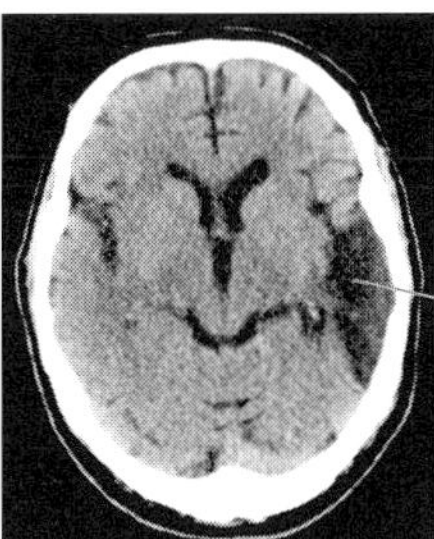

This dark area in the left cerebral hemisphere indicates an old infarction within the vascular territory of the left middle cerebral artery. Infarcted brain eventally necroses to form a fluid filled cyst with this appearance. This stroke will have caused his right sided spasticity, which classically develops several days after the onset of a stroke - initially, a flaccid paralysis is seen.

Since there is an obvious stroke syndrome which came on within the previous 3 hours, this man is a possible candidate for thrombolysis if facilities exist to perform this (in the UK it should only be done at a hyperacute stroke unit (HASU) with neurosurgical backup). Contraindications to thrombolysis include:

(1) Recent/significant bleeding from any body site, e.g. epistaxis, menstrual bleeding, upper or lower GI bleeding

(2) Recent major surgery or trauma

(3) Pregnancy

(4) Coagulopathy—haemophilia or warfarin therapy

(5) Known vascular abnormalities.

If thrombolysis is not possible then this man should be treated with aspirin. If there was any haemorrhage on his CT scan then he should be discussed with neurosurgeons since operations to decrease intracranial pressure may improve prognosis after haemorrhagic stroke.

Standard treatment for any suspected stroke is to make the patient nil by mouth until their swallow is formally assessed, with intravenous fluids being prescribed until then. This patient's high blood pressure should not be treated acutely—this may worsen cerebral perfusion and increase damage to area on the edge of the infarct with borderline levels of perfusion—the so-called 'watershed zone'. After a few days at a HASU, patients are commonly transferred to an acute stroke unit where intensive physiotherapy and speech and language therapy aim to maximize functional performance.

3. Sudden-onset weakness in the right arm and leg imply that this man has had a left-hemisphere stroke. This is also a typical cause of aphasia, particularly in someone who is right handed: in almost all right-handed and 70% of left-handed patients the speech centres are in the left hemisphere. This man has evidence of dense expressive dysphasia: his comprehension as evidenced by his ability to follow instructions remains intact, but he cannot form words or express himself appropriately. **Expressive aphasia** (**Broca's aphasia**), is often caused by left frontal lobe lesions. A **receptive aphasia** (**Wernicke's aphasia**), is commonly caused by more posterior damage to the temporal lobe, and produces an inability to understand speech, leading to a patient speaking fast and fluently but completely unintelligibly using random collections of jargon wards. **Dysarthria** describes a problem with articulation caused by the inability to control the muscles of the larynx, mouth, and tongue, due to facial, vagal, and hypoglossal damage. **Dysphonia** (hoarseness or complete loss of voice) is the inability to produce the sounds required to speak normally. It is invariably caused by local laryngeal pathologies (e.g. vocal cord lesions or paralysis).

This man has had an anterior circulation stroke, probably affecting a branch of the middle cerebral artery. Typically an initial flaccid paralysis is caused, followed over a few days with partial resolution but also the development of spasticity, with increased tone, hyperreflexia, and upgoing plantars. Rehabilitation in this man will be focused on improving mobility and communication. Initially the multidisciplinary team (MDT) would include medical input from specialist stroke doctors, alongside:

- Good nursing care will be essential to prevent the patient from developing complications—for instance, regular turning regimes prevent the development of pressure sores.
- Physiotherapy helps improve mobility and fine motor coordination, relieving spasticity.
- Speech and language therapy improve communication and may help relieve some of the frustration felt by patients who are unable to express themselves.

Once the initial phase is complete, other essential members of the MDT would include psychologist, occupational therapist, social worker, community stroke team, GP, and community nurses.

4. Swallowing is often a major problem after patients suffer a stroke, and can lead to serious problems if an aspiration pneumonia develops as a result of the airway not being protected during eating. Because of this, patients are usually made nil by mouth following a stroke, and are then gradually assessed by speech and language therapists (beginning with sips of water and proceeding to solid foods), aiming for a safe swallow without coughing or spluttering. The best long-term feeding option for patients with an unsafe swallow is a percutaneous endoscopic gastrostomy (a PEG tube), which is inserted endoscopically through the abdominal wall and into the stomach.

Discharge planning should begin early on when patients with strokes are admitted to hospital—read the patient's social history and find out how well they will cope at home with whatever new disability has been caused by the stroke. Writing a problem list can help clarify the progress being made in the rehabilitation of patients, as well as identifying ongoing challenges. The patient's ongoing problems would include (1) dysphagia, (2) dysarthria, and (3) limited mobility. This woman's case poses complex issues around discharge planning and these need to be recognized and planned for from the start of her rehabilitation. The focus of physiotherapy, speech therapy, and occupation therapy should be on preparing the patient for discharge and handing over care to community teams. Occupation therapy aims to aid safe and rapid discharge by modifying the home environment to permit this. An access visit may be undertaken with the patient, and modifications such as a chairlift, handrails, easy-access bath, or changes to sleeping arrangements may be suggested. Social workers can assess how well the patient will cope at home and arrange for carers to visit to help with personal care or household tasks.

Further reading

Guidelines: NICE guidelines on acute stroke or TIA (http://www.nice.org.uk/CG68)

OHCM: 474–481

Acute confusion

This section should be used to clerk patients presenting to hospital with a change in their mental state, or who become acutely confused during an admission to hospital. This is very common in hospital, especially in the elderly. Such confusion may be acute, or it may be acute-on-chronic if there was pre-existing cognitive impairment. Patients with acute confusion may be found on the Medical Admissions Unit or Elderly Care Ward.

Learning challenges

- Why is sedation of acutely confused patients potentially dangerous and best avoided if possible?
- Why are the elderly particularly vulnerable to confusion during acute illness?

History

Comment on

- Known/previous history of cognitive impairment
- Time course of cognitive decline
- Likely causes of acute exacerbation—sepsis, medications, systemic illness
- Changes in behaviour and sleep patterns
- Mental health symptoms—mood, hallucinations, delusions, aggression
- Previous strokes or other intracranial disease
- Pre-morbid and present general level of functioning including activities of daily living (ADL)
- Medications—including antiplatelet medications; exacerbating medications including sedatives and opiates
- Previous alcohol consumption, time of last drink
- Accommodation and carers (formal and informal)

Examination

Well or unwell? Why?

Feet to face:

Vital signs: Temperature Blood pressure Pulse rate Respiratory rate O2 saturations

Clinical clues:

Cardiovascular:

1 2 1

Respiratory:

GCS [ ]E [ ]V [ ]M

Abdominal:

Neurological:

Other:

Comment on

- Signs of causes of delirium—temperature, HR and regularity, BP, CBG, GCS, oxygen sats
- Cardiovascular and stroke risk—stigmata of hyperlipidaemia, CBG, BP, pulse (AF)
- Signs of previous or long-term illnesses—cancers, strokes
- Behaviour
- Full physical examination—signs of infection
- Palpable bladder
- Rectal examination—constipation
- Focal neurological signs—stroke disease, space-occupying lesion

Cognitive testing

Comment on

- AMTS (Abbreviated Mental Test score, out of 10)

Blood tests

Comment on

- FBC–WCC and differential
- U&Es
- Thyroid function tests
- Vitamin B12 and folate levels
- Glucose
- CRP
- Calcium
- Others, including liver function tests, clotting

Microbiology - including urinalysis and MSU; blood cultures

ECG

Comment on

- Arrhythmia (brady- and tachy-), signs of acute ischaemia

Chest X-ray

Comment on

- Infection, malignancy, acute heart failure

CT head

Comment on

- Space-occupying lesions
- Cerebral atrophy
- Intracranial bleeds, e.g. subdural
- Signs of raised intracranial pressure and hydrocephalus

Evaluation

1. Is there an obvious acute medical cause for this patient's confusion? How should it be treated?

Infection?	Space-occupying lesion?	Hypothyroidism?
Renal failure?	Urinary retention?	Constipation?
Electrolyte disturbance?	Hyper/hypoglycaemia?	Depression?

2. Are the features displayed by the patient more in keeping with delirium or dementia? Is there a history of chronic confusion?

Delirium	Dementia
Fluctuating impairment of cognitive function	Permanent cognitive impairment
Fluctuating consciousness (drowsiness and hyperactivity, very distractible)	Normal level of consciousness
Day–night sleep reversal	Normal sleep pattern
Hallucinations and delusions prominent	Memory symptoms predominant
May be frightened, uncooperative or restless, or apathetic and hypoactive	Many be placid and calm, or suspicious and aggressive

3. Once the patient begins to recover from any acute illness, does their cognitive function also improve? If there is chronic cognitive impairment, what is the likely aetiology?

4. What is the patient's baseline level of functioning? What are their care needs? Can these needs be met in the community, by carers or family? If not, would residential or nursing home admission be necessary?

Questions

1. You accompany the on-call junior doctor who has been called to one of the orthopaedic wards in the middle of the night because of a disruptive patient. The patient, a previously fit and well 87-year-old woman, was admitted 2 days earlier after slipping on ice. She sustained a fractured left neck of femur, which had been operatively repaired today. The surgery was uncomplicated and she had returned from recovery with no clinical problems. You find the patient lying in her bed singing loudly and incoherently. She occasionally shouts and seems to be gesturing towards something on the ceiling which is frightening her. The doctor attempts to talk to her but finds it difficult to attract the patient's attention for more than a few seconds at a time. The nurses are concerned because the patient is disturbing all the other patients on the ward, and ask whether she can be given a sedative to calm her down.

(1) What is the generic name given to this presentation?

(2) List five common causes that may be responsible in this patient.

(3) What further information should the doctor try to obtain before agreeing to sedate the patient?

(4) Describe your further management.

2. A 93-year-old woman is admitted to hospital because her family, who normally look after her at home, report that she has become very withdrawn, drowsy, and uncommunicative over the previous 5 days. Her mobility has been markedly decreased for the previous 2 days. She has not complained of any specific symptoms, and the family have not noticed any obvious signs of systemic disease. Two days earlier she fell and injured her left wrist, and since then has been taking tramadol (which they had at home from a previous fall) and a benzodiazepine sedative to help her sleep at night. Previously she was relatively well. She was able to hold a coherent conversation and complete the crossword in the newspaper. She was mobile within her home, walking with two sticks. Her previous medical history includes hypertension, heart failure, and a hysterectomy for menorrhagia (50 years previously). Her only regular medications are bendroflumethiazide 2.5 mg od and furosemide 80 mg od.

On examination she is confused (AMTS of 3/10), and appears clinically dehydrated. Apart from a clinical Colles' fracture of the left wrist, cardiovascular, respiratory, and abdominal examinations (including digital rectal examination) are unremarkable. Her initial blood tests are shown below:

Sodium: 118 mmol/L	Haemoglobin: 13.5 g/dL
Potassium: 3.2 mmol/L	White cells: 8.2 × 10^9/L
Urea: 8.1 mmol/L	Platelets: 311× 10^9/L
Creatinine: 112 μmol/L	CRP: 9 mg/L

(1) List three possible contributing factors to her confusion

(2) Describe the essential steps in your management?

3. An 87-year-old man is admitted to hospital with increasing confusion and hallucinations. Over the previous 2 weeks his son and daughter had become increasingly concerned about his confusion, and him claiming to see and talk to his wife who had died several months earlier.

On arrival in the Emergency Department he is disoriented in time and place, and scores 3/10 on an AMTS. He is pyrexial and complains of lower abdominal pain, and is found to be in urinary retention with a secondary urinary tract infection. He is diagnosed as having an acute delirium secondary to urosepsis and is admitted to the Elderly Care Ward, for urinary catheterization, intravenous antibiotics, and fluids.

Over the course of his 12-day admission to hospital he makes good progress, becoming less confused. After a week his AMTS is 7/10 and he scores 24/30 on a Mini-Mental State Examination (MMSE). His blood tests, which initially revealed evidence of renal failure and sepsis, return to normal. A CT head scan performed 2 days after admission shows mild cerebral atrophy(in keeping with his age) but nothing else of note. However, his family maintain that he is still far from his normal self; they are concerned that he 'is very quiet, uncommunicative, avoids eye-contact, and very low'. He continues to suffer visual hallucinations.

What might explain why this man has not returned to his previous self, and how might he be helped now that he has recovered physically?

4. A 79-year-old man from a residential home is admitted to hospital with increasing confusion over the previous 3 weeks. He was admitted to the residential home 18 months previously because he was not coping at home due to decreased mobility and recurrent falls after suffering a stroke. He is not usually confused, and a month previously scored 29/30 on Mini-Mental State Examination. On admission to the Emergency Department, examination is unremarkable except for obvious confusion (the patient has an AMTS of 4/10), and routine blood tests, chest X-ray, and urine dipstick are normal. The next day he undergoes a CT scan of his head, shown below.

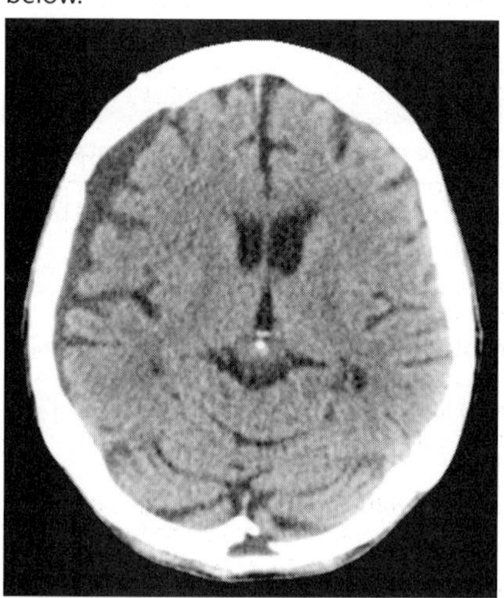

(1) What does the scan show?

(2) What would you do about his discharge?

Presentation

Presented to ______ Grade ______ Date ______

Signed

Remember that you can find large-size, annotated versions of many of the X-rays and ECGs that appear in this book on the book's web site at www.oxfordtextbooks.co.uk/orc/randall/

Answers

1. This presentation is referred to as **acute confusional state**, or **delirium**. It refers to an acute, global decline in neurological function, often with disordered levels of consciousness and distractibility, which is common in the elderly often in response to a illness, pain, or another trigger. A reversal of the day/night sleeping pattern is common. Some patients develop hypoactive delirium where they are drowsy, withdrawn, and vacant, where delirium may be harder to recognize than in this woman.

Sedation should be used only with great caution in elderly confused patients, and only if they pose a risk either to themselves or to other patients. It would only be indicated for this woman if she was, for instance, trying to walk around the ward, was unsteady on her feet and in danger of falling over, or if she was attacking another patient.

The real question to be asking here is why this lady is confused at all. She should be assumed to be delirious rather than to have dementia (until all causes of delirium have been excluded). The patient's notes may be helpful to determine whether she has been noted to be confused before, since in the middle of the night it will be impossible to speak to a relative or family doctor.

It is important to look for a precipitating cause. Surgery itself can cause delirium, but examining the patient, checking her basic observations and blood test results, may reveal, for example, underlying sepsis which should be treated. In the meantime it may be worth suggesting to the nurses that the patient be moved into a side-room where she will be less disruptive to the other patients. A low-stimulation environment is recommended, with a window to allow natural patterns of light and darkness. She should be kept well hydrated and any fever brought down with paracetamol. Pain, constipation, urinary retention, and other obvious triggers should be addressed.

2. The primary reason why this lady is confused is her very low sodium level. Hyponatraemia initially causes confusion and drowsiness, and if severe can also cause seizures, coma, and cardiac arrest. In evaluating hyponatraemia it is important to estimate the patient's fluid balance—hyponatraemia associated with dehydration, euvolaemia, and fluid overload all point to different likely causes. In this case, bendroflumethiazide (a thiazide diuretic) is the likely culprit. This patient appears dehydrated, and has mild pre-renal kidney failure. In the absence of diarrhoea and vomiting, the most likely cause is excessive diuretic use. The bendroflumethiazide should be stopped, as should the furosemide.

All medicines are potentially toxic, and this is especially so in the elderly. This lady's confusion is probably added to by the tramadol (strong opiate) and benzodiazepine she is taking. Confused elderly patients should always have their drug chart reviewed and any unnecessary medicines removed. The same is true with elderly patients who fall, where antihypertensives, sedatives, antidepressants, prostate drugs, and several other classes of medication may all be responsible for producing dizziness or unsteadiness on walking. When prescribing for the elderly always think very carefully about the risks of medication, and the risks of polypharmacy, before adding another drug to an already long list.

3. Delirium can present in a number of ways—as hyperactive psychosis or as a very withdrawn, depressive illness. A psychiatrist's opinion is only of value in the elderly once there is no evidence of physical disease underlying any psychological disturbance. In this case, this man remains withdrawn and suffering with hallucinations once his physical illness has resolved, suggesting that there may be an underlying psychiatric illness.

Depression in older people is common and under-recognized. Many elderly people are lonely, isolated, and afraid of the future. They may (like this man) have been bereaved. Depression may also present with psychotic symptoms in the elderly, including hallucinations or nihilistic delusions such as that their intestines are dead and rotten. It would be unusual for schizophrenia to present for the first time in a man of this age, and depression is a much more likely diagnosis. He may be helped by lifestyle measures (for instance, encouraging visits to a day centre), bereavement counselling, or possibly antidepressants.

4. This man has evidence of a subdural haematoma on CT:

A chronic subdural haematoma, which classically produce this concave shape which may extend right round one half of the brain. Acute haematomas appear hyperdense (whiter) compared to normal brain; haematomas 1-3 weeks old appear isodense (the same colour as brain tissue, making them hard to spot), and haematomas greater than 3 weeks old (like this one) appear hypodense (darker) than normal brain tissue.

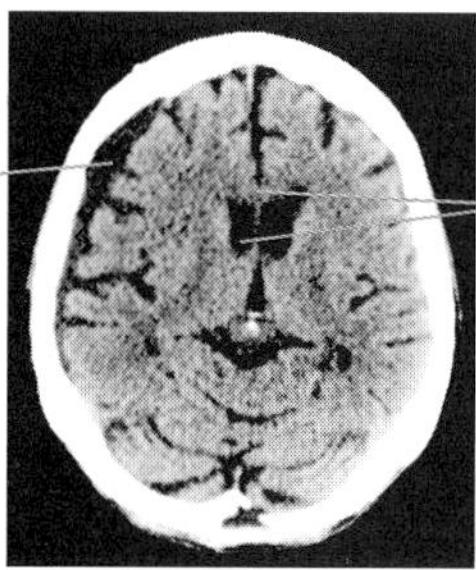

Note some evidence of mass effect affecting the brain. The right lateral ventricle is partially compressed and the falx cerebri (seen as a line running along the midline of the brain) is slightly pushed over to the left hand side.

This CT scan should be discussed with a neurosurgeon. In view of this man's previously good cognitive function, evacuation of the haematoma could produce a good recovery from confusion. CT scans in patients with chronic confusion (dementia) are often similar to the two patterns below, which sadly do not permit any surgical intervention and consequently have little chance of significant recovery of function.

Significant brain atrophy in advanced Alzheimer's dementia. Note how the brain is generally shrunken (especially the temporal lobes), leaving widened sulci and ventricular spaces.

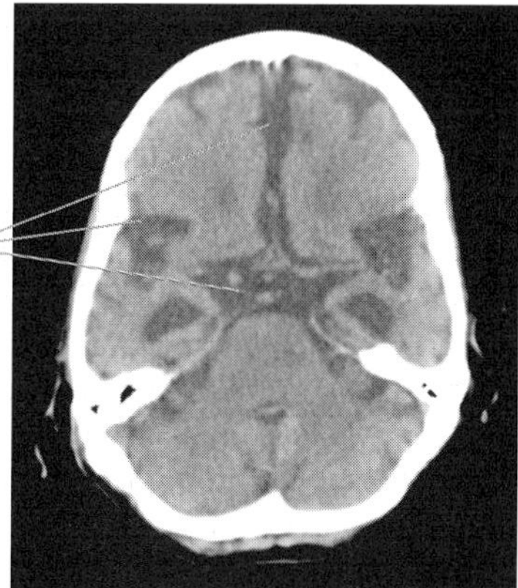

Here the diagnosis is vascular dementia (also known as small vessel disease or multi-infarct dementia). This is caused by multiple strokes of tiny blood vessels supplying structures deep in the brain. Characteristic features seen here include brain atrophy (widened ventricles and sulci), and periventricular lucency (darker areas around the ventricles where brain tissue has been damaged by ischaemia).

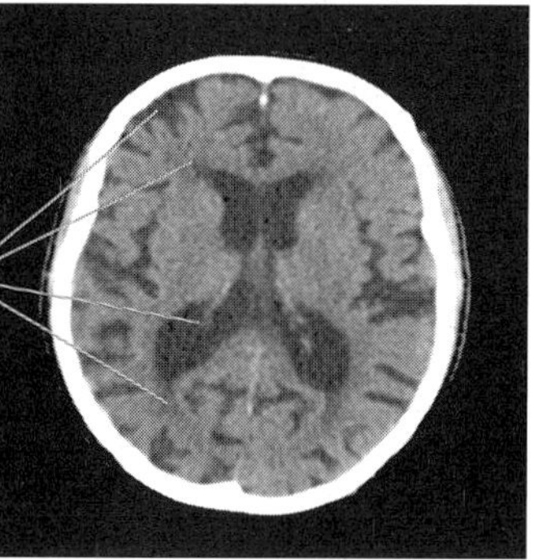

Further reading

Guidelines: British Geriatrics Society guidelines for the prevention, diagnosis and management of delirium in hospital (http://www.bgs.org.uk/index.php?option=com_content&view=article&id=170:clinguidedeliriumtreatment&catid=42:catclinguidelines&Itemid=107)

OHCM: 488–493

Seizures

This section should be used to clerk patients presenting to hospital after suffering a seizure, or who are being investigated for seizures in out-patients. Patients are rarely admitted for long after a seizure, and are discharged (from the Emergency Department or Medical Admissions Unit) once their post-ictal drowsiness has worn-off and any necessary tests are completed.

Learning challenges

- What does the term 'seizure threshold' refer to and how does it help the understanding of secondary seizures and epileptic foci?
- Where in the brain does 'consciousness' lie? Why is it maintained in partial seizures and lost in generalized seizures?

History

Comment on

- Before seizure: sensory, motor, or other neurological phenomena
- During seizure: this will be gathered from eye-witness account:
    - facial colour
    - jerking of limbs, eye rolling, stiffness
    - tongue biting
    - urinary or faecal incontinence
    - duration of seizure
- After seizure: drowsiness; aching and pain in limbs; time to 'return to normal'.
- Systemic illnesses.
- Previous seizures, including in infancy
- Family history of seizures
- Hypoxic birth injury, head injury
- Alcohol consumption
- Adherence to antiepileptic medication (known epileptics)

Examination

Well or unwell? Why?

Feet to face:

Vital signs: Temperature Blood pressure Pulse rate Respiratory rate O2 saturations

Clinical clues:

Cardiovascular:

1 2 1

Respiratory:

CBG

GCS [ ]E [ ]V [ ]M

Abdominal:

Neurological:

Other:

Comment on

- Signs of recent seizure—post-ictal drowsiness, evidence of incontinence or tongue biting
- Focal neurological signs
- Signs of global neurological impairment, e.g. altered level of consciousness
- Signs of systemic illness, e.g. common malignancies (breast, lung, colon, prostate)

CT head

Comment on

- Space-occupying lesion
- Anatomical abnormalities

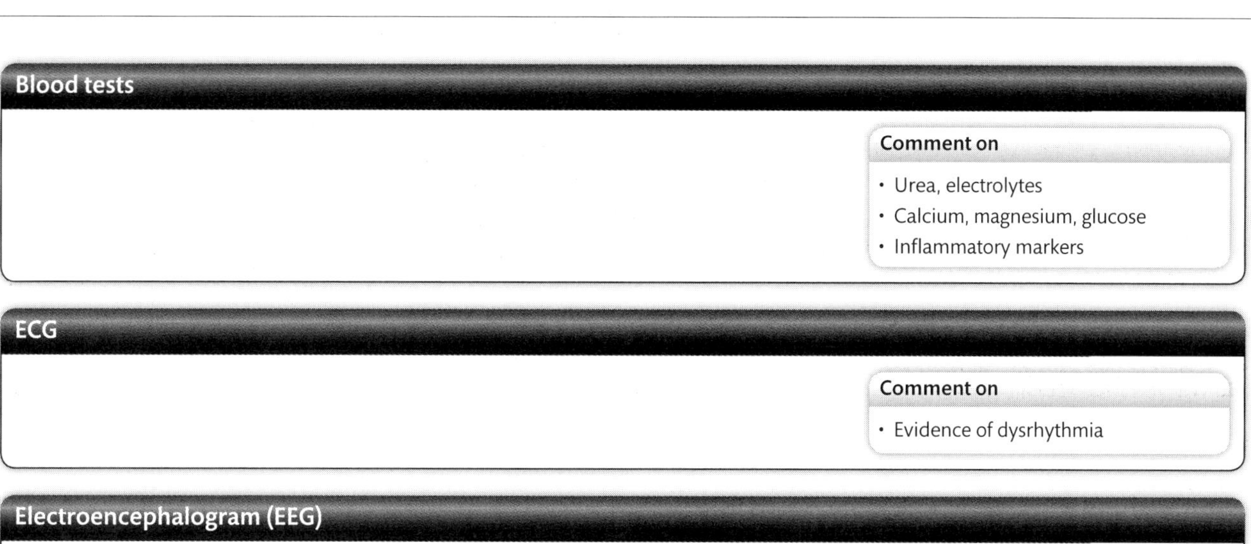

Blood tests

Comment on

- Urea, electrolytes
- Calcium, magnesium, glucose
- Inflammatory markers

ECG

Comment on

- Evidence of dysrhythmia

Electroencephalogram (EEG)

Rarely useful for diagnosis of primary epilepsy but may be useful to exclude secondary causes

Comment on

- Evidence of ongoing seizure activity

MRI head

Comment on

- Hippocampal sclerosis (often associated with 'idiopathic' epilepsy)

Evaluation

1. Is there evidence of ongoing seizure activity? What emergency treatment is needed?

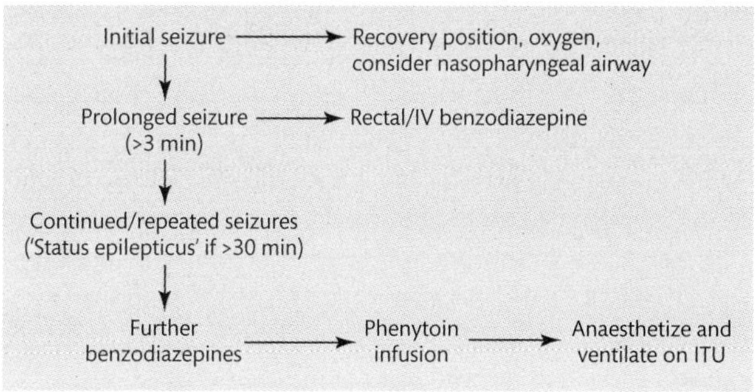

Initial seizure → Recovery position, oxygen, consider nasopharyngeal airway
↓
Prolonged seizure (>3 min) → Rectal/IV benzodiazepine
↓
Continued/repeated seizures ('Status epilepticus' if >30 min)
↓
Further benzodiazepines → Phenytoin infusion → Anaesthetize and ventilate on ITU

See Walker M; Status epilepticus: an evidence based guide. BMJ. 2003. **24**; 331(7518):673–7.

2. Was this a genuine fit?

Consider pseudoseizures, syncope, dysrhythmias, TIA, or hypoglycaemia

3. What pattern of seizure is this most likely to be?

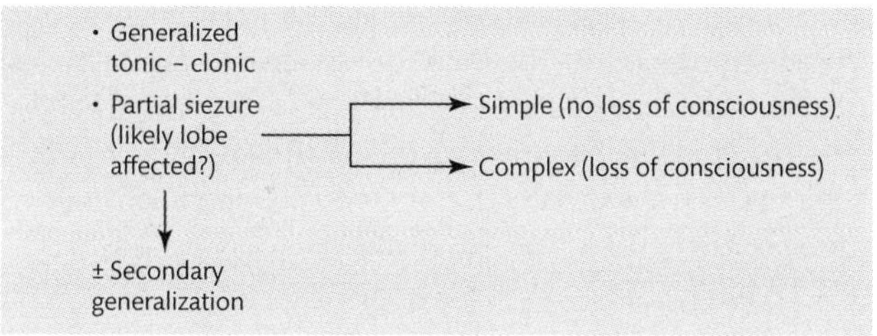

- Generalized tonic - clonic
- Partial siezure (likely lobe affected?) → Simple (no loss of consciousness) / Complex (loss of consciousness)
  ↓
  ± Secondary generalization

4. Is there any evidence of a secondary cause?

5. Is treatment with antiepileptic drugs warranted?

6. What lifestyle advice should be given?

Questions

1. You are a third-year medic attached to a medical firm who are on-call. You are seeing a 27-year-old man with known epilepsy in the Emergency Department who was admitted after suffering a tonic–clonic seizure at work. He is drowsy but rousable and is only able to give a limited history, having poor recollection of the day's events. Whilst you are examining him he begins to fit again. His whole body becoming stiff and then he begins to jerk all over. You are on your own with him in the cubicle.

(1) Describe your immediate actions.

You are joined by the one of your seniors; she manages to gain venous access and gives the man 5 mg of diazepam IV which terminates the seizure.

(2) Why is it so important to note the time at which the seizure began?

(3) What happens if the patient continues to fit despite the intravenous diazepam?

2. A previously fit and well 56-year-old man is brought in to the Emergency Department by ambulance after suffering a seizure, which occurred whilst he was eating dinner with his wife. She described him suddenly letting out a grunting noise, stiffening up, and then beginning to shake all four limbs. He had been incontinent of urine and had bitten his tongue. He has no significant medical history of note and has no history of seizures or head trauma. When he is seen in the Emergency Department he is very drowsy but there are no focal neurological signs. A CT scan of his head performed in the Emergency Department is shown below. What does it show, and what steps should be taken next?

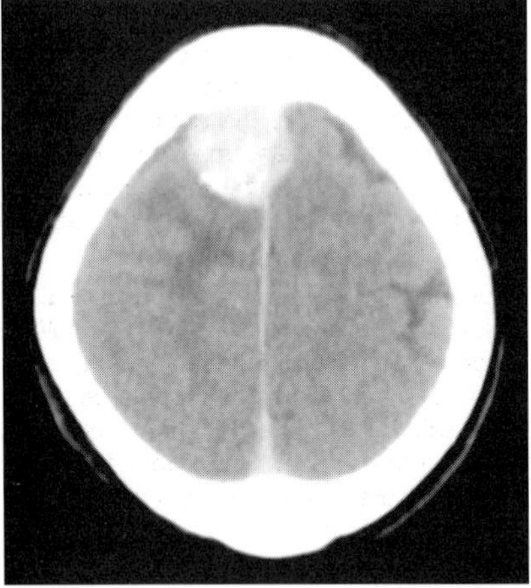

3. A 23-year-old man is referred to the neurology out-patient clinic. He has suffered four or five strange episodes during the previous 4 months. The episodes are random in onset and do not seem to have any clear precipitants. The episodes begin with a strange smell which he describes as 'musty'. He then gets a feeling which he finds hard to describe, but where he feels extremely familiar with whatever situation he finds himself in—as if he had been there before and knows exactly what will happen next. On one occasion this was followed by some jerking of his right arm which he experienced whilst being fully alert and conscious. On a different occasion he lost consciousness and his mother gives a history of seeing him fall to the floor with all four limbs jerking, with eye rolling and foaming of the mouth. He is very worried about his symptoms.

(1) What are the names of the phenomena described and what are their significance?

(2) Describe the further investigations and management of this patient.

4. A 19-year-old woman is brought to hospital after suffering a seizure at work. Whilst being seen by the Emergency Department doctor she closes her eyes and begins to shake all over. All of her limbs flail independently and she makes a low moaning noise. The intensity of the movements fluctuates until the episode finishes after 4–5 minutes without medication and she is lying quietly. There is no incontinence of urine or faeces, but she wakes up several minutes later and asks what happened, complaining that she has bitten her tongue and wonders whether she may have suffered another fit. She goes on to become tearful, saying that she really hopes that she does not have epilepsy because everything bad seems to be happening to her at the moment, since her partner left her a week earlier and she is under pressure at work. She says she really does not want to be admitted to hospital.

(1) What is the likely diagnosis?

(2) Describe your further management

5. A 28-year-old man is seen in the Emergency Department after an observed tonic–clonic seizure at a railway station on his way home from work. He denies ever having an episode like that before and is systemically well. A CT head scan is unremarkable and all blood tests are within normal limits. He makes a full recovery within a couple of hours and is fit for discharge. However, he is full of questions. Is he epileptic? Will he have to take medications? Is he allowed to drive? What should you tell him?

6. A 55-year-old woman with known epilepsy is brought to hospital after suffering her first seizure for 5 years. She is taking phenytoin 300 mg once daily and is generally very well controlled. On direct enquiry about other medicines she is taking she denies any, but says she has recently felt depressed because of being under a lot of pressure at work, and had started taking St John's Wort (a herbal remedy) to help with this because it was 'natural'. Her random blood phenytoin level is 3.8 mg/L (normal 10–20 mg/L).

(1) What is the likely cause of this seizure?

(2) What will you do about her dose of phenytoin?

Presentation

Presented to | Grade | Date

Signed

Remember that you can find large-size, annotated versions of many of the X-rays and ECGs that appear in this book on the book's web site at www.oxfordtextbooks.co.uk/orc/randall/

Answers

1. Observing a seizure can be frightening, but as a medical student you must attempt to stay calm.

- As with all medical emergencies you need to call for help!
- The main priority initially is the patient's safety, and so the sides of the bed should be put up and any immediate hazards removed.
- If possible the patient should be rolled onto their side and put into the recovery position, though this may only be possible once seizure activity has subsided. Do NOT try to physically restrain the patient or to force something between their teeth to stop them biting their tongue.
- Note down the time—subsequent interventions depend on the length of time for which the patient's seizure has lasted.
- Benzodiazepine drugs should be given to any patient who has been in a seizure for more than 2 minutes.

Almost all seizures will self-terminate within a few minutes. If they last any longer than this, then medication should be given to help stop them. If the patient has an intravenous cannula (or one can be inserted) then **lorazepam** or **diazepam** can be given; if not then rectal diazepam is first choice. You should try to keep note of the times seizures begin, and when interventions occur. Patients who suffer prolonged seizures can become hypoxic so they should be placed on high flow oxygen and if possible a nasopharyngeal airway inserted.

If the initial benzodiazepines fail to work then an additional dose can be given after 10 minutes. If these fail to work then a **phenytoin infusion** should be set up and the patient placed on a cardiac monitor (because of the cardiotoxicity). A definitive airway (tracheal intubation) may be required. **Status epilepticus** is defined as ongoing seizure activity (or a further seizure without full recovery) 30 minutes after the initial seizure. Patients with 'status' should be intubated, anaesthetized, paralysed, and placed on a ventilator, and managed on the ICU. Status epilepticus carries a 10–15% mortality.

2. This is a classic history of a true tonic-clonic seizure. The **tonic phase** occurs first, with the whole body stiffening, the patient letting out a cry and incontinence of urine or faeces. Then the **clonic phase** begins with rhythmic jerking of all limbs, which gradually reduce in force until the fit stops and the patient is very drowsy or asleep.

To suffer a first tonic-clonic seizure in middle age raises the suspicion of an intracranial pathology. This CT head scan reveals:

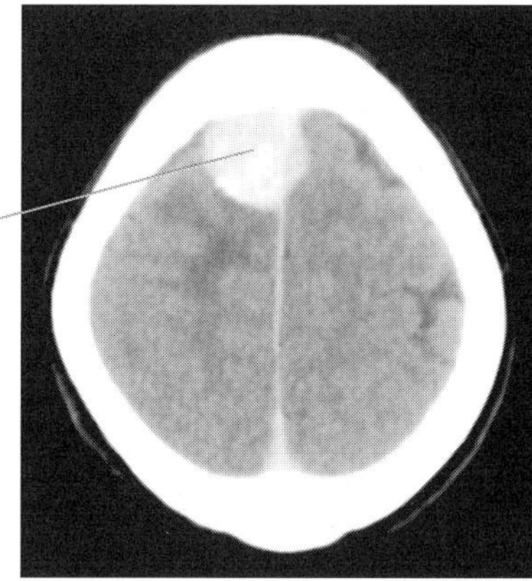

This tumour enhances avidly with intravenous contrast. The appearances suggest a right frontal meningioma - a benign tumour arising from the meninges which may serve as a focus of epileptic activity.

A proportion of seizures will prove to be secondary to an underlying epileptic focus. Common foci include primary and metastatic brain tumours, arteriovenous malformations, meningeal tumours, areas of brain damaged after a stroke or head injury, and areas (often in the hippocampus) damaged due to birth asphyxia. Surgical removal of the affected area may resolve seizure activity. All patients suffering a first seizure in adulthood should receive a scan of their brain.

3. This man describes features consistent with complex partial seizures. Such seizures have epileptic activity focused in a single area of the brain—commonly causing what is described as an '**aura**', which may then go on to produce generalized seizure activity. Strange smells are characteristic of frontal lobe partial seizures, limb jerking suggests involvement of the motor cortex, visual symptoms suggest the occipital cortex, and personality change or feelings of familiarity with a situation (**déjà vu**) suggest temporal lobe activity. It is possible that this man has an epileptic focus in his frontal lobe, which also produces local effects in the motor cortex and temporal lobe before on one occasion producing secondary generalization. The investigation of choice is head MRI which may reveal the epileptic focus and reveal whether neurosurgery is appropriate. If symptoms come sufficiently frequently then electroencephalography (EEG) may catch seizure activity and localize it within the brain. Otherwise seizure activity can be controlled by antiepileptic drugs.

4. A major differential diagnosis for epileptic seizures is **pseudoseizures**, which may represent an expression of inner psychological disturbance. Several features of this episode suggest a pseudoseizure rather than a true epileptic seizure: closed eyes, moaning, fluctuating intensity, flailing limbs rather than jerking or shaking, and the lack of significant post-ictal drowsiness, incontinence, or clear evidence of tongue biting.

A serum prolactin level may help to differentiate the causes of this patient's presentation. In true seizures, prolactin may rise 20-30-fold in the post-ictal period. If she remains well, she may be discharged but should be referred to a neurologist for further investigation and management. Further support and review should be arranged to ensure all her personal issues are addressed.

5. After a 'first fit', patients should be investigated to exclude all secondary, treatable causes. Epilepsy is defined as the 'tendency to seizures' and therefore a single seizure is not classifiable as epilepsy. However, patients should be told that they are more likely to have further episodes and if this is the case they may then be told they have developed epilepsy. Lifestyle changes to reduce the tendency to seizures, including reducing alcohol intake or the taking of illicit drugs, should be encouraged. Intervention with antiepileptics should be reserved for people who have suffered multiple seizures that have had serious impact on their daily activities. He should be discharged and followed up by his doctor. However, he should be counselled about driving—in UK law he should inform the DVLA and not drive for at least a year (he can return to driving a year afterwards in the absence of further seizures). He should not operate any heavy machinery. He should also be advised to take showers rather than baths because of the risk of drowning, and to keep the bathroom door unlocked whilst he does so. Hobbies such as scuba diving or sky diving should be ceased until seizure-free.

6. This patient has probably had a seizure because her phenytoin level is subtherapeutic. This in turn has been caused by St John's Wort, which induces the cytochrome P-450 enzymes that are responsible for the breakdown of phenytoin. Increased metabolism causes reduced serum levels of the drug. The solution is to stop the St John's Wort rather than to change the (previously sufficient) phenytoin dose. If there was no obvious reversible cause for the low phenytoin level then the dose could be increased slightly—for instance to 400 mg once daily. After any changes in dose, levels should be rechecked after steady state has been reached (usually after 1 or 2 weeks), since phenytoin has a narrow therapeutic window with toxic effects occurring at concentrations only slightly above therapeutic levels.

Further reading

Guidelines: NICE guidelines on epilepsy (http://guidance.nice.org.uk/CG20)

OHCM: 464, 494–497, 502–503, 836

Headache

This section should be used to clerk patients admitted to hospital with headache—which implies that an admitting doctor suspects one of the sinister causes of headache, such as a subarachnoid haemorrhage, meningitis, or a space-occupying lesion. Patients are admitted to the Admissions Unit and then either discharged or transferred to a specialist unit or even intensive care as appropriate.

Learning challenges

- Where are the pain receptors in the central nervous system? How do commonly occurring causes of headache actually lead to pain?
- Why are headaches caused by space-occupying lesions worse in the mornings or on straining?

History

Comment on

- Method of onset, similar previous episodes
- Exacerbating factors
- Features of meningism
- Seizures, visual disturbance
- Vomiting
- Focal neurological deficit
- Fever, rash
- Risks for intracranial haemorrhage—anticoagulation, antiplatelet medications, recent head injury

Examination

Well or unwell? Why?

Feet to face:

Vital signs: Temperature Blood pressure Pulse rate Respiratory rate O2 saturations

Clinical clues:

Cardiovascular:

1 2 1

Respiratory:

GCS [ ]E [ ]V [ ]M

Abdominal:

Neurological:

Other:

Comment on

- GCS
- Blood pressure, HR (Cushing's reflex—hypertension and bradycardia, occurs with raised intracranial pressure), temperature
- Meningism, rash
- Scalp tenderness
- Papilloedema
- Focal neurological deficit—cranial nerves and limbs

Blood tests

Comment on

- FBC—evidence of bleeding, infection, normal platelet count
- Clotting screen
- ESR

CT head

Comment on

- Raised intracranial pressure
- Intracranial bleed
- Space-occupying lesion
- Hydrocephalus

Lumbar puncture

Comment on

- White and red cell counts
- Gram stain
- Glucose and protein
- Xanthochromia
- PCR for rapid microbiological diagnosis

Evaluation

1. **Are there features of the history or examination to suggest that this is an emergency (meningitis, subarachnoid haemorrhage, temporal arteritis)?**

Worrying features:
- Acute onset
- Low GCS
- Meningism
- Fever/rash
- Fits
- Scalp tenderness
- Raised CRP/white cell count/ESR

2. **Is a CT head scan indicated? If performed, does it aid the diagnosis?**

3. **Is lumbar puncture indicated? Is it safe to perform one? If carried out, does it aid diagnosis?**

4. **What emergency treatment is needed?**

5. **How can this patient's headaches be treated in the longer term to maximize quality of life?**

Questions

1. A 35-year-old woman with no significant medical history presents to the Emergency Department with an acute, severe headache. The headache is occipital, with no radiation. She describes it as coming on very suddenly that morning whilst she was on the toilet, and has suffered nothing like it before. She has vomited twice since the headache came on.

On examination she is apyrexial but looks unwell. Her GCS is 15. She has a very stiff neck and is avoiding bright lights, wanting to lie down quietly in a dark room. There is no focal neurological deficit. Blood tests are all within normal limits. A CT head scan is arranged, and this is reported as normal as well. The decision is made to perform a lumbar puncture, and the results of CSF examination are below.

	CSF values	Normal CSF values
Red cells	9000/mm³ in all three bottles	Should reduce in each consecutive bottle taken
White cells	In proportion to red cells	<5/mm³
Protein	0.4 g/L	0.2–0.4 g/L
Glucose	3.8 mmol/L (matched capillary blood glucose = 4.2 mmol/L)	50–66% of serum
Gram stain	No organisms seen	No organisms seen

(1) What does the presentation and CSF results suggest as the likely diagnosis?

(2) Describe five essential steps in the further management.

2. A 43-year-old woman presents to her GP for the third time in a month, complaining of a worsening headache. During this period the headache has insidiously worsened, now being present almost all the time. It is particularly bad first thing in the morning when she wakes up, bends over, or when she strains or coughs. For the past week she has felt slightly nauseated but has not vomited. She has also felt 'unsteady' on occasion whilst walking. Neurological examination is unremarkable except for a slightly ataxic gait. On ophthalmoscopy she has bilateral papilloedema. She is admitted to hospital where a CT scan is performed, shown below.

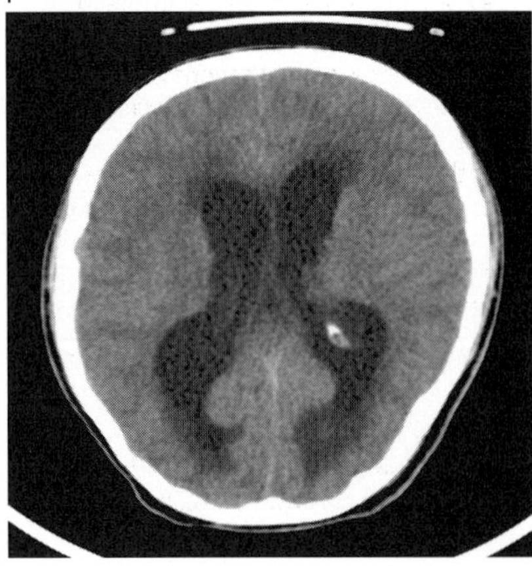

(1) What does the history suggest about her headache?

(2) What is the main abnormality shown on the scan?

(3) What is the unifying diagnosis?

3. A previously fit and well 74-year-old man is admitted to hospital with an acute headache that has developed progressively over the previous 24 hours. It is worst over the right temple, where the pain is so severe that it even hurts when the patient brushes his hair. He is otherwise systemically well and has had no associated neck stiffness or visual impairment, though the patient has noticed some 'cramps' in his jaw muscles whilst eating. Over the past few months he has noticed his shoulders and hips being painful and stiff in the mornings, which he had attributed to his age.

On examination his temperature is 37.4°C, and his right temple is exquisitely tender to touch. There is no meningism, photophobia, or rash, and examination of the cranial nerves is unremarkable. In particular, his visual acuity is 6/6 in both eyes. Blood tests reveal a very raised ESR of 92 mm/hour (normal for this man <42 mm/hour) and a CRP of 178 mg/L (normal <10 mg/L).

(1) What is the likely underlying diagnosis?

(2) What immediate management would you instigate?

(3) Why is it essential to start the therapy before the diagnosis is confirmed?

(4) How would you attempt to confirm the diagnosis?

4. A fit and well 20-year-old student is admitted to hospital with a 12-hour history of severe headache. It began the previous evening and has worsened through the night. The pain has been accompanied by vomiting, rash, and drowsiness. He is on no regular medications.

On examination he is drowsy with a GCS of 13/15 and a temperature of 38.9°C, heart rate of 124 bpm and blood pressure of 110/74 mmHg. He is lying with his arm over his eyes, and mumbling about the brightness of the lights. His has marked neck stiffness and there is a widespread non-blanching purpuric rash over his body.

(1) What is the likely diagnosis?

(2) List five essential investigations

(3) List five essential management steps in this case.

5. A 27-year-old woman presents to the Emergency Department with a severe headache. The pain came on rapidly around 2 hours earlier and was preceded by her seeing flashing lights in front of her eyes, and a tingling sensation in her left arm. The headache, which she describes as 'pulsating', began on the left hand side of her head but has now generalized. She has vomited twice and is feeling nauseated. There is no history of head injury and she is otherwise well. When examined she is apyrexial, photophobic, and irritable when the door to the cubicle is opened and light comes in. No focal neurological deficit is found and there is no meningism. Blood tests including FBC, U&Es, and CBG are all normal.

(1) What is the likely diagnosis?

(2) Given her presentation and investigations should this patient have a CT head scan?

Presentation

Presented to ______ Grade ______ Date ______

Signed

Remember that you can find large-size, annotated versions of many of the X-rays and ECGs that appear in this book on the book's web site at www.oxfordtextbooks.co.uk/orc/randall/

Answers

1. This woman has had a subarachnoid haemorrhage. This presentation is classical, with **acute onset** of very **severe headache**, which may come on whilst **physically straining.** Such haemorrhages are caused by arterial bleeding into the subarachnoid space, often from a ruptured aneurysm of the circle of Willis or from an arteriovenous malformation. CT scanning of the head may reveal fresh blood in the subarachnoid space, a berry aneurysm, or another vascular abnormality (see below). However, CT may be normal, and lumbar puncture is required to look for red cells or xanthochromia (a yellowish discoloration of the CSF caused by breakdown of haemoglobin).

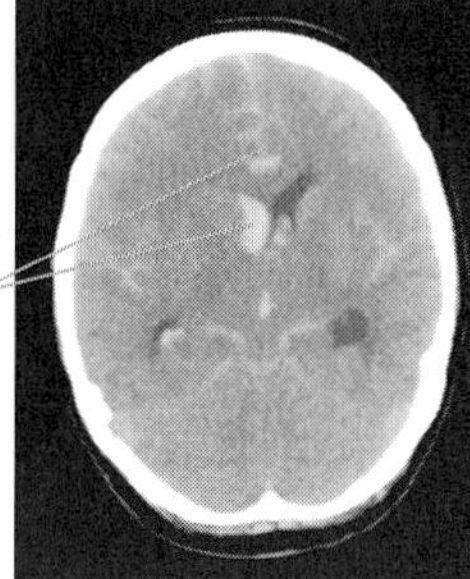

Fresh blood (which appears hyperdense on CT - whiter than brain tissue), may be seen anywhere within the subarachnoid space (where CSF circulates). Here, fresh blood is especially prominent in the anterior horn of the right lateral ventricle and in the interhemispheric fissure.

CT in subarachnoid haemorrhage may also give evidence of what has caused the bleed - for instance evidence of trauma (such as skull fracture), or a berry aneurysm or arteriovenous malformation. Hydrocephalus may be present as a consequence of blood clot blocking the normal flow of CSF.

Patients presenting acutely with subarachnoid haemorrhage are at very high risk of subsequent bleeds within 24 hours that lead to raised intracranial pressure and death. They require transfer to a neurosurgical centre, vascular imaging (such as a CT angiogram), and then either open arterial surgery (to clip a berry aneurysm or excise an arteriovenous malformation), or repair by interventional radiologists (where wire coils are introduced into aneurysms leading to thrombosis). In the meantime blood pressure should be controlled and laxatives given to prevent straining at stool. Nimodipine is a calcium channel blocker specifically used in patients with subarachnoid haemorrhage to prevent secondary vasospasm and bleeding.

2. This presentation is typical of the headache of raised intracranial pressure. Such headaches are constant and dull, and are exacerbated by things that raises the pressure within the head, e.g. lying flat for a prolonged period (hence they are often worse on waking from sleep) or straining at stool. The commonest causes of raised intracranial pressure include the condition idiopathic intracranial hypertension (which predominantly affects young women who are overweight), space-occupying lesions (such as primary or secondary tumours), or intracranial bleeds. In the case of this patient, though, a rarer cause is to blame. Her CT scan reveals hydrocephalus, with markedly enlarged ventricles and a decrease in visible sulci around the brain.

Hydrocephalus describes an increased volume of CSF within the CNS. This may result from: (1) **Obstruction to CSF flow**—causes include obstruction secondary to blood, or tumour; this is known as **non-communicating hydrocephalus**, where the flow between the ventricles and subarachnoid space is interrupted. (2) **Increased CSF production** or (3) **reduced absorption**, which are both examples of communicating hydrocephalus, where the flow between the ventricles and subarachnoid space is maintained.

Clinically, hydrocephalus may present with headache, nausea and vomiting, symptoms of raised intracranial pressure, cognitive impairment, and gait disturbance. Whatever the cause, in appropriate circumstances patients with hydrocephalus require neurosurgical intervention with placement of a subcutaneous shunt to drain CSF from the enlarged ventricles into the peritoneum (**V-P shunt**). This woman will also require investigation of the cause of her hydrocephalus, looking particularly for lesions (such as tumours) obstructing the flow of CSF.

3. This patient has presented with classical features of temporal or giant cell arteritis (GCA). This is a large-vessel vasculitis where there is inflammation of the superficial temporal artery (which runs along the temporal scalp roughly along the hair line) and the ophthalmic artery. It may be associated with polymyalgia rheumatica, a more widespread vasculitis of large arteries which characteristically produces shoulder and hip girdle pain.

The combination of unilateral headache with scalp tenderness is classical. In this case it is associated with jaw claudication, malaise, and fever, with a markedly raised ESR (often >100 mm/hour). It is a medical emergency because involvement of the ophthalmic artery can lead to irreversible blindness (missed temporal arteritis is a significant cause of medical negligence claims). Treatment is with oral steroids (prednisolone at a minimal dose of 1 mg/kg/day). The diagnosis may be confirmed by surgical biopsy of the superficial temporal artery. In biopsy proven GCA the prednisolone dose should be increased to 80–100 mg per day. More recently aspirin 75 mg od has also been recommended to prevent loss of vision and strokes. Steroids should be slowly reduced in dose in response to the ESR and clinical symptoms.

4. Where there is evidence of infection along with confusion, drowsiness, or coma, the diagnosis of acute bacterial meningitis has to be considered. This is especially true here where the patient has obvious meningism along with a purpuric rash associated with meningococcal septicaemia. This man is gravely unwell and will die unless treatment is initiated rapidly, as cerebral oedema leads to an increase in intracranial pressure whilst sepsis leads to a fall in systemic blood pressure. Together these lead to underperfusion of the brain (as shown by this patient's reducing level of consciousness) and death by widespread brain injury.

The only reason to delay giving antibiotics is if facilities are available immediately to perform a lumbar puncture to confirm the organism (which later allows antibiotic choices to be altered). If there will be any delay in performing a lumbar puncture (or if to do so will be unsafe—perhaps in this man if raised intracranial pressure is possible), then antibiotics should be given empirically. Blood cultures taken from the intravenous cannula inserted to give antibiotics provide an alternative source of microbiological information. Broad-spectrum antibiotics such as a third-generation cephalosporin should be given to cover all likely organisms. Patients are often treated on ICUs where invasive monitoring of blood pressure can allow cerebral perfusion to be maximized. After antibiotics are given, other key investigations in confirming the diagnosis include FBC and inflammatory markers, renal function tests, and a CT scan of the brain.

5. This patient is suffering from an episode of migraine. Classical migraines present with an aura (of flashing lights or other neurological symptoms), throbbing unilateral headache (which may generalize), vomiting, and prostration with photophobia. However, there is some overlap between migraine and tension headaches and presentations may be more variable. There is no need for a CT scan of the head at this stage of the presentation but atypical features, neurological deficit, or reduced level of consciousness are indications for a scan.

The symptoms of migraine are likely to be caused by intracranial vasodilatation, probably linked to abnormalities of serotonin metabolism. In some patients there is an obvious precipitant, for instance chocolate or cheese. Acute interventions include adequate analgesia, intravenous fluids, rest in a dark, quiet room, use of an antiemetic and specific therapies, for instance a triptan drug (e.g. sumatriptan) which acts as a serotonin agonist.

Further reading

Guidelines: Scottish Intercollegiate Guidelines Network guidelines on management of headache in adults (http://www.sign.ac.uk/guidelines/fulltext/107/index.html)

OHCM: 460–463, 482, 794, 832–835

Spinal and peripheral nerve lesions

This section should be used to clerk patients complaining of motor or sensory symptoms which do not fit with a presentation of acute stroke (which generally causes focal, unilateral symptoms). Rapidly progressive neurological symptoms such as weakness are a medical emergency. Such patients are often assessed in the Emergency Department, the Medical Assessment Unit or on the General Medical Ward whilst a diagnosis is reached, but may also be found in the ICU or specialist neurological rehabilitation units.

Learning challenges

- How is the architecture of tracts in the spinal cord arranged? What functional losses are experienced in cord hemisection, syringomyelia, and infarction of the anterior spinal artery?
- What are the five main nerves of the arm? How would you test the function of each?

History

Comment on

- Muscle groups affected—myotomes
- Sensory deficits—dermatomes
- Time course, progression, previous episodes
- Problems with gait and posture
- Dysphagia or dysarthria
- Back pain
- Bowel and bladder symptoms
- Multisystem diseases
- Alcohol intake, diet
- Medications

Examination

Well or unwell? Why?

Feet to face:

Vital signs: Temperature Blood pressure Pulse rate Respiratory rate O2 saturations

Clinical clues:

Cardiovascular:

1 2 1

Respiratory:

GCS [ ]E [ ]V [ ]M

Abdominal:

Neurological:

Other:

Comment on

- Evidence of wasting
- Degree of power loss
- Reflexes
- Sensation, vibration, joint position sense
- Swallow
- Anal tone and sensation
- Gait

Blood tests

Comment on

- Vitamin B_{12} and folate levels
- Blood glucose
- Other routine blood tests

Head CT/MRI

Comment on

- Ischaemic lesions
- Demyelination

Nerve conduction studies and electromyography

Comment on

- Nerve conduction velocity
- Motor latency

Cerebral evoked potentials

Comment on

- Speed of central transmission

CSF

Comment on

- Protein
- Oligoclonal bands

Spirometry/arterial blood gas analysis

Comment on

- Respiratory compromise

Evaluation

1. Where is the lesion likely to be?

Upper motor neuron
- → Cerebral cortex (unilateral symptoms, higher functional losses)
- → Brainstem (altered consciousness, bulbar signs)
- → Spine (back pain, sensory level)

Lower motor neuron
- → Spinal roots (spinal dermatome /myotomal losses)
- → Peripheral nerve lesion (specific patterns)
- → Demyelinating /neuromuscular/muscle disease (generalized symptoms)

2. Does this patient require urgent investigation or management? Is there respiratory compromise?

3. What is the likely nature and cause of the patient's symptoms?

4. What is the prognosis? Is there any specific treatment?

Questions

1. A 57-year-old man attends the Emergency Department complaining of weakness in his legs which began the day before in his left leg and is now affecting his right leg as well. He first noticed it when he stumbled climbing the stairs the day before, but now it has progressed to be noticeable on walking. He also complains that both legs feel numb and 'heavy'. For the previous 6 months he has been being treated by his family doctor for sciatica affecting primarily his left leg; he has also over this time suffered intermittent lower back pain which has become more severe over the previous 2 days. Examination of the cranial nerves and arms are normal, but examination of the lower limbs revealed increased tone throughout, reduced power (4/5) in all muscle groups, and brisk patellar and ankle reflexes bilaterally with equivocal plantars. Light touch sensation felt 'fluffy' bilaterally up to the level of the inguinal ligament. Sensation was also altered over the perineum, and digital rectal examination revealed decreased anal tone. On catheterization of the bladder, 800 ml of clear urine drained immediately. An urgent MRI scan of the spine was requested which is shown below.

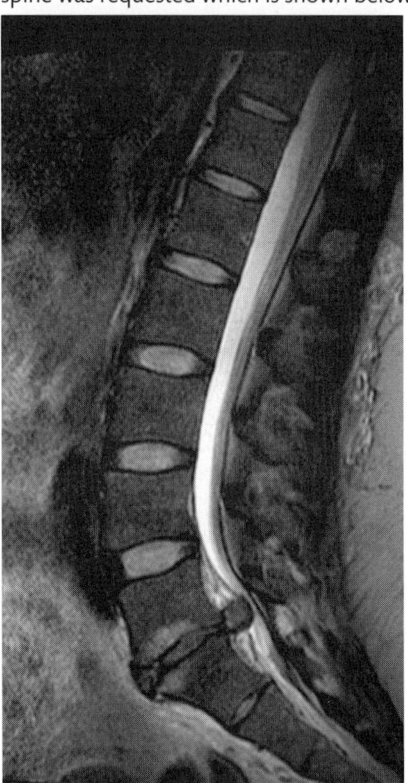

(1) What does the MRI show?

(2) What is the clinical syndrome being described and how should this patient be managed?

2. A previously fit and active 30-year-old man presents to the Emergency Department with a 2-day history of progressive weakness and numbness in both legs, which this morning he describes as paralysis. He admits to having suffered from a mild diarrhoeal illness several weeks earlier but is otherwise well, with no medical history of note. The onset was insidious over the preceding 48 hours with no associated pain. Examination confirms a flaccid paralysis of both lower limbs, with power 2/5 proximally and 0/5 distally. Ankle reflexes and plantars are absent and knee reflexes diminished. There is also weakness (grade 4/5) in his upper limbs with sensory loss extending from the legs up the trunk and into both arms. Spirometry and arterial blood gas analysis are performed (see below).

Arterial blood gas analysis	Spirometry
pH 7.31	FVC 1.5 L
pCO_2 6.81 kPa	FEV_1 1.35 L
pO_2 9.5 kPa	FEV_1/FVC 0.9
HCO_3^- 30	

(1) What is the likely unifying diagnosis?

(2) Why is it now a medical emergency?

(3) What urgent interventions are required?

3. A 23-year-old woman is seen at the hospital Emergency Department complaining of weakness in her right upper limb. The problem began a week earlier when she experienced a feeling of numbness and tingling in the left arm, with weakness of the right arm developing over the course of the week. She was otherwise well and had no other symptoms. A year previously she had suffered some blurring of vision in her right eye, associated with mild eye pain, which resolved spontaneously after 6 weeks. On examination all cranial nerves are normal, but the right trapezius muscle is noted to be weak. Her right upper limb is globally weak (power 3/5 proximally, 4/5 distally), with a brisk biceps reflex and normal sensation. Her left upper limb is neurologically normal except for an absence of pain and temperature sensation. Light touch sensation is preserved. An MRI of her cervical spine was arranged which is reported below.

> There is a hypodense area on the right side of the cervical cord at the level of C3–C5 which is likely to represent demyelination. Vertebral architecture is normal and there is no evidence of disc prolapse or cord compression. No other lesion is seen.

(1) What is the likely diagnosis?

(2) List three possible therapeutic interventions.

4. A 34-year-old woman is referred to the neurology out-patient clinic for investigation of a 2-month history of 'generalized weakness'. She has experienced difficulty in rising from a chair, carrying bags of shopping, and standing for prolonged periods of time. In each case she feels that her muscles 'rapidly tire'. Her jaw 'tires' when chewing for a prolonged period, and she has felt her eye-lids droop as if she is excessively tired. She was previously well and has no other medical problems. Examination reveals bilateral ptosis, power initially 5/5 in all limbs but which rapidly fatigues and weakens with repetitive movement. Her reflexes are initially normal but after repeated stimulation become reduced and then absent. Investigations reveal a normal FBC, U&Es, glucose, ESR, and creatine kinase. Electrophysiological studies reveal normal nerve conduction velocities, but decreasing muscle action potentials on repeated stimulation. Chest X-ray revealed an upper mediastinal mass.

(1) What is the unifying diagnosis, and the mass?

(2) What class of drug forms the mainstay of treatment?

Remember that you can find large-size, annotated versions of many of the X-rays and ECGs that appear in this book on the book's web site at www.oxfordtextbooks.co.uk/orc/randall/

Answers

1. This MRI shows:

This is a T2 weighted sagittal MRI of the lumbar spine. MRI scans produce images based on the behaviour of hydrogen ions in a strong magnetic field. The data gained can be synthesised by a computer to produce T1 weighted images (particularly used for identifying tissues with different fat concentrations - for instance grey and white matter in the brain), and T2 weighted images (particularly used for identifying differences in water concentration - for instance, where oedema occurs around an area of tissues damage).

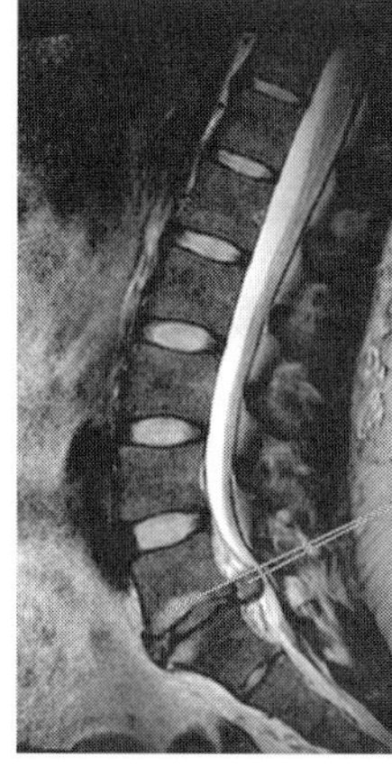

This MRI reveals a loss of disc space at L5/S1, with changes in the inferior endplate of L5 and the superior endplate of S1. There is a large posterior disc bulge at this level which is significantly compressing the cauda equina.

This clinical presentation is classical for the **cauda equina syndrome**, which is an orthopaedic emergency. Without urgent decompression of the free nerve roots, paralysis will become irreversible within hours. The key features that should never be missed are back pain, leg weakness, saddle anaesthesia, decreased anal tone, and urinary retention.

Cauda equina syndrome may be caused by anything which causes compression of the nerve roots in the lumbar spine. The commonest causes are intervertebral disc prolapse, compression from a metastatic malignant deposit, or spinal trauma. Patients displaying the features outlined above require immediate MR imaging of the spine, with transfer to a spinal centre for urgent surgery.

2. This man has a restrictive deficit of spirometry and has type II respiratory failure—he is retaining CO_2, which based on the history and examination findings is likely to be because of weakness of his respiratory muscles. He should be reviewed by the intensive care team with a view to receiving ventilatory support.

The likely diagnosis here is **Guillain-Barré syndrome**, which causes an ascending lower motor neuron polyneuropathy. It may only cause symptoms in the lower limbs or it may ascend to involve the upper limbs and the respiratory muscles. Guillain-Barré syndrome is caused by an autoimmune attack on the myelin sheaths around peripheral nerves. The suggested mechanism is molecular mimicry, where an infectious agent (both *Campylobacter jejuni* and Cytomegalovirus have been implicated) causes production of an autoantibody targeted against an antigen present in myelin sheaths. The diagnosis can be confirmed by nerve conduction studies showing slowed impulse velocities, and by lumbar puncture revealing raised CSF protein. The only agent shown to improve prognosis is pooled intravenous immunoglobulin. If there is respiratory compromise then mechanical ventilation may be required until the patient recovers. The disease develops over the course of days or weeks, and then regresses over a similar period, though it sometimes leaves a residual deficit.

3. Central nervous system demyelination is often caused by multiple sclerosis (MS). This condition is poorly understood, but results in 'plaques' of demyelination which may occur throughout the brain and spinal cord and produce a range of symptoms. In this case, the demyelination seems to be affecting the right-sided spinothalamic tract and corticospinal tract—because fibres of the spinothalamic tract decussate at the level of entry of the cord, whereas fibres of the corticospinal tract decussate in the brainstem, motor and sensory phenomena can occur on opposite sides of the body. In this case the dorsal columns seem unaffected, as light touch sensation is spared. The weakness of the trapezius muscle is likely to be as a result of damage to the spinal root of cranial nerve XI.

MRI of the brain and spinal cord in MS may show multiple plaques throughout the central nervous system which are asymptomatic. Common clinical manifestations include optic (or retrobulbar) neuritis, sensory or motor phenomena in the limbs, and a bulbar palsy causing problems with speech or swallowing. Most MS follows a relapsing and remitting course, eventually becoming secondarily progressive, though primary progressive MS occurs in 20% of cases.

4. The initial differential diagnosis here based on history and examination would include:

- widespread polyneuropathy,
- problems with transmission at the neuromuscular junction, or
- primary disease of muscle.

The normal nerve conduction studies suggest that this is not a neuropathy, and the normal creatine kinase and initial muscle action potentials suggest the muscles are normal. This woman has myasthenia gravis—a disease of the neuromuscular junction caused by autoantibodies to the acetylcholine receptor of the post-synaptic membrane. The key clinical feature is fatiguability of muscle power and reflexes. Myasthenia gravis is associated with tumours of the thymus in the anterior mediastinum, as in this case. The thymoma should be surgically resected. Treatment of myasthenia is with the acetylcholinesterase inhibitor pyridostigmine. A rare paraneoplastic myasthenic syndrome (Lambert-Eaton syndrome) may occur with small cell carcinoma of the lung. The auto-antibody is directed against voltage gated calcium channels (VGCC).

Further reading

Guidelines: NICE guidelines on multiple sclerosis (http://guidance.nice.org.uk/CG8)

OHCM: 456–459, 470–471, 500–501, 504–511, 514–517, 520

Parkinsonism and movement disorders

This section should be used to clerk patients with suspected or confirmed Parkinson's disease, parkinsonism, or those who experience difficulty in controlling, coordinating, or initiating movement. Such patients may be seen on the Medical Admissions Unit or Neurological Ward, but more commonly are managed in primary care, elderly care, or neurology out-patient clinics.

Learning challenges

- What are the roles of the primary motor cortex, the basal ganglia, the cerebellum, and the spinal cord in initiating: (a) a planned action, (b) a well-practised action, and (c) a reflex action?
- What is 'deep brain stimulation'?

History

Comment on

- Symptoms experienced
- Time course and progression
- The classical triad—'bradykinesia, rigidity, and tremor'
- Changes in gait, falls, trips, and instability
- Changes in speech and language
- Problems with bowel or bladder function
- Dysphagia or dysarthria
- Medications—antidopaminergic drugs, e.g. antipsychotics, antiemetics
- Disability—effects on activities of daily living
- Social background—home layout, carers

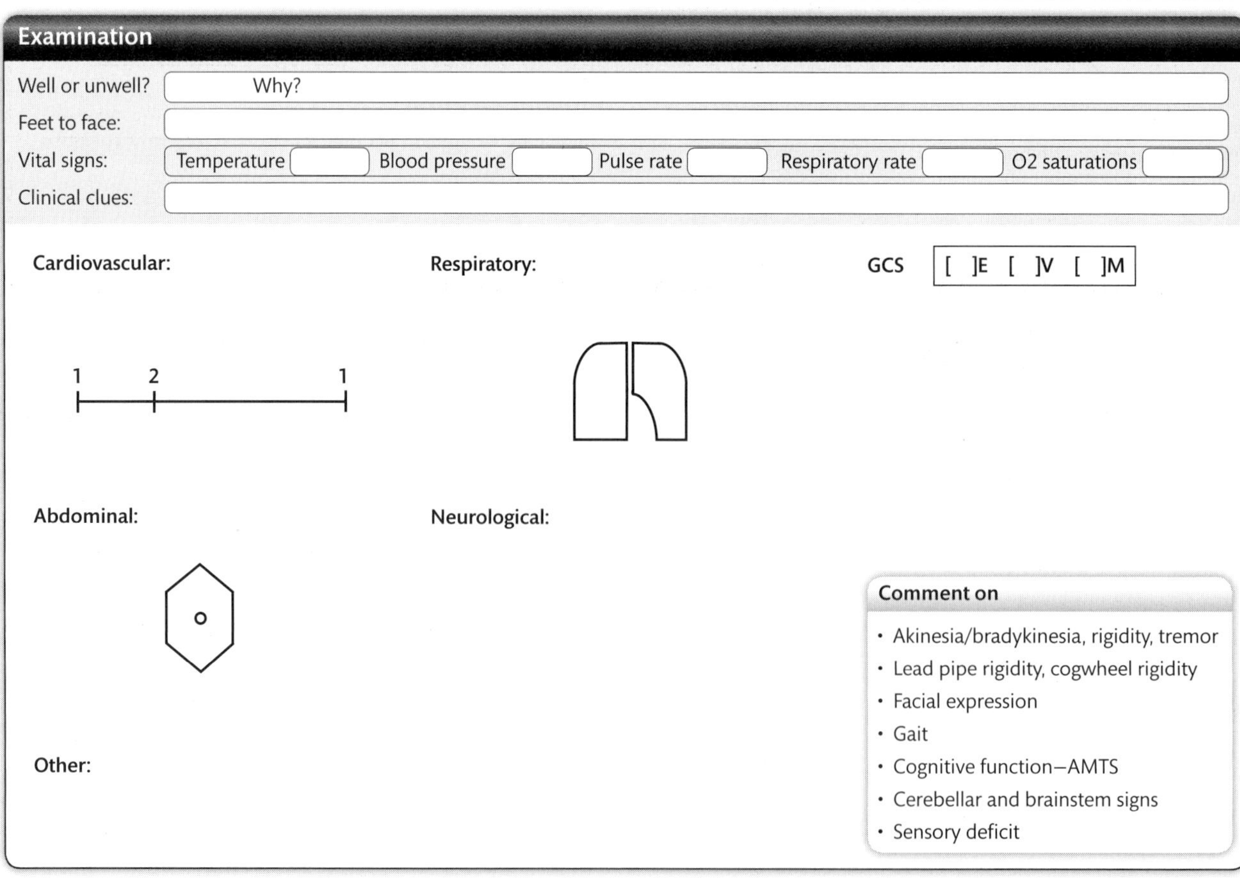

Examination

Well or unwell? Why?

Feet to face:

Vital signs: Temperature | Blood pressure | Pulse rate | Respiratory rate | O2 saturations

Clinical clues:

Cardiovascular:

Respiratory:

GCS [ ]E [ ]V [ ]M

Abdominal:

Neurological:

Other:

Comment on

- Akinesia/bradykinesia, rigidity, tremor
- Lead pipe rigidity, cogwheel rigidity
- Facial expression
- Gait
- Cognitive function—AMTS
- Cerebellar and brainstem signs
- Sensory deficit

CT/MRI

Comment on

- Basal ganglia lesions
- Cerebellar lesions
- Old strokes
- Cerebral atrophy

Evaluation

1. **How severe is this patient's disease?**

Objective clinical assessment:

Reported ability to cope at home:

2. **Is there evidence of non-motor complications of Parkinson's disease?**

Lewy-body dementia:

Parkinson's-plus syndromes:

3. **What is the likely cause of the parkinsonism?**

Idiopathic	Drug induced
Vascular	A 'Parkinson's plus syndrome'

4. **Any side-effects of medication?**

5. **What options exist to control symptoms? What is the goal of treatment for this patient?**

Questions

1. A 56-year-old woman attends her GP's surgery because she is concerned about feeling 'stiff and slow' all the time and struggling to perform tasks around the house. The GP was initially concerned about whether an arthritis could be causing her symptoms, but on closer questioning she denied any pain in her joints—she described the problem as 'not being able to tell my body to move itself'. She also complained about tremor which was particularly bad when she was sitting still. Over the previous few weeks she had fallen over twice. On examination she seemed well, but had a 'mask-like face' and spoke in a monotone voice. She had a resting tremor of her left hand, which was making 'pill-rolling' movements of the thumb across the fingers, at a frequency of approximately 5 per second. Her arm displayed increased tone, consistent throughout the full range of flexion and extension at the elbow, with cogwheel rigidity at the wrist. She was referred up to a neurological out-patient clinic at her local hospital.

List the key features you would elicit in the history to prove the likely diagnosis and exclude the differentials.

2. A 74-year-old man with idiopathic Parkinson's disease is reviewed in the neurology out-patient department. Since his last clinic appointment his symptoms have been worsening—he suffers from regular episodes where he 'freezes' and is unable to initiate movement. He has also noticed that he makes involuntary, jerking movements several hours after taking his previous dose of medication, which usually resolve after his next dose. On examination he displays generalized stiffness with a mild resting tremor worse on the right-hand side. His facial expression is impassive and he has a shuffling, narrow-based gait with absent arm swinging. He has been taking co-careldopa for 4 years, and had his dose increased the year before.

(1) What is likely to account for that fact his symptoms now seem to be less well controlled than before?

(2) What is the 'jerking' due to?

3. An 84-year-old woman lives in a residential home because of significant vascular dementia. She is brought in to the Emergency Department because staff at the home are concerned by an acute deterioration in her balance. She can usually mobilize independently with the use of a walking stick, but today was extremely unsteady on her feet. She denies feeling light-headed or dizzy at rest, but on trying to walk is noticeably ataxic. There is no obvious limb weakness or sensory deficit on examination, and reflexes are normal; however, coordination of movements is noted to be impaired.

What specific signs should be examined for to identify the presence of cerebellar disease?

4. A 45-year-old man with chronic schizophrenia is managed in the community with regular intramuscular injections of the antipsychotic drug risperidone. When he is seen by his psychiatrist in clinic he complains that he feels constantly restless and is always moving his legs. On examination he is continually moving his legs and making chewing movements with his mouth, and will occasionally break off the consultation to walk around the room to 'stretch his legs'. He reports that his psychiatric symptoms are well controlled. The psychiatrist records in the patients notes the presence of 'extrapyramidal symptoms', and reduces the man's risperidone dose as well as prescribing a low-dose beta-blocker for symptomatic relief.

(1) To what does the term 'extrapyramidal' refer, and how does this relate to Parkinson's disease?

(2) Which classes of medications commonly cause extrapyramidal side-effects?

6 Neurology

Presentation

Presented to		Grade		Date	
Signed					

Answers

1. The history is highly suggestive of parkinsonism. Any complex motor disease including tremor and falls should be distinguished from cerebellar disease, vestibular disease of the inner ear, and disease of the peripheral nervous system or muscle (that may produce muscle fasciculation which is misinterpreted as tremor).

Secondary causes for parkinsonism should then be sought. Although most parkinsonism is put down to idiopathic Parkinson's disease (caused by destruction of dopamine-secreting cells in the basal ganglia, of unknown aetiology), some will be secondary to other disease processes, including:

- **Vascular** parkinsonism caused by multiple small-vessel brain infarctions.
- **Drug-induced** parkinsonism caused particularly by antipsychotic and antiemetic medications.
- '**Parkinson plus**' syndromes or neurological degeneration, such as multisystem atrophy, olivo-ponto-cerebellar degeneration, and supranuclear palsy. These are parkinsonian syndromes with added or extra features including blood pressure instability, bowel or bladder dysfunction, dysphagia, and eye movement problems. They are incurable, progressive, and invariably fatal. They do not generally respond to levodopa therapy.
- **Toxic** parkinsonism caused by environmental toxins or copper in Wilson's disease.
- **Post-traumatic or post-infective** parkinsonism.

A careful, expert neurological history and examination is necessary to reach a confident diagnosis. The next big challenge is choosing the therapeutic interventions. Patients with parkinsonism are best cared for by an expert multidisciplinary team who can give advice and support to patients and their carers. Unfortunately the most effective antiparkinsonian drug, levodopa, shows a marked reduction in effect with prolonged use, and so often (especially in younger patients) it is not started immediately if the effect of the disease on the patient's quality of life is not too severe. Dopamine agonists such as rotigotine, or the MAO-inhibitor selegiline, may be used to delay commencing levodopa.

2. The symptoms of Parkinson's disease are related to an inability to initiate voluntary movements, producing **akinesia or bradykinesia**, **rigidity**, and **tremor**. This is caused by destruction of dopamine-secreting neurons in the basal ganglia. The most effective treatment is dopamine supplementation with levodopa (given with a decarboxylase inhibitor to reduce side-effects); however, this treatment gradually becomes unpredictable and side-effects develop. One common problem is that the response to levodopa becomes unpredictable and variable, the effects suddenly 'wearing-off'—leaving the patient 'frozen' and unable to move. Another common problem is the development of involuntary movements (dystonias), which occur as 'late-dose' effects, as the effect of the levodopa is wearing off. These problems can be difficult to address, and neurologists may use various strategies in an attempt to combat them. Doses can be increased, or brought closer together; alternatively a second agent such as selegiline (a monoamine-oxidase-B inhibitor) can be added. Patients need to be informed that Parkinson's disease is a progressive, incurable disease and may become increasingly difficult to treat over time. The management of patients with Parkinson's disease can often prove complex. Thus management should be initiated and followed up wherever possible by a specialist Parkinson's disease multi-disciplinary team.

3. The cerebellum supervises movement and posture, using 'motor programmes' learned from previous experiences of performing actions to improve subsequent performance. The 'cerebellar signs' described below (using the acronym 'DANISH') are all examples of poor coordination in performing actions that usually would come as second nature. Neurons in the cerebellospinal tract do not decussate and so cerebellar lesions produce ispilateral signs.

- **D**ysdiadochokinesia—the inability to alternately pronate and supinate the hand whilst clapping.
- **A**taxia—a staggering and unsteady gait.
- **N**ystagmus—flickering eye movements caused by an inability to maintain focus on a particular visual stimulus on lateral gaze.
- **I**ntention tremor—for instance leading to past-pointing when the patient is asked to touch their finger from their nose to the examiner's finger.
- **S**canning speech—a halting, stammering dysarthria.
- **H**ypotonia and **H**yporeflexia.

A sensitive test is to ask the patient to hold out both hands in front of them and to close their eyes. When one hand is pushed down, in cerebellar disease a reciprocal upwards movement is overactive and overshoots the position of the other arm.

Causes of a unilateral cerebellar lesion include stroke (most likely in this case), demyelination, and primary or secondary brain tumours.

Causes of bilateral cerebellar signs (often called a 'cerebellar syndrome') include all of the unilateral causes (though it is rare for, say, a stroke to affect both sides equally as a single, synchronous event), toxins (alcohol and drugs, antiepileptics), paraneoplastic syndromes commonly associated with gynaecological, and less commonly prostatic, cancers (defined by the auto-antibody anti-Yo), and congenital disease—including fairly rare conditions such as Dandy-Walker syndrome and Friedrich's ataxia.

4. The term 'extrapyramidal side-effects' refers to motor symptoms that are not related to the 'pyramidal' part of the motor system. The pyramidal system consists of the primary motor cortex, the internal capsule, medullary pyramids, and the corticospinal tract, which is involved with the immediate control of motor function. Disease in any part of this system cause upper motor neuron symptoms including weakness and spasticity such as that seen in acute stroke.

Extrapyramidal symptoms usually refer to symptoms of basal ganglia disease. The basal ganglia function to initiate movement, and so extrapyramidal symptoms include parkinsonism (where there is poverty of initiation of movement), and symptoms of abnormal movement initiation (dyskinesia). Antipsychotic and antiemetic medications (for instance metoclopramide and prochlorperazine) are significant secondary causes of parkinsonism due to their antidopaminergic effects. Acute dystonias and oculogyric crisis, where there is fixed upward gaze, are a common side-effect of the antiemetics, particularly in young women. Both the acute and chronic extrapyramidal effects should be treated with procyclidine or benzhexol.

The restlessness displayed by this man is known as akathisia, though repetitive movements that develop late in the course of treatment with antipsychotic drugs are called tardive dyskinesias, and can include muscle spasms, tremor, or tics.

Further reading

Guidelines: NICE guidelines on Parkinson's disease (http://guidance.nice.org.uk/CG35)

OHCM: 472, 490, 498–499

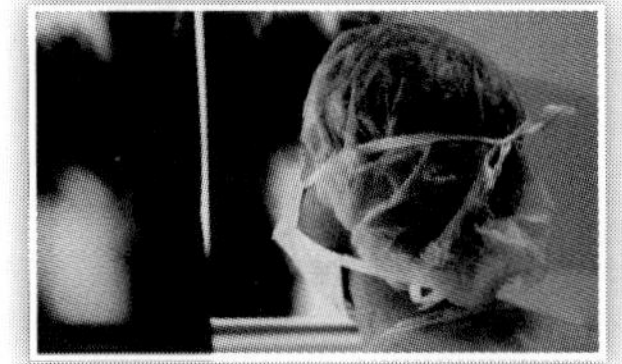
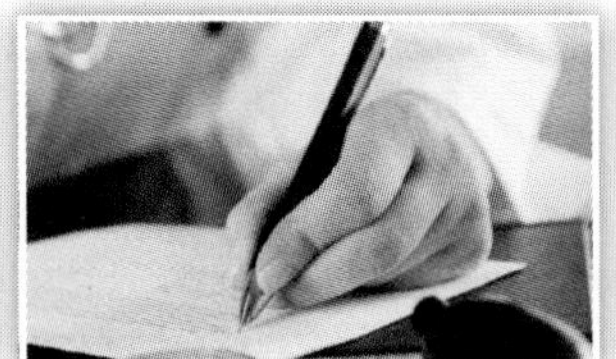
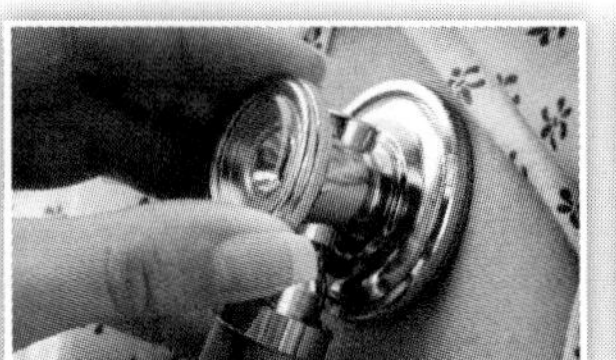
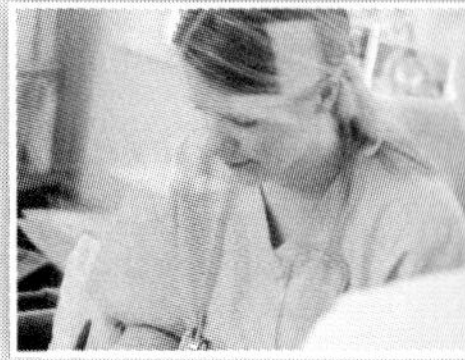

Unit 7
Multisystem diseases

This unit covers a range of complex, multisystem conditions including rheumatological, haematological, dermatological, and infectious disorders. Their complexity means they often require specialist management, but you may encounter such patients on acute medical takes. This unit should help you recognize these patients and help you understand the basis of their conditions and their initial management.

Key learning objectives in multisystem diseases include:

- **Developing an appropriate, systematic approach to patients presenting with non-specific multisystem symptoms.**
- **Understand the fundamentals of inflammatory conditions and recognize common manifestations such as rashes, arthritides, eye, and renal conditions.**
- **Understand common abnormalities of the full blood count , deriving common differential diagnoses from these abnormalities.**
- **Develop a systematic approach to assessing patients presenting with acute arthritis.**
- **Understand how to investigate patients with evidence of infection of unknown source.**

Tips for learning about multisystem diseases on the wards:

- Take an interest in complex 'mystery patients' with no obvious unifying diagnosis; use computer resources and the hospital library to research possible causes.
- Perform a competent assessment of all joints of the upper and lower limbs, and the spine.
- 'Anaemia is not a disease, it's a sign of a disease'—make sure you try to work out why patients are anaemic.
- Visit the medical day unit (or equivalent) where patients with haematological conditions often attend for transfusions or chemotherapy.
- Take an appropriate systematic history, including travel, HIV risk factors, sexual, and contacts from a patient presenting with a febrile illness with no obvious cause.

History

It is common for patients to present with non-specific symptoms such as 'feeling tired all of the time'. Such vague symptoms have broad and disparate differential causes, ranging from mental health problems such as depression, to malignancy, endocrine problems, uraemia, anaemia and other haematological disorders, neurological conditions, infectious diseases, cardiorespiratory problems, and a range of musculoskeletal disorders. This unit includes various complex disorders that commonly present in this manner. They synchronously affect a number of different systems and initially it may not be simple to find the unifying diagnosis. As a doctor you must develop the humility to accept your own limitations and ask others for help when you are unable to make the diagnosis yourself.

The 'review of systems' or 'systemic enquiry'

These questions are very useful for screening purposes in patients presenting with vague, general symptoms such as tiredness. In such patients they may form the basis of your history of the presenting complaint. They may be less relevant in patients presenting with a well-defined single pathology but are always useful to ensure that the patient's general health is unaffected.

Mental health:
- Mood
- Abnormal thoughts (delusions)
- Abnormal perceptions (hallucinations)
- Anxiety

Cardiovascular:
- Chest pain
- Syncope
- Palpitations
- Orthopnoea or paroxysmal nocturnal dyspnoea
- Swollen ankles

Haematological:
- Dizziness palpitations, syncope, breathlessness
- Bruising
- Recurrent infections
- Lymphadenopathy
- Vague abdominal pains secondary to hepatosplenomegaly

General health:
- Tiredness
- Level of function
- Changes in weight
- Appetite

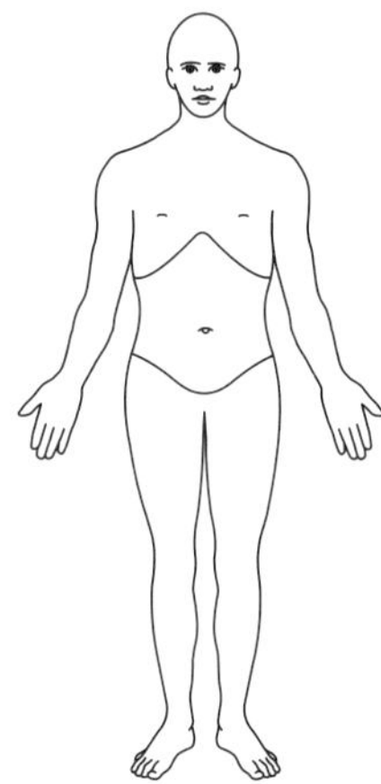

Dermatological:
- Skin rashes
- Pruritis

Neurological:
- Fits
- Limb weakness
- Paraesthesia

Respiratory:
- Breathlessness (quantify)
- Cough
- Haemoptysis

Gastrointestinal:
- Abdominal pain
- Nausea and vomiting
- Diarrhoea
- Jaundice

Musculoskeletal:
- Pain in limbs, neck or back
- Function – such as their ability to mobilize, transfer, climb stairs, wash and dress

Taking a travel history

This is an important part of assessing patients who present non-specifically unwell where there is no obvious diagnosis—particularly in those with presentations in keeping with infectious disease. A knowledge of the patient's ethnic origin may also help in raising the probability of various genetic diseases. A full history will include country of birth and all countries visited since, including the time spent in each, whether the patient stayed in rural or urban locations, and whether they undertook any risky activities whilst there—for instance unprotected sex or blood transfusions (blood-borne viruses), eating salad or other foods (hepatitis A and E, bacterial dysentery), or even swimming in lakes (schistosomiasis).

Time course is important: some diseases have short incubation periods (<10 days, including dysentery and dengue fever), some have slightly longer incubation periods of up to a month after exposure (such as falciparum malaria and typhoid fever), whereas others may not present for weeks, months, or years after they are contracted (including HIV, non-falciparum malaria, tuberculosis, schistosomiasis, and viral hepatitis). A rudimentary knowledge of geography is helpful in knowing which conditions are common in different parts of the world. The website http://www.fitfortravel.scot.nhs.uk/home.aspx is run by the Scottish National Health Service and offers advice to travellers on health risks in different countries.

World malaria map

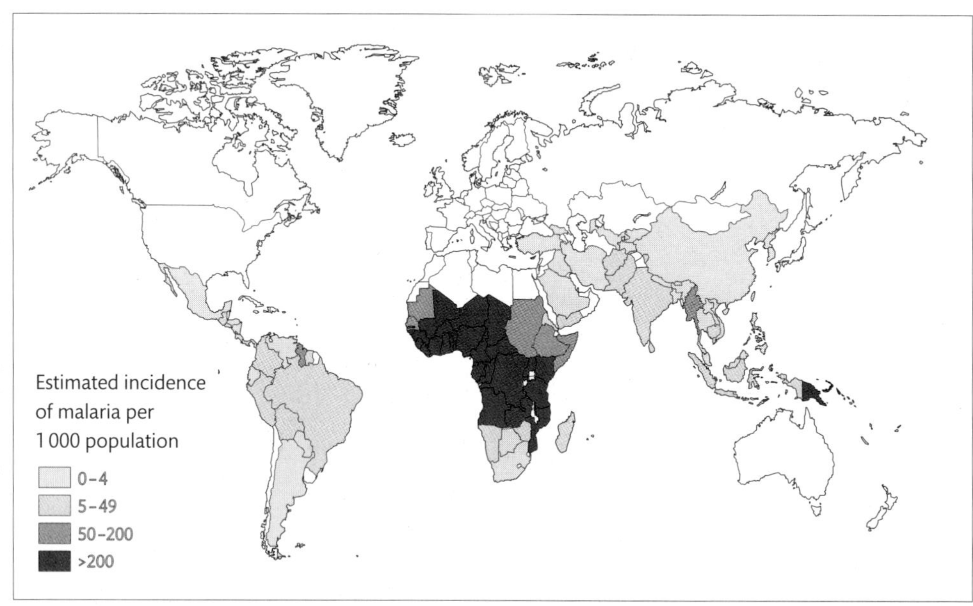

World TB map

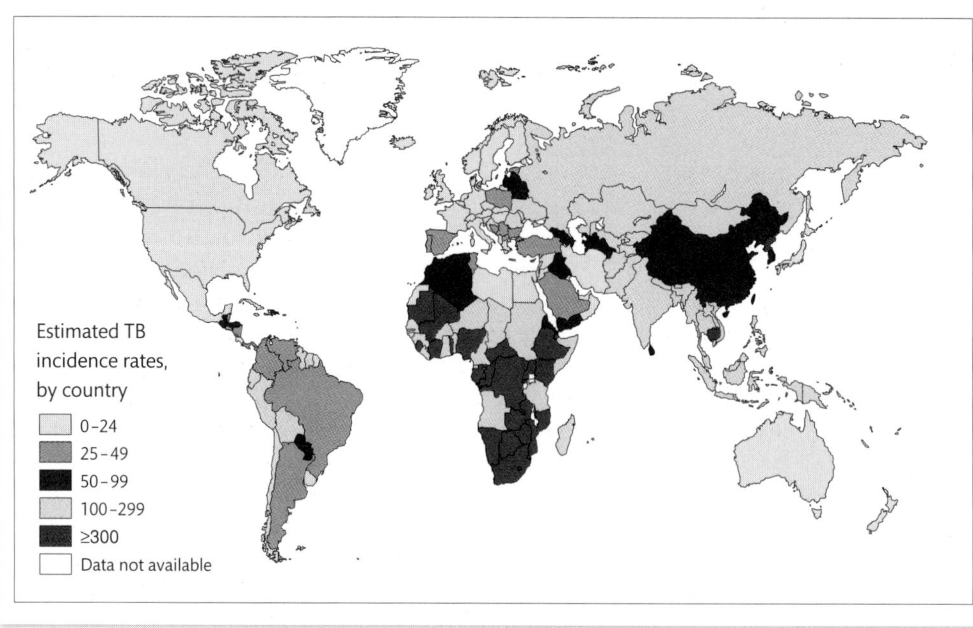

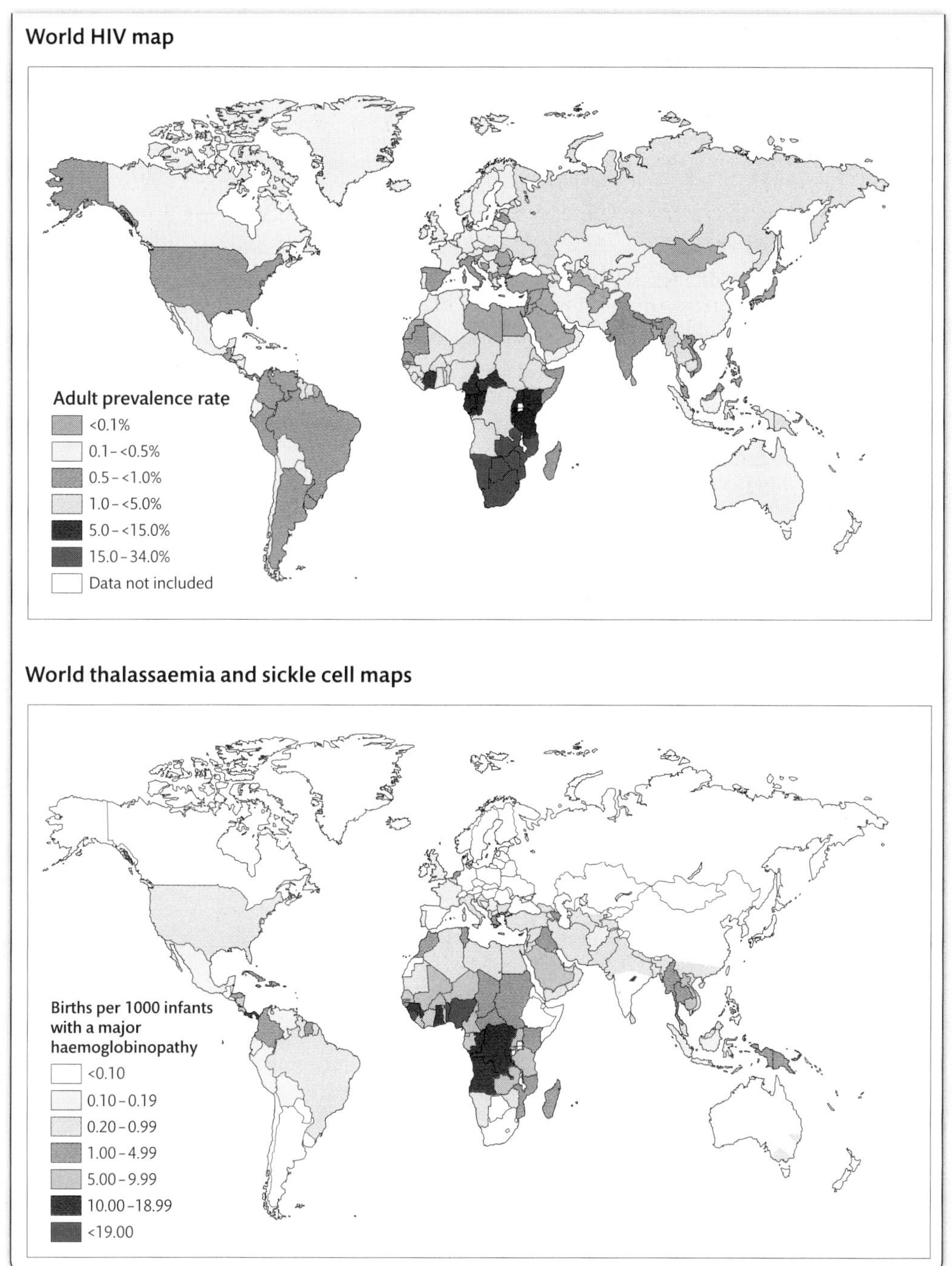

Diagrams re-drawn from World Health Organization data, available online from http://gamapserver.who.int/mapLibrary/

Pyrexia of unknown origin

This is a term applied to patients who are objectively pyrexial but in whom no cause can be found. Eventual diagnoses in these patients fall into three major categories: **infectious diseases** (including the tropical diseases outlined above as well as viral illnesses, bacterial endocarditis, and hidden collections of pus), **inflammatory conditions** (for instance rheumatoid arthritis, systemic lupus erythematosus, sarcoidosis, or a vasculitis), and **cancers** (such as Hodgkin's and non-Hodgkin's lymphoma, renal cell carcinoma, and occasionally others). A pragmatic approach to these patients involves performing an array of investigations including bacterial cultures from multiple sites, CT scanning (if necessary of much of the body), and biopsies of any amenable tissues (e.g. enlarged lymph nodes). Often a trial of empirical broad-spectrum antibiotics is given, after which a trial of steroids is given if there is no response. Sometimes everything settles and no cause is found. Occasionally a 'drug fever' is caused (for instance by a long course of antibiotics) and the patient becomes better once the drug is stopped, though this can be a difficult decision to make as the presence of fever may suggest that an infection is still active.

Examination

Examination of a joint

Remember that pain in the limbs can be referred—so always examine the joint above and below the joint in which the patient is complaining of pain. The basic sequence for examining a joint is in three stages: **look, feel, and move**.

Look

- Swelling
- Bony deformity
- Bruising
- Erythema or cellulitis
- Muscle wasting

Feel

- Tenderness—define exactly where the tenderness is worst
- Effusion—fluid (fluctuant swelling) within the joint capsule
- Temperature—a hot, red, and swollen joint is likely to be acutely inflamed

Move

- Range of active (patient-initiated) movement
- Range of passive movement (where the examiner moves the joint)
- Tests for ligament or tendon stability

You should also assess the **function** of the limb affected, by asking the patient to perform actions requiring use of the joint in question—for instance doing up a button.

Describing skin lesions

The table below suggests phrases that can be used to provide basic descriptions of single skin lesions or more widespread rashes. Describing rashes precisely allows clear communication in the patient's absence, and may also suggest the likely diagnosis by putting the rash in a particular category.

	Rashes	Single (or multiple) individual lesions
Distribution	**Flexural** (on the inside of joints or in skin folds) **Extensor** (on the extensor surfaces of joints) **Localized** or **widespread**	'On the anterior aspect of...' (body region) 'Overlying... ' (deeper structure)
Appearance	**Macular**—flat lesions **Papular**—raised lesions **Maculopapular** (small flat and raised lesions, often red in colour) **Purpuric** or **petechial** (purple and non-blanching cause by skin haemorrhages) **Urticarial** (itchy raised areas of dermal oedema) **Cellulitic** (red, swollen, and hot—skin infection)	**Macule** (flat skin lesion) **Papule** or **nodule** (raised lesions) **Ulcer** (area of full thickness skin erosion) **Vesicle** or **bulla** (small or large blisters) **Pustule** (pus-filled vesicle) **Abscess** (localized pus collection) **Crusted** (flaky dried exudates over lesion)
Edges	**Confluent** (one area runs into the next) **Spreading** (invading neighbouring regions)	**Well demarcated**
Effect on patient	**Pruritic** (itchy) **Painful** **Exudative** (weeping fluid)	

Examination of the haematological patient

On general examination look for signs of **anaemia** (pallor, seen most obviously in the conjunctivae), **bruising** (possibly a sign of thrombocytopenia or another clotting disorder), and signs of **infection** or **immunosuppression** (see below). Then examine for lymph nodes and splenomegaly:

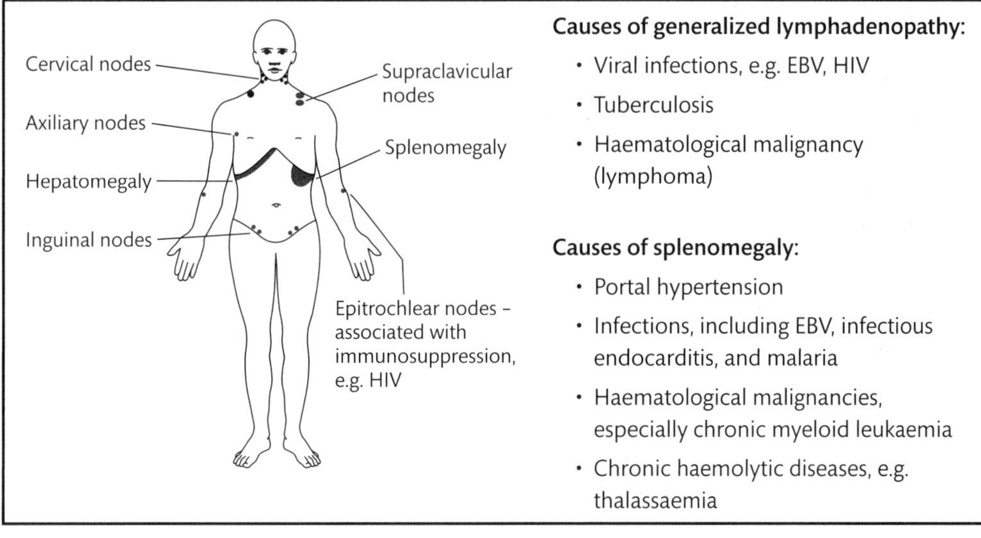

Causes of generalized lymphadenopathy:

- Viral infections, e.g. EBV, HIV
- Tuberculosis
- Haematological malignancy (lymphoma)

Causes of splenomegaly:

- Portal hypertension
- Infections, including EBV, infectious endocarditis, and malaria
- Haematological malignancies, especially chronic myeloid leukaemia
- Chronic haemolytic diseases, e.g. thalassaemia

Signs of immunosuppression and advanced HIV infection

With the increased availability of antiretroviral drugs, most known HIV-positive patients rarely display overt signs of immunosuppression and AIDS. However, a proportion of undiagnosed patients may present acutely unwell with advanced HIV/AIDS displaying the clinical signs below. If the clinical context is appropriate then the diagnosis of HIV should be suspected and the patient tested for the disease.

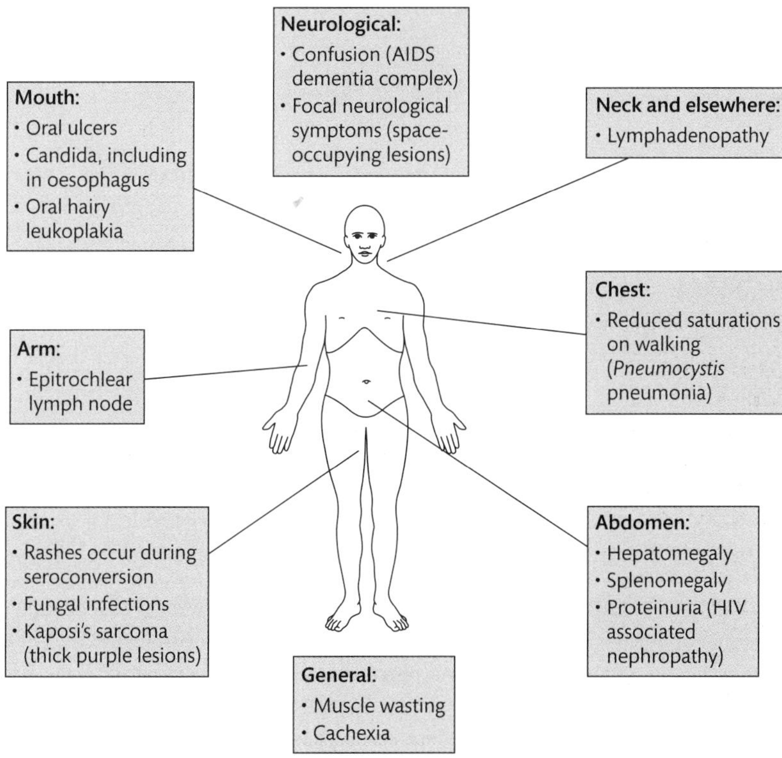

Investigations

Understanding the full blood count

Anaemia denotes a low haemoglobin, and should always be described in terms of the mean corpuscular volume (the average size of red blood cells), which suggests possible causes:

- **Microcytic anaemias (MCV < 80 fL)**
  - **Iron deficiency** is the commonest cause of microcytosis, usually as a result of chronic gastrointestinal or gynaecological blood loss which can be confirmed by abnormal haematinics: low serum iron level, low ferritin, and a high total iron-binding capacity (TIBC).
  - **Thalassaemia**, an inherited disorder of haemoglobin common in those from the Mediterranean.
  - **Other causes**—anaemia of chronic disease and sideroblastic anaemia.
- **Normocytic anaemias (MCV 80–96 fL):**
  - **Chronic disease** is the commonest cause of normocytic anaemia. The mechanism is believed to be due to reduced secretion of erythropoietin by the kidney.
  - **Acute haemorrhage**—chronic blood loss causes a microcytic anaemia but acute haemorrhage does not allow any time for the MCV to fall.
- **Macrocytic anaemias (MCV > 96 fL):**
  - **Vitamin B_{12} or folate deficiencies** cause a megaloblastic anaemia—megaloblasts (seen on blood film) are immature red cells produced if there is inadequate DNA synthesis.
  - **Alcohol excess** or **liver disease** produce non-megaloblastic macrocytosis (and a raised MCV is a good marker of alcohol excess).
  - **Haemolytic anaemia** (where there is a high level of destruction of red cells) produces a macrocytic anaemia because of a high proportion (>2%) of immature red cells called reticulocytes. The bilirubin is raised (a haemoglobin breakdown product), if severe giving a pre-hepatic jaundice.

White blood cells rise in number during infection. Levels are kept low by bone marrow suppression, e.g. in leukaemias or after chemotherapy, when the patient may be susceptible to opportunistic infection.

- **Neutrophils:** Neutrophil levels rise in bacterial infection, especially if it is widespread. The term **neutropenia** refers to a dangerous fall in neutrophil numbers, often due to the effects of drugs (e.g. chemotherapy) or viral infection. It renders patients extremely vulnerable to bacterial sepsis, and patients require broad-spectrum antibiotic treatment until their neutrophil count recovers.
- **Lymphocytes:** Lymphocyte levels are raised in viral infections and chronic bacterial infections, e.g. TB. They may be reduced in advanced HIV infection.
- **Eosinophils:** These cells have a role in allergy, and may be raised in hypersensitivity reactions (e.g. to drugs) or in parasitic infections (e.g. hookworm).
- **Monocytes:** Monocytes may only circulate in the blood for several hours before entering tissues to become macrophages. Their levels are raised in chronic infections such as TB or infective endocarditis.

Platelets are small cell fragments that have important roles to play in coagulation. Their deficiency, **thrombocytopenia**, can worsen haemorrhage and may produce easy bruising or a purpuric rash. Platelet numbers are commonly reduced with conditions causing splenomegaly, e.g. chronic liver disease producing portal hypertension, or in bone marrow dysfunction, e.g. myeloma.

Looking further

After initial, simple assessment, further investigations of the full blood count are conducted by a haematologist. These investigations can include a **blood film** (a microscope slide of peripheral blood cells) or a **bone marrow biopsy**, taken (often from the iliac crest) under local anaesthetic for microscopy of the bone marrow. More recently genetic testing has become routine in the investigation of haematological malignancies.

Markers of rheumatological diseases

These tests are used in patients who present with symptoms suggestive of a multisystem rheumatological disease, for instance arthritis, a vasculitic rash, a glomerulonephritis, or interstitial lung disease.

- **Rheumatoid factor (RF):** this is an antibody directed against IgG. It leads to the production of immune complexes that in turn lead to the many of the manifestations of rheumatoid disease. RF is raised in 70% of patients with rheumatoid disease, and may also be raised in other rheumatological conditions. Anticyclic citrullinated peptide (anti-CCP) is a newer, more specific, test for rheumatoid arthritis.
- **Antinuclear antibodies (ANA):** these are raised in a number of autoimmune diseases, and are used as a screening test for systemic lupus erythematosus (SLE).
- **Antidouble-stranded DNA antibodies (anti-dsDNA):** if raised these are a specific marker of SLE.
- **Antineutrophil cytoplasmic antibodies (ANCA):** these are particularly associated with vasculitides (diseases caused by autoimmune attack on blood vessels) such as Wegener's granulomatosis.
- **Complement:** C3 and C4 levels fall when they are being 'used up'—this is commonly used as a marker of immune complex formation and indicates active disease in patients with SLE or rheumatoid disease.
- **Other autoantibodies:** various other markers exist such as anti-Jo-1 or anti-topoisomerase-1, which may suggest other connective tissue diseases such as systemic sclerosis or Sjögren's syndrome.

Investigating infections

The diagram below shows how to examine and investigate patients suspected of having infection (for instance with a fever and raised inflammatory markers) but no obvious source. If no infection is found after full initial investigations then the patient may be decided to have pyrexia of unknown origin (described earlier).

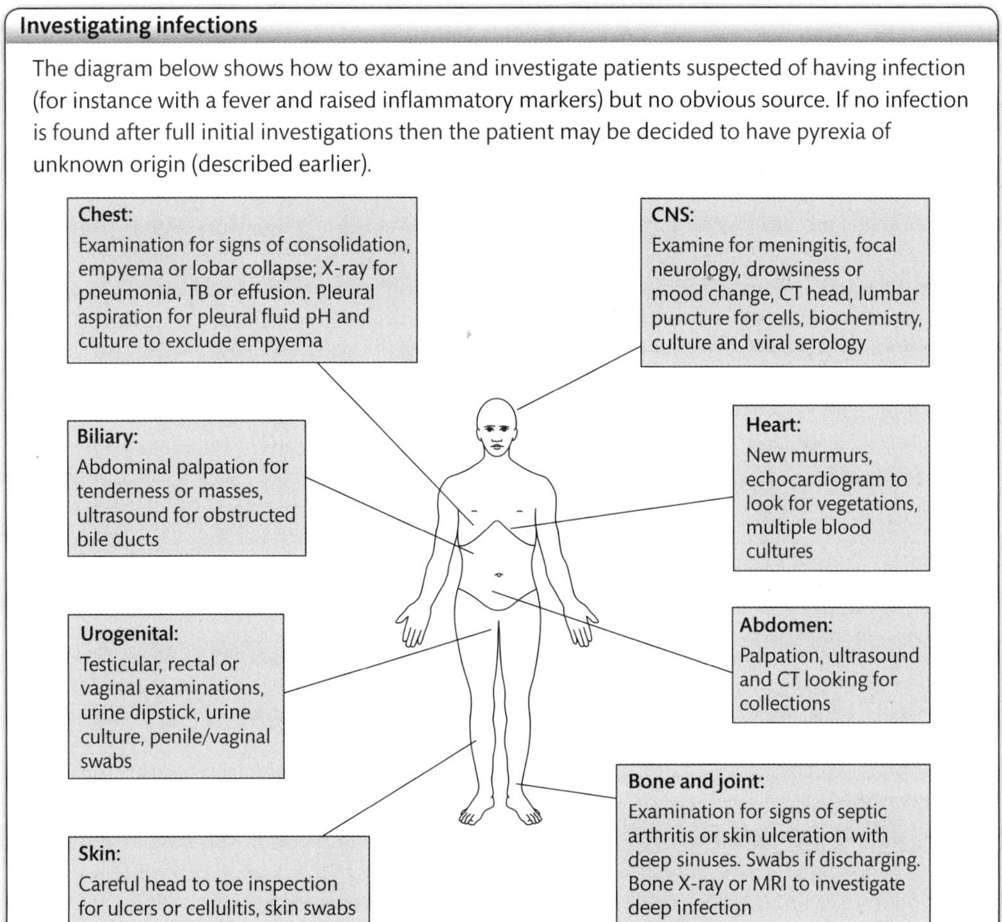

Interventions

Principles of antibiotic therapy

There are dangers of both overtreating and undertreating infections. Overtreatment leads to the emergence of antibiotic resistance in microorganisms, and the use of inappropriately broad-spectrum antibiotics may lead to the development of *Clostridium difficile* diarrhoea, especially in the elderly. However, research from the Surviving Sepsis campaign (http://www.survivingsepsis.org/) links death from infection closely with delay in administering antibiotics. The following principles are useful guidelines in trying to avoid both overtreating and undertreating infection:

- If the source of infection is known, treat with the narrowest spectrum antibiotic possible that will cover all likely organisms.
- If the source of infection is unknown and the patient displays signs of systemic sepsis then rapidly take cultures of blood, urine, sputum, and relevant others before giving broad-spectrum antibiotics.
- If the source of infection is unknown but the patient is not systemically unwell, hold off antibiotics and perform cultures and investigations to determine the likely source. Monitor the patient and treat empirically if they become unwell. This may not be followed in elderly patients, as they can decompensate rapidly if one is wrong about the diagnosis of sepsis.
- Amend antibiotic choices once the organism and its sensitivities are known.

Most hospitals now have antibiotic policies that suggest which antibiotics should be used for which types of infection, e.g. gentamicin (which is very effective against Gram-negative organisms but has limited efficacy against Gram positives) is often used for urinary sepsis where the commonest organisms are Gram-negative rods.

Principles of chemotherapy and radiotherapy

Antibiotics target features of bacteria which are not present in human cells (e.g. cell wall synthesis) and therefore generally produce few toxic effects. Anticancer drugs target abnormal host cells, and therefore have fewer targets to aim at: many target all fast-growing cells and so consequently produce significant side-effects. This must be borne in mind when starting patients on chemotherapy. Chemotherapy is sometimes given with curative intent (usually only in haematological malignancies); otherwise it is given to prolong survival. The likely benefits should be explained to patients so that they can weigh these against the often significant side-effects.

Radiotherapy also often makes patients feel very unwell because of chemical mediators released as cells die. It may also cause collateral damage to neighbouring healthy tissue, e.g. radiation colitis or radiation pneumonitis. Radiotherapy may be used palliatively (e.g. to reduce pain in bony metastases), to debulk tumour mass (e.g. if tumours are obstructing other structures), or, very rarely, with curative intent.

Principles of immunosuppressive therapy

Immunosuppressants are commonly used in long-term inflammatory conditions. There may be a dramatic improvement in symptoms, but side-effects of treatments always need to be taken into account.

- **Steroids** are often used to induce remission in inflammatory conditions, and sometimes to maintain remission, but long-term steroid use risks development of a cushingoid syndrome including osteoporosis, gastric erosion, hypertension, diabetes, weight gain, and skin changes.
- **Steroid-sparing agents** such as azathioprine or methotrexate are often preferred for long-term use, though these have their own particular toxic side-effects (such as bone marrow suppression or pulmonary fibrosis) which require monitoring.
- **New biological agents** such as infliximab or etanercept oppose the action of the cytokine TNF-α and often have striking efficacy in improving symptoms in rheumatoid disease and other inflammatory diseases.

The danger with any medication which suppresses the immune system is of overwhelming infection. This is particularly true with the new anti-TNF-α drugs (see above). Patients should be screened for TB before the treatment is commenced.

Medications for rheumatological, haematological, and infectious diseases

Class	Examples	Mechanism	Indications	Contraindications	Side-effects	Special notes
Oral steroids						
Intravenous steroids						
Steroid-sparing immunosuppressants						
Disease modifying antirheumatoid drugs						
Anti-TNFα drugs						
NSAIDs						
Weak opioids						
Combination analgesics						
Xanthine-oxidase inhibitor						
Blood						
Platelets						
Fresh frozen plasma						
Penicillins						
Cephalosporins						
Macrolides						
Aminoglycosides						
Sulphonamides						
Quinolones						
Antiretroviral agents						
Systemic antifungal agents						

Acute arthritis

This section should be used to clerk patients being admitted to hospital with one or more acutely painful or swollen joints. The focus is on diagnosing the cause of the acute arthritis and instituting appropriate initial management. Some acute arthritis will be part of a wider systemic disorder and require specialist rheumatological management. Patients with acute arthritis are often seen and stabilized on the Medical Admissions Unit and then transferred to specialist care, either as an in- or out-patient.

Learning challenges

- What are immune complexes and why are they formed in many systemic arthritic conditions? What common manifestations do they produce in different organ systems?
- What is HLA-B27 and which disease associations does it explain?

History

Comment on

- Pattern of joint involvement—small joints, large joints, spine
- Symmetry of involvement
- Symptoms of acute arthritis—hot, painful, acutely swollen joints
- Systemic features—fevers, rigors, lethargy, malaise
- Exacerbation, e.g. with activity or with immobility
- Relieving factors—rest, activity, analgesia
- Full systems review—especially eyes, respiratory, skin, renal tract
- Medications
- Effect on activities of daily living (ADL), i.e. disability

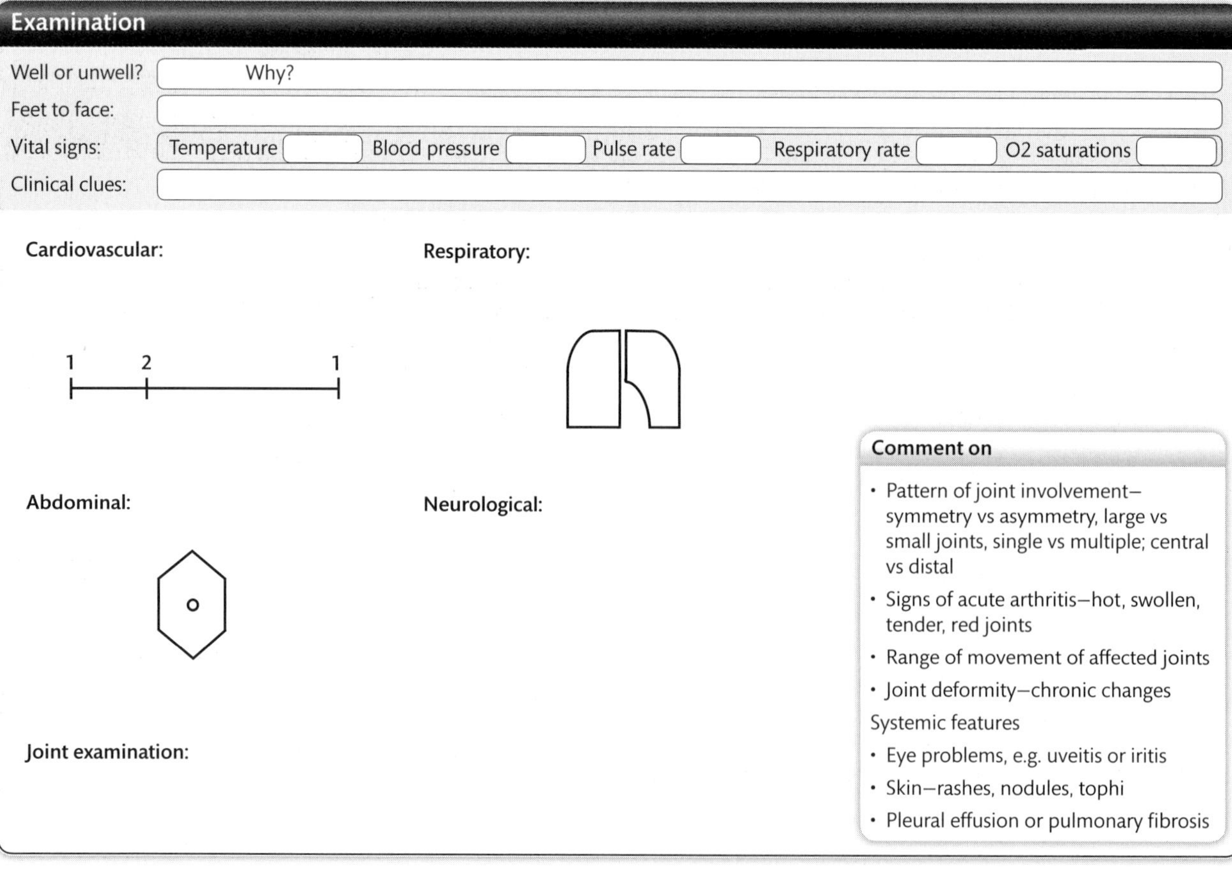

Examination

Well or unwell? Why?

Feet to face:

Vital signs: Temperature | Blood pressure | Pulse rate | Respiratory rate | O2 saturations

Clinical clues:

Cardiovascular:

1 2 1

Respiratory:

Abdominal:

Neurological:

Joint examination:

Comment on

- Pattern of joint involvement—symmetry vs asymmetry, large vs small joints, single vs multiple; central vs distal
- Signs of acute arthritis—hot, swollen, tender, red joints
- Range of movement of affected joints
- Joint deformity—chronic changes

Systemic features

- Eye problems, e.g. uveitis or iritis
- Skin—rashes, nodules, tophi
- Pleural effusion or pulmonary fibrosis

Blood tests

Comment on

- FBC—Hb/MCV, WCC and differential, platelets
- U&Es
- ESR and CRP
- Autoantibodies, e.g. rheumatoid factor, anti-dsDNA, ANA
- Complement levels

Radiology

Comment on

- X-ray of involved joints—signs of acute vs chronic arthritis
- Specific signs of arthritis—deformity, loss of joint space, erosions, sclerosis, osteopenia, effusions, calcinosis

Joint aspiration

Comment on

- Appearance—clear or turbid
- Crystals—positive and negative birefringence under polarized light
- Cells
- Microbiology—organisms

Urine dipstick

Comment on

- Proteinuria

Evaluation

1. How many joints are involved? What are the likeliest diagnoses?

Monoarthritis	Oligoarthritis (<5 joints)	Polyarthritis
Crystal arthropathy – gout and pyrophosphate	Crystal arthropathy	Rheumatoid arthritis
Septic arthritis	Psoriatic arthropathy	Osteoarthritis
Osteoarthritis	Reactive arthropathy	SLE or other connective tissue diseases
Trauma—haemarthrosis	Osteoarthritis	Reactive arthritis
	Septic arthritis	

2. Is urgent joint aspiration indicated? Are the results diagnostic?

3. What pain control is most appropriate?

4. Is immunomodulatory therapy appropriate?

5. What is the likely prognosis? Will the patient require joint replacement surgery in the future?

Questions

1. A 37-year-old woman presents to her GP complaining of feeling lethargic and generally unwell for several months. She tells the GP that she has been suffering with painful joints in her fingers and toes and has also had some pain in her chest, made worse on deep inspiration. She noticed that her symptoms got worse 3 weeks ago after a holiday abroad when she got badly sunburned.

On examination the joints of her hands, wrists, ankles, and knees are all mildly tender to touch, with slight surrounding 'bogginess', but they are not erythematous or hot to touch. The GP arranges X-rays of her hands and some routine blood tests, and refers her to the rheumatology out-patient department. Both hand X-rays are reported as being normal. The results of her blood tests are shown below:

Sodium: 139 mmol/L	Haemoglobin: 12.1 g/dL
Potassium: 4.2 mmol/L	White cells: 3.9 × 10^9/L
Urea: 5.2 mmol/L	Platelets: 136 × 10^9/L
Creatinine: 89 μmol/L	ESR: 72 mm in first hour
CRP: 8 mg/L	INR: 1.0
Rheumatoid factor: Negative	
Antinuclear antibody (ANA): Postive	
Antidouble-stranded-DNA (anti-dsDNA): Positive	
Antiextractable nuclear antigen (anti-ENA): Negative	
Antineutrophil cytoplasmic antibodies (ANCA): Negative	
Complement C3 and C4 levels: Reduced	

(1) What is the suggested diagnosis?

(2) List three drugs used in the treatment of this condition

2. A 54-year-old man presents to hospital complaining of an extremely painful left big toe, which began to hurt 6 hours before. It is exquisitely tender, and he is unable to walk on it or put on his socks or shoes. He suffers from hypertension, for which he was started on bendroflumethiazide a week previously by his GP. He regularly drinks three pints of strong beer a night (around 70 units per week). From his records the GP notes he is 1.65 m tall and weighs 98.8 kg. On examination his temperature is 37.8°C, his heart rate is 84 bpm, and his blood pressure 156/78 mmHg. The first metacarpophalangeal joint of his right foot is red and inflamed and exquisitely tender on palpation. No movement is possible.

(1) What is the likely diagnosis?

(2) How will you prove the diagnosis?

(3) What is the acute and long term management?

3. A 67-year-old man complains of worsening pain in his hips and knees on walking. The pain is particularly severe in his right knee and is worst when he walks, improving dramatically with rest. He has been taking occasional paracetamol to help with the pain; however, he is still very restricted in terms of his ability to leave the house and engage in normal day to day activities. He has been unable to play his beloved golf for months. An X-ray of his right knee is shown below:

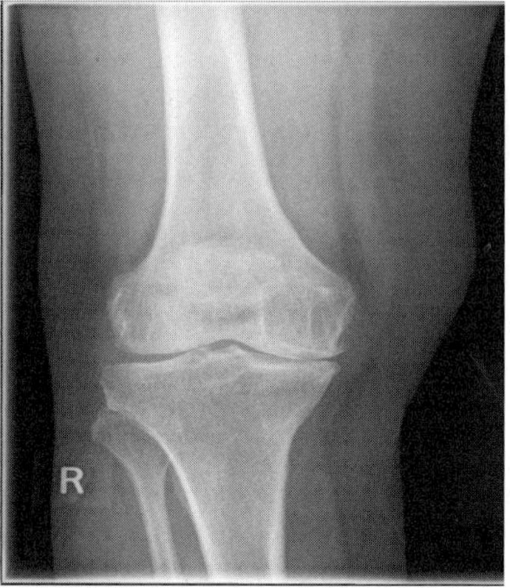

(1) What does the radiograph show?

(2) List five essential steps in the management of this patient

4. A 29-year-old woman presents to the hospital complaining of an acutely swollen and painful right knee joint, with symptoms developing over the previous 12 hours. There was no history of trauma. She does not disclose any other medical problems, and is not taking any medications. On examination she is pyrexial (38.9°C) and tachycardic (120 bpm). Her blood pressure is maintained at 115/65 mmHg. Her right knee is red and swollen, warm to the touch, and very tender. A moderate effusion is palpable. Movement is severely restricted to only a few degrees of flexion and extension. Blood tests reveal a white cell count of 23.8 × 10^9/L and a CRP of 276 mg/L. Turbid fluid is aspirated from the joint, which on microscopy contains large numbers of polymorphic leucocytes. Gram stain reveals Gram-negative cocci.

(1) What other relevant history should be sought in this case?

(2) What is the likely diagnosis?

(3) What is the essential, immediate management in this case?

Remember that you can find large-size, annotated versions of many of the X-rays and ECGs that appear in this book on the book's web site at www.oxfordtextbooks.co.uk/orc/randall/

Answers

1. This patient has systemic lupus erythematosus (SLE). A classic feature of SLE is raised ESR with normal CRP. SLE is a true multisystem disease which is diagnosed by having four out of the eleven diagnostic criteria drawn up by the American Rheumatological Association:

Serositis (pleuritic/pericarditic/peritoneal pain)
Oral ulceration
Arthritis—usually non-deforming
Photosensitivity (rashes which are worse after sun exposure)
Haematological abnormalities (e.g. anaemia, leucopenia, thrombocytopenia)
Renal failure, glomerulonephritis
ANA positive
Other immunological abnormalities, e.g. anti-dsDNA, antiphospholipid antibodies
Neuropsychiatric disorder (e.g. seizures or psychosis)
Malar rash
Discoid rash

SLE is a complex condition caused by autoimmune inflammation of uncertain aetiology. Most clinical manifestations are caused by the production of immune complexes where different autoantibodies clump together with native antigen. These may be deposited in the skin (producing the various rashes associated with SLE), in the kidneys (causing a glomerulonephritis), in the joints (producing arthritis), or in blood vessels causing them to become inflamed (a vasculitis). There may also be problems in other organ systems. Deposition of immune complexes causes activation of the complement system, so depletion of complement is a non-specific marker of disease activity. SLE can present in many different ways and may mimic a number of other conditions.

Management of SLE is similarly complex. Patients should avoid the sun, which can worsen symptoms. If appropriate, aspirin and other cardiovascular drugs should be started to reduce the (raised) cardiovascular risk. Arthritis may be helped with non-steroidal anti-inflammatory drugs (NSAIDs), and rash and general malaise by the antimalarial drug hydroxychloroquine. If symptoms are severe, immunomodulatory drugs or steroids may be required, and particularly resistant disease may be helped by monoclonal antibody drugs such as rituximab.

2. This presentation is characteristic of gout. Uric acid crystals are deposited in the joint causing intense pain and inflammation. Factors predisposing to hyperuricaemia include male sex, family history, high protein intake, consumption of alcohol, and obesity. Often, crystal deposition precipitating an acute attack is triggered by dehydration, with thiazide diuretics being common culprits. Overeating or alcohol binges may also trigger an acute attack.

The major differential diagnoses here are pyrophosphate arthropathy and septic arthritis. The diagnosis of gout is suggested by a raised serum uric acid. It can be confirmed by aspiration of the joint, when negatively birefringent crystals are seen. Pyrophosphate arthropathy or 'pseudogout' is caused by crystals of calcium pyrophosphate which are positively birefringent, and affects a wider spectrum of patients than gout.

It is important to differentiate gout and pyrophosphate arthropathy because the long-term management is very different. Acutely, NSAIDs and colchicine may be used, but long term the prophylactic medication allopurinol is used in patients with gout. Patients should also be advised to avoid obvious precipitants.

3. Osteoarthritis is caused by gradual wearing away of the cartilage, with subsequent reaction of the underlying bone. The process is accelerated by any process that leads to unusual load being placed on the joint - for instance obesity or after a fracture involving the articular surface of the joint:

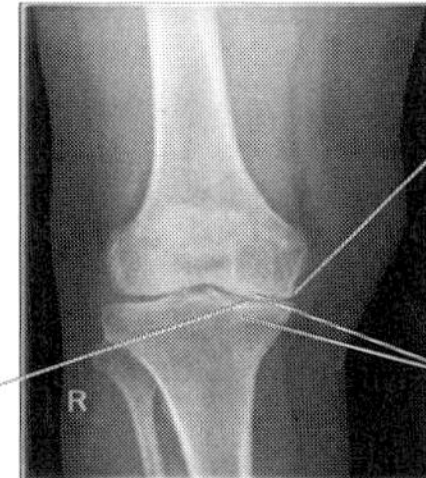

This x-ray demonstrates early changes of osteoarthritis.

Note that the joint space is narrowed, especially on the medial side of the joint. This is caused by wear-and-tear erosion of the cartilage lining the articular surfaces of the bone.

Osteophytes are classically a feature of osteoarthritis, where spurs of new bone form at the margins of affected joints. They have begun to form here.

Another common feature of osteoarthritis seen here is osteosclerosis - thickening of the bone adjacent to the joint in response to the erosion of the joint cartilage. This is seen as a bright rim at the bone edge. Sometimes, bone cysts form below this.

Osteoarthritis is a major cause of morbidity but the course of the disease cannot be altered by medication. Therapy is therefore palliative, focused on symptom control. This man should be given stronger pain killers as suggested by the World Health Organisation's 'analgesic ladder', shown below.

Rung 3: Strong opioid e.g. morphine plus non-opioid

Rung 2: Weak opiod e.g. codeine plus non-opioid

Rung 1: Non-opioid e.g. paracetamol or NSAID

Adjuncts: may be added at any rung, include:

- Antidepressants
- Steroids
- Physiotherapy
- Hot/cold pads

Many patients eventually require joint replacement for painful, deformed joints.

4. This woman has clinical evidence of sepsis, which in the context of an acutely inflamed joint should be treated as septic arthritis. Young patients may have dramatic presentations (as here); in older patients the joint may not be so obviously hot, painful, and swollen, so a high index of suspicion is required. This is especially the case in patients with previous joint disease (e.g. rheumatoid arthritis) who are already predisposed to septic arthritis because of their abnormal joint anatomy. Septic arthritis may be mistaken for a flare-up of the underlying disease, leading to dangerous delays in starting antibiotics.

The commonest cause of septic arthritis in younger patients is *Neisseria gonorrhoeae*, which infects the joint through haematogenous spread after contraction of gonorrhoea via sexual contact. Thus taking a sexual history is very important in young patients being admitted with an acute mono- or oligoarthritis. Treatment is with an extended course of antibiotics which should initially be given intravenously. Broad-spectrum antibiotics can be narrowed down once the causative organism and its sensitivities are known. Complications include bone destruction and infection (osteomyelitis), and surgical drainage of the joint can be performed to prevent these from occurring. Infection of a prosthetic joint is especially serious and often requires further surgery to remove infected metalwork.

Further reading

Guidelines: British Society for Rheumatology guidelines on managing hot swollen joints (http://www.rheumatology.org.uk/includes/documents/cm_docs/2009/m/management_of_hot_swollen_joints_in_adults.pdf)

OHCM: 541, 546–552

Anaemia

This section should be used to clerk patients with unexplained anaemia—which always requires investigation to identify a likely cause. They may present in general practice or to hospital with symptoms of tiredness and breathlessness, and no obvious diagnosis. These patients may be found on any general medical ward, though especially those for gastroenterology or haematology patients.

Learning challenges

- What different types of blood products are available for transfusion in most hospitals? What is the difference between 'group and save' and 'cross-match' requests?
- What leading cause of iron-deficiency anaemia is common in the developing world but rarely seen in richer countries?

History

Comment on

- Symptoms of anaemia, e.g. exertional dyspnoea, reduced or limited exercise tolerance, lethargy and malaise; onset and duration
- Overt blood loss, including: GI—haematemesis, melaena, bleeding per rectum; menorrhagia or post-menopausal vaginal bleeding; haematuria, epistaxis
- Symptoms of bone marrow dysfunction—increased Infections, bruising and easy bleeding
- Systemic features of haematological malignancy—night sweats, lymphadenopathy, weight loss, lethargy, malaise, bony pain (myeloma)
- Racial background, family history—haemoglobinopathies
- Gallstones, leg ulcers (sickle cell disease)
- Medications—especially NSAIDs and antiplatelet medications; any new or changed medications
- Alcohol consumption

Examination

Well or unwell? Why?

Feet to face:

Vital signs: Temperature | Blood pressure | Pulse rate | Respiratory rate | O2 saturations

Clinical clues:

Cardiovascular:

1 2 1

Respiratory:

Abdominal:

Neurological:

Other:

Comment on

- Pallor, lymphadenopathy, jaundice
- Bruising, petechiae
- Koilonychia, glossitis, angular stomatitis
- Systolic 'flow' murmur
- Hepatomegaly, splenomegaly, abdominal masses
- Rectal examination: melaena or fresh blood

Blood tests

Comment on

- Haemoglobin, MCV
- White cell count and differential
- Platelet count
- Clotting screen
- Bilirubin
- Haemetinics—iron studies, vitamin B_{12}, folate
- Anti-tissue transglutaminase antibodies (coeliac disease)

Blood film

Comment on

- Red cell morphology
- Reticulocytes
- White cell morphology

Bone marrow aspirate

Comment on

- Cellularity
- Infiltration
- Iron stores

Gastrointestinal endoscopy

Comment on

- Bleeding
- Atrophic gastritis
- Coeliac disease/inflammatory bowel disease

Evaluation

1. What is the likely cause of this anaemia?

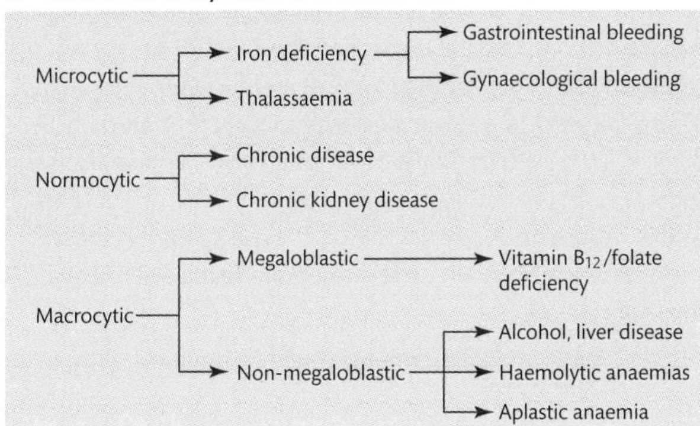

2. Does this patient require transfusion? How much?

3. How should the underlying condition be managed?

Questions

1. An 80-year-old woman is referred to hospital after routine blood tests organized by her GP reveal a haemoglobin of 7.7 g/L, with a MCV of 104 fL. She had attended her doctor complaining of gradually increasing fatigue and breathlessness on exertion over the previous 2 months. She also complained of weakness in her legs and tingling in her feet. Her medical history includes Graves' disease and Addison's disease. On examination she is pale, with few positive findings except for loss of distal light touch and joint position sensation in the legs, with absent ankle reflexes and brisk knee reflexes bilaterally. Additional blood tests ordered to try to explain her anaemia are below:

Ferritin: 178 μg/L (normal 10–250)
Iron: 24 μg/L (normal 10–32)
Total iron binding capacity: 32 μg/L (normal 45–82)
Vitamin B_{12}: 47 pg/mL (normal 74–516)
Folate: 18 nmol/L (normal 7–36)
Peripheral blood film: multiple megaloblasts seen

(1) What is the diagnosis?

(2) What is the further management of this patient?

2. A 24-year-old Nigerian man with known sickle cell disease presents to hospital complaining of severe pain in his left hip. The pain had come on over the previous 6 hours and was constant and severe (rated 9/10 in severity by the patient). He had been mildly unwell for the previous 2 days with symptoms consistent with a viral upper respiratory tract infection. His previous medical history includes sickle cell disease, with painful crises roughly every 3 months, and gallstone disease, for which he had a cholecystectomy 2 years before. He has never suffered an acute chest crisis. On examination he is clearly in pain, and is tachycardic (105 bpm); his other observations are within normal ranges. It is noticed that his fingers are of very different lengths. Examination of the chest and abdomen are normal, and although the patient complains of pain in the left hip joint, it is only mildly tender and has a full range of movement. X-ray of his chest and hip are likewise unremarkable. The patient's blood tests are shown below:

Sodium: 143 mmol/L	Haemoglobin: 6.8 g/dL
Potassium: 4.3 mmol/L	MCV: 97 fL
Urea: 5.4 mmol/L	White cells: 5.8 × 10^9/L
Creatinine: 71 μmol/L	Platelets: 480 × 10^9/L
CRP: 4 mg/L	Bilirubin: 31 μmol/L

Blood film: High numbers of reticulocytes are seen (15% of total red cells). Sickle cells are seen. The presence of irregularly contrasted cells and Howell–Jolly bodies is suggestive of hyposplenism.

(1) List the abnormalities and a reason for each.

(2) What is the unifying diagnosis?

(3) List three essential steps in the patient's immediate management.

(4) What long-term medication should patients with this condition be taking?

3. Mr Adam Smith (hospital number 05849352, date of birth 6 November 1960), attends his local Emergency Department after an episode of chest pain and tightness that occurred on climbing a flight of stairs at home. He gives a 6-week history of extreme fatigue and breathlessness, with his exercise tolerance now limited by shortness of breath to 50 m on the flat (previously 800 m). During this period he has also suffered dizzy spells and several episodes of palpitations. His past medical history includes osteoarthritis of his knees and a myocardial infarction 2 years previously with associated heart failure. He is taking regular diclofenac, aspirin, perindopril, and simvastatin.

On examination he is extremely pale but has no lymphadenopathy. Vital signs reveal: respiratory rate 20 breaths/min, HR 108 bpm, BP 128/76 mmHg and oxygen sats 97% on air. Further examination reveals a soft systolic murmur in the aortic area but cardiorespiratory examination is otherwise normal. Routine investigations reveal:

FBC: Hb 4.9 g/dL, MCV 66 fL, WCC 6.9 × 10^9/L (normal differential), platelets 223 × 10^9/L
Blood film: microcytic and hypochromic red cells.

A presumed diagnosis of chronic upper gastrointestinal bleeding is made (secondary to his non-steroidal inflammatory drugs and aspirin), and he is admitted to the Medical Admissions Unit under the care of Dr Sadiq (one of the gastroenterology team), awaiting an endoscopy the following day.

(1) Using a sample fluid chart downloaded from the Online Resource Centre, write up an appropriate blood transfusion schedule for this man.

(2) List the acute and chronic risks of transfusion.

4. A 27-year-old man from Greece is a known to suffer with homozygous beta-thalassaemia (thalassaemia major), and has been receiving transfusions every 6 weeks since the age of 2. A splenectomy was performed at the age of 6, and he takes regular folic acid and penicillin V. The previous year he was diagnosed with type 1 diabetes mellitus and was started on insulin. He is seen in the haematology out-patient clinic where he complains of increasing shortness of breath on exertion over the previous 2 months. On examination he has short stature and appears developmentally immature, with lack of male pattern hair growth, small testis, and smooth, pale skin. His haemoglobin concentration is 6.4 g/L and his mean corpuscular volume is 59 fL (4 weeks after his most recent transfusion). An echocardiogram reveals restrictive cardiomyopathy.

(1) What is the underlying cause of his multiple clinical problems?

(2) What is done to limit this complication?

Blood tests

Comment on

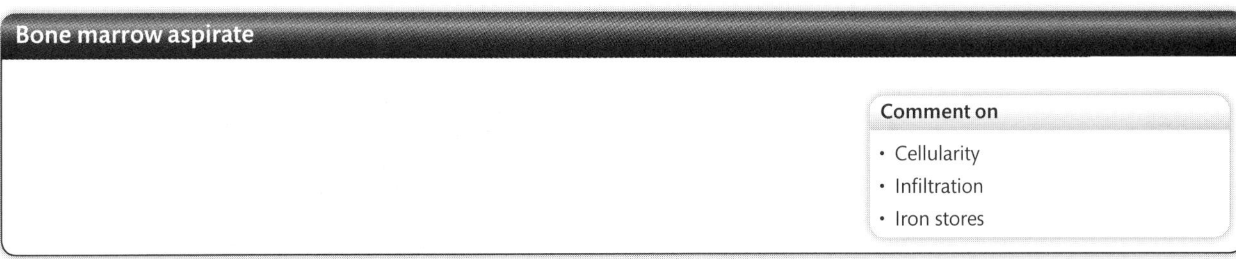

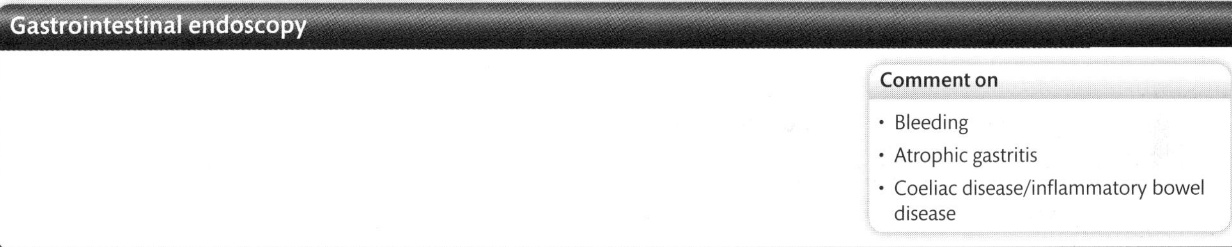

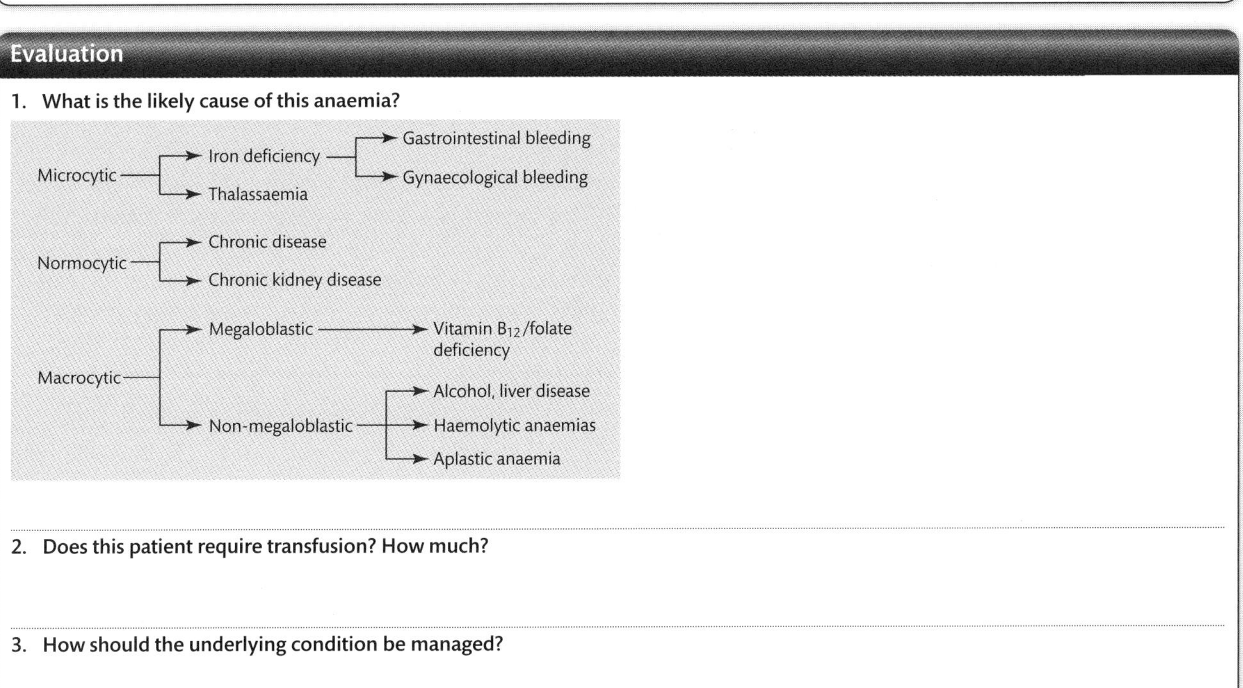

Answers

1. This patient has severe vitamin B_{12} deficiency. Along with folic acid, vitamin B_{12} is an essential B vitamin playing an important role in cellular DNA formation, neuronal myelin synthesis, and erythrocyte production. Moderate to severe deficiency leads to inadequate formation of mature erythrocytes, and central and peripheral neuropathy.

Ineffective erythropoiesis leads to immature red cell precursors, megaloblasts (hence, **megaloblastic anaemia**), being released into the circulation. These lead to an increase in the average size of circulating red cells producing a macrocytosis.

Vitamin B_{12} deficiency also produces subacute combined degeneration (**SACD**) of the spinal cord. This manifests itself over weeks to months as peripheral numbness and tingling, followed by motor weakness, loss or exaggeration of reflexes, and eventually dementia. The early stages of this condition are reversible with vitamin B_{12} supplementation.

Vitamin B_{12} may be lacking in very strictly restricted diets, for instance in vegans. Additionally any cause of intestinal malabsorption can cause vitamin B_{12} deficiency. However, the commonest cause in adults is **pernicious anaemia**, an autoimmune condition (associated with thyroid disease and Addison's disease) where autoantibodies are formed against the parietal cell receptor Intrinsic Factor (IF), (responsible for the uptake of vitamin B_{12} from the gut), or the B_{12}:IF complex itself.

To treat vitamin B_{12} deficiency, supplements are initially given intramuscularly every other day for 1 week; it is then given by intramuscular injection every 3 months for the rest of the patient's life. If folate deficiency is diagnosed it is important to exclude concomitant B_{12} deficiency, as replacing folate without first correcting the low B_{12} levels may precipitate a rapid onset of the neurological complications associated with B_{12} deficiency.

2. Sickle cell disease is caused by a mutation in the gene encoding for the beta-globulin chain of haemoglobin. When the patient is subjected to a stressor, e.g. hypoxia, low temperatures, dehydration, acidosis, or sepsis, this abnormal haemoglobin polymerizes, distorting the shape of red blood cells (into characteristic sickles), which can then occlude small blood vessels leading to tissue ischaemia. This is what causes the characteristic painful crises. Immediate management is with opiate analgesia, intravenous, or oral rehydration, maintaining the normal body temperature, and, where indicated, antibiotics.

'Sickled' red cells have a short half-life, being constantly broken down by the spleen. There is a chronic haemolytic anaemia, with raised reticulocytes as the bone marrow struggles to produce enough red cells to maintain a normal haemoglobin (since reticulocytes are larger than normal red blood cells, the MCV is raised). Sickle cell patients tolerate mild to moderate anaemia very well and do not routinely require transfusion. Most crises are caused by tissue ischaemia and can be treated conservatively as described above. However, there are several major acute and chronic complications associated with this condition, that need medical intervention.

Complication	Causes	Management
Chest crisis	Infection, fat embolism, lung infarction	Oxygen, ventilation, exchange transfusion
Severe anaemia	Splenic sequestration of red cells, parvovirus suppressing bone marrow	Transfusion
Gallstones	Caused by excess bile pigment from haemolysis	Cholecystectomy
Leg ulcers	Skin ischaemia	Dressings, elevation
Hyposplenism	Multiple small splenic infarctions	Penicillin V prophylaxis
Chronic renal failure	Multiple small renal infarctions	Dialysis
Osteomyelitis	Infection in infarcted bone	Antibiotics
Blindness	Proliferative retinopathy	Laser treatment

This man should receive regular folic acid to support his bone marrow, and penicillin prophylaxis against infection.

3. This man has presented with a symptomatic microcytic anaemia. Each unit of blood will raise his haemoglobin by approximately 1 g/L, so three or four units should be given (transfusion is usually only performed when the haemoglobin is less that 8.0 g/L, with the aim of restoring the level up to 8.0–10.0 g/L). If his haemoglobin had dropped due to acute gastrointestinal bleeding then he is likely to be volume depleted, and aggressive fluid resuscitation is indicated (with the first unit of blood going in as fast as possible). However, as this is an insidious presentation, this man is likely to be euvolaemic, and fast fluids, especially with a history of heart failure, may cause pulmonary oedema. An appropriate schedule is shown below, with blood given as slowly as possible and furosemide to prevent volume overload:

Date	Time	Fluid type	Infusion rate	Signature
17/12	10.00	Packed red cells	4 hourly	DR
17/12	14.00	Furosemide 20 mg	Stat	DR
17/12	14.00	Packed red cells	4 hourly	DR
17/12	18.00	Furosemide 20 mg	Stat	DR
17/12	18.00	Packed red cells	4 hourly	DR
17/12	2200	Furosemide 20 mg	Stat	DR
18/12	0800	Packed red cells	4 hourly	DR

Blood transfusion must be carried out with scrupulous attention to detail to ensure that the right patient gets the right blood—that no errors are made in taking blood for cross-matching, in the lab, or in administration of the blood. There are immediate risks of anaphylaxis and death if a patient is given incompatible blood. Non-anaphylactic febrile reaction can occur (to antigens on white cells) if whole blood is given, but this is rare now where only packed red cells are used. Large-volume transfusion can cause problems with fluid overload, hypothermia (blood should be warmed), and coagulopathy (platelets and clotting factors should also be replaced). Infection should now be screened for.

4. Thalassaemia is a relatively common genetic haemoglobinopathy leading to an imbalance in the production of haemoglobin alpha and beta chains. Patients who are homozygous for the condition present a few months after birth with severe failure to thrive. Left untreated they suffer with recurrent infections and bone fractures, as the bone marrow increases in size in order to increase erythropoieisis. Folic acid is given to augment erythropoieisis, and patients are regularly transfused partly to avoid anaemia and partly to suppress erythropoiesis outside bones (for instance in the liver).

One of the consequences of regular transfusion (as in this case) is **iron overload.** This is also seen in hereditary haemochromatosis, a primary disorder of iron metabolism. Excess iron is laid down in the liver (causing cirrhosis), the heart (causing a cardiomyopathy), and in the endocrine organs—especially the pancreas (causing diabetes) and the pituitary (causing hypopituitarism and delayed or abnormal development). Damage caused is often irreversible. Iron overload can be treated with the chelating agent **desferrioxamine** but this is painful when injected and only serves to prevent further damage—it cannot reverse pre-existing injury.

Further reading

Guidelines: Blood Transfusion Service Transfusion Handbook (http://www.transfusionguidelines.org.uk/Index.aspx?Publication=HTM&Section=9&pageid=1129)

OHCM: 318-323, 326-337, 342-343

Haematological malignancies

This section should be used to clerk patients with any of the leukaemias, lymphoma, or myeloma. Management of these conditions is complex and usually directed by specialists and carried out in haematology units or on medical day units. However, the diagnosis of a haematological malignancy is often first made on a General Medical Ward during an acute admission.

Learning challenges

- What are the Philadelphia chromosome and the BCR:abl oncogene, and how do they lead to cancer formation?
- What is a 'pathological fracture'?

History

Comment on

- Symptoms of cell lineage dysfunction/bone marrow failure
  - Red cells—anaemia or polycythaemia
  - White cells—recurrent infections (too few cells or many, dysfunctional cells)
  - Platelets—bleeding and bruising
  - Lymphatic system dysfunction: lymph node enlargement or splenomegaly (abdominal pain and discomfort)
- Bone pain
- Systemic features—weight loss, night sweats, malaise

Examination

Well or unwell? Why?

Feet to face:

Vital signs: Temperature | Blood pressure | Pulse rate | Respiratory rate | O2 saturations

Clinical clues:

Cardiovascular:

1 2 1

Respiratory:

Abdominal:

Neurological:

Other:

Comment on

- Signs of anaemia
- Bruising, petechiae
- Lymphadenopathy—sites and character of the enlargement
- Hepatosplenomegaly
- Bony tenderness

Blood tests

Comment on

- Hb—anaemia/polycythaemia
- WCC—absolute white cell count and differential; leucocytosis/leucopenia; abnormal counts
- Platelets—thrombocytopenia/thrombocytosis
- Anaemia + leucopenia + thrombocytopenia = **pancytopenia**
- CRP
- Renal function
- Plasma immunoglobulins—monoclonal bands
- Serum calcium, LFTs, LDH, ESR

Blood film

Comment on

- Abnormal white cells, e.g. blast cells
- Abnormal numbers of immature cells, e.g. reticulocytes

Bone marrow aspirate

Comment on

- Cellularity
- Abnormal cells

Lymph node biopsy

Comment on

- Malignant cells

Radiology

Comment on

- Lytic lesions
- Pathological fractures

Evaluation

1. **What type of disorder is likely to be responsible for this patient's presentation?**

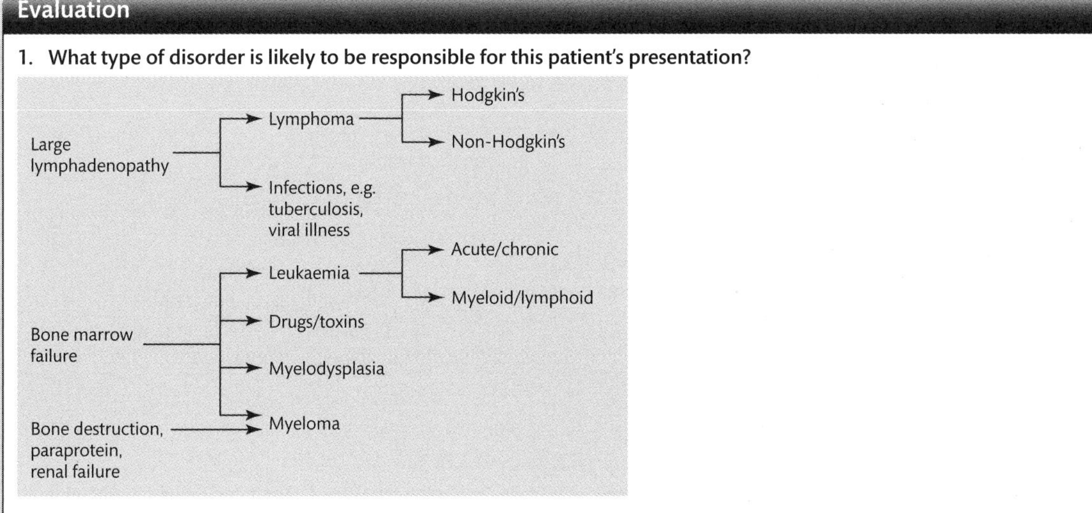

2. **Are there acute issues, e.g. neutropenia or thrombocytopenia, requiring urgent treatment?**

3. **Is chemotherapy appropriate for this patient, and what are their feelings about it?**

4. **What is the likely prognosis?**

Questions

1. A 23-year-old woman is referred to the ear, nose, and throat surgical out-patient clinic after presenting to her doctor complaining of a swelling in her neck. This swelling had grown rapidly over the preceding month, and although unsightly did not cause any pain. She gave a history of occasional fevers and night sweats over this period, and said that she had unexpectedly lost around 5 kg in weight. Examination revealed a smoothly enlarged painless lymph node in the anterior triangle of the neck, measuring 5 cm across. There was no evidence of airway obstruction or dysphagia. There was no other palpable lymphadenopathy but she had 5 cm splenomegaly below the left costal margin on examination of her abdomen. Of note, routine blood tests revealed:

- FBC: Hb 14.9 g/dL, MCV 88 fL, WCC 9.5 × 10^9/L (normal differential), platelets 209 × 10^9/L
- ESR: 123 mm in the first hour.

Her chest X-ray is shown below.

(1) What does the chest X-ray demonstrate? What is the likely cause in this patient?

(2) Her lymph node biopsy reveals Reed–Sternberg cells. What are these cells and what conditions are they seen in?

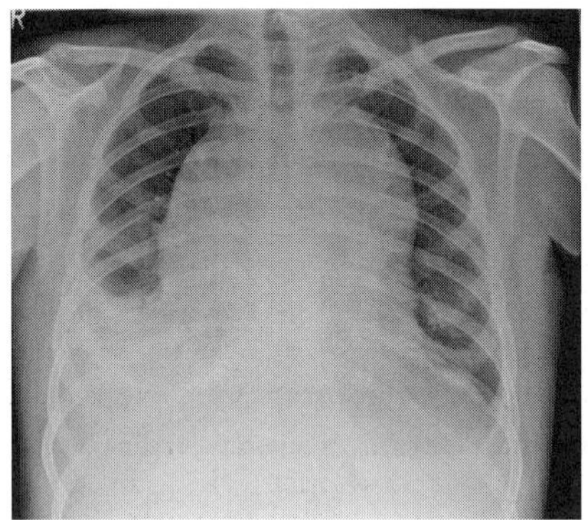

2. A 57-year-old woman presents to her GP with a 2-month history of feeling tired and fatigued: 'I'm just washed out, with no energy doctor'. She has also noticed a vague sensation of fullness in her abdomen which she describes as a discomfort but not actually painful. Examination revealed a grossly enlarged spleen with no associated signs of liver disease or lymphadenopathy. Her full blood count is shown below:

- Hb: 10.8 g/dL (normal 11–16 g/dL)
- White cells: 70.8 × 10^9/L ((4–11) × 10^9/L)
  - Neutrophils: 68% (40–60%)
  - Lymphocytes: 5% (20–40%)
  - Monocytes: 0.5% (2–8%)
  - Eosinophils: 18% (1–4%)
  - Basophils: 11% (0.5–1%)
- Platelets: 132 × 10^9/L (150–400 × 10^9/L)

(1) List five causes of a moderate to grossly enlarged spleen.

(2) What is the likely underlying cause in this patient?

(3) What factors determine the prognosis of this condition?

3. A 44-year-old woman is receiving chemotherapy for acute myeloid leukaemia (AML). Her last cycle of therapy was 11 days ago. She now presents to her local Emergency Department feeling unwell, having suffered fevers and rigors for the past 12-hours. She has a slight cough and sore throat but no other systemic symptoms. Physical examination reveals: temperature 38.9°C, heart rate 105 bpm, blood pressure 105/67 mmHg. There are no localizing signs of infection. Of note there is no lymphadenopathy, hepatosplenomegaly, anaemia, or bruising. Her FBC is: Hb 9.4 g/dL, MCV 87 fL, WCC 1.9 × 10^9/L (neutrophils 0.1 × 10^9/L), platelets 79 × 10^9/L.

(1) What does the full blood count demonstrate? Which abnormality is the most concerning?

(2) What is the likely underlying diagnosis?

(3) List five three essential management steps in this case.

4. A 62-year-old woman is admitted to hospital after falling and suffering a mid-shaft fracture of the left femur, requiring internal fixation. The orthopaedic surgery team request that the patient is reviewed by the on-call medical team because they are concerned that the fracture was 'pathological' (the radiograph shows large lytic lesion through which the fracture has occurred).

Reviewing the patient, she complains of feeling generally 'run down' and being tired for several months before her admission. Physical examination is unremarkable except for the presence of the fracture.

Routine pre-operative investigations reveal:

- FBC: Hb 7.6 g/dL, MCV 112 fL, WCC 3.1 × 10^9/L (neutrophils 2.8 × 10^9/L), platelets 81 × 10^9/L
- U&Es: Na^+ 146 mmol/L, K^+ 4.2 mmol/L, urea 12.6 mmol/L, creatinine 134 μmol/L
- ESR: 116 mm in first hour
- Corrected calcium: 3.56 mmol/L
- ECG: Normal sinus rhythm

(1) What is the likely unifying diagnosis?

(2) List three further diagnostic investigations for this patient.

Presentation

Presented to ______ Grade ______ Date ______

Signed

Remember that you can find large-size, annotated versions of many of the X-rays and ECGs that appear in this book on the book's web site at www.oxfordtextbooks.co.uk/orc/randall/

Answers

1. This chest X-ray reveals evidence of gross mediastinal lymphadenopathy (there is also a right-sided pleural effusion). Together with cervical lymphadenopathy and splenomegaly the most likely diagnosis is lymphoma; less likely diagnoses include infections (such as infective mononucleosis or tuberculosis), other haematological malignancies (such as acute leukaemias), and secondary cancers. A definitive diagnosis as in this case is made through a lymph node biopsy of one of the enlarged neck lymph nodes. Sternberg-Reed cells are giant, abnormal lymphocytes (usually B-cell derived) with characteristic bilobed nuclei, or multinucleated cells. They are characteristic (but not pathognomonic) of Hodgkin's lymphoma, also being found in infections such as EBV and occasionally in non-Hodgkin's disease.

The lymphomas are cancers of lymphocytes which may present primarily with lymphadenopathy, or in other sites containing lymphoid tissue such as the brain, the eye, or the stomach. The classification of lymphomas is extremely complex, but they are divided on histological grounds into **Hodgkin's** and **non-Hodgkin's** disease. Generally, the prognosis depends on the speed of growth: high-grade tumour divide and spread rapidly but tend to be far more chemosensitive, and therefore have a better prognosis, than slower-growing, less aggressive tumours.

2. Mild to moderate splenomegaly has a number of causes, including infection (e.g. malaria or bacterial endocarditis), inflammatory diseases (e.g. rheumatoid arthritis or sarcoidosis), portal hypertension (e.g. secondary to liver cirrhosis), or other rarer conditions such as amyloidosis. **Massive**, or **giant splenomegaly** has five classical causes listed below:

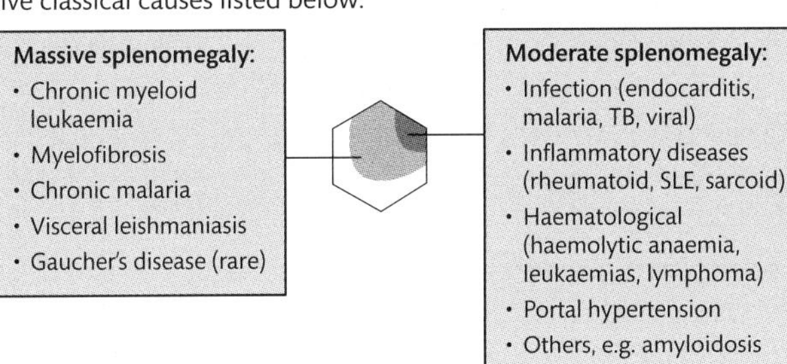

This woman's massive splenomegaly, in the presence of extremely high white cell counts (>30 × 10^9/L) raise the possibility of a haematological malignancy, especially in the absence of other causes of leucocytosis, such as acute sepsis. This woman has raised levels of neutrophils, eosinophils, and basophils—all granulocytes, of myeloid lineage. The diagnosis here is likely to be **chronic myeloid leukaemia**, which is often an incidental diagnosis in asymptomatic individuals. The mild anaemia and thrombocytopenia are likely to be as a result of bone marrow infiltration. The diagnosis can be confirmed on the basis of bone marrow biopsy, with cells testing positive for the **BCR:abl oncogene** associated with the **Philadelphia chromosome**.

Chronic myeloid leukaemia begins insidiously with a chronic phase lasting for several years. It then transforms into a more aggressive acute phase, with increasing symptoms and death within a few months without treatment. The prognosis of CML has been transformed recently by the new antibody drug imatinib, which offers the real possibility of a complete cure.

3. The most concerning abnormality here is the very low neutrophil count, contributing to a low overall white cell count. Neutrophils are the mainstay of the body's defence against bacterial infection and so neutropenia renders a patient susceptible to overwhelming sepsis.

This lady has **neutropenic sepsis**, which is a medical emergency. Left untreated she could die of bacterial sepsis and multiorgan failure. After blood, urine, stool, and sputum cultures are taken, she needs rapid treatment with broad-spectrum antibiotics, e.g. piperacillin and vancomycin. **Neutropenia** often occurs 10–14 days after a course of chemotherapy, in a predictable and dose-dependent way. The bone marrow recovers after a few days. If the patient remains septic on antibiotics then other organisms should be considered, for instance atypical pathogens (like mycoplasma or fungi).

Chemotherapy is generally poorly selective, and works by attacking any rapidly dividing cells. Hence common side-effects include hair loss (hair follicle cells affected), gastrointestinal symptoms (bowel mucosa affected), and bone marrow suppression. Because of the relatively long half-life of red cells and platelets, the most profound effects are seen on white cells, and especially neutrophils. The use of **granulocyte colony-stimulating factor (GCSF)** may lead to a reduction in recurrent cases of neutropenia in such patients.

4. The most likely diagnosis here is multiple myeloma. This is a malignancy of plasma cells: B-lymphocytes are located in the bone marrow and which provide immunological memory of previous infections. Clinical features of the disease arise predominantly from several parallel processes:

- **Bony destruction**, causing bone pain, pathological fractures of long bones or crush fractures of vertebrae, and raised serum calcium. Myeloma should be suspected in any middle-aged or older person presenting with new onset lower back pain.
- **Paraproteinaemia**: The clonal expansion of plasma cells leads to production of large amounts of antibody (immunoglobulin), shown on plasma electrophoresis. Typically, one line of immunoglobulin is present in excess, whilst other lines are suppressed: in the example below, gamma globulins are present in excess—a class which includes many immunoglobulins. Alongside albumin, the alpha and beta globulin peaks on this diagram include other serum proteins such as lipoproteins, transferrin, and complement.

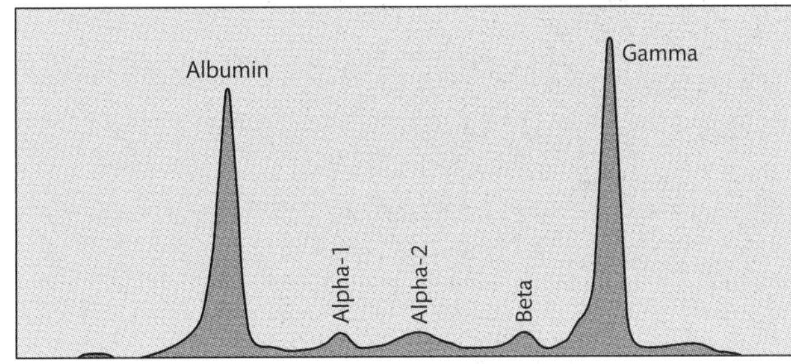

- **Bone marrow infiltration**: This causes suppression of all bone marrow progenitor cells, causing pancytopenia.
- **Renal impairment**: This has a variety of causes, known collectively as '**myeloma kidney**'; the five causes are immune-mediated glomerulonephritis, obstruction of the tubules by light chains, nephrocalcinosis (due to hypercalcaemia), UTIs and dehydration, and secondary amyloidosis.

Myeloma is incurable; however, a phase or remission called the 'plateau phase' can be induced with chemotherapy and maintained with thalidomide, prolonging mean survival by several years.

In this patient, investigations would include:

- a series of X-rays of the whole skeleton (the 'skeletal survey'), looking for evidence of **lytic lesions** where bone destruction has been caused by plasma cell expansion
- urine analysis for free antibody light chains (**Bence-Jones protein**)
- plasma electrophoresis to look for paraprotein bands.

Further reading

Guidelines: British Committee for Standards in Haematology guidelines on the investigation of lymphoma (http://www.bcshguidelines.com/pdf/draft_Lymphoma_main_042010.pdf)

OHCM: 346–365

HIV and AIDS

This section should be used to clerk patients admitted to hospital with HIV-related disease, who may be found on a General Medical Ward or specialist HIV unit. HIV should be considered as one of the differential diagnoses in patients who present with an unusual or atypical infection, or complex multisystem problems, regardless of whether they are perceived to be high risk for transmission.

Learning challenges

- Why has the prevention of HIV transmission become so controversial? What evidence exists for different proposed strategies?
- Why has development of a vaccine against the HIV virus proved so difficult?

History

Comment on

- History of presenting complaint
- Full sexual history
- Travel history
- Blood transfusions, intravenous drug use
- Previous antiretroviral treatment
- Pregnancy

Examination

Well or unwell? Why?

Feet to face:

Vital signs: Temperature Blood pressure Pulse rate Respiratory rate O2 saturations

Clinical clues:

Cardiovascular:

1 2 1

Respiratory:

Abdominal:

Neurological:

Other:

Comment on

- Cachexia, lipodystrophy
- Skin lesions and rashes
- Oral ulceration, candidiasis, and oral hairy leucoplakia
- Lymphadenopathy, including epitrochlear nodes
- Examination of all systems
- Oxygen desaturation on exercise

Blood tests

Comment on

- FBC, U&Es, LFTs
- HIV1 and -2 antibodies
- CD4 count
- HIV viral load
- Markers of infection

Microbiology

Comment on

- Viral hepatitis screen
- CMV antibody
- Toxoplasmosis serology
- Syphilis serology
- Test for other sexually transmitted infections

Chest X-ray

Comment on

- In classical **Pneumocystis** *carinii* (now called **P. jiroveci**) ***pneumonia*** you 'hear nothing–see nothing'; i.e. the patient looks very unwell but there is little or nothing to hear on auscultation of the chest, and little or nothing to see on the chest X-ray
- Bilateral hilar lymphadenopathy
- Evidence of TB
- Bilateral interstitial shadowing

CT scanning

Comment on

- Space-occupying lesions in the head
- Lymphadenopathy
- Collections/neoplasms elsewhere in body

Evaluation

1. **Does this patient have HIV? How might they have contracted it?**

2. **Where are they in the natural course of infection?**

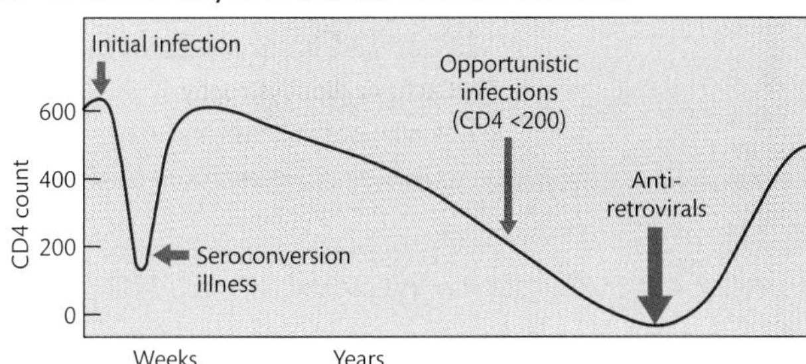

3. **Is there evidence of opportunistic infection or cancer?**

4. **Is there evidence of HIV-associated organ damage?**

5. **Should antiretroviral drugs be considered in the patient at the current time?**

Questions

1. A 34-year-old man from Zimbabwe attends his GP complaining of a 6-week history of persistent watery diarrhoea. During this period he has felt generally unwell, with nausea, vomiting, and anorexia. He has had mild general abdominal pain. He was previously well, with no known medical conditions. Examination revealed a thin man with no obvious lymphadenopathy or signs of dehydration. He was apyrexial and basic observations were within normal ranges. The abdomen was slightly tender on palpation but was soft with no guarding or rebound tenderness. A stool sample was sent for microbiological investigation which revealed cysts of *Cryptosporidium parvum*, a protozoan parasite which can cause short-lived self-limiting diarrhoea in normal individuals but more prolonged symptoms in the immunocompromised.

(1) List the important steps in the discussion the GP should have with the patient regarding the diagnosis, the likely underlying cause, and how consent may be obtained for HIV testing.

(2) Why might this patient be reluctant to be tested?

2. A 52-year-old man who has sex with men, and is known to be HIV positive, is brought into the Emergency Department after having suffered a seizure. He has never before required antiretroviral medication, but has failed to attend his previous two out-patient clinic appointments. His partner, who is with him, reports that for several days the patient has complained of feeling feverish and unwell, and has also been unusually clumsy around the house. Today whilst eating dinner he lost consciousness and began to convulse, with shaking in all limbs, tongue biting, and urinary incontinence. There was no history of epilepsy or any other medical condition, and the patient had never suffered seizures before. On examination the patient was very drowsy and difficult to rouse making formal neurological assessment difficult. An urgent CT scan was booked, a frame from which is shown below after intravenous contrast was given.

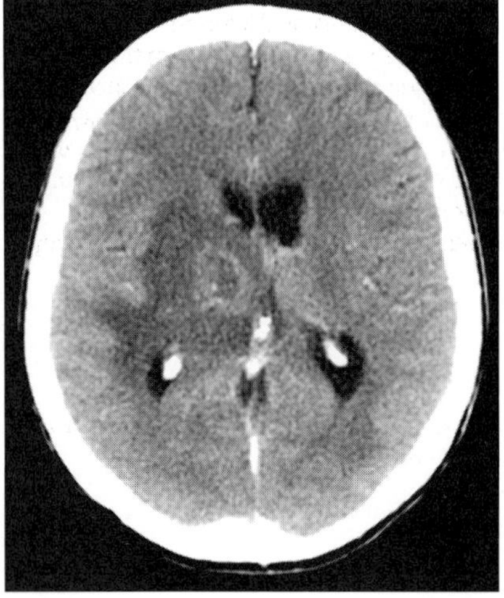

(1) What does the scan show?

(2) List the differential diagnosis of these appearances.

3. A 44-year-old man who is HIV positive presents to his GP complaining of extensive small purplish lumps over his lower left leg, as well as bleeding in his mouth. These lesions had developed over the previous 4 weeks, and the patient had initially put them down to bruising, though there was no history of trauma. The patient is on antiretroviral drugs and his last CD4 count, 2 weeks earlier, was 188 cells/μL. Examination revealed multiple small purplish non-tender papules and plaques which are well demarcated and distributed over the left leg below the knee, where there is also some pitting oedema. Several similar plaques with evidence of recent bleeding were noted inside the mouth on the hard palate.

(1) What are the lesions described?

(2) Describe the further investigation and management of this patient.

4. A 33-year-old man from Russia presents to hospital with a 2-week history of fever, dry cough, and breathlessness, especially on exertion. There is no chest pain. He is otherwise well with no known medical problems. On examination, he was pyrexial (temperature 39.7°C) with saturations of 95% on air. Examination of the chest was unremarkable. After being asked to walk up and down in the department he became very breathless, and his post-exercise oxygen saturations were recorded at 88%. Initial investigations revealed raised inflammatory markers, and a chest X-ray which is shown below. Based on the appearance of the chest X-ray he had an urgent HIV test which was positive, and his CD4 count was revealed to be 156 cells/μL.

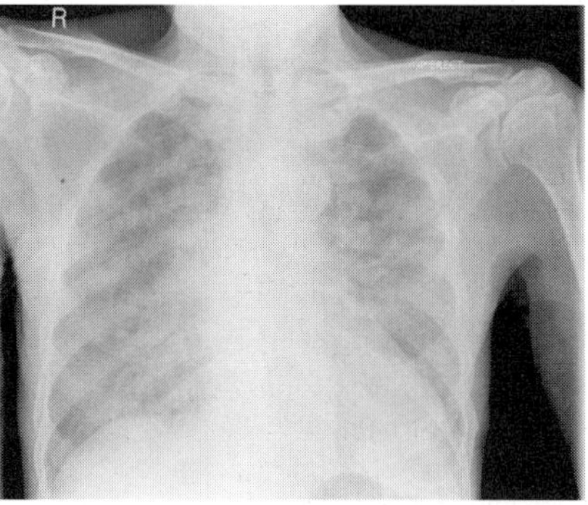

(1) What does the image of the chest show?

(2) What is the likely diagnosis?

(3) Describe the further management.

5. A nurse treating a hospital in-patient accidentally stabs herself with a needle, and presents to the hospital Emergency Department very worried about developing HIV infection. How might the doctor seeing her decide on whether or not she should receive post-exposure prophylaxis to prevent this?

Presentation

Presented to		Grade		Date	
Signed					

Remember that you can find large-size, annotated versions of many of the X-rays and ECGs that appear in this book on the book's web site at www.oxfordtextbooks.co.uk/orc/randall/

Answers

1. Despite many public health campaigns to increase awareness about HIV disease, its transmission, and prognosis, there is still considerable fear and prejudice around being HIV positive. This stigma stems partly from its association with sexual behaviours and partly because of fear about it being untreatable and rapidly fatal (as it was before the advent of antiretroviral drugs).

In the context of traditional African cultural beliefs, this stigma may be heightened. AIDS may be seen not as caused by a viral infection but rather as a punishment from God for sin or as a curse from evil spiritual forces. There is a tragically widespread belief in sub-Saharan Africa that HIV can be cured by having unprotected sex with a virgin.

The doctor treating this patient needs to proceed very carefully. The likelihood that this man is HIV positive is high, and confirming the diagnosis would allow his immune status to be monitored and antiretroviral drugs to be commenced as necessary. He should be told about the possibility of HIV infection, and asked about his understanding of the disease. He should be told about the benefit of being tested, and the dangers of undiagnosed HIV infection. He should also be told that whilst not being curable, with modern drugs HIV infection now generally has a good prognosis and a life expectancy similar to that of the uninfected population. He should be reassured that the results of the tests will be completely anonymous. Hopefully he will give consent to testing and then if positive can be managed by a secondary care sexual health physician.

2. This CT scan reveals:

This CT scan reveals what is described in radiology as a 'ring enhancing lesion' – an abnormality with increased contrast uptake around its periphery. This has acted as a focus of epileptiform activity and triggered the patient's seizure.

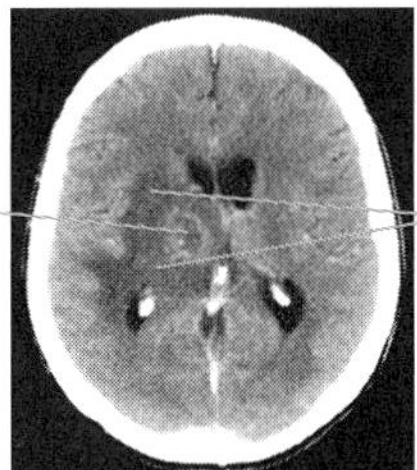

The scan also reveals evidence of vasogenic cerebral oedema surrounding the mass – seen here as a darker area which is producing a mass effect on neighbouring brain tissue with midline shift and some effacement of the ventricles. This can also be seen around malignant brain tumours and may be reduced by oral steroids such as dexamethasone.

The most likely diagnosis is toxoplasmosis, with other possibilities including tuberculosis, central nervous system lymphoma, and focal cryptococcal infection. Further investigations include CD4 count, *Toxoplasma* serology, lumbar puncture with CSF analysis, and MRI to better characterize the lesions. If the diagnosis remains unclear then brain biopsy is indicated.

All of these possible differential diagnoses are AIDS-defining illnesses in the presence of HIV infection. AIDS-defining illnesses include general opportunistic infections and cancers. The different infections commonly occur at different levels of CD4 cell depletion (see the table below). *Toxoplasma* is a protozoan parasite which is excreted from its definitive host, the cat, in faeces. The seroprevalence of the condition ranges widely between different countries from 25–80%. After an initial infection, which is often subclinical, it can reactivate in the presence of immunosuppression and produce focal brain lesions, chorioretinitis, and severe fetal damage in pregnant women.

CD4 count	Common opportunistic infections
200–300	Protozoal diarrhoeal infections, candida
100–200	Tuberculosis, pneumocystisis, toxoplasmosis
50–100	Atypical mycobacteria
<50	Cytomegalovirus causing colitis and retinitis

3. This description is characteristic of Kaposi's sarcoma, a cancer of the vascular epithelium with very rare sporadic incidence but which is common in those living with HIV. It can cause skin, gastrointestinal, and respiratory lesions, which can bleed or ulcerate producing a wide range of symptoms and signs. It often responds well to chemotherapy.

Kaposi's sarcoma is caused by human herpesvirus 8. There are a number of malignancies associated with HIV infection which share a viral aetiology, including non-Hodgkin's lymphoma (Epstein-Barr virus) and invasive cervical and anal squamous cell carcinoma (human papilloma virus).

4. This X-ray shows bilateral perihilar hazy shadowing:

A classic feature of pneumocystis pneumonia is that patients appear far more ill than would be suggested by their chest x-ray. However, if you look closely here there is bilateral ground glass shadowing diffusely within the lung fields, but centered on the hila.

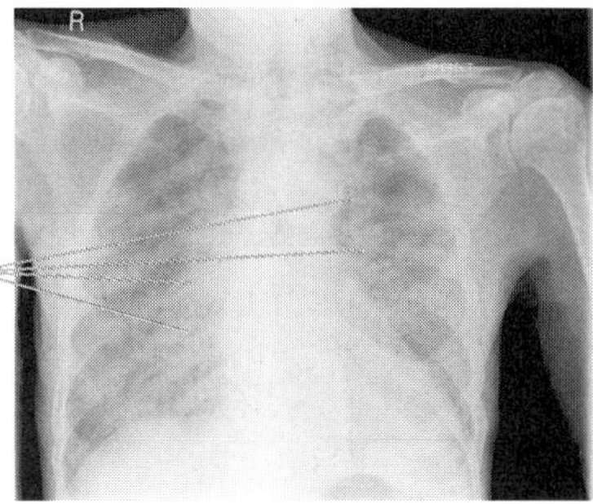

With clinical evidence of pneumonia and the classic sign of exertional desaturation, the most likely diagnosis is *Pneumocystis jiroveci* pneumonia (formerly *P. carinii* pneumonia or PCP). This is a fungal lung infection, the commonest opportunistic infection associated with HIV, and is an AIDS-defining illness. The nature of the X-ray shadowing can be confirmed by a chest CT scan, and the diagnosis confirmed by bronchoalveolar lavage and cytology. Treatment is with high-dose co-trimoxazole, with oral corticosteroids if infection is severe.

Other HIV-associated lung diseases include tuberculosis, atypical mycobacterial infection (such as *Mycobacterium avium intracellulare*), aspergillosis, or pulmonary Kaposi's sarcoma.

5. Antiretrovirals are very unpleasant to take, and so post-exposure prophylaxis (PEP) is only offered if there is a significant risk of HIV infection after a needlestick injury. A risk assessment should be carried out, based on the likelihood of the patient having HIV or other blood-borne viruses (according to their known risk factors), and the nature on the injury (injuries with significant penetration by a hollow needle increase the chance of transmission; gloves decrease the chance). Blood should be taken from both the patient and the healthcare worker for urgent HIV testing. The situation is complicated by the 'window period' for seroconversion: it can take up to 3 months before the HIV test becomes positive in an individual infected with HIV. If the initial test from the patient is negative, and the chance of them having recently acquired HIV is low, then a decision not to commence PEP may be taken. However, if there is a chance that the patient may have recently developed HIV then PEP should be continued for several months until the healthcare worker is definitively tested. The chances of developing a needlestick injury (or splash injury) are greatly reduced by following universal precautions when dealing with body fluids.

Further reading

Guidelines: British HIV Association guidelines on HIV testing (http://www.bhiva.org/HIVTesting2008.aspx)

OHCM: 408–415

Skin ulcers

This section should be used to clerk patients presenting with ulcers—either in primary care or (if the ulcers are severe or there are complicating factors such as cellulitis) in hospital. Patients with ulcers can be found on any wards, but especially on diabetic, elderly care, and vascular surgery wards.

Learning challenges

- What causes of chronic venous disease and what can be done to improve its symptoms?
- What are the indications for the following type of ulcer dressings: dry dressings, iodine-soaked dressings, liquid paraffin dressings, and alginate dressings?

History

Comment on

- Onset and duration of symptoms
- Changes in ulcer—size, pain, bleeding, surrounding tissues
- Symptoms of PVD including claudication or rest pain
- Symptoms of rheumatological disease—arthralgia, eye problems, rashes
- Venous disease, including previous DVT and varicose veins
- Trauma
- Other risks—sickle cell disease (where appropriate), diabetes mellitus, rheumatological diseases
- Systemic sepsis—fevers, rigors

Examination

Well or unwell? Why?

Feet to face:

Vital signs: Temperature | Blood pressure | Pulse rate | Respiratory rate | O2 saturations

Clinical clues:

Cardiovascular:

1 2 1

Respiratory:

CBG

Abdominal:

Neurological:

Other:

Comment on

- Vitals—temperature, HR, BP, CBG
- Ulcer: size, shape, location, base, edges, exudate
- Description of surrounding skin—evidence of cellulitis
- Peripheral pulses
- Evidence of venous disease—varicose veins, chronic venous changes
- Peripheral sensation
- Inguinal masses/lymphadenopathy

Blood tests

Comment on

- Inflammatory markers
- Blood glucose
- Renal function
- Albumin
- Vasculitic screen
- Blood cultures

X-ray

Comment on

- Evidence of underlying osteomyelitis

Ankle:brachial pressure index (ABPI)

(ratio of ankle:arm blood pressures)

Doppler ultrasound

Comment on

- Deep vein thrombosis

Blood cultures and wound swab

Comment on

- Causative organism

Evaluation

1. **Is there evidence of systemic sepsis? How should the patient be resuscitated? Are antibiotics indicated?**

2. **What is the likely aetiology of the ulcer? What specific management is indicated?**

Type of ulcer	Clinical evidence	Specific management
Venous ulcer	Varicose veins, haemosiderin deposition, lipodermatosclerosis, venous eczema	Compression bandaging, elevation
Arterial ulcer	Decreased pulses, decreased ABPI	Dressings, revascularization
Pressure ulcer	Over heels or sacrum, immobility, malnutrition, institutionalization	Turning regimes, pressure-relieving mattresses, cushions
Neuropathic ulcer	Over areas of trauma, reduced sensation, diabetes	Foot care, well-fitting shoes, cleaning and dressing ulcer
Vasculitic ulcer	Non-blanching rash, raised inflammatory markers, systemic disease, autoantibodies	Treatment of underlying disease, e.g. steroids

3. **Is a skin biopsy required to make a diagnosis?**

4. **Should this patient see the tissue viability nurse/dermatologist/plastic surgeon?**

5. **What dressings and subsequent wound care are appropriate? Can this be arranged outside hospital?**

Questions

1. An 89-year-old woman is brought to the hospital's Emergency Department after developing community-acquired pneumonia at the nursing home where she lives. She is admitted to hospital for intravenous fluids and antibiotics. On admission the nursing home staff report that she has a pressure ulcer over her sacrum which has been dressed for several months by the district nurse who visits every other day. On examination it is 5 cm × 3 cm in size, and extends through the superficial tissue layers to the deep tissues below. No bone is visible. The base of the ulcer appears to be clean and granulating, with no exudates, slough, or surrounding erythema. Two days after admission the patient seems to have responded well to fluids and antibiotics, and is apyrexial and haemodynamically stable. Wound swabs taken from the ulcer sent for culture and sensitivities are reported as growing methicillin-resistant *Staphylococcus aureus* (MRSA), which also grows from routine swabs taken from the patient's nose and perineum.

(1) What is the grade of this pressure ulcer?

(2) List the generic steps in managing a patient with a sacral pressure ulcer.

(3) What is the difference between colonization and infection?

(4) How does the new discovery of MRSA affect the further management of this patient?

2. A 79-year-old woman has suffered with chronically swollen legs for a number of years. She is brought to hospital by ambulance after her daughter visited her at home and found her drowsy and confused. Her daughter reports that she is allergic to penicillin, having suffered a severe rash when given it for a chest infection many years ago. On examination basic observations reveal a temperature of 38.2°C, heart rate of 114 bpm, blood pressure of 104/60 mmHg, a respiratory rate of 24 breaths/min, and oxygen saturations of 98% on room air. Examination of the chest and abdomen is unremarkable. Both legs are very swollen, with an 'inverted champagne bottle' shape. The skin is thickened and tough, with a brownish tinge and small white scarred areas. There is an 8 cm × 4 cm area of superficial ulceration overlying and superior to the medial malleolus of the left ankle, producing a smelly yellowish-green sloughy exudate. The skin surrounding the ulcer appears red, tense, and shiny. Initial investigations are shown below:

Sodium: 136 mmol/L	Haemoglobin: 13.4 g/dL
Potassium: 5.5 mmol/L	White cells: 14.4 × 10^9/L
Urea: 15.1 mmol/L	Platelets: 451 × 10^9/L
Creatinine: 136 μmol/L	
Lactate: 4.4 mmol/L	
CRP: 280 mg/L	

(1) What do the FBC, U&Es, and other test results suggest?

(2) How do the examination findings suggest a likely underlying diagnosis?

(3) List the essential steps in the short- and long-term management of this patient.

3. An 80-year-old man with type 2 diabetes mellitus is reviewed by a community podiatrist. The patient is unaware of any problems with his feet, and feels he is generally in good health. On inspection the podiatrist notices a small area of ulceration on the plantar aspect of the foot overlying the first and second metatarsophalangeal joints of the right foot. The ulcer appears punched out with clear edges and a pink, granulating base. A small sinus is found into which a sterile swab can be inserted to a depth of 1.5 cm. The underlying bone is easily felt with the tip of the swab. A small amount of cream-coloured pus exits the wound after this probing. The patient is referred to hospital where blood tests reveal mildly elevated inflammatory markers (CRP 25 mg/L, white cells 11.1 × 10^9/L), and a plain X-ray of the foot is suggestive of chronic osteomyelitis.

List three essential therapeutic interventions in this patient.

4. A fit and well 86-year-old man with no chronic medical problems presents to his GP to complain about an area of ulceration on his forehead. Several months before he noticed a skin-coloured lump on the right side of his forehead that slowly grew in size. A week ago the skin overlying it broke down and has formed an unsightly ulcer. On examination there is a circular lesion 2 cm across on the patient's forehead, with central ulceration. There is no pus, exudate, or surrounding cellulitis. The edges of the ulcer appear 'rolled'—flesh-coloured ridges surrounding the central ulceration. The lesion is painless of touch. The doctor reviewing the patient arranged an urgent out-patient appointment with the hospital dermatologist who reviewed the patient and arranged for an excision-biopsy.

(1) List the 'sinister' features of the ulcer that made the GP refer this patient so urgently.

(2) What is the likely diagnosis?

5. A 44-year-old woman is referred to the hospital's Emergency Department urgently because of a rash and fever, suggesting she may need intravenous antibiotics. Both have developed over the previous 2 days. She does not have a headache but complains of vague joint aches, and reports having recently suffered an upper respiratory tract infection. She has no previous medical history and takes no medications. On examination she is alert and well oriented, with pyrexia (temperature 38.1°C), but is otherwise haemodynamically stable. There are irregular purple slightly raised lesions measuring between 5 and 10 mm in diameter over her lower legs and feet which are non-painful and which do not blanch when pressed. They look like small purple bruises. Several have begun to ulcerate forming dry erosions with no surrounding erythema.

(1) What name is given to this kind of rash?

(2) Why did the doctor who initially saw this patient refer her urgently for intravenous antibiotics?

(3) What is the differential diagnosis for this kind of rash and how should this woman be investigated?

Presentation

Presented to ______ Grade ______ Date ______

Signed

Answers

1. Pressure ulcers are a major problem in the immobile elderly, being caused by ischaemic necrosis over areas where pressure between bony prominences and the bed or chair does not allow adequate blood flow to skin and underlying tissues. The grading system below allows their severity to be assessed:

Grade 1	Non-blanching erythema of intact skin. In patients with dark skin, warmth, oedema, or hardness of the skin may be indicators
Grade 2	A blister or abrasion, with loss of epidermis or dermis only
Grade 3	Full-thickness skin loss and damage to subcutaneous tissues. Underlying fascia not breached
Grade 4	Extensive destruction with damage to bone, muscle, and other deep structures

Management of pressure ulcers is essentially based around good nursing, with regular turning, cleaning and dressing of ulcers, and attention paid to urinary and faecal incontinence. Patients entering hospital should be assessed for the probability that they will develop pressure ulcers based on risk factors. Scoring systems such as the **Waterlow score** use factors such as immobility, frailty, hypoalbuminaemia, and steroid use to predict the chances of developing a pressure ulcer. Patients at high risk should have a pressure-relieving mattress.

There is a big difference between colonization and infection with MRSA:

Colonization: Presence of MRSA in or on tissue with no symptoms or evidence of tissue damage. Does not warrant treatment.

Infection: Presence of MRSA in or on tissues with evidence of disease: pain, inflammation, fever, raised inflammatory markers. Should be treated with antibiotics.

This patient may be heavily colonized—including at the ulcer site—but not be clinically infected. This patient should not be treated for MRSA infection with antibiotics. As far as possible she should be isolated (for instance in a ward side-room) and barrier nursing should be employed to prevent transmission of MRSA to other patients. A decontamination regime involving topical antiseptic agents (for instance chlorhexidine body wash and nasal spray) can be used to eradicate MRSA carried asymptomatically.

2. This woman has systemic sepsis as a result of cellulitis surrounding her ulcer. The high lactate is a marker of anaerobic respiration and proves that her blood pressure is inadequate to fully oxygenate her tissues. She requires management with fluid resuscitation and intravenous antibiotics. The antibiotic combination of choice would be flucloxacillin and benzyl penicillin, but in the presence of penicillin allergy, alternatives such as vancomycin or clindamycin (see also local antibiotic policies) should be used.

Her ulcer is likely to be due to chronic venous insufficiency. Valves on the perforating veins draining superficial veins into the deep venous system fail, so blood pools in the subcutaneous tissues. Chronic venous hypertension produces extravasation of fluid and deposition of haemosiderin, giving skin a characteristic thickened, pigmented appearance, known as **lipodermatosclerosis**. The 'inverted champagne bottle' shape of this woman's lower leg is characteristic of chronic venous insufficiency.

Once the sepsis is treated management will involve **compression bandaging** (as long as there is no evidence of peripheral arterial disease) and **elevation of the lower limbs** when in bed or relaxing at home. Together the measures improve venous return in the legs, decreasing venous pressures and allowing the ulcer to heal. Around 80% will heal within 6 months, after which long-term pressure stockings should be worn to prevent recurrence.

3. Management of chronic osteomyelitis is based around long courses of antibiotics (to cover pathogens including staphylococci, streptococci, and anaerobes) along with possible debridement of infected bone by an orthopaedic surgeon. Deep-seated bony infections can prove extremely difficult to treat, especially in diabetics where the vascular supply to the foot may be compromised. In severe cases amputation may be required.

The two commonest aetiologies for foot ulcers in diabetics are arterial disease and peripheral sensory neuropathy. This patient's pulses and ankle:brachial pressure index should be assessed, with referral to a vascular surgeon if blood supply to the foot is limited (since this will prevent healing). It is likely that there is a degree of neuropathy present in this patient since he was unaware that the ulcer had developed, and since the ulcer has developed over a pressure area—this could be confirmed by assessing light touch, joint position sense, and vibration sensation in the feet. Providing this patient with well-fitting shoes can reduce pressure over these bony areas and reduce ulcer formation.

4. Unusual ulcers require further explanation. Sinister features of skin lesions that require urgent dermatological assessment include:

- **A**symmetry
- **B**order irregularities—jagged or ill-defined edges
- **C**olour irregularities—such a lesion containing white, brown and black areas
- **D**iameter—lesions >7 mm in diameter require investigation
- **E**volution—any rapidly changing lesions require rapid assessment

In the case of this patient, the likely diagnosis based on the description offered is a basal cell carcinoma (or 'rodent ulcer'), one of the commonest forms of skin cancer which hardly ever metastasizes and which is readily curable by excision.

In the absence of clear evidence of trauma, arterial insufficiency, venous hypertension, or pressure necrosis, ulcers require an alternative explanation. Certain well-described patterns of ulceration may suggest the presence of another systemic disease. **Pyoderma gangrenosum**, large gangrenous ulcers which form rapidly in otherwise normal skin, may be linked to inflammatory bowel disease or liver disease; **erythema nodosum**, painful bruising and ulceration over the shins, may be linked to streptococcus infection, tuberculosis, or sarcoidosis; and **erythema multiforme**, the combination of concentric ring lesions on the arms with oral ulceration, may be linked to herpes simplex infection or various drugs.

5. This rash is best described as **purpuric**—the description classically given to areas of purplish discoloration which do not blanch with pressure. Larger confluent areas of purpura are known as **ecchymoses**. Purpura is caused by blood leaking out of vessels and into the skin. This lady was referred as an emergency to hospital because one of the causes of a purpuric rash is meningococcal septicaemia as a complication of meningitis.

The differential diagnosis for a purpuric rash includes any process which damages vessel walls or predisposes to bleeding, including:

Infectious diseases: meningococcal disease, viral haemorrhagic fevers, bacterial toxins

Haematological disease: low platelets of any cause, for instance idiopathic thrombocytopenic purpura

Vasculitis: many rheumatological diseases including SLE or Henoch-Schönlein purpura

Drugs: may cause a particular type of vasculitis called leucocytoclastic vasculitis

Key investigations in this woman include:

Inflammatory markers: rule out bacterial septicaemia

Platelet count: look for thrombocytopenia

Renal function and urine dipstick: many vasculitides also produce acute glomerulonephritis

Rheumatological investigations: the autoantibody ANCA is positive in several systemic vasculitides including Wegener's granulomatosis or Churg-Strauss disease. Antistreptolysin-O titres (ASOT) suggest a vasculitis secondary to streptococcal disease. Raised serum IgA levels suggest Henoch-Schönlein purpura

Further reading

Guidelines: Association for the Advancement of Wound Care venous ulcers guidelines (http://www.guideline.gov/summary/summary.aspx?ss=15&doc_id=7109&nbr=4280)

OHCM: 204–205, 564, 658, 660–663

Tropical diseases

This section should be used to clerk patients presenting to hospital unwell after recent travel to tropical areas. The differential diagnoses in such patients include common and more unusual tropical infections, e.g. malaria or tropical sprue, as well as common disorders presenting incidentally after foreign travel, e.g. malignancy. These patients may be found on medical admissions units or specialist infectious diseases wards.

Learning challenges

- What are the predicted effects on the distribution of infectious diseases as a result of climate change, antibiotic overuse, and mass migration? Which diseases may re-emerge in the developed world as a result?
- What does the term 'the neglected diseases' refer to?

History

Comment on

- History of presenting complaint. Duration and progression
- Place of travel (the country and areas visited—rural or urban?)
- Mosquito and other insect exposure, e.g. ticks
- Activities whilst abroad—unprotected sex, blood transfusion, animal contact
- Precautions taken regarding food and water
- Antimalarial prophylaxis. Vaccinations before trip
- Contacts with similar symptoms
- Systems review

Examination

Well or unwell? Why?

Feet to face:

Vital signs: Temperature Blood pressure Pulse rate Respiratory rate O2 saturations

Clinical clues:

Cardiovascular:

1 2 1

Respiratory:

Abdominal:

Neurological:

Other:

Comment on

- Fever, haemodynamic stability
- Lymphadenopathy
- Rashes
- Organomegaly
- Signs of serious systemic illness—confusion, reduced level of consciousness, cardiac, renal, or hepatic impairment

Blood tests

Comment on

- FBC—WCC and differential (eosinophilia may imply parasitaemia, thrombocytopenia may imply malaria)
- CRP
- Glucose
- Renal function
- Liver function tests

Blood film

Comment on
- Malarial parasites
- Degree/percentage of parasitaemia

Blood cultures

Urine, sputum, CSF cultures

(where clinically indicated)

Stool

Comment on
- Cultures
- Ova, cysts, and parasites (O,C&P)

Chest X-ray

Comment on
- Tuberculosis

Serology

Comment on
- For specific infections

Evaluation

1. **Is this patient so unwell as to warrant empirical treatment? What are the likeliest causes of their illness? (Think about discussion with an expert in infectious diseases.)**

2. **If the presentation is primarily with fever and few localizing symptoms, which particular disease is most likely? What specific investigations and treatments are required?**

Disease	Clinical features	Diagnostic test	Management
Malaria (falciparum malaria may run a rapid, malignant course)	High fever, renal failure, dark urine, drowsiness or coma, splenomegaly	Thick and thin blood films—species, percentage parasitaemia	IV quinine. May require treatment on intensive care unit
Typhoid (enteric fever)	High fever, headache, abdominal pain, leucopenia, maculopapular rash, hepatosplenomegaly	Blood cultures, stool cultures	Ciprofloxacin
Tuberculosis	Fevers, sweats, weight loss, cough, ascites, effusion, lymphadenopathy	Microscopy or culture or sputum, body fluid or culture	Long course of antituberculous antibiotics
Dengue	High fever, headache and retro-orbital pain, backache, haemorrhage and shock	Clinical; serology	Supportive

3. **If one group of symptoms are predominant (e.g. gastrointestinal or dermatological), which diagnoses are most likely?**

4. **Still unsure? Are there any particular diseases affecting the area to which the patient travelled? (Look on relevant websites and take expert advice.) Consider non-infectious causes of fever, and diseases presenting incidentally that have nothing to do with travel.**

Questions

1. A 34-year-old man of Nigerian origin is brought to hospital by ambulance. His wife had become worried because during the evening he had become increasingly confused and drowsy and didn't recognize her. They had returned to London after a 2-week holiday in Nigeria a week earlier, during which time they had visited a rural part of the country. They had not received any vaccinations before leaving or taken malaria prophylaxis whilst there. For the previous 2 days the patient had complained of feeling feverish and unwell, with no localizing symptoms. On arrival in the Emergency Department basic observations include temperature 40.1°C, heart rate 120 bpm, blood pressure 122/67 mmHg, and GCS 9/15. His pupils are poorly reactive to light. There is no neck stiffness, rash, or lymphadenopathy. The chest is clear and heart sounds are normal. The abdomen is soft and non-tender with a palpable spleen. Initial blood tests are shown below:

Sodium: 141 mmol/L	Haemoglobin: 10.2 g/dL
Potassium: 4.8 mmol/L	MCV: 86 fL
Urea: 22.3 mmol/L	White cells: 10.2 × 10^9/L
Creatinine: 204 μmol/L	Platelets: 88 × 10^9/L
CRP: 20 mg/dL	
Bilirubin: 54 μmol/L	
ALP: 98 IU/L	
ALT: 23 IU/L	
Albumin: 35 g/L	

(1) What is the likely diagnosis?

(2) What complications of this condition have arisen?

(3) What is the management of such a patient?

2. A 23-year-old gap-year student presents to the hospital's Emergency Department 2 days after returning from travelling in India. Since her return she has experienced abdominal pain and bloating, anorexia, and diarrhoea, passing stool three or four times per day. The stool is profuse and watery but does not contain any blood or mucus. She had spent 3 weeks in India, installing water pumps for villages, during which time she had lodged with local families with whom she ate regularly. She had not experienced any health problems whilst there. On examination she is apyrexial and there are no sign of dehydration. The patient is able to tolerate oral fluid, and she is haemodynamically stable. Apart from mild, diffuse abdominal tenderness, examination is unremarkable.

(1) What is the likely diagnosis?

(2) What is the management in this case?

3. A 34-year-old man consults his GP with a week-long history of haematuria. He has been passing urine with normal frequency and without pain, but the urine, especially at the end of voiding, has been noticeably blood stained. He has otherwise been well and has no other medical problems. He works as an engineer, and 2 months previously had spent a month in Malawi, swimming in the lake several times.

Given his travel history, what is the most likely diagnosis, and why is it important to treat it effectively?

4. A 39-year-old journalist presents to the hospital's Emergency Department 4 weeks after returning from Southeast Asia where she had stayed in local lodging houses whilst filming. She had not taken precautions regarding her diet. She had not received any vaccinations prior to departure. Since returning she had felt generally unwell, nauseated, having no appetite and a distaste for cigarettes, of which she had previously smoked 20 per day. The last 2 days she had become increasingly jaundiced. Her liver function tests are shown below:

Bilirubin: 94 μmol/L
ALP: 291 IU/L
ALT: 791 IU/L
Albumin: 39 g/L
INR: 1.1

(1) What is the most likely diagnosis?

(2) What tests would prove the diagnosis?

(3) What is the treatment?

Answers

1. This man is extremely unwell. The combination of fever, decreased consciousness, recent travel, renal failure, and thrombocytopenia (this secondary to splenic enlargement) makes the most likely diagnosis cerebral malaria, though bacterial meningitis, viral encephalitis, and TB meningitis are amongst the other diagnoses that should be considered. Urgent investigations should include thick and thin blood films for malarial parasites (and if present the degree of parasitaemia), CT head scanning, lumbar puncture (unless contraindicated by raised intracranial pressure), blood glucose measurement, and an HIV test. In the meantime he requires care in a high-dependency area, with close monitoring and management of his airway. He may require intubation if his GCS drops further. If there is evidence of raised intracranial pressure on CT then intravenous corticosteroids can help to reduce this. Good fluid management is required to prevent further deterioration in renal function, though patients with serious malaria often require haemofiltration.

Falciparum malaria causes an acute febrile illness which can be fatal. Severe disease is defined by a parasitaemia of >1% (i.e. >1% of red cells infected). Two common complications are cerebral malaria (causing seizures, reduced level of consciousness, and coma) and 'blackwater fever' (where massive intravascular haemolysis leads to dark-coloured urine and renal failure). Other complications include severe anaemia (due to acute sequestration of red cells in an enlarged spleen), pre-renal kidney failure which along with pulmonary oedema can make fluid management very challenging, hypoglycaemia, and secondary bacterial sepsis. Treatment of severe malaria is with intravenous quinine.

2. The history of this diarrhoea makes it highly likely to be of infective origin. Infective diarrhoea can be **secretory** (as here), where fluid is (sometimes copiously) secreted into the bowel lumen as a result of bacterial toxins (for instance, the diarrhoea produced in cholera or most *E. coli* infections). It can also be **inflammatory**, where organisms (such as *Salmonella* or *Shigella* species) invade the bowel wall producing diarrhoea containing blood and mucus. Stool microscopy (for ova, cysts, and parasites) along with culture (for bacteria) may reveal the cause in this case.

The management of infective diarrhoea is based largely on preventing dehydration. This is best done with oral fluid rehydration unless the diarrhoea is severe or the patient is unable to swallow, when intravenous fluids may be required. In the absence of any signs of dehydration or significant vomiting (preventing drinking), this patient does not require admission to hospital. Oral antibiotics have some role to play, with ciprofloxacin shortening the duration of symptoms in *Salmonella* and *Shigella* infections. Sometimes tropical diarrhoea can be longer lived, with amoebiasis or giardiasis diarrhoea presenting several weeks after initial infection, and sometimes progressing to cause a long-term malabsorption syndrome. They are treated with high-dose metronidazole.

3. Painless haematuria in a man of this age would normally be suggestive of urological malignancy or intrinsic renal disease and require urgent investigation (urine cytology, cystoscopy, and ultrasound or CT scanning) to determine the cause. However, in this case, the travel history makes the most likely diagnosis schistosomiasis. Schistosomes are parasitic worms whose larvae multiply in their intermediate host, water snails (being especially prevalent in the Great Lakes of central and eastern Africa). They can pierce the skin of swimmers, migrating via the patient's lung to mature and pair up, before lying in the blood vessels of the bowel or bladder wall for many months or years producing thousands of eggs. These may be passed in urine or stool, or may lodge in the bladder or bowel wall, producing chronic inflammation. Some become lodged in the liver producing a characteristic pattern of periportal fibrosis, which can lead to portal hypertension, ascites, and oesophageal varices.

The disease is simple to treat with the antihelminthic medication praziquantel. Chronic, undiagnosed infection predisposes to bladder and bowel cancer, as well as producing portal hypertension as discussed above.

4. Jaundice may be:

(1) **Pre-hepatic**—this is suggested by an isolated rise in bilirubin without derangement of the other enzymes. For example, malaria-induced haemolysis leads to a rise in bilirubin due to increased breakdown of red cells.

(2) **Intrahepatic**—caused by direct damage to the hepatocytes within the liver. This damage releases the transaminases, AST and ALT. A disproportionate rise in transaminases compared with the other enzymes is suggestive of 'hepatic' jaundice. This is classically caused by the viral hepatitides.

or

(3) **Post-hepatic or obstructive**—caused by obstruction of the biliary tree, producing a predominant rise in alkaline phosphatase (ALP).

In this case the LFTs demonstrate a disproportionate rise in the ALT, in keeping with an intrahepatic jaundice. The two most likely causes of an acute intrahepatic jaundice in an otherwise healthy individual are viral infection and drugs. In this case serology for hepatitis A, B, C, D, and E viruses may well reveal the source of the infection. Hepatitis A or E infection is probably most likely; these are common in the developing world and spread faeco-orally. However, the patient should be asked about sexual practices, intravenous drug use, or blood transfusions which may allow the transmission of hepatitis B and C. Hepatitis A and E occasionally produce a fulminant hepatitis that can be fatal; more commonly they produces a self-limiting illness lasting weeks to months where the patient feels unwell and becomes jaundiced but does not develop serious complications. They (unlike hepatitis B and C) never progress to cause chronic liver disease.

This patient requires close monitoring over the next few days to ensure that the derangement in her LFTs resolves and does not develop into decompensated liver failure—the INR may be a particularly useful marker here as it measures the liver's synthetic function. If the patient is compliant and not systemically unwell, this monitoring could be done as an out-patient. Her LFTs may not normalize for several months, during which time she may feel generally very unwell. She and any others living with her should observe meticulous food hygiene to prevent further spread of the infection.

Further reading

Guidelines: British Infection Society guidelines for fever in the returning traveller (http://www.britishinfectionsociety.org/drupal/sites/default/files/FeverReturnDraftBISNov08.pdf)

OHCM: 377, 386–389, 394–406

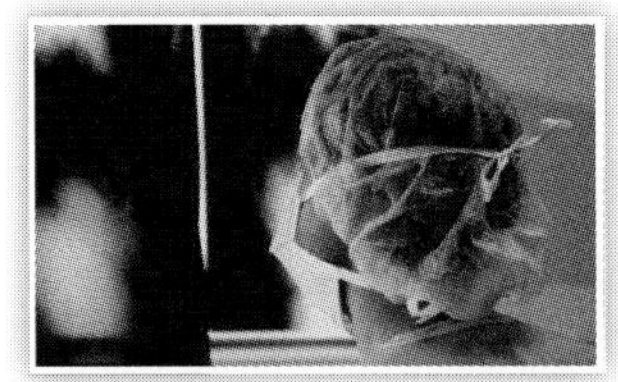 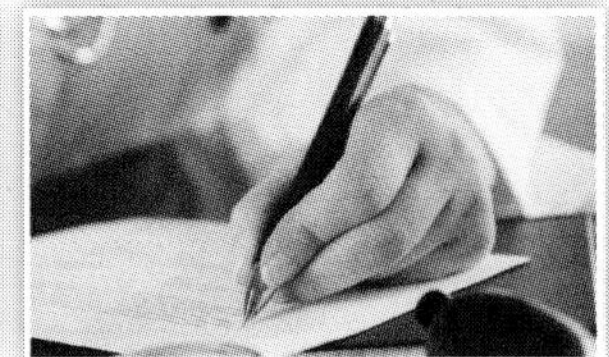 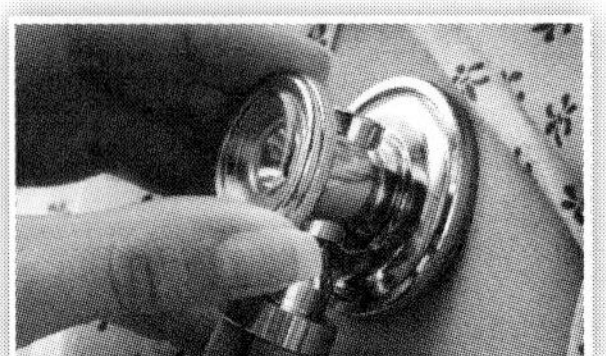 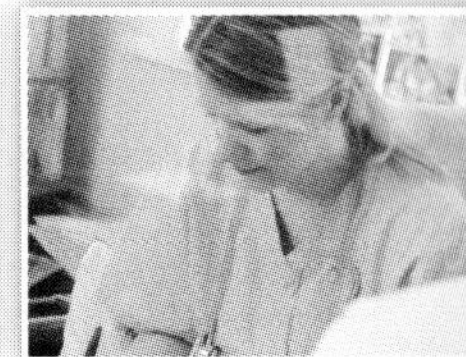

Unit 8
Surgery

Key learning outcomes in surgery include:

- **Performing a thorough assessment of a patient with acute abdominal pain, including suggesting a likely diagnosis and commencing appropriate initial management.**
- **Understanding the principles of caring for sick surgical patients, particularly with reference to fluid balance and in the resuscitation of trauma patients.**
- **Understanding the role and limitations of surgery in treating a number of common cancers, including cancer of the colon, breast, stomach, prostate, and urinary tract.**
- **Understanding the principles of modern surgery and become competent at 'scrubbing up' and assisting in theatre.**
- **Reflecting on the ethics of surgery, particularly thinking about issues of consent and about balancing the risks and benefits of surgical interventions.**

Tips for learning surgery on the wards:

- Clerk new surgical admissions to the hospital and devise initial management plans for patients—present them to a senior and see if their impression agrees with yours.
- Surgical ward rounds are often very quick—there is often not time to present patients, but with each patient try to review either their observations, their fluid chart, or their drug chart, to gain familiarity with reading these. Try to identify what leads senior surgeons to be worried about patients or to be happy with their progress.
- Go to theatre. Early on, ask one of the theatre staff to teach you how to 'scrub up', and then whenever theatre is not too busy (for instance, during routine operating lists), ask if you can assist.
- Attend 'pre-admission clinics' (often run by junior doctors or specialist nurses), where patients due to be admitted for elective surgery are assessed for suitability for anaesthetic. These are excellent opportunities to clerk and examine patients under supervision.
- Learn procedures—surgical patients often require regular blood tests, intravenous cannulation, urethral catheterization, and placement of nasogastric tubes. Helping out with routine ward jobs will create the time for junior doctors to observe and teach you these procedures.

History

Acute abdominal pain

This is one of the commonest surgical presentations to hospital with a broad range of possible diagnoses. The initial history should follow the 'SOCRATES' acronym common to all presentations of pain:

- **S**ite: **Visceral pain** (e.g. from the intestines) will be referred to the midline in one of three regions:

Epigastric pain is referred from structures originating from the embryonic foregut including the stomach, oesophagus, duodenum, gall bladder and pancreas

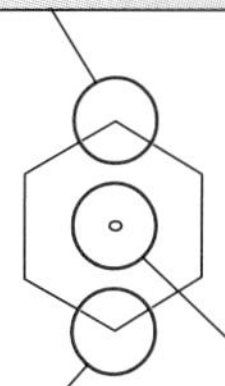

Suprapubic pain may be caused by disease of the pelvic organs (e.g. by cystitis or gynaecological problems), or by disease of the embryological hindgut, from the transverse colon to the anal canal.

Peri-umbilical pain is referred from structures originating from the embryonic midgut, including all structures from the third part of the duodenum to the mid transverse colon (including the appendix)

  Peritonitic pain may be generalized or localized to **one area of the abdomen** (e.g. the right iliac fossa).

- **O**nset: Sudden onset may indicate a mechanical event, e.g. perforation or rupture of a structure. Onset over hours or days suggests developing obstruction or inflammation.
- **C**haracter: Sharp pain may be caused by peritoneal irritation. Colicky pain (which comes and goes in waves) is associated with obstruction to peristalsis, e.g. through the bowel or the biliary or renal tract.
- **R**adiation: Pain from the urinary tract may be felt anywhere from the **loin** to the **external genitalia**. Pain from irritation of the diaphragm may radiate to the **tip of the shoulder** (**C3,4,5 dermatome**). Pain in retroperitoneal structures (such as the pancreas or the abdominal aorta) radiates to the **back**.
- **A**lleviating factors: Some causes of upper gastrointestinal pain may be alleviated by eating or drinking (or conversely these activities may worsen the pain). Constipation (or pain from irritable bowel syndrome) may be alleviated by defaecation.
- **T**ime course: Intermittent pain suggests an intermittent cause, for instance a gallstone that occasionally moves to obstruct the cystic duct, exacerbations of inflammatory bowel disease, or stress-related symptoms in irritable bowel disease.
- **E**xacerbating factors: Peritonitic pain is worse on movement, so the patient will lie very still. Biliary colic or cholecystitis is often worse shortly after eating. Patients with renal colic may be uncomfortable on lying still, gaining limited relief from moving around.
- **S**everity: Renal colic may cause a particularly severe pain. Colicky pain will fluctuate in intensity whilst pain from inflammatory causes, e.g. acute appendicitis, will generally build in intensity.

Remember to ask about:

- Vomiting—this may be caused by simply being unwell, but always bear in mind intestinal obstruction.
- Bowel habit—complete constipation implies obstruction, but non-obstructive constipation is a significant source of abdominal pain.
- Urinary symptoms - UTI is a common cause of lower abdominal pain.
- Menstrual history - this is absolutely crucial in the assessment of abdominal pain in women aged 10-55.

Symptoms of prostate disease

See the introduction to Unit 4 (Renal medicine) for how to distinguish irritant lower urinary tract symptoms (caused by infection) from obstructive lower urinary tract symptoms (caused by bladder outflow obstruction—usually (in men) due to prostate disease).

Symptoms of peripheral vascular disease

There are lots of causes of pain in the legs, and the history is by far the best way of determining whether the pain patients are describing is of vascular origin. Occlusive disease in the arteries of the legs may cause three main syndromes: intermittent claudication, rest pain, and acute ischaemia.

Intermittent claudication	Rest pain	Acute ischaemia
Cramping pain in the calves, thighs, or buttocks brought on reproducibly by exercise and relieved by rest (within 1 or 2 minutes). Determine what the patient's 'claudication distance' is in metres. Buttock claudication and impotence is called Leriche's syndrome and is a symptom of iliac disease	Similar pain to the pain of intermittent claudication, but it occurs at rest. It is often especially bad at night (since the leg is elevated so gravity does not assist with perfusion), and patients may sleep in a chair to reduce the pain. There may be ulceration or gangrene of the toes	Sudden onset of severe pain in a leg, often on a background of known peripheral vascular disease. Features include: pain, paraesthesia, paralysis, pallor, pulselessness, perishing cold

Pre-operative assessment

Even the simplest surgical procedure is potentially hazardous, and full planning and preparation are essential in making it as safe as possible. For elective surgery, all patients are seen at 'pre-admission clinics' a few days before their operation to assess their fitness for anaesthetic and to identify potential problems. For emergency theatre this assessment may only be done hours or minutes before the operation, but is essential to avoid and prepare for potential anaesthetic complications. Key parts of a pre-operative assessment include:

- **The indication for surgery**—if surgery is elective make sure the patient's condition has not vastly worsened or improved in the time between when the operation was booked and the present time. Any changes should be discussed with the surgeon as a different operation (or no operation) may now be indicated.
- **Previous medical history**—especially any conditions affecting the airway (e.g. arthritis of the cervical spine affecting ease and risk of tracheal intubation), breathing (e.g. COPD), or circulation (e.g. previous heart attacks, poorly controlled hypertension, or bleeding disorders). Further investigations, e.g. chest X-ray, echocardiogram, or spirometry may be required to ensure that anaesthesia can be planned safely.
- **Known surgical risks**—previous reactions to general anaesthetic. Previous DVT or PE. A family history of anaesthetic reactions such as malignant hyperpyrexia or other conditions like porphyria.
- **Drugs**—some should be stopped or substituted (e.g. a heparin infusion is used perioperatively for patients on warfarin as it has a shorter half-life, and an insulin sliding scale with intravenous dextrose written up for insulin-dependent diabetics). Other medications should be increased, e.g. steroids
- **Preparation for surgery**—the patient should be nil-by-mouth for 6 hours before the operation. Bowel preparation may be required (laxatives and enemas) in bowel surgery. Prophylactic antibiotics may be given.
- **Consent**—this should explain the benefits of surgery as well as commonly-occurring or serious risks. Consent should not be rushed and should not be coercive. Questions should be answered and alternatives explained. If the patient lacks capacity to consent (e.g. cannot understand, retain, and repeat the information required to make the decision), then they should be treated according to their best interests—a decision made by their clinicians usually in partnership with the patient's relatives.

Examination

Examination of the patient presenting with an acute abdomen

Begin in the same way as with all examinations:

- **Well or unwell?** If unwell why? Give analgesia before proceeding if the patient is in pain.
- **Feet to face assessment**—look for signs of chronic diseases, e.g. liver disease. Look for pallor (upper GI bleed?) and jaundice (biliary obstruction?). Feel for peripheral temperature and capillary refill time (decreased if the patient is shocked). Look for scars that betray a previous surgical history.
- **Vital signs**—is the patient shocked? Give fluids early as resuscitation is almost always required before surgery commences.
- **Clinical clues**—alcohol is a major cause of pancreatitis (has the patient been drinking?). Look for stomas, drains, oxygen, fluids, and intravenous medications.

Remember to examine the cardiovascular and respiratory systems, to exclude alternative diagnoses (for instance, a right lower lobe pneumonia may cause right upper quadrant pain) and to identify comorbidities that may affect fitness for surgery.

Then examine the abdomen, **inspecting** for scars or signs of illness, **palpating** for tenderness, guarding, rebound tenderness, organomegaly, and masses, **percussing** for ascites and organomegaly, and **auscultating** for bowel sounds.

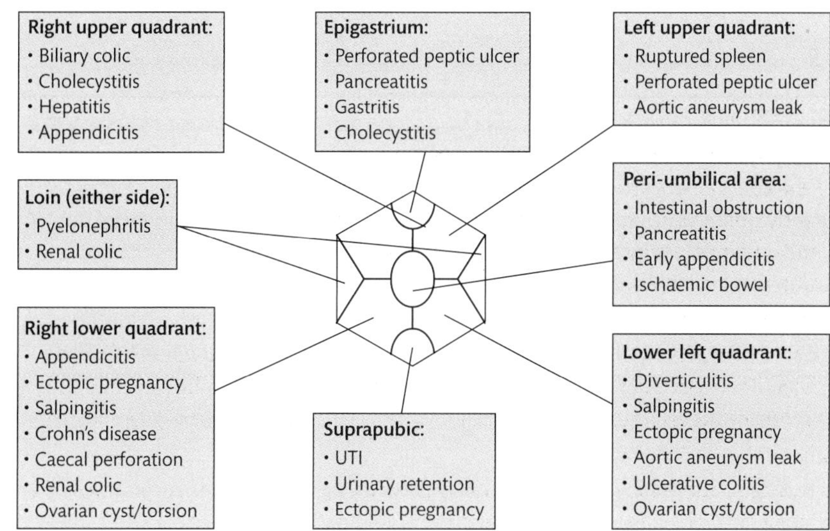

The key to most acute surgical abdomens is time: patients should be nil by mouth, have intravenous fluids, and adequate analgesia and then be re-examined in a few hours. Pain that worsens or fails to settle often requires an operation.

Digital rectal examination

This is essential in making a number of surgical diagnoses, including assessment for rectal bleeding (fresh blood or evidence of piles), upper GI bleeding (melaena), intestinal obstruction (empty rectum), and prostate disease (enlarged prostate, craggy or smooth). It is potentially embarrassing for both the patient and the doctor, so ensure privacy, take a chaperone of the same sex as the patient, and explain clearly why the examination is necessary.

- Ask the patient to remove the necessary clothing and lie in the left lateral position.
- Inspect the perianal area for abscesses, fissures, skin tags, haemorrhoids, or bleeding.
- Lubricate your right index finger and insert it into the rectum. Sweep around inside the anal canal assessing for stool (is it hard or soft?) and for masses or breaches in the epithelium.
- Assess the prostate (in men)—does it feel large (bulging into the rectum)? Is the surface smooth or rough and irregular?
- Look at your glove—is there fresh blood? Melaena? Stool?
- Cover the patient and explain your findings to them.

Examination of a lump

Most of this is done by inspection and palpation, though percussion and even auscultation and transillumination can have a role in certain situations. The aims of the examination are: (1) to be able to describe the lump using precise and concise medical terminology and (2) to be able to suggest the likely diagnosis or a list of differentials.

Comment on each of the following features:

- **Site**: describe exactly where the lump is, with reference to surrounding structures, e.g. 'overlying...', 'just medial to...', 'on the anterior border of...'
- **Size**: in centimetres
- **Shape**: round, cylindrical, irregular
- **Consistency**: hard, firm, fluctuant (where fluid can be squeezed from one part to another)
- **Surface**: smooth, irregular, craggy
- **Relations**: where does the lump seem to be arising from or tethered to? The skin? The muscle? Other organs?
- **Lymph nodes**: always assess for local lymphadenopathy, particularly if the lump has any sinister features

Breast examination involves inspection of the breasts (and especially the nipples), including when the woman raises her arms or pushes down on her hips, and thorough palpation of all breast quadrants and the axillary tail for lumps. The axillae should be palpated on all four walls for lymphadenopathy.

Examination of peripheral pulses

First **inspect** the legs for colour, ulceration, gangrene, and scars from previous vascular surgery. **Palpate** first for the abdominal aortic pulse, and note whether the pulse is simply pulsatile (normal) or expansile (potentially aneurysmal). Then palpate for the femoral (mid-point of the inguinal ligament), popliteal (against the posterior border of the upper tibia), posterior tibial (posterior to the medial malleolus), and dorsalis pedis pulses (lateral to the extensor hallucis longus tendon). Comment on whether they are present, reduced, absent, or aneurysmal. A handheld Doppler ultrasound probe can be used to assess for impalpable pulses, and can be used with a sphygmomanometer to measure the ankle:brachial pressure index. Buerger's test can be performed (see section on vascular surgery).

Investigations

General surgery remains a very clinical speciality, with the decision for surgery often depending on symptoms and signs and their changes over a period of time. However, various investigations have an important role to play in identifying key surgical emergencies:

Plain radiography

This chest radiograph reveals a large amount of air under the diaphragm – likely to have been caused by perforation of the stomach or small or large intestine, where subdiaphragmatic air is seen in up to 90% of patients.

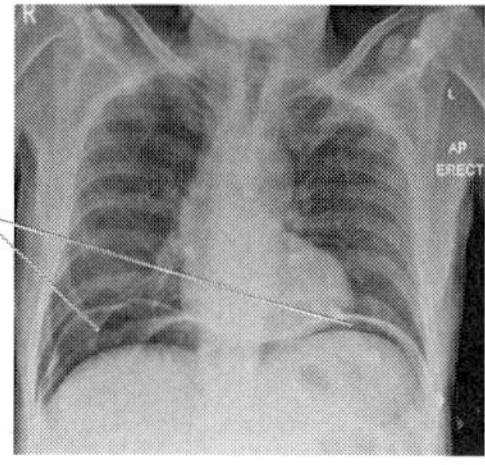

Other key uses of plain chest radiography in medicine include in and assessing fitness for surgery (for instance in patients with known heart or lung disease), in looking for pulmonary metastases from intra-abdominal malignancies or in assessing post-operative patients who become breathless.

This x-ray reveals distended loops of small intestine. These are sometimes said to resemble stacked coins. Note the valvulae conniventes which cross the whole width of the bowel lumen, confirming this is small rather than large bowel. Sometimes fluid levels form within loops of distended bowel so that multiple dome-shaped radiolucent areas are seen on x-ray.

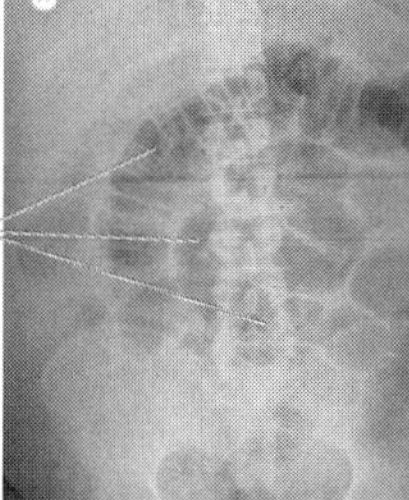

Abdominal x-rays have a useful role in general surgery in diagnosing (or excluding) intestinal obstruction, for instance in a patient with vomiting and constipation. They can be used to diagnose faecal impaction in constipated patients, to monitor for acute colonic distension in acute colitis and can be used pre- and post contrast when performing an intravenous urogram to look for stones and ureteric obstruction in renal colic.

Abdominal ultrasound

This is extremely useful in assessing right upper quadrant pain or jaundice, where dilated bile ducts are diagnostic of obstructive jaundice. Gallstones or a pancreatic mass may be seen. Ultrasound is also used to diagnose ureteric obstruction and hydronephrosis, and can be used as an initial investigation for most abdominal masses. It is also used in a trauma setting to assess for free fluid within the abdomen which may indicate intestinal perforation or intra-abdominal haemorrhage.

Abdominal CT scanning

This is increasingly being used to investigate acute abdominal pain, abdominal masses, and urological problems such as biliary colic. Generally all scans are reviewed by specialist radiologists, but it is helpful for all doctors to be able to identify basic structures:

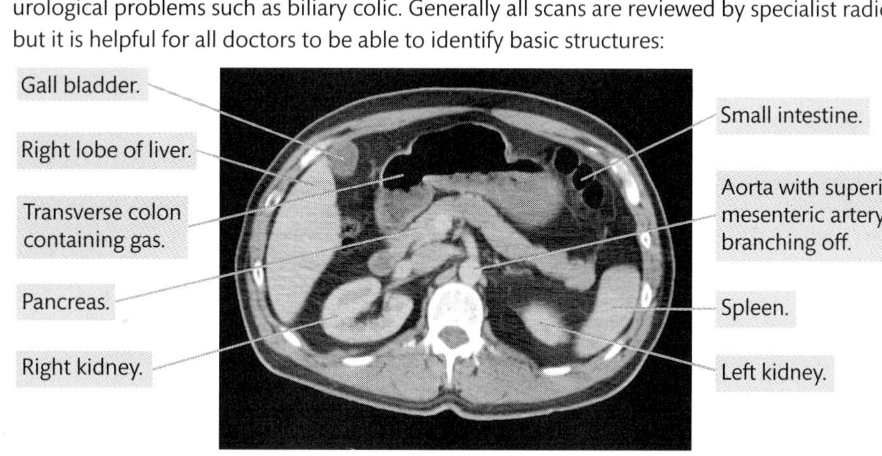

Remember that you can find large-size, annotated versions of many of the X-rays and ECGs that appear in this book on the book's web site at www.oxfordtextbooks.co.uk/orc/randall/

Vascular imaging

Imaging of blood vessels is crucial in the evaluation of peripheral vascular and cerebrovascular disease. Three main techniques exist, which aim to identify the degree and location of vessel stenosis, so that the need for surgery and the particular surgical approach can be decided on.

Conventional angiography

In this technique a vascular catheter is inserted into one of the femoral arteries or veins and used to instil contrast directly into whichever blood vessel is being imaged. Serial images captured after the injection of contrast are subtracted from those captured before (digital subtraction angiography or DSA) to remove bone and soft tissue from the images and to produce clear pictures of the blood vessels.

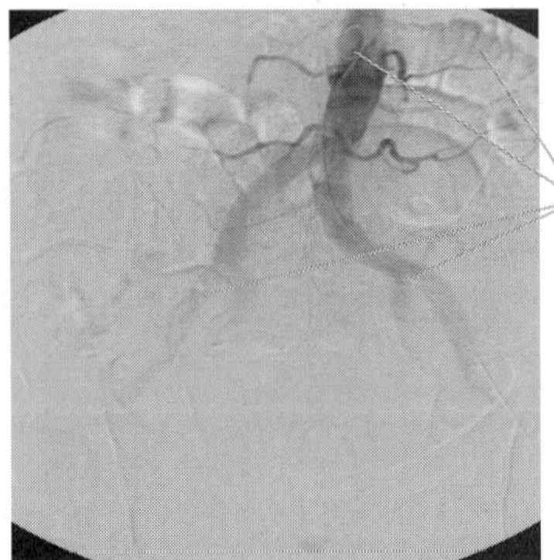

A femoral angiogram. A cannula has been passed into the femoral artery and on into the abdominal aorta (where the tip can be seen curled up, with small intestine visible above this). An angiogram like this can be used to investigate the aorta (though less invasive investigations such as ultrasound are preferred for this), to investigate the renal and splanchnic vessels as well as investigate the arteries of the pelvis and lower limbs. Here the bifurcation of both iliac vessels is clearly visible.

Duplex ultrasonography

Here conventional ultrasound scanning of blood vessels is combined with Doppler scanning (which measures blood flow) to produce a clear picture of vessels and the flow through them, illustrating areas of stenosis or occlusion. Doppler imaging is especially used for the investigation of strokes and TIAs, where >70% stenosis of the carotid arteries is an indication for surgical endarterectomy.

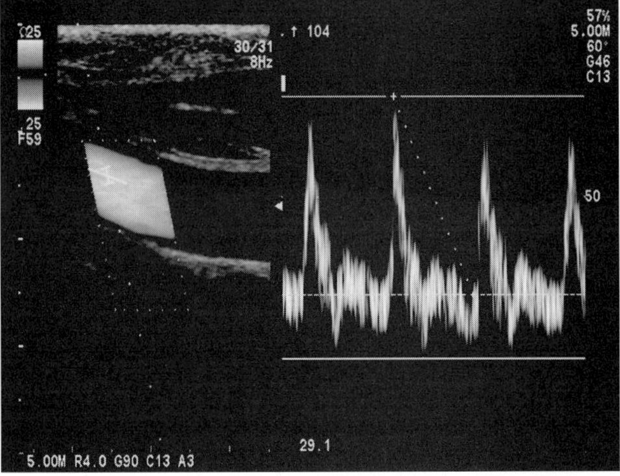

In the image on the left, the black and white outline to the blood vessels is created using conventional ultrasound. Bright colours are created using Doppler technology to give an idea of the direction and speed of flow through the artery. The screen on the right displays graphically the wave form of blood flow through the artery highlighted. This waveform can be used to calculate the extent of stenosis in the vessel.

CT or MR angiography

This is carried out with contrast injected through a peripheral cannula, making it safer than conventional angiography, which requires direct access to central arteries and veins. Risks of CT angiography include contrast toxicity and radiation exposure.

Both CT and MR angiography allow the creation of complex reconstructions of vascular structures that can be rotated and examined from different angles on the computer desktop. Here the whole aorta can be seen, curving upwards from the heart and descending through the thorax and abdomen to bifurcate in the pelvis.

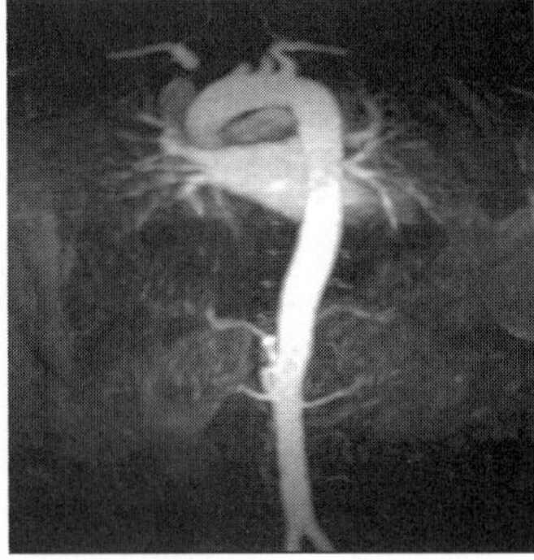

Remember that you can find large-size, annotated versions of many of the X-rays and ECGs that appear in this book on the book's web site at www.oxfordtextbooks.co.uk/orc/randall/

Mammography

Mammograms are x-rays taken of the breast. They are examined by specialist radiographers who look for particular patterns of lucency (such as small areas of calcification) which are particularly associated with cancer. They are then classified according to the **BIRADS score** according to the clinical probability of cancer. This score, together with findings on clinical examination, is used to guide the need for biopsy, further observation or regular follow-up.

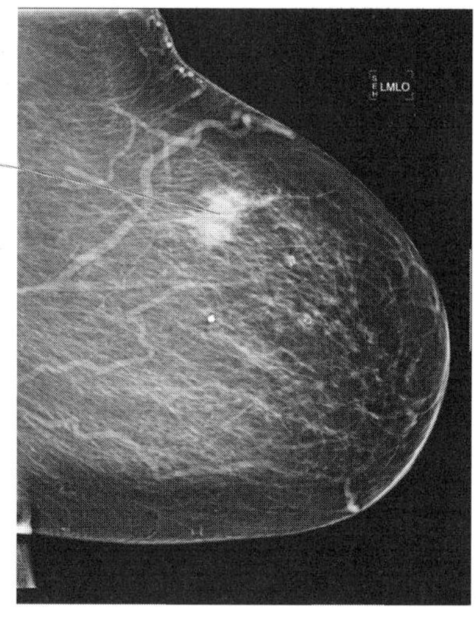

Lesion consistent with breast carcinoma.

Interventions

Surgical terminology

The following terms are put together to create some of the complex terminology used to describe surgical procedures.

Body part		Body part		Procedure	
Angio-	Blood vessel	**Laparo-**	Abdomen	**-otomy**	Opening
Chole-	Related to bile	**Litho-**	Stone	**-ectomy**	Removal
Colp-	Vagina	**Nephro-**	Kidney	**-ostomy**	Artificial opening
Cyst-	Bladder	**Colo-**	Large bowel	**-gram**	Imaging
Entero- or ilio-	Small bowel	**Splene-**	Spleen	**-scopy**	Visualizing
Gastro-	Stomach	**Thoraco-**	Chest	**-pexy**	Fixing in place
Hystero-	Uterus	**-docho-**	Duct	**-plasty**	Reshaping

So a gastrectomy involves removal of the stomach, a laparotomy involves opening the abdomen whilst a laparoscopy involves only looking inside it, a colostomy is an abnormal opening of the large bowel, and a choledocholithotomy involves the removal of a stone from the bile duct.

Surgical incisions

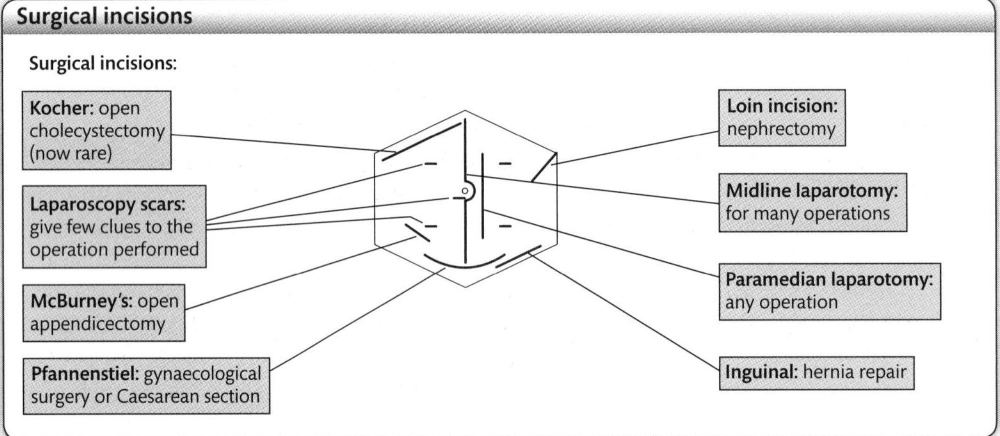

Anaesthesia

The aim of anaesthesia is to induce hypnosis, analgesia, and muscle relaxation. Drugs given to a typical patient undergoing a major operation may include:

- **Pre-medication:** Anxiolytics to relieve anxiety, analgesia if the patient is in pain, antiemetics if the patient feels nauseous and is at risk of vomiting and aspiration.
- **Induction:** Often with an intravenous agent such as thiopental or propofol
- **Muscle relaxation:** to allow intubation. Often a depolarizing agent such as suxamethonium is used. This may be followed by a longer-acting muscle relaxant such as vecuronium.
- **Maintenance of anaesthesia:** A gaseous volatile anaesthetic (such as isoflurane) is usually used.
- **Reversal of anaesthesia:** Inhaled anaesthetics are replaced by oxygen, muscle relaxation is reversed (for instance by atropine), and secretions are controlled by antimuscarinics (e.g. neostigmine). The endotracheal tube is carefully removed once the patient is spontaneously breathing, and after suctioning the oropharynx to prevent secretions entering the lungs.

Perioperative care

Performing an operation on someone under general anaesthesia involves disrupting almost all of their body's natural homeostatic mechanisms, and so great care must be taken to ensure their safety:

- **Fluids:** Patients are usually made nil by mouth from the night before their operation, and for a period afterwards if the operation involved their bowel. Such patients require intravenous fluid administration: as a rule 2.5–3 L of fluid is given over a 24-hour period. If there are high fluid losses (for instance from a high-output stoma), then fluid is commonly given to equal the previous day's output + 500 ml for insensible losses. Urine output should be at least 0.5 ml/kg/hour, roughly 35 ml/hour for a person of average size.
- **Glycaemic control:** Diabetic patients may be prone to hyperglycaemia due to the stress of surgery, or hypoglycaemia whilst they are nil by mouth. To allow for these fluctuations in insulin requirements, in most centres diabetic patients stop their insulin the day before surgery and receive an insulin infusion according to a sliding scale until they have recovered and are eating and drinking properly. Wherever possible, diabetic patients should be placed first on the operating list.
- **Thromboprophylaxis:** Major surgery and the immobility it entails is a major risk for the development of deep vein thrombosis. **Thromboembolic deterrent (TED) stockings** and 'Flotron' boots are used to support the deep venous and lymphatic systems. Thromboprophylaxis with low-dose molecular weight heparin can be used, but this may impair blood clotting and raise the risk of haemorrhagic complications of surgery. Patients on oral anticoagulants should generally stop these before surgery (consider starting a heparin infusion, which is rapidly reversible in those at high risk).
- **Antibiotics:** Surgery on non-sterile sites (such as the bowel) carries a significant risk of post-operative wound infection. Each hospital has its own policy to prevent this, but commonly a single dose of broad-spectrum antibiotic is given 1 hour before surgery (or three doses given, one before and two after). This significantly reduces post-operative infections.
- **Nutrition:** Up to 25% of hospitalized patients may be malnourished, and surgical patients are often especially at risk because of being placed nil by mouth for prolonged periods of time (for instance, awaiting surgery, because of nausea and vomiting or the need to 'rest' bowel which has been operated on). Clinicians should always consider the nutritional status of the acutely ill, or patients with serious long-term conditions. Options for feeding include encouraging the patient to eat (giving adequate antiemetics, providing appetizing food, and helping patients with disabilities to feed themselves), feeding nasogastrically (if the patient's swallow is unsafe), or feeding intravenously (total parenteral nutrition). Involving a dietician will help manage patients' nutritional needs.

Principles of operative surgery

- **Sterilization:** Of the operating equipment, the patient's skin and the surgeon's hands, together with draping around the site of incision.
- **Incision:** The skin incision should be as small as possible whilst being big enough to allow adequate access to the relevant underlying structures.
- **Haemostasis:** Bleeding points caused by the incision should be tied off or cauterized with electrical diathermy to allow good visualization of the relevant structures.
- **Dissection:** Of all relevant anatomy so that structures are clearly identified and not confused with each other. This is often the lengthiest part of the operation.
- **Operative procedure:** The aim of the operation is carried out.
- **Skin closure:** After full haemostasis is achieved and the aims of the operation have been achieved, the incision is closed in layers (e.g. peritoneum-muscle-skin) with sutures or staples.

Acute abdominal pain

This section should be used to clerk patients with acute abdominal pain being managed by surgical teams. Patient pathways usually lead from the Emergency Department to the Surgical Assessment Unit and General Surgical Ward, where patients are observed for a period of time before a decision is reached for conservative or operative management.

Learning challenges

- How might the syndromes of organ rupture, generalized peritonitis, localized peritonitis, and colic be differentiated? Which are likely to require surgery?
- List five medical conditions which produce acute abdominal pain and must always be considered alongside surgical causes.

History

Comment on

- Site of pain, radiation
- Duration—constant or intermittent?
- Nature of pain—sharp, achy, colicky, tearing, burning
- Previous episodes
- Exacerbating/relieving features
- In women—menstrual history, pregnancy
- Associated features—vomiting and nausea, fever, constipation, diarrhoea, anorexia

Examination

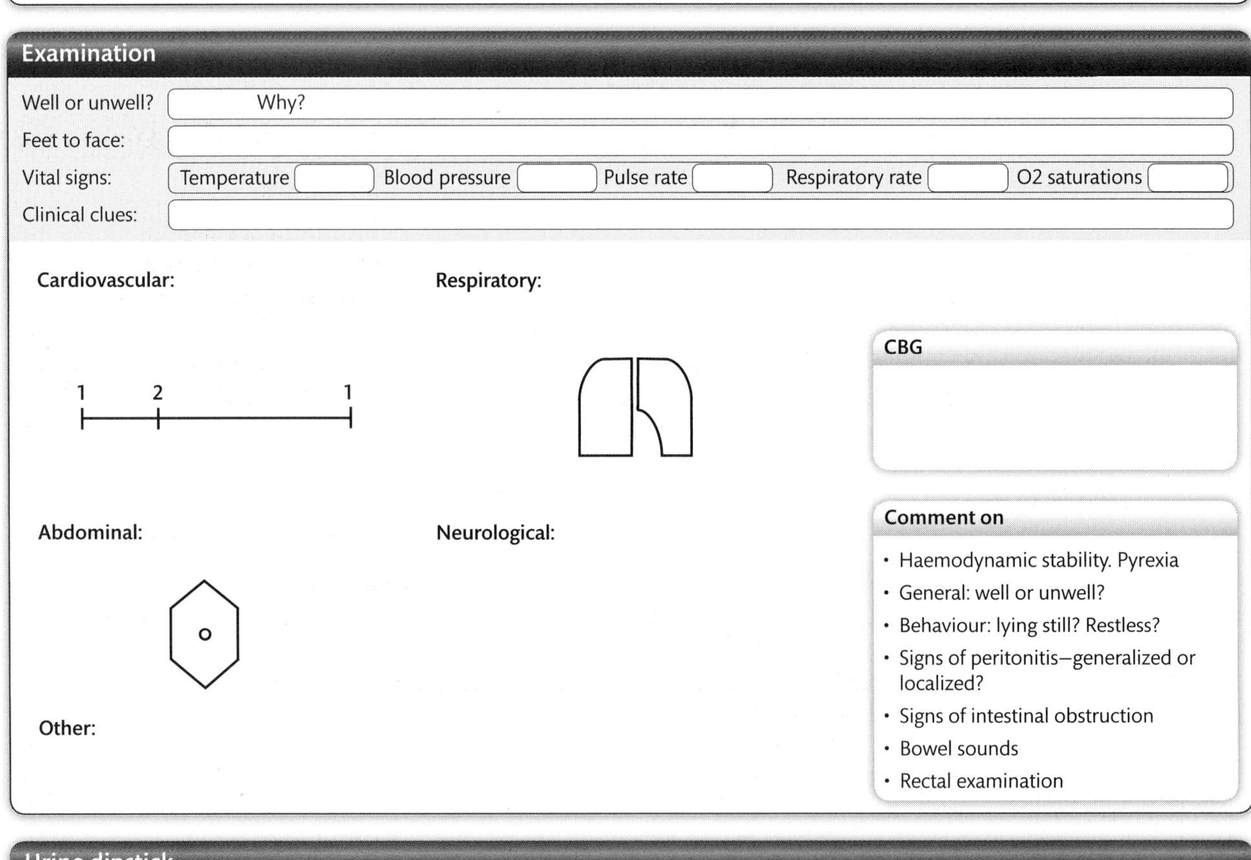

Well or unwell? Why?

Feet to face:

Vital signs: Temperature | Blood pressure | Pulse rate | Respiratory rate | O2 saturations

Clinical clues:

Cardiovascular:

Respiratory:

CBG

Abdominal:

Neurological:

Other:

Comment on

- Haemodynamic stability. Pyrexia
- General: well or unwell?
- Behaviour: lying still? Restless?
- Signs of peritonitis—generalized or localized?
- Signs of intestinal obstruction
- Bowel sounds
- Rectal examination

Urine dipstick

Comment on

- Evidence of infection, e.g. nitrites, leucocytes
- Pregnant?

Blood tests

Comment on

- Evidence of infection
- Liver and renal function
- Clotting
- Group and save (or cross-match)

Erect chest X-ray

Comment on
- Air under diaphragm?

ECG

Comment on
- Ischaemia
- Atrial fibrillation

Blood gases

Comment on
- Metabolic acidosis

Abdominal X-ray

Comment on
- Obstruction
- Constipation

Abdominal ultrasound

Comment on
- Free fluid in abdomen
- Gallstones, bile duct dilatation
- Renal stones, hydronephrosis

Evaluation

1. **Before proceeding: does this patient need urgent fluid resuscitation? Has analgesia been given?**

2. **What is in the differential diagnosis based on the site and nature of the pain?**

Right upper quadrant Biliary colic Cholecystitis Hepatitis Pneumonia	**Epigastric** Perforation Pancreatitis Myocardial infarction Gastritis	**Left upper quadrant** Pneumonia Large bowel obstruction Tender splenomegaly
	Generalized Intestinal obstruction Bowel ischaemia Inflammatory bowel disease Gastroenteritis	
Right lower quadrant Appendicitis Ectopic pregnancy Ovarian torsion UTI/renal colic	**Suprapubic** Urinary retention UTI Dysmenorrhoea Endometriosis	**Left lower quadrant** Diverticular disease Ectopic pregnancy Ovarian torsion UTI/renal colic

Radiating to back: think pancreatitis, aortic dissection, ruptured aortic aneurysm
Loin to groin pain: think renal colic
Intermittent pain: think visceral obstruction
Others: diabetic ketoacidosis, irritable bowel syndrome

3. **Does this patient need urgent surgery, or is conservative initial management appropriate?**

4. **How should they be prepared for surgery? What other management is indicated?**

Questions

1. A 76-year-old woman presents with severe central abdominal pain of 6 hours' duration, which had started suddenly. She had previously been feeling completely well. The pain was constant in nature and not affected by simple oral analgesia or by changing position. She has not been vomiting. She opened her bowels 1 hour ago and noticed her stool was loose, and mixed with some fresh blood. Past medical history includes a myocardial infarction 3 years previously. On examination she appears unwell and very uncomfortable. Basic observations include temperature 36.8°C, respiratory rate 28 breaths/min, blood pressure 133/87 mmHg, and pulse 124 bpm, irregularly irregular, with oxygen saturations 96% on room air. The chest is clear, and her heart sounds are normal but irregular. The abdomen is generally tender on palpation, with some guarding and rebound tenderness. Bowel sounds are present but reduced. Arterial blood gas analysis is performed (below).

(1) What does the blood gas demonstrate?

(2) What is the likely diagnosis?

pH: 7.18
pCO_2: 4.02 kPa
pO_2: 13.6 kPa
HCO_3^-: 18.1 mmol/L
Base excess: −10.6 mmol/L
Lactate: 9.4 mmol/L

2. A 24-year-old woman is admitted complaining of gradually developing lower abdominal pain, worse on the right-hand side, which began 8 hours earlier. The pain has been eased by morphine, and is also helped if she lies still on her back. She has previously been feeling well and has no other medical problems. On examination she appears uncomfortable and is lying as motionless and as flat as possible on the bed. Her basic observations include temperature 37.5°C, heart rate 114 bpm, and blood pressure 105/74 mmHg. On palpation she is tender in the right iliac fossa and suprapubically, with guarding and rebound tenderness. The rest of the abdomen is soft, and bowel sounds are heard. Rovsing's sign is negative.

(1) What other important information must you find out about this patient, and what bedside test could you perform to help you with this?

(2) What is the differential diagnosis?

(3) What is Rovsing's sign?

3. A 62-year-old man is admitted with acute upper abdominal pain. On examination his abdomen is rigid to palpation throughout, with completely absent bowel sounds. His erect chest X-ray is shown below. He is taken to theatre where a laparotomy is performed, and a perforated duodenal ulcer with peritoneal soiling is discovered. The small 1 cm perforation is repaired with an omental patch which is sutured into place over the hole. During the operation the patient becomes increasing tachycardic despite receiving 3 L of intravenous fluid. Inotropic support is required to maintain his blood pressure. Intraoperative blood loss is minimal. A diagnosis of refractory septic shock secondary to gross bacterial soiling of the peritoneal cavity is made.

(1) What does the X-ray show?

(2) What interventions are necessary to increase this man's chances of survival?

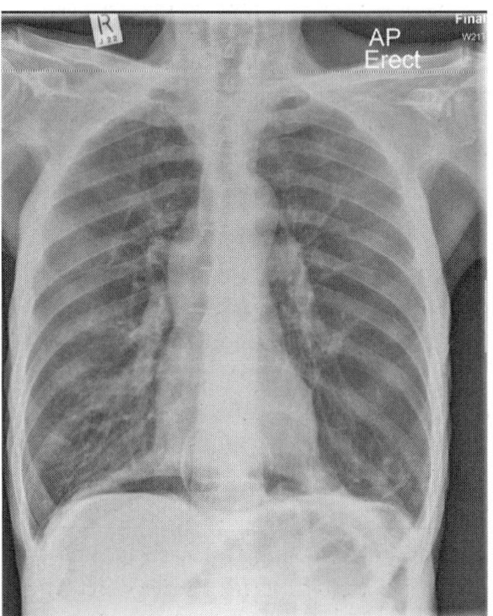

4. A 46-year-old Caucasian woman is admitted because of acute upper abdominal pain, which is worse on the right-hand side and radiates in a band round to her back. The pain is described as coming and going in waves. An ultrasound several months before (organized by her GP as she had suffered abdominal cramps), had revealed the presence of stones in her gall bladder. She is apyrexial, slightly tachycardic (104 bpm), and normotensive. On examination there is moderate right upper quadrant tenderness, with no hepatomegaly or palpable masses. Murphy's sign is negative. Blood tests reveal CRP of 8 mg/L, white cells of 7 × 10^9/L, amylase of 90 IU/dL, and normal liver function.

(1) What is the diagnosis?

(2) Why is it important that all of the tests mentioned above should be checked in the presence of known gallstones?

(3) What is Murphy's sign?

Answers

1. The blood gas shows a metabolic acidosis. This is demonstrated by the low bicarbonate, negative base excess, and raised lactate. The low $PaCO_2$ shows there is some attempted respiratory compensation, as the patient hyperventilates in an attempt to produce a respiratory alkalosis. Therefore the arterial blood gas reveals a lactic metabolic acidosis with partial respiratory compensation.

In this instance, the lactic acidosis is most likely to be caused by hypoperfusion of tissue, leading to increased anaerobic metabolism and a consequent increase in lactate. In this patient, the most likely cause is ischaemic bowel due to an embolus in the mesenteric vessels secondary to her atrial fibrillation.

The biggest risk factor for developing ischaemic bowel, or mesenteric infarction, is atrial fibrillation. Emboli from the fibrillating atria can be ejected into the circulation and occlude one of the mesenteric arteries, blocking blood supply to part of the bowel. The bowel will rapidly become swollen and oedematous, and then necrotic, causing death without intervention. Patients present with severe central abdominal pain (sometimes with only minimal tenderness on direct palpation), with or without rectal bleeding. Initial management is with fluid resuscitation, antibiotics, and analgesia, whilst optimizing the patient for surgery. Surgery will involve laparotomy, resection of the ischaemic portion of bowel, and anastomosis. A stoma will be considered to divert bowel contents from the anastomosis in order to give the best chance of healing. The stoma may be reversible at a second operation at a later stage, or may become permanent.

2. The two principal differential diagnoses in this patient are appendicitis and ruptured ectopic pregnancy. Any female patient of childbearing age presenting with abdominal pain should be asked the date of their last menstrual period and whether they may be pregnant. A urine dipstick analysis for beta-human chorionic gonadotrophin (beta-hCG) is a rapid and reliable pregnancy test. If this patient has a positive pregnancy test then she should be referred to the gynaecology team for urgent abdominal ultrasound scanning. Ectopic pregnancies can rupture and lead to massive haemorrhage and death, and urgent surgical intervention may be required.

If this patient's pregnancy test is negative and she has had a recent menstrual period, then appendicitis is the more likely diagnosis. Others to consider would include urinary tract infection, renal colic, and ovarian torsion. Urine dipstick (for nitrites and leucocytes in UTI, or blood in renal colic), abdominal ultrasound and CT KUB (kidneys, ureter, bladder) may be used to help narrow down the differential. Appendicitis is a clinical diagnosis, treated with appendicectomy. However, when the diagnosis is not certain, and when patients are reasonably well with their symptoms, a decision to admit for observation may be taken prior to deciding whether to proceed with appendicectomy or arrange further investigations. They should be nil by mouth and maintained with intravenous fluid, analgesia, and antibiotics. If symptoms do not improve, open or laparoscopic appendicectomy may be undertaken.

Rovsing's sign is demonstrated by pain reported at the right iliac fossa in response to palpation on the left side of the abdomen. This may be a feature of appendicitis and the patient should always be asked whereabouts they feel the pain whenever they report tenderness on palpation.

3. This X-ray reveals:

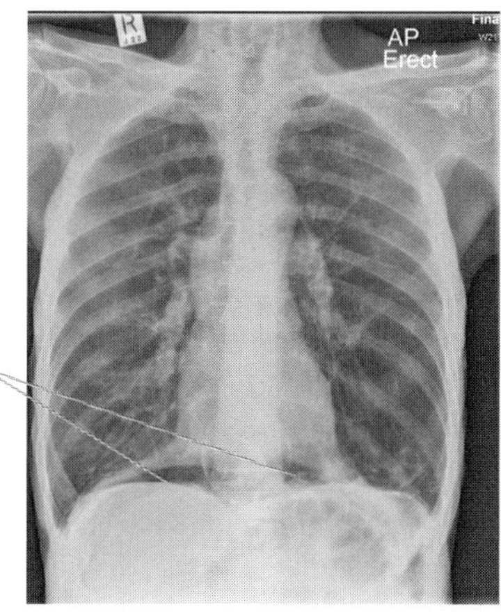

Free gas can be seen underneath both hemidiaphragms here. It is of little significance in this patient since his operation has only just ended, when many patients who have had a laparotomy would be expected to have some air within their peritoneum, which will be absorbed slowly over several days or weeks. A patient presenting to hospital with acute abdominal pain and an x-ray like this requires an urgent laparotomy.

This patient has suffered a severe septic insult, and the subsequent release of inflammatory mediators has produced widespread vasodilatation and capillary leak, causing compensatory vasoconstriction and tachycardia, which is inadequate to maintain blood pressure, hence the need for inotropic support. He is extremely unwell. The most important part of his management will be completing a thorough peritoneal washout. According to the old aphorism, '**the solution to pollution is dilution**', and many litres of warmed saline should be used to remove as much contaminant as possible from the peritoneal cavity. One or several drains may be sited which can be put on suction to help eliminate further waste after the initial operation.

Broad-spectrum intravenous antibiotics should be given, along with intravenous fluids and continuing inotropes. The patient should be managed on the ICU, with invasive monitoring of blood pressure (with an arterial line), central venous pressure (central venous catheter), and urine output (with a urinary catheter). This invasive monitoring allows interventions to be tailored to optimize the patient's physiological parameters—for instance, central venous pressure monitoring guides fluid resuscitation, allowing fluid depletion to be fully treated without causing fluid overload and pulmonary oedema.

4. Much right upper quadrant pain is related to gallstones, which can cause different clinical problems depending on where they impact. This is why the answer to the question, 'What are gallstones?' is 'They are dangerous' (**Maclean's rule**). Below is a schematic diagram of the gall bladder and biliary tree, with numbers indicating the different clinical problems caused by gallstones in different places:

(1) Stones in the body of the gall bladder cause no symptoms. They can be detected in asymptomatic individuals on ultrasound examination. Occasionally they may move upwards and obstruct the outflow to the gall bladder, producing an attack of biliary colic. This is often preceded by eating fatty food, which causes the gall bladder to contract to release bile. An attack of biliary colic produces intense right upper quadrant pain, which may be colicky or constant. Blood tests are normal and the pain usually subsides after several hours. The woman in this question is suffering with biliary colic and requires analgesia, buscopan (to relax smooth muscle), and observation to make sure that the pain subsides. Elective laparoscopic cholecystectomy may be offered to prevent the problem recurring.

(2) Gallstones impacted in the cystic duct cause pain similar to that of biliary colic. However, bile in the gall bladder can stagnate, leading to infection (acute cholecystitis). Inflammatory markers are raised and there may by physical signs of infection. Murphy's sign is positive—there is intense pain when the examiner's hand is placed on the patient's right upper quadrant as the patient breathes in. These patients require intravenous antibiotics, and scheduling of a cholecystectomy, usually after the initial infection has settled.

(3) A gallstone which is obstructing the common bile duct will lead to an obstructive jaundice (with abnormal liver function tests—especially a raised bilirubin and alkaline phosphatase). Complete obstruction of the biliary drainage system will lead to ascending cholangitis, as infections tracks back up the cystic and hepatic ducts to the liver and gall bladder. These patients can be extremely unwell, requiring intravenous antibiotics as well as emergency stone removal, generally by endoscopic retrograde cholangiopancreatography (ERCP).

(4) A gallstone stuck in the ampulla of Vater may produce pancreatitis in addition to ascending cholangitis and obstructive jaundice. The patient will have raised serum amylase and may exhibit the various signs and symptoms of acute pancreatitis. Urgent stone removal is imperative to allow resolution.

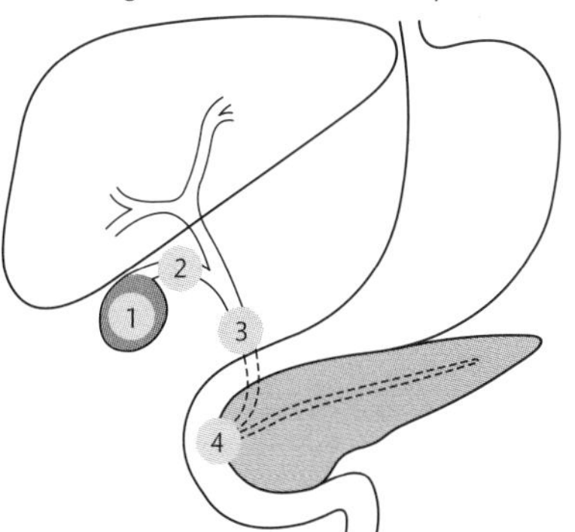

Rarely gallstones may pass directly from the gallbladder into the small bowel (through a fistula) and may impact in the terminal ileum leading to 'gallstone ileus' and intestinal obstruction.

Further reading

Guidelines: National Institute for Health Research Health Technology Assessment clinical review of decision making tools in acute abdominal pain (http://www.hta.ac.uk/project/1130.asp)

OHCM: 608–611, 622, 626, 630, 636–639, 640, 654, 656

Intestinal obstruction

This section should be used to clerk patients admitted with acute intestinal obstruction. These patients are usually initially managed conservatively on a General Surgical Ward, before a decision is made as to whether they require emergency surgery.

Learning challenges

- Why do patients with acute obstruction often become severely hypovolaemic and require aggressive fluid resuscitation?
- What are trichobezoars and phytobezoars?

History

Comment on

- Abdominal pain—character, duration
- Constipation: stool and flatus?
- Vomiting: nature of vomitus—faeculent?
- Feeling of abdominal distension or bloatedness
- Previous abdominal surgery
- History of hernia
- Change in bowel habit, weight loss
- Medications

Examination

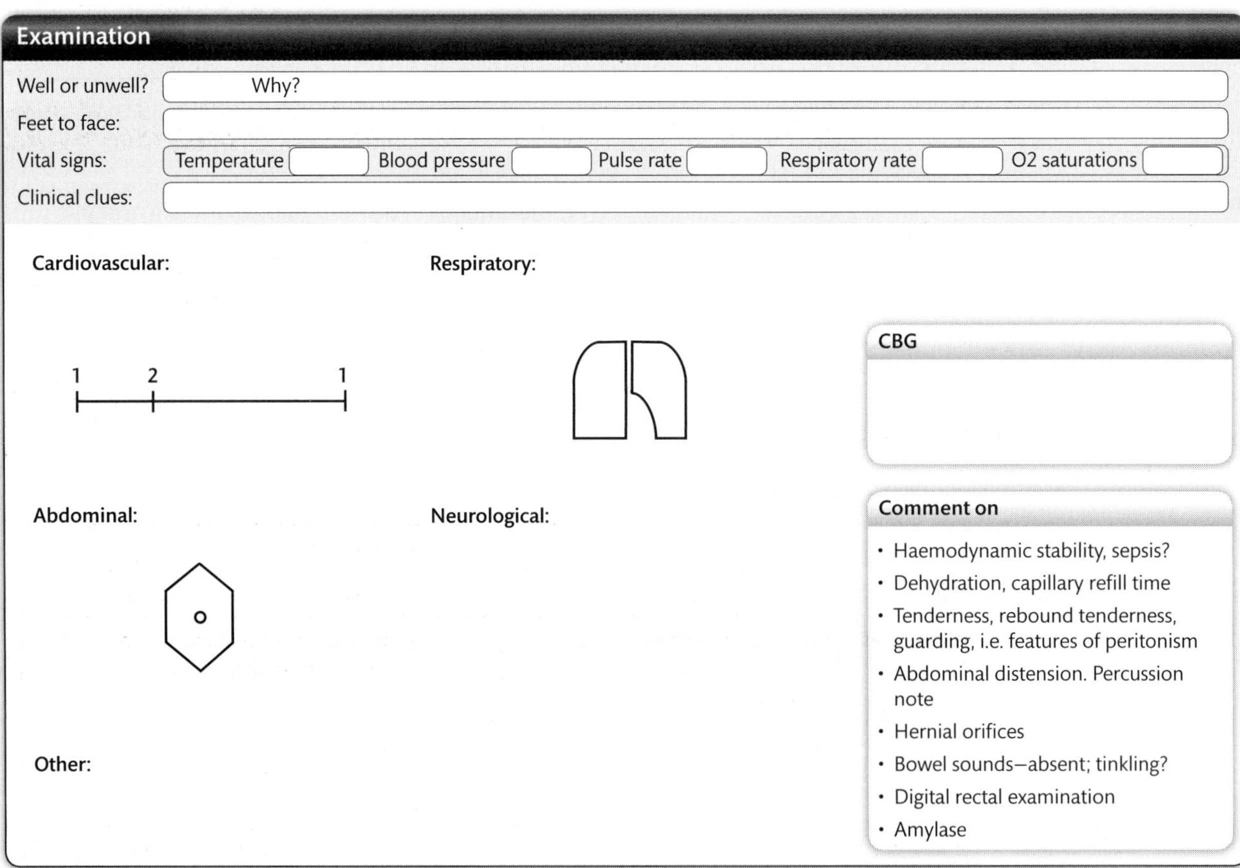
Well or unwell? Why?
Feet to face:
Vital signs: Temperature Blood pressure Pulse rate Respiratory rate O2 saturations
Clinical clues:

Cardiovascular:

Respiratory:

CBG

Abdominal:

Neurological:

Other:

Comment on

- Haemodynamic stability, sepsis?
- Dehydration, capillary refill time
- Tenderness, rebound tenderness, guarding, i.e. features of peritonism
- Abdominal distension. Percussion note
- Hernial orifices
- Bowel sounds—absent; tinkling?
- Digital rectal examination
- Amylase

Blood tests

Comment on

- Evidence of dehydration
- Anaemia?
- Electrolyte imbalance
- Evidence of infection

Abdominal X-ray

Comment on

- Distended small/large bowel
- Thickened bowel wall?
- Faecal loading

Erect chest X-ray

Comment on

- Air under diaphragm?

Arterial blood gas analysis

Comment on

- Metabolic acidosis from dehydration?
- Metabolic alkalosis from vomiting?

Urine output

Comment on

- Should be >0.5 ml/kg/hour

Evaluation

1. **How severely dehydrated is this patient? Is fluid resuscitation indicated?**

2. **Is this patient obstructed or just constipated? What might be causing this?**

High intestinal obstruction	Low intestinal obstruction	Constipation
Vomiting: copious, may contain bile	Vomiting: appears late, may be faeculent	Vomiting: rare. May be nauseous
Constipation: may still pass small amounts of stool for some time	Constipation: complete, to solids and gas	Constipation: intermittent, may pass small-volume hard motions or have 'overflow' diarrhoea
Signs: distended abdomen, generally tender, tympanic to percussion, 'tinkling' bowel sounds	Signs: distended abdomen, generally tender, tympanic to percussion, 'tinkling' bowel sounds	Signs: possibly distended, mildly tender, palpable faecal impaction, sluggish bowel sounds
PR: may be small amount of stool initially, then empty	PR: empty rectum	PR: loaded with stool. May be hard like pellets or mushy
X-ray: dilated small bowel	X-ray: dilated small or large bowel	X-ray: faecal loading

3. **How urgently should surgery be performed?**

4. **What initial management should be instituted?**

Questions

1. A 49-year-old woman presents to hospital complaining of abdominal pain and vomiting which had begun that morning. The pain was felt in the upper and central abdomen and came in waves. She had vomited five times, initially stomach contents and then dark green bile. Her stomach felt bloated. She has no active medical problems. Three years ago she underwent total abdominal hysterectomy for painful fibroids, and 7 years before she had undergone a laparoscopic cholecystectomy. On examination she appeared dehydrated. Her heart rate was 118 bpm and her blood pressure 104/77 mmHg. Her abdomen was distended, generally tender, and produced a note like a drum on percussion, with high pitched active bowel sounds on auscultation. The rectum was empty on digital examination. An abdominal X-ray was performed and is shown below.

(1) What does it show and what are the likely causes?

(2) How should this woman be managed?

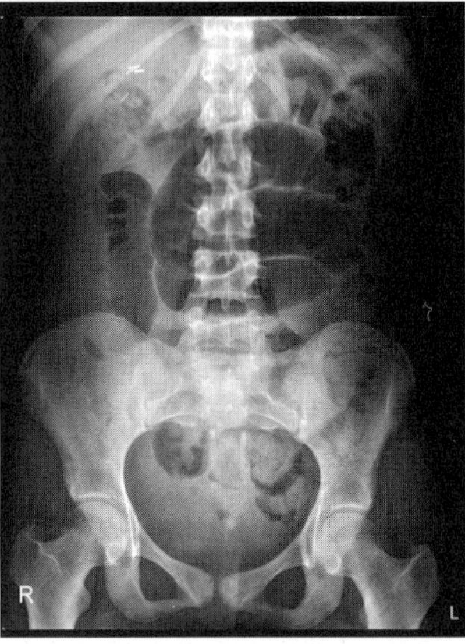

2. A 79-year-old man is referred to hospital by his doctor. He complains of a week-long history of vomiting. He had been diagnosed with a duodenal ulcer a month before after suffering epigastric pain, and had been treated with triple therapy leading to some improvement in his symptoms. For the past week he had been feeling generally well and not nauseous, but had vomited shortly after each meal or whenever he drank fluids. The vomiting was forceful and contained most or all of the meal he had just eaten. Previous medical history included a myocardial infarction and congestive cardiac failure. On examination he is severely dehydrated, with a dry mouth, very decreased skin turgor, no visible jugular venous pressure, and sunken eyes. His abdomen was soft and not tender; however, a succussion splash was heard over the epigastrium. His rectum was empty. Arterial blood gas measurement and basic blood tests were performed, with the results shown below.

pH: 7.64	Sodium: 144 mmol/L
pCO_2: 6.22 kPa	Potassium: 2.1 mmol/L
pO_2: 9.98 kPa	Urea: 28.9 mmol/L
HCO_3^-: 36.6 mmol/L	Creatinine: 166 µmol/L
Base excess: 7.9 mmol/L	Haemoglobin: 17.1 g/dL
Chloride: 88 mmol/L	White cells: 6.6 g/dL
	Platelets: 564 g/dL

(1) What do these test result indicate, and what is the most likely diagnosis?

(2) How should this man be managed?

3. An 82-year-old woman is brought into hospital from a residential home complaining of abdominal pain. Staff at the home report that she has not opened her bowels for 6 days. She also complains of feeling nauseous though she has not actually vomited. Her medical history includes primary hyperparathyroidism, Parkinson's disease, and osteoarthritis, and her regular medication includes co-dydramol and senna. On examination she appears uncomfortable and confused (staff from the nursing home report that this is worse than usual for her). She has an AMTS of 6/10. All basic observations are within normal ranges. Her stomach is soft but tender (especially on the left-hand side). Bowel sounds are present but reduced. Digital rectal examination reveals hard impacted stool in the rectum. Her abdominal X-ray is shown below.

(1) What does the X-ray show?

(2) What are the likely causes of this problem in this particular patient?

(3) How should she be managed?

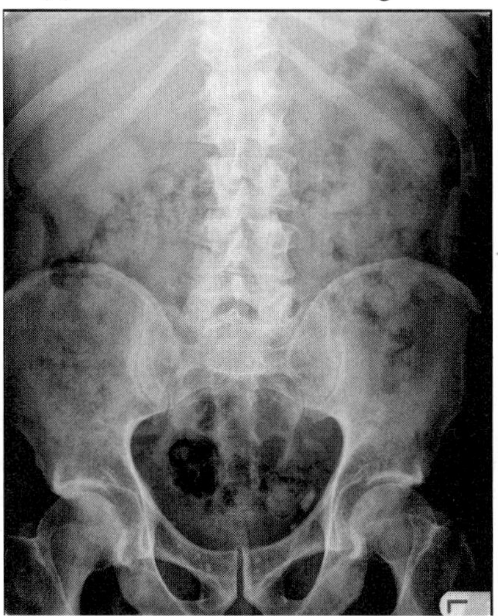

4. A 64-year-old woman is admitted electively for a right hemicolectomy for colorectal carcinoma of the ascending colon. Five days after surgery her bowels have not opened. For the previous 2 days oral feeding has been introduced; however, she has suffered nausea and vomiting and complains of increased abdominal swelling. On examination she has a low-grade fever (temperature 37.8°C) and is slightly tachycardic (108 bpm), but other observations are within normal ranges. Examination of the chest is unremarkable, but the abdomen is slightly distended. There is moderate tenderness around the site of the incision, and the abdomen is quite firm but there is no guarding or other features of peritonism. Bowel sounds are absent. Blood tests reveal normal electrolytes and renal function, and inflammatory markers are not raised. Abdominal X-ray reveals distended loops of both small and large bowel, with a small amount of air visible under the diaphragm.

What are the possible diagnoses, and what would be a sensible course of action?

Remember that you can find large-size, annotated versions of many of the X-rays and ECGs that appear in this book on the book's web site at www.oxfordtextbooks.co.uk/orc/randall/

Answers

1. This X-ray reveals the classic appearances of small bowel obstruction:

There are several features here to explain why this is small bowel obstruction rather than large bowel obstruction:

1. The loops of distented bowel are in the centre rather than the peripheries of the abdomen.
2. The lumen of the bowel is narrower than that of the large bowel.
3. The valvulae conniventes can be seen completely crossing the whole width of the bowel. Colonic haustra do not cross the bowels width.

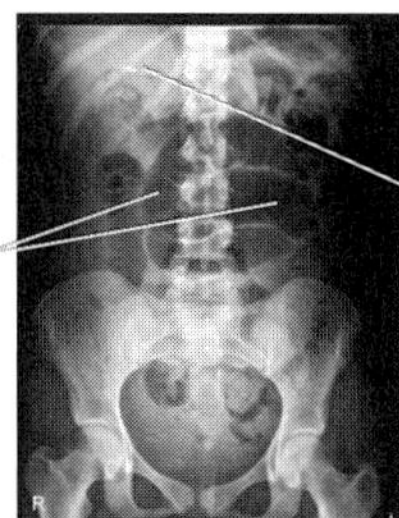

Did you notice the cholecystectomy clips? This operation may have caused intra-abdominal blood loss which has led to the formation of adhesions, which are causing obstruction.

The most common causes for bowel obstruction are listed in the table below:

Small bowel (75%)	Large bowel (25%)
Adhesions (60%)	Cancer (70%)
Hernias (20%)	Diverticular strictures (10%)
Tumours (10%)	Sigmoid volvulus (5%)

This woman is most likely to have adhesional obstruction, secondary to her previous surgery. The examination findings documented above do not include hernial orifices: these should be examined (especially for a small obstructing femoral hernia since these are commoner in women).

Management involves nasogastric drainage, to decompress the upper gastrointestinal tract proximal to the obstruction, and intravenous fluids. Copious amounts of fluid may be secreted into the proximal bowel, leading to hypovolaemia, electrolyte imbalance, and dehydration. Approximately 50% of adhesional obstruction settles with conservative management, though there is a risk of recurrence, which nonetheless increases with each abdominal operation. Surgery is indicated when perforation or strangulation are suspected, or where symptoms do not improve with conservative management.

2. This man has quite pronounced metabolic alkalosis, with a degree of respiratory compensation. A common cause of metabolic alkalosis is acid loss through persistent vomiting. Since gastric acid is hydrochloric acid, regular vomiting results in loss of hydrogen ions (producing alkalosis) and loss of chloride ions (which also contributes to alkalosis). There is also evidence of significant dehydration, due to fluid loss through vomiting and the inability to tolerate oral rehydration. Potassium depletion commonly accompanies gastrointestinal fluid loss, whether through vomiting or diarrhoea, and if severe can produce arrhythmias. His raised haemoglobin and platelets are due to haemoconcentration.

This man's presentation is likely to be due to gastric outflow obstruction. Commonly this occurs where a peptic ulcer in the gastric pylorus or early duodenum heals and produces a fibrotic stricture. A 'succussion splash' can be demonstrated when the examiner auscultates over the epigastrium whilst shaking the patient gently from side to side. The diagnosis is confirmed either by barium meal or by endoscopy. The initial management priority in this man is fluid rehydration and correction of electrolytes, for instance using intravenous saline with added potassium. Gastric outflow obstruction may be treated with endoscopic dilatation, but sometimes surgical reconstruction is needed (for instance, a gastrojejunostomy).

3. The X-ray reveals classic features of constipation:

This abdominal x-ray reveals extensive constipation. This mottled appearance represents faecal impaction, which extends here from the rectum right up through the descending and transverse colon into the ascending colon.

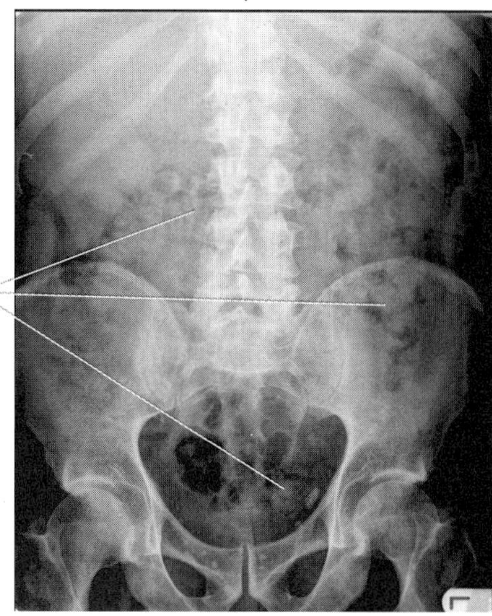

Constipation is an important and often overlooked cause of acute confusion in the elderly. Its incidence rises with age. Factors here which may be contributing to constipation include opiate analgesia (co-codamol), autonomic nervous system dysfunction (which may be present in Parkinson's disease), and electrolyte imbalance (this woman is likely to be hypercalcaemic due to her primary hyperparathyroidism).

Constipation in this woman is best tackled 'from the top and the bottom'—with a combination of oral laxatives and rectal enemas. Glycerine suppositories, or a phosphate enema, along with a stimulant laxative (such as movicol) and possibly a stool softener (such as lactulose) should lead to good resolution. Ideally her opiate analgesia should be changed and her hypercalcaemia addressed. Regular laxatives should prevent this problem recurring.

4. This woman has features consistent with ileus, a form of pseudo-obstruction caused by transient paralysis of the intestine. It is very common after abdominal surgery and usually resolves after 72 hours. It is characterized by constipation, nausea and vomiting, a soft abdomen with no signs of peritonitis, and absent bowel sounds. Common causes which should be looked for include electrolyte imbalances, drugs such as opiates or anti-muscarinics, or retroperitoneal injury.

Other possible causes of this woman's presentation include genuine intestinal obstruction, an anastomotic leak causing localized peritonitis, or an intra-abdominal abscess or collection. She should be managed with close observation, being nil by mouth, nasogastric suction, and intravenous fluid management. Blood tests should be undertaken regularly to observe for trends in inflammatory markers, and biochemical abnormalities. If the symptoms persist, a CT scan or abdominal ultrasound may aid diagnosis.

Further reading

Guidelines: Eastern Association for the Surgery of Trauma small bowel obstruction guidelines (http://www.east.org/tpg/archive/html/sbo.asp)

OHCM: 612–613

Pancreatitis

This section should be used to clerk patients with pancreatitis, which is often a mild illness requiring observation for a few days on a General Surgical Ward, but which may produce very serious disease requiring ITU management and prolonged hospitalization with major complications.

Learning challenges

- Why does disease of the pancreas have the potential to wreak such havoc inside the abdomen?
- Why is cholecystectomy one of the most commonly performed operations in the Western world despite having a significant risk of complications?

History

Comment on

- Careful description of abdominal pain and radiation
- Vomiting, nausea, pallor, sweating
- Previous pancreatitis
- Gallstone disease
- Alcohol
- Drugs

Examination

Well or unwell? Why?

Feet to face:

Vital signs: Temperature Blood pressure Pulse rate Respiratory rate O2 saturations

Clinical clues:

Cardiovascular:

1 2 1

Respiratory:

Abdominal:

Neurological:

Other:

CBG

Comment on

- Haemodynamic stability
- Dehydration
- General appearance, jaundice
- Abdominal tenderness and guarding
- Periumbilical or flank bruising

Blood tests

Comment on

- Amylase
- White cells, CRP, haematocrit
- LFTs—obstructive jaundice?
- Renal function—dehydration?
- Calcium
- Glucose

ECG

Comment on

- Myocardial infarction?

Erect chest X-ray

Comment on

- Air under diaphragm?

Abdominal X-ray

Comment on

- 'Sentinel loop' of small intestine in the upper abdomen

Arterial blood gas

Comment on

- Acidosis, hypoxia

Abdominal ultrasound

Comment on

- Gallstones, dilated common bile duct
- Collections, pseudocyst

Abdominal CT or MRI scan

Comment on

- Confirms diagnosis?

Evaluation

1. **Does this patient have pancreatitis (clinical presentation, amylase)?**

2. **What is the severity? (this scoring system only applies to acute pancreatitis)**

Ranson criteria

At initial presentation	48 hours post-admission:
Age >55 years	Haematocrit falls >10%
White cells >16 g/L	Urea increase of >1.8 mmol/L despite fluids
Blood glucose >10 mmol/L	Calcium <2.0
AST >250 IU/L	pO_2 <6.0
LDH >350 IU/L	Base excess below −4
	Estimated fluid sequestration >6 L

Score < 3, low risk of severe pancreatitis.

Score > 3 – high risk of severe pancreatitis

3. **What is the likely cause?**

4. **Do any of these issues need to be addressed, and how?**

Fluid loss	
Oral intake and nutrition	
Removal of gallstone or other obstruction	
Secondary infection	
Drainage of collections	

5. **Is there evidence of exocrine or endocrine pancreatic insufficiency?**

Questions

1. A 38-year-old man is admitted after becoming acutely unwell that morning. He complains of severe upper abdominal pain which radiates to his back, and has vomited several times. He has never had anything similar before, and has no previous medical history of note. He regularly drinks half a bottle of wine each day (5 units), but the day before had been celebrating a promotion at work and had consumed a lot of alcohol—he estimates around 25–30 units. On examination he is pale and sweaty. His basic observations include temperature 37.8°C, heart rate 126 bpm, blood pressure 103/66 mmHg, respiratory rate 24 breaths/min, and oxygen saturations 95% on room air. His hands feel cool and clammy. Examination of the chest and praecordium is unremarkable, but his abdomen is diffusely tender, with generalized guarding and rigidity. Bowel sounds are absent. Ecchymoses are visible around the umbilicus. ECG is normal. Arterial blood gas analysis reveals a metabolic acidosis with respiratory compensation. Initial blood tests are below. What are the most important steps in managing this patient?

Sodium: 137 mmol/L	Haemoglobin: 12.2 g/dL
Potassium: 4.3 mmol/L	White cells: 18.5 g/dL
Urea: 13.3 mmol/L	Platelets: 231 g/dL
Creatinine: 112 μmol/L	Glucose: 8.3 mmol/L
CRP: 271 mg/L	
Amylase: 4087 IU/dL	

2. A 44-year-old woman with a prior history of biliary colic presents to hospital with upper abdominal pain. She is pyrexial (temperature 38.9°C), sweaty, tachycardic, and has intermittent rigors. The abdomen is tender in the epigastrium and right upper quadrant. Blood tests reveal deranged LFTs, including an alkaline phosphatase of 403 IU/L and serum amylase of 1704 IU/L. An urgent abdominal ultrasound scan is arranged, which reveals a dilated common bile duct and the presence of a 10 mm gallstone in the distal pancreatic duct. An urgent endoscopic retrograde cholangiopancreatogram (ERCP) is arranged. The initial endoscopy reveals a normal upper gastrointestinal tract. The sphincter of Oddi is identified, and a catheter is introduced and contrast instilled into the ampulla of Vater. The image below is obtained.

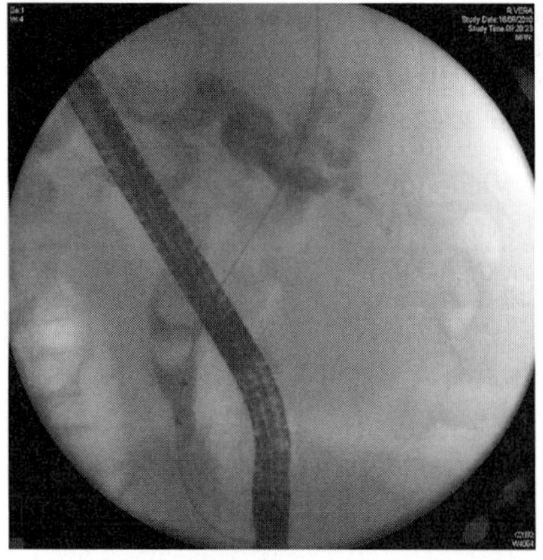

(1) What does it show?

(2) If you were the endoscopist performing the ERCP, what procedure would you now consider performing?

(3) In what ways is the management of gallstone pancreatitis different from the management of pancreatitis of a different cause?

3. A 61-year-old man develops acute abdominal pain after undergoing a diagnostic ERCP. He is diagnosed with severe pancreatitis, and after 3 days of ward-based care is admitted to the hospital's ICU for respiratory and inotropic support. After admission to the ICU the doctors looking after him are concerned to address his nutritional requirements. They discuss with the hospital's gastroenterologists the options for feeding. The gastroenterologists ask about the patient's albumin, phosphate, potassium, calcium, and magnesium levels.

(1) Why are these values important?

(2) What are the options for feeding this man?

4. A 61-year-old man who has suffered with several previous bouts of acute pancreatitis requiring hospital admission visits his GP complaining of a dull epigastric ache which has been troubling him on and off for several months. It radiates to his back and he has noticed that it is exacerbated after drinking alcohol. When the pain is particularly severe he also feels nauseous and frequently vomits. He has also noticed that his stool is always loose, fatty in consistency, and difficult to flush away. He has lost 5 kg in weight over the previous 2 months. Two months earlier he had been diagnosed with diabetes mellitus. He drinks around 40 units of alcohol per week. On examination he is thin and appears malnourished. The abdomen is soft with mild central abdominal tenderness. Basic blood tests, including serum amylase, are normal. What is the likely diagnosis, and how can his symptoms be controlled?

5. A 60-year-old man is admitted to hospital after becoming jaundiced over a short period of time. He had suffered no abdominal pain, no change in bowel habit, and had not been vomiting. He had no other symptoms and otherwise reported feeling well, except for having lost 5 kg in weight over the previous 2 months. There was no previous medical history of note. On examination he appears well but is markedly jaundiced. The abdomen is soft and not tender but a distinct upper abdominal mass in felt. His initial LFTs suggest an obstructive jaundice. What might be an appropriate sequence of investigations to determine the cause of this man's symptoms?

Presentation

Presented to ______ Grade ______ Date ______

Signed

Remember that you can find large-size, annotated versions of many of the X-rays and ECGs that appear in this book on the book's web site at www.oxfordtextbooks.co.uk/orc/randall/

Answers

1. This man almost certainly has acute pancreatitis as evidenced by his history and examination findings. However, an erect chest X-ray should be arranged to exclude perforation of a peptic ulcer (which can also raise the serum amylase, though not usually to this extent). At present he is at the stage where his body is compensating for the pathological changes in his physiology—so he is compensating a metabolic acidosis by increasing his respiratory rate, and is compensating hypovolaemia by increasing his heart rate to maintain blood pressure. If the inflammatory process in his pancreas continues or becomes more severe these compensatory mechanisms will begin to fail and he will become even more unwell.

Initial management has three goals. Firstly to minimize ongoing pancreatic damage—this can be achieved to some extent by making the patient nil by mouth (so that gastrointestinal enzymes stimulating the pancreas are no longer released in response to food), and if the cause is obstructive (e.g. gallstones) by removing the obstruction.

Secondly, optimizing fluid management is essential. Large amounts of fluid can be lost into the peritoneum, either through inflammatory exudation or haemorrhage (in this patient, periumbilical ecchymoses (Cullen's sign), indicate pancreatic haemorrhage into the peritoneum). This patient's urea is raised, indicating that he is already dehydrated. Patients may need up to 6 L of fluid in the first 24 hours after presentation, with fluid balance being guided by central venous pressure and urine output.

Thirdly, this patient needs attention to his symptoms. Non-morphine-based strong analgesia is used (for instance pethidine or tramadol), along with antiemetics and nasogastric suction to relieve nausea. Because of the potential severity of acute pancreatitis, patients with severe disease should be managed on high-dependency or intensive care units.

2. This image, taken during ERCP, shows:

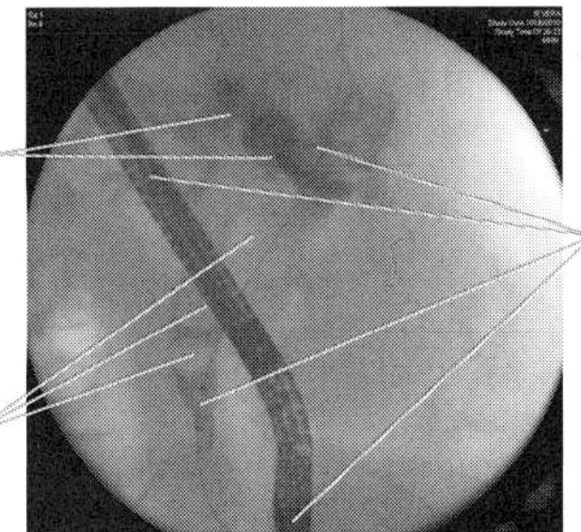

These intra-hepatic bile ducts are dilated, a feature which will be visible on liver ultrasound making it key to diagnosing obstructive jaundice.

Contrast has been injected into the common bile duct and three stones in the distal duct are seen here as filling defects.

A small cannula over a flexible wire is passed into the pancreatic or biliary duct via the ampulla of vater using a side-viewing endoscope. The endoscope itself remains within the duodenum.

A stone causing obstruction of the pancreatic duct may have already passed into the duodenum. An appropriate procedure to perform now would be a sphincterotomy, where a knife or wire is used to create a cut in the sphincter of Oddi to allow a gallstone (or biliary sludge) to drain easily into the duodenum. Complications of this procedure include bleeding from the sphincterotomy wound (which may be severe), localized perforation, and pancreatitis.

All cases of pancreatitis should have abdominal ultrasound, especially where LFTs are abnormal, to exclude an obstructive cause. ERCP with sphincterotomy (or stent insertion if there is a non-gallstone cause of obstruction) is indicated if there is an obstruction, or if the common bile duct is dilated. Gallstone pancreatitis may also warrant early antibiotics, which are not indicated in uncomplicated pancreatitis. This woman may also have an ascending cholangitis (since she has rigors, a high-grade pyrexia, and deranged LFTs), a common companion to gallstone pancreatitis.

3. The reason why these blood tests are important in this man is because he is at significant risk of malnutrition after not having been fed for several days. Malnutrition becomes a serious issue after 5 days without oral intake. Serum **albumin** levels fall in malnutrition, but can also be affected by a number of other factors, including liver disease. In the absence of liver disease, hypoalbuminaemia is a marker of malnutrition. Serum **potassium**, **phosphate**, **magnesium**, and **calcium** levels should always be monitored in malnutrition when a patient is being fed after a period of prolonged starvation, to prevent 'refeeding syndrome'. This syndrome occurs due to recommencement of cellular metabolism on refeeding, leading to rapid intracellular shifts in electrolytes, causing serum levels to drop. If not corrected, this can lead to multiorgan failure and death.

An important component of the management of pancreatitis is restricting oral intake (making the patient 'nil by mouth')—this serves to reduce stimulation of the pancreas which normally occurs in response to eating. A patient with severe pancreatitis may need to remain nil by mouth for weeks or months until the inflammation has subsided, and addressing nutritional requirements is mandatory. One option is total parenteral nutrition (TPN), where patients receive a sterile nutrition infusion through a peripheral or central venous catheter. However, this carries a high risk of infection if continued for prolonged periods. Another option is to feed enterally, but bypassing the stomach and duodenum, using a naso-jejunal tube (inserted endoscopically). This is generally preferred in pancreatitis since it eliminates the infection risks associated with total parenteral nutrition.

4. This patient has chronic pancreatitis. Chronic pancreatitis may develop after recurrent episodes of acute pancreatitis. The commonest cause is alcohol. It is characterized by constant (or recurrent) severe abdominal pain with vomiting, as well as failure of both endocrine pancreatic function (hormone production) and exocrine pancreatic function (digestive enzymes). The patient may lose weight, develop diabetes (with difficult glycaemic control due to failure of both insulin and glucagon production), and have chronic steatorrhoea due to intestinal malabsorption. The mainstay of treatment is with replacement of pancreatic enzymes (for instance, Creon preparations), as well as insulin, analgesia, and antiemetics.

5. Painless obstructive jaundice should raise the suspicion of pancreatic cancer, especially in the context of weight loss and an upper abdominal mass. This patient requires urgent radiological investigation of his upper abdomen, either by abdominal ultrasonography followed by CT scanning or by proceeding directly to CT scanning. MRI is also often used for investigation of biliary disease, with magnetic resonance cholangiopancreatography (MRCP) increasingly replacing ERCP for diagnostic purposes, to reduce the risks from instrumentation (especially pancreatitis) due to ERCP. If imaging suggests a pancreatic tumour then histological confirmation can be obtained by biopsy at ERCP. Endoscopic ultrasound may also be used to define the extent of any tumour and the presence of lymphadenopathy. Pancreatic tumours often produce few symptoms until they are very large, by which time they are often inoperable. Palliative procedures such as biliary stenting (performed at ERCP) may improve quality of life by allowing bile to drain and relieving the symptoms of jaundice such as severe itching.

Further reading

Guidelines: UK Working Party on Acute Pancreatitis guidelines on the management of acute pancreatitis (http://www.bsg.org.uk/pdf_word_docs/pancreatic.pdf)

OHCM: 280, 636–639

Hernias

This section should be used to clerk patients undergoing hernia repair. This is often done as an out-patient when patients can be found in hospital day stay units, though sometimes patients are admitted acutely to a General Surgical Ward if they develop complications such as obstruction or strangulation.

Learning challenges

- What is the embryology of the testicle? Revise the anatomy of the spermatic cord and the different layers acquired from the anterior abdominal wall. What defines the inguinal canal?
- What are the advantages and disadvantages of laparoscopic hernia repair, and how is this achieved?

History

Comment on

- Duration of hernia
- Tenderness or skin changes over the lump
- Can the patient reduce the hernia? What makes it come out again?
- Symptoms of bowel obstruction, e.g. vomiting, absolute constipation, absence of flatus
- Risk factors—heavy lifting, chronic cough, urinary obstruction, chronic constipation, previous hernia
- Fitness for surgery

Examination

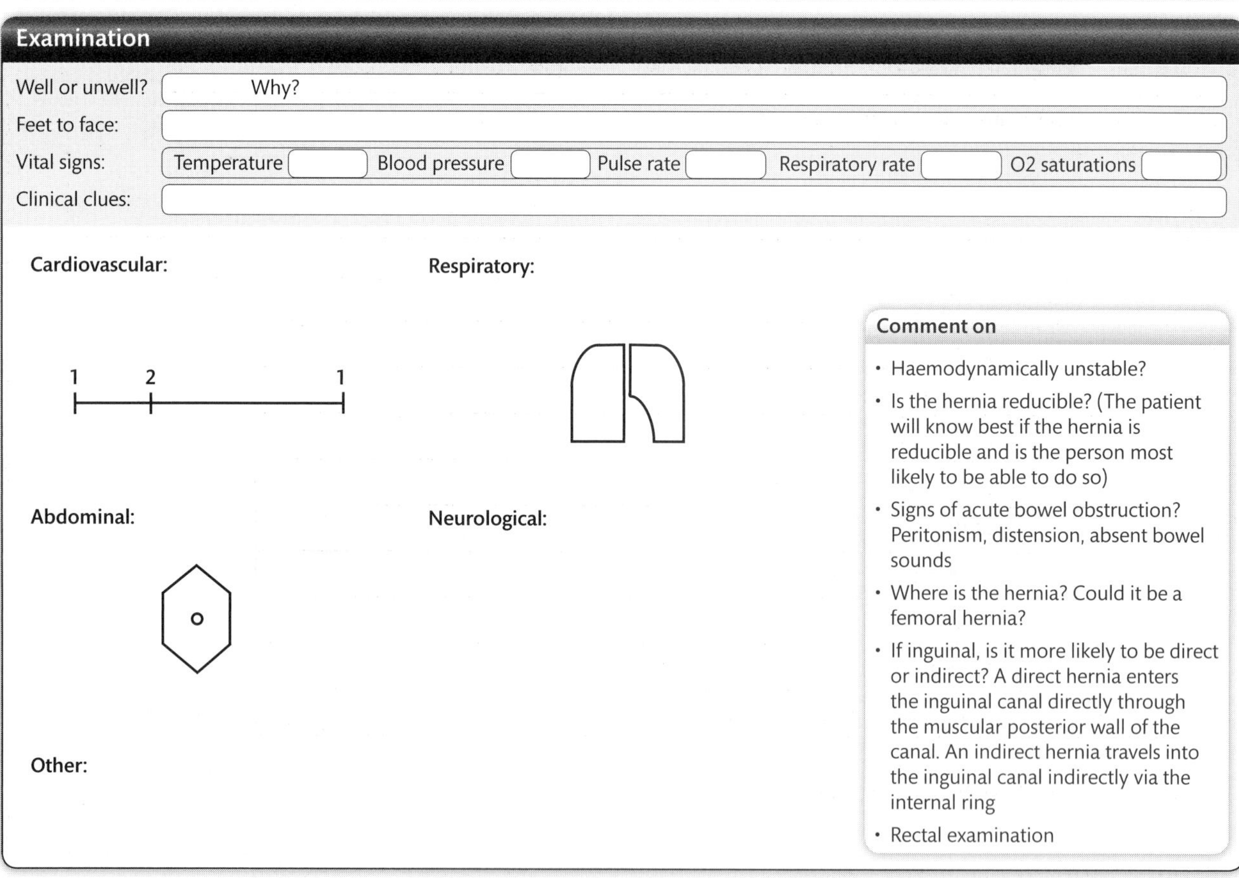

Comment on

- Haemodynamically unstable?
- Is the hernia reducible? (The patient will know best if the hernia is reducible and is the person most likely to be able to do so)
- Signs of acute bowel obstruction? Peritonism, distension, absent bowel sounds
- Where is the hernia? Could it be a femoral hernia?
- If inguinal, is it more likely to be direct or indirect? A direct hernia enters the inguinal canal directly through the muscular posterior wall of the canal. An indirect hernia travels into the inguinal canal indirectly via the internal ring
- Rectal examination

Abdominal X-ray

Comment on

- Signs of bowel obstruction

Blood tests

Comment on
- Dehydration, renal function
- Inflammatory markers—evidence of strangulation
- Clotting
- Group and save sent?

Arterial blood gas

Comment on
- Metabolic acidosis

Operative report

Comment on
- Findings
- Method of fixation
- Skin closure used
- Post-operative plan

Evaluation

1. **Is this patient haemodynamically stable? Do they require fluid resuscitation?**

2. **Is this lump in the groin (or elsewhere) definitely a hernia? Have other possibilities been excluded?**

Other conditions which may mimic inguinal hernias
- Lymphadenopathy
- Femoral artery aneurysm
- Abscess

3. **How would you classify this hernia?**

Site	Inguinal: direct or indirect
	Femoral
	Incisional
	Umbilical/paraumbilical
	Other
Other	Reducible
	Irreducible (incarcerated)
	Strangulated (blood supply compromised)
	Obstructed (obstructed bowel)

4. **Is this patient a good candidate for operative repair?**

5. **Have all preoperative requirements been met?**

- Consent gained [ ]
- Area marked [ ]
- Blood tests (may include G&S, clotting) [ ]
- Nil by mouth for 6 hours [ ]

Questions

1. An 18-year-old man is admitted for elective repair of an inguinal hernia. He first noticed it when he was 12 years old but decided at the time not to have it operated on because he was afraid of undergoing surgery. He is feeling well, opened his bowels that morning and has no nausea, vomiting, or abdominal pain. He has no other medical problems and is at college studying law. On examination he has a reducible right-sided inguinal hernia. Reduction can be maintained by pressure over the deep inguinal ring, which when released whilst the patient is standing up causes the hernial contents to descend down into the patients scrotum. Both testis are easily palpated and are non-tender, and the skin over the hernia sac appears normal and is non-tender.

(1) How would you classify this hernia?

(2) Why do children develop these hernias?

(3) What other risk factors are there for developing inguinal hernia?

2. A 90-year-old man is referred to surgical out-patients for advice on management of an inguinal hernia. The hernia had been noticed by staff at the residential care home where he is living. It is unclear for how long it had been present. The patient has a history of ischaemic heart disease with congestive cardiac failure, type 2 diabetes, and a previous fractured neck of femur. He mobilizes indoors with a frame and requires help with dressing, but is fully continent and can feed himself. He has mild to moderate cognitive impairment. Examination reveals a large direct inguinal hernia in a well-looking elderly man. The hernia can be fully reduced on lying down with gentle pressure over the sac, but recurs immediately when the patient stands up and pressure over the groin is released. What factors should influence the decision-making process about the best management of this hernia?

3. Whilst attached to a general surgical team, you (a medical student) are asked by one of the surgeons to audit the hospital's performance in implementing prophylaxis against venous thromboembolism in patients admitted for elective hernia repair. She directs you to guidelines from the National Institute of Health and Clinical Excellence (NICE) on the subject (available from http://www.nice.org.uk/guidance/index.jsp?action=byID&o=12695), where two key criteria for good practice in patients admitted for gastrointestinal surgery are: (1) placing all patients on mechanical thromboembolism prophylaxis (e.g. compression stockings) and (2) assessing all patients for their risk of bleeding before considering anticoagulation (e.g. prophylactic dose of low-molecular-weight heparin).

(1) How would you begin to perform this audit?

(2) What is the 'cycle of audit'?

(3) How is audit different from research? Will this project require ethical approval?

Presentation

Presented to ______ Grade ______ Date ______

Signed

Answers

1. This patient is likely to have an indirect inguinal hernia. It is fully reducible, with no signs of incarceration (another term for irreducibility), bowel obstruction, or strangulation (loss of blood supply producing ischaemia and necrosis).

Direct inguinal hernias occur when abdominal contents traverse the deep inguinal ring, and travel with the spermatic cord in the inguinal canal. The hernia sac is formed from the remnants of the processus vaginalis, an embryological structure allowing the testis to descend from the abdominal cavity into the scrotum before birth. This normally obliterates, but may remain patent predisposing some patients to the development of inguinal hernias.

Direct hernias tend to affect older patients. The hernia pierces the muscle that forms the posterior wall of the inguinal canal (it does not pass through the internal ring). Anatomically, direct hernias originate medial to the inferior epigastric vessels while indirect hernias originate lateral to them. This fact may be used to attempt to differentiate the two by seeing if reduction of a hernia can be maintained by pressure over the internal inguinal ring. This is, however, often unreliable.

Both types of hernia are associated with activities or physical illnesses that lead to repeated increases in intra-abdominal pressure—for instance heavy lifting, straining at stool (in constipation), or recurrent coughing. After hernias are repaired efforts should be made to address the risk factors (e.g. by changing job) to avoid recurrence.

In practice, the difference is of little clinical significance as patients with hernias of either type will benefit from their repair in the same way. The difference between a direct and an indirect inguinal hernia may only be apparent during the operation, when the defect is seen under direct vision. Although various techniques are practised, the defect is closed and a prosthetic mesh is generally applied over the area to prevent recurrence. Many hernias are repaired laparoscopically with good outcomes and low rates of recurrence.

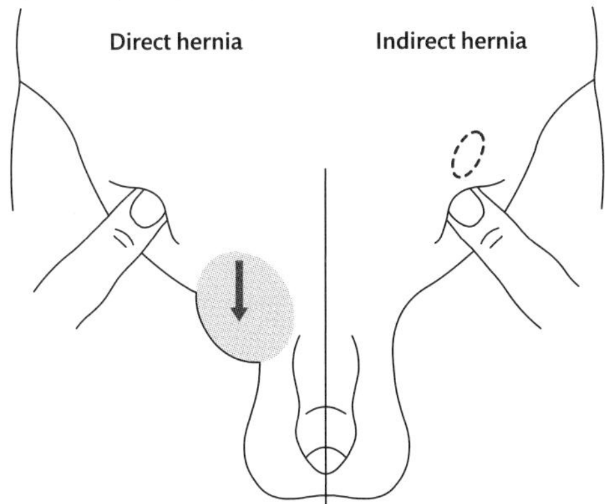

On both sides, the examiner is applying pressure over the deep inguinal ring

2. Surgery can be hazardous, especially in the elderly, and making decisions about the best course of action can be challenging. A key principle of medical ethics is encapsulated in the Latin phrase *primum non nocere*—first do no harm. The benefits of surgery to each patient must be balanced with the possible risks, and the likelihood of complications occurring. The pre-operative morbidity must be carefully considered, and in this patient the risks of complications at surgery would be significantly increased by his history of ischaemic heart disease, heart failure, and diabetes. Even though there is a risk that his inguinal hernia may worsen symptomatically, or even strangulate, it appears that he is relatively comfortable living with the hernia, and a conservative approach may be better advised. A truss, or support, can be provided which keeps the hernia reduced and may prevent further problems.

Of course, should this man be seen in the emergency setting with an obstructed or strangulated hernia the decision must be tackled again. In spite of his pre-morbid conditions, surgery in this instance may be life saving and the argument for advising surgery is compelling. However, in cases where the pre-morbid quality of life is poor, and the likelihood of surgery leading to a good outcome is low, a palliative approach may be considered, with close communication with family and all the medical teams involved.

Anaesthetists use the ASA (American Society of Anesthesiologists) scoring system to help stratify risk according to pre-operative morbidity (reproduced below). At present this patient is ASA physical status 3; were he to come in as an emergency with intestinal obstruction secondary to his hernia then he would be ASA physical status 5E.

Physical Status 1 (PS-1)	A normal healthy patient
Physical Status 2 (PS-2)	A patient with mild systemic disease
Physical Status 3 (PS-3)	A patient with severe systemic disease
Physical Status 4 (PS-4)	A patient with severe systemic disease that is a constant threat to life
Physical Status 5 (PS-5)	A moribund patient who is not expected to survive without the operation
Physical Status 6 (PS-6)	A declared brain-dead patient whose organs are being removed for donor purposes

'E' is added to the status (e.g. PS-4E) if the operation is being carried out as an emergency.

3. Audit is very different from research. The classic research technique evaluates new ways of managing patients (for instance, a new surgical technique for hernia repair), comparing the new treatment with the existing gold standard in a randomized controlled trial. In contrast, audit assesses how well an existing treatment is being delivered. Audit does not require ethical approval whilst research does (though audits should be registered with the hospital's research and audit department). Audit is all about improving standards of care, and is an important part of clinical medicine. There are several stages involved in the cycle of audit (see below):

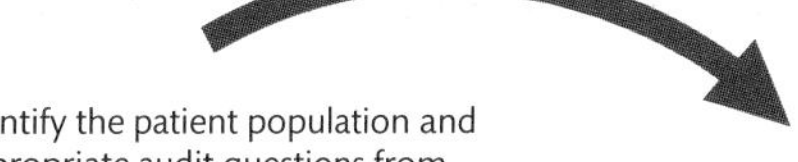

1. Identify the patient population and appropriate audit questions from widely accepted guidelines for the management of that condition. In this case the audit population might be all patients admitted for hernia repair within the last six months, and appropriate questions from the NICE guidelines may be (a) prescription of mechanical thromboembolism prophylaxis to all patients, (b) documentation of a thromboembolism and bleeding risk assessment, with appropriate prescription or pharmacological thromboembolism prophylaxis, and (c) adherence to prescribed prophylaxis - whether or not stockings are actually worn and anticoagulation is actually given.
2. Gather data and analyse them to answer the audit questions. Request notes from the hospital's medical records department for all patients to be included. Fill in a proforma for each patient assessing whether each outcome was achieved. Put the information from all proformas into a spread-sheet and analyse the data.

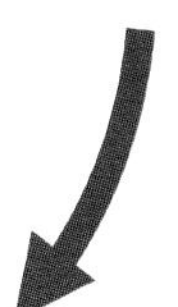

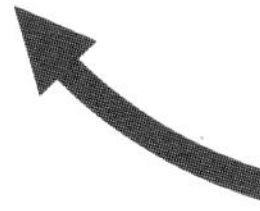

3. Assess the performance of the department and publicize the results, identifying areas for improvement. Which outcomes are being met, and which can be improved upon? Perhaps compression stockings are being prescribed on drug charts, but not actually being put on patients by nursing staff? Perhaps a bleeding risk assessment is not being carried out, and so no patients are receiving pharmacological thrombo-embolism prophylaxis? Present the findings at a departmental meeting and discuss changes to implement. After implementation, repeat the audit to see if there are improvements in the performance of the department as a result of the changes suggested.

Further reading

Guidelines: NICE technology assessment for laparoscopic repair of inguinal hernias (http://guidance.nice.org.uk/TA83)

OHCM: 614-617

Colorectal carcinoma

This section should be used to clerk patients with suspected or confirmed colorectal carcinoma at any stage of their disease. Patients are initially referred urgently to a colorectal surgery clinic (as out-patients) for rapid endoscopy or sometimes present acutely to hospital with intestinal obstruction or rectal bleeding. Post-operative patients can commonly be found on general surgical wards.

Learning challenges

- What do the terms 'well differentiated', 'poorly differentiated', and 'anaplastic' refer to when describing the histology of colon cancers?
- How might colorectal cancer demonstrate (1) direct invasion, (2) lymphatic spread, (3) haematogenous spread, and (4) transcoelomic spread?

History

Comment on

- Altered bowel habit—looser, more frequent stool or pain on defaecation; tenesmus—feeling of incomplete voiding after defaecation
- Rectal bleeding—identify clearly what the patient has experienced
- Mucus with stool
- Weight loss
- Symptoms of anaemia
- Family history of bowel cancer
- Smoking

Examination

Well or unwell? Why?

Feet to face:

Vital signs: Temperature | Blood pressure | Pulse rate | Respiratory rate | O2 saturations

Clinical clues:

Cardiovascular:

1 2 1

Respiratory:

Abdominal:

Neurological:

Other:

Comment on

- Signs of bowel obstruction
- Cachexia, pallor
- Masses on abdominal palpation
- Hepatomegaly
- Digital rectal examination: masses, blood, mucus

Blood tests

Comment on

- Anaemia, microcytosis
- Deranged liver function
- Hypercalcaemia

Colonoscopy

Comment on

- Was complete examination to caecum possible?
- Masses
- Polyps
- Patency of lumen

Abdominal CT

Comment on

- Site of tumour
- Signs of local invasion
- Lymphadenopathy
- Distant metastases (commonly liver and lung)

Histology

Comment on

- Tumour type
- Degree of differentiation
- Degree of bowel wall invasion

Evaluation

1. Does this patient have colorectal cancer? What kind of tumour is it and where is it located?

2. What is the staging? (use either Duke's classification or the TNM system)

Duke's staging system	TNM staging system
• **Stage A:** Tumour confined to bowel wall • **Stage B:** Tumour invades through bowel wall • **Stage C:** Local lymph nodes involved • **Stage D:** distant metastases For example 'Duke's C disease'	• **Tumour:** Confined to submucosa (T1), invades muscle (T2), invades subserosa (T3), breaches peritoneum (T4) • **Nodes:** No lymphadenopathy (N0), three or fewer nodes involved (N1), four or more nodes involved (N2) • **Metastases:** No distant metastases (M0), metastases present (M1) For example 'T2, N0, M0' or 'T4, N2, M1'

3. What is the intention of treatment (curative or palliative)? What surgical approach should be used if surgery is possible? Should chemotherapy be offered?

4. How can this patient be helped to cope with their diagnosis? Think about pain relief, troubling symptoms, emotional and spiritual support, and, if relevant, help with stomas.

Questions

1. A 64-year-old man attends his doctor complaining of diarrhoea. When the doctor takes a careful history, the patient complains of passing loose stool two to three times per day for the past 6 weeks, where previously he opened his bowels every other day. He has occasionally noticed streaks of blood on the surface of the stool. He does not regularly monitor his weight, but when pressed, said that he thinks that his clothes feel looser now than they have recently. Examination, including rectal examination, is unremarkable. Blood tests reveal a low haemoglobin (10.2 g/dL) with a slight microcytosis (MCV 75 fL), with no other abnormalities. He is referred for colonoscopy, where a 7 cm diameter area of ulceration causing luminal narrowing is discovered in the lower descending colon. Two small polyps are discovered (one at the splenic flexure and the other in the ascending colon), both of which are removed endoscopically, and the ulcerated lesion is biopsied. He is reviewed in the out-patient department by one of the hospital's colorectal surgeons, who reviews the histology report on the biopsy specimens received (reproduced below).

(1) What steps should be taken next in managing this man?

(2) What is the significance of the colonic polyps discovered, and how are they related to the formation of malignant disease?

Department of Histopathology
Biopsy report
Specimens received:
Specimen A: 2 cm pedunculated polyp from ascending colon
Specimen B: biopsy of sessile polyp from distal transverse colon
Specimens C and D: biopsy specimens from ulcerated area in distal descending colon

Clinical details: altered bowel habit, blood in stool, weight loss

Histological findings:
Specimens A and B both reveal mucosal hyperplasia with no evidence of malignancy or ulceration.
Specimens C and D reveal malignant changes in keeping with signet ring cell adenocarcinoma. The tumour is moderately differentiated with evidence of vascular invasion. It invades through the muscularis mucosa into the subserosa though no evidence is seen of breach of the visceral peritoneum.

2. A 55-year-old woman presents to the Emergency Department with a brisk bleed of fresh blood from her rectum. The patient remains systemically well and no transfusion is required. A rigid sigmoidoscopy is performed, where an irregular growth with evidence of fresh bleeding is discovered in the upper part of her rectum. She is subsequently diagnosed with a well-differentiated signet cell adenocarcinoma, which is staged as T2, N0, M0 (Duke's A). Imaging of her abdomen does not reveal evidence of any local invasion, lymphadenopathy, or distant spread. She has no other medical problems and is considered fit for surgery. A plan is made to perform an anterior resection with primary anastomosis and formation of a defunctioning loop ileostomy.

(1) What does this mean?

(2) Complete the table below defining the terminology used to describe surgical procedures used for colorectal cancer.

Term used	Definition
End colostomy	
Defunctioning ileostomy	
Primary anastomosis	
Reversal of ileostomy	
Hartmann's procedure	
Abdominal perineal ('AP') resection	
Anterior resection	
Hemicolectomy	
Hartman's procedure	
Lymphadenectomy	

3. A 34-year-old man presents to his GP complaining of difficulty in passing faeces. He complains of anal pain on defaecation, streaks of blood on the surface of stool, and of fresh blood which drips into the toilet pan and on the toilet paper after defaecation. He is currently extremely uncomfortable because he has not opened his bowels for 4 days because of fear of pain. The problem has been developing for 3 weeks. He is extremely worried about the symptoms because his father contracted bowel cancer aged 67.

(1) What are the likely causes of his symptoms?

(2) What would be a sensible way to proceed in managing this man?

4. A 59-year-old woman is referred for an urgent colonoscopy after she presents to her GP reporting an episode of rectal bleeding. The blood was dark red and clotted and trickled out for around 10 minutes after she passed stool. She estimated that around one small cup (200 ml) of blood was passed. She was otherwise well, with no change in bowel habit and no change in weight. Blood tests ruled out anaemia. Based on her symptoms, a flexible sigmoidoscopy was performed, and the colon visualized as far as the splenic flexure. Several large diverticula were seen, one with a prominent submucosal blood vessel visible. Histology revealed no evidence of malignancy or of bowel wall inflammation.

(1) What is diverticular disease and what other clinical presentations might it cause?

(2) What options exist for visualizing the lower gastrointestinal tract?

Answers

1. This man has confirmed colorectal cancer. The urgent priority is to stage the cancer so that treatment can be planned. So far the patient can be confirmed to have at least T3 disease (or Duke's C disease), based on histological evidence of subserosal invasion. Vascular invasion may suggest metastatic spread, but to prove this requires a CT scan of the chest, abdomen, and pelvis. The particular focus will be on the presence of lymphadenopathy and metastases in the liver or lung. The CT scan below shows multiple liver metastases. Curative surgery is not possible if the tumour is locally invasive (for instance, if a rectal tumour invades the sacrum) or if it is widely metastatic. A single metastasis to the liver or lung which can be fully excised does not prohibit surgery with curative intent.

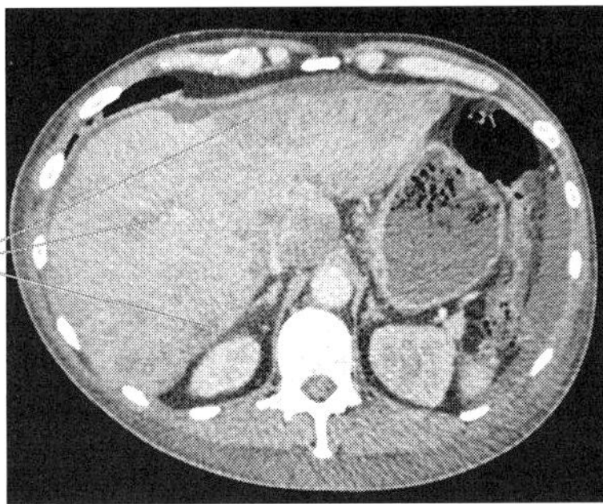

The key abnormality here is the presence of multiple low intensity lesions within the liver. Given the patient's history the likely diagnosis is metastases, however if the nature of these lesions were in doubt (e.g. if there was only a single, small lesion), then liver biopsy could be used to obtain a diagnosis. The fact that these metastases are throughout the liver precludes operability.

Adenocarcinomas are by far the commonest form of cancer affecting the colon and rectum. They are classified according to their histological appearance (signet ring, mucinous, anaplastic) and according to their degree of differentiation—well, moderately, and poorly differentiated, with poorly differentiated tumours carrying a poor prognosis. There is a well-described progression from normal bowel mucosa through benign adenoma formation with increasing dysplasia until frank cancer develops. Benign adenomas may appear as pedunculated or sessile polyps at colonoscopy, and are biopsied to assess the level of dysplasia, i.e. how close they are to malignant transformation.

2. This cancer is potentially curable with complete excision. The operation described here involves removing the upper rectum via a lower abdominal wall incision, joining the two ends together (with staples or conventional sutures), and then bringing out a loop of small intestine to defunction, or 'rest' the newly created join. A good working knowledge of the terminology used in colorectal cancer is required for all doctors:

Term used	Definition
End colostomy	An end -ostomy is where part of the bowel (in this case the colon) is brought out through the skin via a stoma, with what is left of the bowel distal to this being sewn shut
Defunctioning loop ileostomy	A loop, in this case of small bowel, is brought out through the skin so that faeces do not travel through the bowel distal to this—usually to protect a primary anastomosis whilst it heals
Primary anastomosis	After a section of bowel is resected, the two cut ends are rejoined. These are prone to 'anastomotic leak', especially in the rectum, and so are often 'defunctioned' with a proximal loop ileostomy
Reversal of ileostomy	A subsequent procedure, where a loop ileostomy or colostomy is closed and the bowel sutured shut, or an end ileostomy or colostomy is joined onto what is left of the distal bowel
Hartmann's procedure	Resection of the rectosigmoid colon with closure of the rectal stump and formation of a colostomy. This colostomy can later be reversed ('reversal of Hartmann's')
Abdominal peroneal ('AP') resection	For tumours in the lower rectum. Working from both abdominal and peroneal incisions, the whole of the rectum and anus is removed and an end colostomy created
Anterior resection	For tumours high in the rectum. Working from an abdominal incision, the tumour is resected and a primary anastomosis formed, often with a loop ileostomy to protect the join
Hemicolectomy	Removal of half of the colon—either a right hemicolectomy for ascending/ proximal transverse colon tumour, or a left hemicolectomy for distal transverse or descending colon tumours. Often with an end ileostomy (which can later be reversed), or primary anastomosis and defunctioning loop ileostomy
Lymphadenectomy	Extensive dissection with removal of local lymph nodes—essential in a 'cancer operation'.

3. Fresh blood passed rectally, with blood on the toilet paper or dripping into the pan and anal pain, is suggestive of anal pathology. Common causes for this man's symptoms include haemorrhoids, an anal fissure (tear), or a first presentation of inflammatory bowel disease (e.g. ulcerative colitis). Digital examination of the rectum should easily differentiate these, though if no obvious cause can be found then referral for further investigations may be necessary. Haemorrhoids are managed initially with steroid-containing creams, local anaesthetic topical preparations, and with band therapy or surgical excision if symptoms continue. Anal fissures are extremely painful and are often helped by stool softeners and rectal nitrate cream (producing anal dilatation) to reduce further damage on defaecation and promote healing. Despite a positive family history, colorectal cancer is unlikely in this man because of his age. However, if there is no evidence on examination of perianal disease, or if his symptoms fail to settle with the management outlined above, then referral for colonoscopy may be appropriate.

4. Diverticula are outpouchings in the bowel wall and develop with age due to collagen breakdown. They are highly prevalent and usually asymptomatic. Common presentations relating to diverticula include:

- acute diverticulitis—where a diverticulum becomes inflamed and infected, presenting with left iliac fossa pain, tenderness, peritonism, and evidence of acute inflammation,
- rectal bleeding,
- stricture formation which can lead to intestinal obstruction,
- perforation and abscess formation.

The disease itself is managed by recommending a high-fibre diet. Acute diverticulitis usually settles with intravenous antibiotics. Bowel resection is generally reserved for cases with recurrent symptoms or perforation.

Proctoscopes are 15 cm long and are useful for investigating disease of the anal canal and lower rectum, for example allowing elastic bands to be placed over haemorrhoids. A rigid sigmoidoscope is 30 cm long and allows visualization of the whole rectum and lower sigmoid colon. A flexible sigmoidoscope functions like a conventional endoscope, and can be inserted up to 1 m from the anus, allowing visualization and biopsy of left-sided colonic lesions. A colonoscope can visualize the whole colon (up to 2 m), and a full colonoscopy should include examination of the terminal ileum.

Further reading

Guidelines: NICE colorectal cancer guidelines (http://guidance.nice.org.uk/CSGCC)

OHCM: 618–619, 630–634

Lumps and bumps

This section should be used either to clerk patients being investigated for lumps of unknown origin that are suspicious for serious disease, who may commonly be seen in surgical out-patient clinics (e.g. general surgery or ear, nose, and throat surgery clinics), or to clerk patients having lumps and bumps removed who often undergo minor surgical procedures as out-patients in hospital day-stay units.

Learning challenges

- What is the difference between a cyst and an abscess, and between a fistula and a sinus?
- Describe the operative steps involved in removing a suspected lipoma

History

Comment on

- Duration
- Changes over time; skin changes; discharge
- Pain, symptoms related to neighbouring structures
- History of trauma or previous disease at this site
- General health
- Social history including HIV risk factors/sexual history/foreign travel

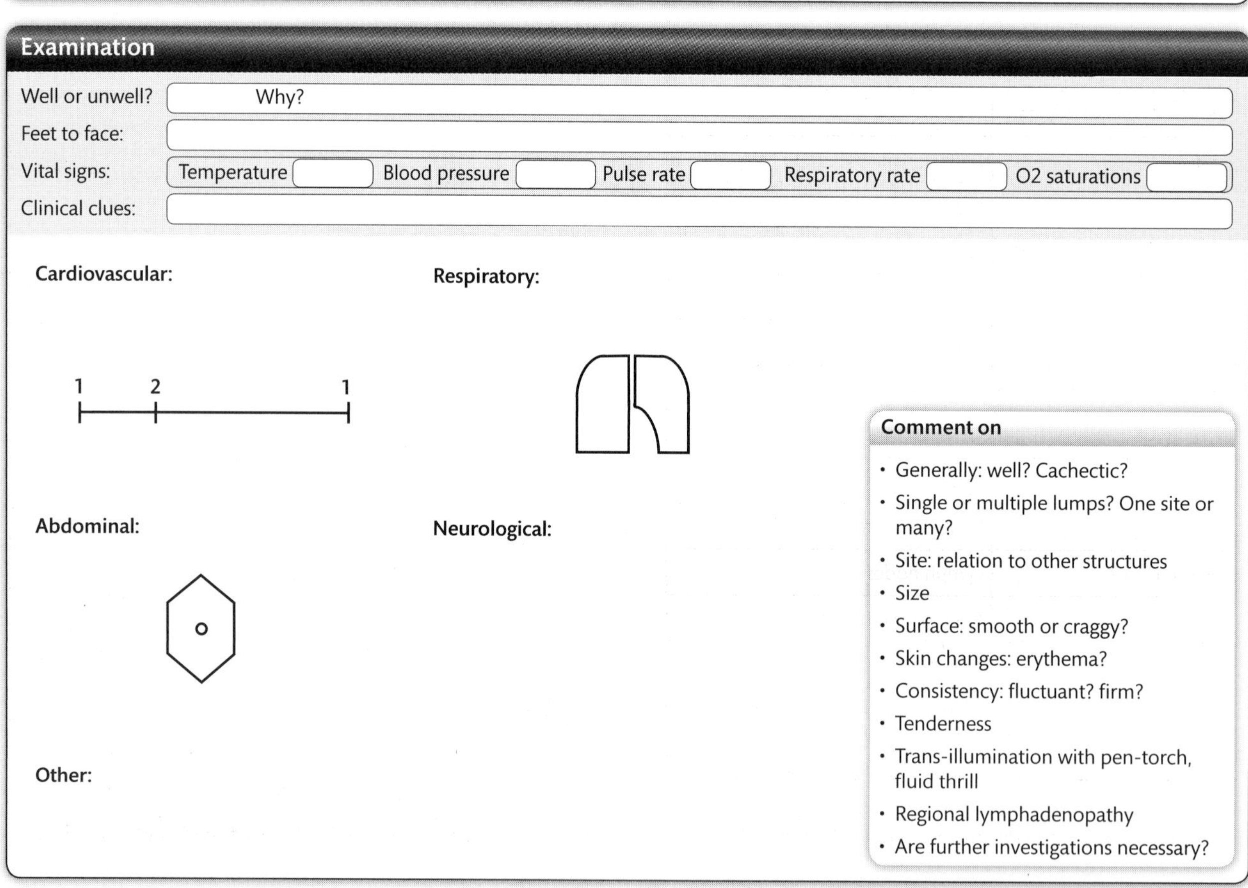

Examination

Well or unwell? Why?

Feet to face:

Vital signs: Temperature | Blood pressure | Pulse rate | Respiratory rate | O2 saturations

Clinical clues:

Cardiovascular:

1 2 1

Respiratory:

Abdominal:

Neurological:

Other:

Comment on

- Generally: well? Cachectic?
- Single or multiple lumps? One site or many?
- Site: relation to other structures
- Size
- Surface: smooth or craggy?
- Skin changes: erythema?
- Consistency: fluctuant? firm?
- Tenderness
- Trans-illumination with pen-torch, fluid thrill
- Regional lymphadenopathy
- Are further investigations necessary?

Ultrasound

Comment on

- Solid or cystic?
- Anatomical relations

8 Surgery

CT or MRI

Comment on

- Involvement of local structures
- Other lumps, metastatic spread, primary cancers
- Is this lump resectable?

Aspiration cytology

Comment on

- Nature of cells. Malignant cells?

Biopsy/excision biopsy

Comment on

- Tissue classification
- Malignant? Complete excision? Invasion of other tissues?

Evaluation

1. **What is the likely nature of this lump?**

Type	Example
Congenital/embryological	
Malignant	Primary (e.g. lymphoma)
	Metastatic
Structural	Hernias
	Hydrocoele
	Duct blockage
Infective	Abscesses
	Tuberculosis
	Parasitic
	Secondary infection
Inflammatory	Lymph nodes
	Rheumatoid nodules
Vascular	Aneurysm
	Arteriovenous malformation
Calcification	

2. **Considering the location of this lump, what important differential diagnoses need to be considered? Can these be confidently excluded?**

3. **Is there likely to be significant underlying disease responsible for producing this lump? How should this be managed, and by whom?**

4. **Can the lump be safely excised? What are the patient's wishes? Have the risks and benefits of surgery been well explained to them?**

Questions

1. A 23-year-old air steward presents to her doctor to complain about a lump on her forehead, just above her left eyebrow. She has noticed it growing gradually for a number of months, during which time it has not caused her any pain or other symptoms, except for looking unsightly. Examination reveals a single 8 mm diameter well circumscribed spherical lump which feels smooth and firm. The skin overlying it is not erythematous, but contains a small punctum in the centre of the lesion. There is no fluctuance and the lesion is tethered to the skin. The patient has no other health problems.

(1) What is the likely diagnosis?

(2) What factors should be explained to her in deciding on management of this lump?

2. A 44-year-old man presents to the Emergency Department of the hospital complaining of a painful swelling in his left axilla. It has developed over the previous 2 days, with the patient having experienced no previous problems in that area. Apart from type 2 diabetes mellitus, the patient has no other medical problems. On examination there is a 3 cm tender, fluctuant swelling in the medial wall of the left axilla. The skin overlying it is red and inflamed, but surrounding skin appears normal. There is no regional lymphadenopathy. The patient is apyrexial and haemodynamically stable, but blood results indicate a mild inflammatory response with slightly raised white cells and CRP. A diagnosis of an axillary abscess is made and the patient is admitted by the general surgical team for incision and drainage. Consent is obtained and the patient is transferred to theatre and anaesthetized. One of the junior doctors on the surgical team is offered the opportunity to perform the procedure under senior guidance.

(1) What is the operative technique (write a list of what he should do)?

(2) The wound will be left to heal by secondary intention. What does this mean, and how is it different from closure by primary intention?

3. A patient is referred to the ear, nose, and throat surgeons in their out-patient clinic for evaluation of a neck lump. How might each of the clinical features listed below, if present, help to differentiate between different kinds of neck swelling?

Clinical feature	Suggestive of...
Present for a few days	
Slowly growing over several months	
Present for as long as the patient can remember	
In the midline	
Moves with swallowing	
Moves when the tongue is protruded	
Just anterior to the upper third of the sternocleidomastoid muscle	
Associated with symptoms and signs of hyperthyroidism	
Colicky pain when eating	

4. A 24-year-old man is referred urgently to the urology outpatient clinic after presenting to his family doctor having noticed a lump on his right testicle. He noticed it on self-examination after seeing a television advert raising awareness of testicular cancer. He is not sure for how long before this the lump had been present. He is otherwise fit and well. His past medical history includes surgery aged 7 months old for maldescent of the same testicle. Examination revealed a painless, hard, irregular swelling on the surface of the right testicle, approximately 1 cm in size. He is extremely worried about the possibility of cancer.

(1) List two other examination findings and three investigations that are likely to be crucial in evaluating this man's testicular swelling.

(2) What should he be told about the likely cause and prognosis of this swelling at this stage?

5. A 73-year-old man is admitted to hospital after complaining of general ill-health, aches and pains, weight loss, anorexia, and fatigue. He also complains of various lumps and bumps about his body. He has no relevant medical history, is not on any medications, has smoked 20 cigarettes per day for all of his adult life, and has had no recent foreign travel. On examination, he appears pale and cachectic. Several lumps are felt in the anterior triangle of his neck, in his axillae, and in his groin, ranging from 2 cm to 5 cm in diameter. The lumps are hard and irregular, have a rubbery consistency, and are tender. A surgical biopsy is arranged, and one of the lumps sent for histology. Initial microscopy reveals a poorly differentiated adenocarcinoma of unknown origin.

(1) Based on the initial presentation, what were the possible differential diagnoses?

(2) After the initial histology results, how can the patient be further investigated to 'hunt for the primary'? What is the value in doing this?

6. A 47-year-old man is referred to the general surgical out-patient clinic with a left-sided scrotal swelling. He has noticed the swelling gradually increasing over the previous month. There is no pain and he is otherwise well, except for having some difficulty in walking because of the degree of swelling. Examination reveals marked swelling to the left hemiscrotum, approximately the size of an apple. It is soft, fluctuant, painless, and cannot be reduced. The testicle itself cannot be felt. The right testicle feels normal, though it is pushed to the side of the scrotum. A pen torch is held up behind the swelling, which lights up brightly and appears to glow with an orange light (trans-illumination). What is the diagnosis, and how can this man be managed?

Answers

1. Asymptomatic, slow-growing skin lumps are common, and 'lump and bump' excision day surgery lists make up a significant proportion of minor day-case surgery. The two commonest causes for this presentation are lipoma (small benign tumours of fatty tissue, which characteristically form smooth, lobulated subcutaneous swellings that slip easily under the skin surface) and sebaceous cysts (caused by blockage to the lumen of a skin follicle, leading to formation of small spherical cysts which are tethered to the skin surface and which have the punctum of the original follicle overlying). The diagnosis here is likely to be a sebaceous cyst.

Both small lipomas and sebaceous cysts are easily removed under local anaesthetic, either in local health centres by specially trained general practitioners or in day-case surgery by general surgeons. Complications included recurrence and scarring. Scars are inevitable with most forms of surgery, but some patients may develop keloid or hypertrophic scars, which may be more unsightly than the original lesion. Keloid scar formation is particularly common in Afro-Caribbeans, and forms as a result of excessive scar tissue formation in response to the healing process. Because of the cosmetic implications of scarring for this patient, she should be warned carefully about this pre-operatively and the procedure should be carried out by an experienced surgeon, perhaps using subcuticular sutures to minimize scarring.

2. Operative technique for incision and drainage of a simple abscess:
   - The patient should be consented for the procedure, and warned of serious and commonly occurring complications.
   - Abscesses may be drained under local or general anaesthesia depending on their site, size, and other patient factors.
   - The overlying skin should be thoroughly cleaned with antibacterial skin wash, and drapes applied to create a sterile operating field.
   - An incision should be made into the abscess to drain the pus it contains. Often, a cruciate incision (crucifix shaped) is used. Pus is then expressed from the cavity.
   - A gloved finger should be inserted and swept around the abscess cavity to break down any loculations and ensure all pus is fully drained.
   - A sample of pus should be taken, using a sterile swab, and sent for microscopy, culture, and sensitivities.
   - Once fully drained, the abscess cavity should be irrigated well (with either sterile saline, hydrogen peroxide, or an antibacterial solution) and packed with sterile gauze or similar.
   - The wound should be left open, and dressings changed daily or every other day until the cavity has fully healed. Adequate analgesia should be given post-operatively.

Wound closure by primary intention involves closing the skin (by sutures, glue, or adhesive dressings) after the primary procedure is completed. It is appropriate for sterile procedures such as most elective surgery. Closure by secondary intention involves leaving the skin incision open and packing the wound with gauze. It is used for grossly contaminated surgery such as abscess drainage. Closure by delayed primary intention (where the skin is left open for a few days and then closed), or closure by primary intention but with surgical drains left *in situ*, can be used where there is considerable contamination but where skin closure is important to allow quicker healing (for instance, after a laparotomy following bowel perforation).

3. The clinical features are suggestive of the following conditions:

Clinical feature	Suggestive of...
Present for a few days	Acute process such as abscess or haematoma formation
Slowly growing over several months	Suggests malignancy, gradual cyst formation or a chronic inflammatory process
Present for as long as the patient can remember	Suggests a congenital or embryological origin
In the midline	Suggests a congenital or embryological origin, e.g. a thyroglossal cyst
Moves with swallowing	Lump is linked to the thyroid gland, for instance a thyroid cyst or nodule
Moves when the tongue is protruded	The classic feature of a thyroglossal cyst, which is linked by a tract to the back of the tongue
Just anterior to the upper third of the sternocleidomastoid muscle	The classic position of branchial cysts
Associated with symptoms and signs of hyperthyroidism	Suggests a thyroid swelling, such as a toxic multinodular goitre
Colicky pain when eating	Suggests a problem of the salivary glands. May be associated with swelling or tenderness under the jaw

4. The history and examination findings are suggestive of a testicular tumour. The most common forms are seminoma, germ cell tumours (teratomas), and yolk sac tumours (rare). It is important to confirm the diagnosis and to assess whether the tumour has spread. Examination should also include the groin and abdomen for evidence of lymphadenopathy. Important investigations include serum alpha-fetoprotein (AFP), raised in yolk sac tumours, and beta-human chorionic gonadotrophin, (β-hCG), raised in seminoma and teratoma. Ultrasound of the testicle will assess if the swelling is solid or cystic, and confirm that it is arising from the testicle, and CT scanning of the chest and abdomen will look for lymphadenopathy and metastases.

Testicular cancer generally has an excellent prognosis, even if it has spread. If there is no spread then treatment is by orchidectomy alone; if there is spread then orchidectomy plus chemotherapy is offered. At this stage, the patient should be told that he is being investigated for cancer, and he should be told that if he does have cancer of the testicle, various management options exist and the prognosis is generally good.

5. The patient presented with weight loss, feeling generally unwell and with generalized large lymphadenopathy. The differential diagnosis at this stage would include primary lymph node cancer (lymphoma), infection (particularly tuberculosis), and metastatic cancer. A tissue diagnosis is imperative and so surgical biopsy is crucial.

The term 'poorly differentiated adenocarcinoma' refers to cancer originally from epithelial glandular tissue, but which has disorganized microarchitecture poorly reflective of the tissue that the tumour originally derived from. Possible primary cancers in this man include prostate, colon, oesophagus, stomach, lung, and pancreas, with breast and cervix possible in women with a similar presentation. Poorly differentiated cancers generally have poor prognosis.

Some cancers present in this way, with multiple metastases but no obvious primary tumour. It is useful to identify the location of the primary tumour so that management can be planned accordingly. Some tumours are more responsive to chemotherapy, whilst others respond better to radiotherapy. Whole-body CT scanning may be appropriate to find the primary, as may further testing of the biopsy specimen using immunofluorescence with labelled markers specific to antigens of different body tissues.

6. This presentation is classic for a hydrocoele, where fluid accumulates in a sac in the lining around the testis. It may present in childhood as a result of incomplete closure of the processus vaginalis, perhaps alongside an indirect inguinal hernia, or in later life. It is almost always benign, though the testis and groin should be examined for signs of malignancy or infection. In this man, the fluid in the hydrocoele can be drained percutaneously using a needle and syringe and local anaesthetic. This will both improve symptoms and allow the testicle to be examined, but is associated with high recurrence rates. More definitive surgical management includes incision and drainage of the hydrocoele and fixation of the sac within which the fluid has collected.

Further reading

Guidelines: Sydney Head and Neck Cancer Institute diagnostic guide for neck lumps (http://www.medicineau.net.au/directory/documents/228/SHNCI_NL_BKLET_tiny.pdf)

OHCM: 596–603, 652–653, 656

Breast lumps

This section should be used to clerk patients being investigated or managed for breast cancer. Most hospitals run specialist breast cancer clinics where women have all of their 'triple assessment'—physical examination, mammography, and fine-needle aspiration—done in one session. After discussion at cancer multidisciplinary meetings, they may then be admitted to a Female Surgery Ward for operative management or receive out-patient chemo- or radiotherapy.

Learning challenges

- Why are multidisciplinary team meetings so central to the UK cancer strategy? Which professionals should be present at a multidisciplinary meeting?
- What is the difference between cytology and histology, and why does histology generally give more useful information?

History

Comment on

- Presence of lump; duration; has it 'always been there'?
- Nipple abnormalities and discharge
- Breast pain
- Systemic health, changes in weight, other symptoms
- Family history of breast cancer
- Obstetric history—number and timings of pregnancies, previous breast feeding
- Gynaecological history—dates of menarche and menopause, hormone replacement therapy

Examination

Well or unwell? Why?

Feet to face:

Vital signs: Temperature Blood pressure Pulse rate Respiratory rate O2 saturations

Clinical clues:

Cardiovascular:

1 2 1

Respiratory:

Abdominal:

Neurological:

Other:

Comment on

- Full description of lump: size, shape, surface, mobility
- Attachments of lump: to chest wall, skin, or surrounding breast tissue
- Skin: dimpled (peau d'orange), ulcerated
- Nipple: deviation, inversion, symmetry, discharge
- Signs of inflammation
- Axillae: lymphadenopathy. Number of nodes, consistency, mobility

Mammography

Comment on

- Mass seen?
- Micro- or macrocalcifications? Pattern of calcifications
- BI-RADS category
- Suggested further action

Needle aspiration

Comment on

- Fluid? Clear, bloody, pus? Lump still present?
- Solid—send for cytology

Blood tests

Comment on

- Evidence of metastasis, e.g. raised ALP or calcium
- Evidence of infection

Cytology or histology

Comment on

- Malignant cells?
- Grade and stage
- Oestrogen receptors present?

Sentinel node biopsy

Comment on

- Evidence of spread?

Evaluation

1. **From the information available to you, how likely is it that this lump is cancerous? What additional investigations are needed? Is simple resolution possible with drainage (abscesses and cysts)?**

2. **If cancer is likely or proven, is there evidence of lymph node involvement or distant metastasis?**

3. **Which cancer treatments are likely to be appropriate?**

Surgery	Hormone therapy	Chemotherapy	Radiotherapy
Wide local excision (small peripheral lump), **mastectomy** (large or central lump), ± **axillary node sampling**, **clearance** or **sentinel node biopsy**	Oestrogen receptor blockers, e.g. **tamoxifen**. Used in all oestrogen receptor-positive disease, including metastatic disease	For example **epirubicin** + **5-FU** + **cyclophosphamide** + **methotrexate**. For any disease at high risk of metastasis	**To breast:** reduces local recurrence after surgery. **To axilla:** if evidence of spread and incomplete surgical clearance. **To metastases:** to improve symptoms

4. **What is the prognosis? Is symptom control needed? What about emotional and spiritual support?**

Questions

1. A 62-year-old woman attends her local hospital as part of the national breast cancer screening programme. She is fit and well and has not noticed any problems with her breasts; however, both her mother and her maternal aunt had suffered with breast cancer. She undergoes a mammogram. The radiologist's report is strongly suggestive of malignancy, and recommends urgent cytological investigation (see mammogram below).

(1) What is the role of mammography within breast cancer screening programmes?

(2) How should this woman be further managed?

(3) What causes breast cancer to run in families?

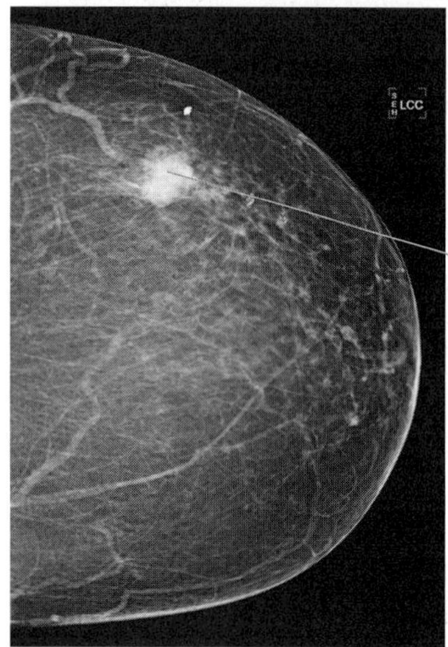

This cranio-caudal mammogram reveals a large, dense, spiculated mass in the outer part of the breast which is very suggestive of carcinoma. The term 'spiculated' can refer to lesions seen on a variety of imaging modalities (e.g. on CT scan), and refers to an irregular edge containing points or spikes. It is suggestive (but not diagnostic) of malignancy.

2. A 55-year-old woman attends her GP after having noticed a lump in her right breast. On examination the doctor notes a hard irregular mass measuring 3 cm in diameter in the lower outer quadrant. It is painless, irregular, and immobile within the surrounding breast tissue, but is not tethered to the skin or attached to the chest wall. No axillary lymphadenopathy is felt, and otherwise a full physical examination is unremarkable. She is referred urgently to the breast cancer out-patient clinic. After both mammography and cytology indicated malignancy, a wide local excision (lumpectomy) is carried out with sentinel node biopsy, after which the patient recovered well. Urgent histology reveals a well-differentiated invasive ductal carcinoma, with clear excision markers and no evidence of vascular invasion, and which tested positive for oestrogen receptors, and no evidence of spread to the sentinel node.

(1) What is the prognosis on the basis of this information?

(2) Should the patient receive any further treatment?

(3) What is sentinel node biopsy?

3. A 25-year-old woman gave birth to her first child 4 weeks previously, and has been breast feeding the baby since. She presents to the hospital Emergency Department complaining of an acutely painful left breast. She is otherwise well and has not felt feverish or sweaty. On examination the right breast is normal. The left breast has a painful, red, tender, swollen lump measuring 2.5 cm in length just lateral to the nipple. The patient reports that this has developed over the previous 24 hours.

(1) What is the likely diagnosis and how should she be managed?

(2) What are the implications for breast feeding?

4. An 87-year-old woman was diagnosed with breast cancer a year earlier after noticing a lump in her breast. Unfortunately, cytology had revealed aggressive invasive disease, and palpation of the axilla had revealed multiple enlarged lymph nodes. After all options were discussed with the patient (and her family), she elected not to undergo surgery or chemotherapy, and decided instead to be managed with tamoxifen monotherapy. For the past year she has been relatively well; however, the GP was asked to review her at home by the family who were concerned about her becoming increasingly confused and breathless over the previous 2 weeks. On examination the patient appears cachectic, uncomfortable, and breathless. She is drowsy and confused. The right breast is almost entirely taken up by tumour mass which has ulcerated and fungated through the skin. The breast is extremely tender to touch. She is tachypnoeic (respiratory rate 30 breaths/min) with good bilateral air entry throughout the chest but a notably elevated jugular venous pressure. The doctor arranges emergency admission to hospital, where she is found to be hypotensive (94/67 mmHg) and tachycardic (122 bpm). As part of her emergency assessment a limited echocardiogram is carried out (image shown below).

(1) What does this image reveal?

(2) Write a problem list for this patient and suggest how her symptoms might be addressed.

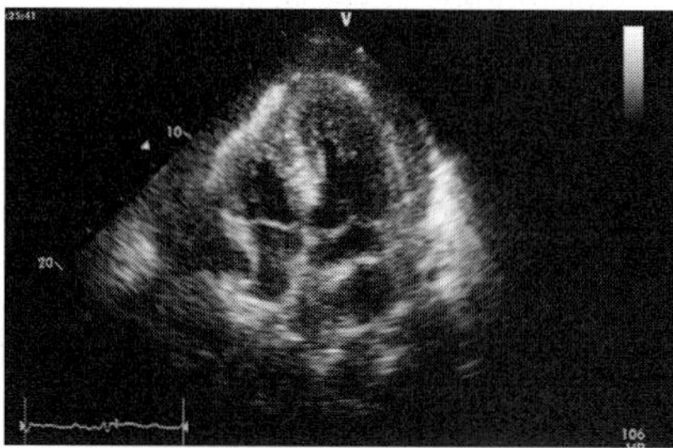

5. A 34-year-old woman visits her GP to complain about lumpy, uneven breasts which cause her pain. For several years she has suffered with painful breasts, which are especially painful during her menstrual period. She has noticed that her breasts have an uneven lumpy texture, and that the left breast appears bigger than the right. For the past month she has noticed an especially prominent lump just below the nipple of the left breast, which aches vaguely and is moderately tender to touch. She is otherwise well and her weight is stable. On examination, both breasts do feel generally lumpy with a particularly prominent lump below the left nipple which feels smooth but firm. There is no axillary lymphadenopathy.

(1) What is the likely diagnosis, and the management if this is confirmed?

(2) Does this woman need investigation for cancer?

Remember that you can find large-size, annotated versions of many of the X-rays and ECGs that appear in this book on the book's web site at www.oxfordtextbooks.co.uk/orc/randall/

Answers

1. Breast cancer screening aims to identify early cancers or carcinoma-in-situ at a stage where the disease is curable by surgical and medical therapy. Assessment is by mammogram, looking for masses (especially spiculated lesions) and microcalcification. Mammograms are categorized using the BI-RADS scoring system according to features found on the scan, with different categories requiring different follow-up:

Category 0	Incomplete scan
Category 1	Negative
Category 2	Benign findings
Category 3	Probably benign
Category 4	Suspicious abnormality
Category 5	Highly suspicious of malignancy
Category 6	Known malignancy from previous biopsy

Patients with suspicious lesions, such as the woman in this question, are recalled for 'triple assessment'—a full physical examination of the breast, radiological assessment with mammography or ultrasound, and pathological assessment with aspiration cytology or biopsy.

Overall, the false negative rate of mammography (radiologically undetectable cancer) is 10%, and over a 10-year period the false positive rate (suspicious mammogram with benign breast disease) is 25%. Critics of screening argue that it causes considerable and unnecessary anxiety in women, and that unnecessary, destructive operations are performed on women with ductal carcinoma-in-situ (the earliest form of breast cancer) which may never go on to become invasive. However, advocates of screening point to evidence of an absolute reduction in mortality in populations that are screened.

Breast cancer is strongly associated with certain known genetic defects, including the *BRCA1* and *BRCA2* genes, which may lead to an 85% lifetime risk of breast cancer, with patients occasionally undergoing bilateral mastectomy in early adulthood in view of the high risk of developing breast cancer. However, 95% of breast cancer is sporadic in incidence, or due to unknown genetic factors.

2. This woman has a good prognosis, with a well-differentiated oestrogen-responsive tumour, with no evidence of vascular invasion, and which has been completely excised. The Nottingham Prognostic Index is used to estimate prognosis in breast cancer, calculated as below. This patient's score is 2.6, putting her well within the 85% 5-year survival cohort. She should receive tamoxifen to further reduce the chances of recurrence, but does not require radio- or chemotherapy.

Nottingham prognostic index = [0.2 × S] + I + N + G	Interpretation: score and 5-year survival:
• **S**ize: size of index lesion in cm	• ≥2.0 to ≤2.4: 93%
• **I**nvasion: absent = 0, present = 1	• >2.4 to ≤3.4: 85%
• **N**odes involved: 0 = 1, 1–3 = 2, >3 = 3	• >3.4 to ≤5.4: 70%
• **G**rade: grade I = 1, grade II = 2, grade III = 3	• >5.4: 50%

The procedure of sentinel node biopsy is used to assess for the spread of cancer into draining lymph nodes. Before operating, radiolabelled dye and/or blue dye is injected into the breast. A gamma probe or Geiger counter (and visual assessment if blue dye is used) is used to assess which node (or nodes) is the primary or 'sentinel' node draining the breast (which is expected to have the highest concentration of dye). This is then biopsied and assessed for the presence of metastatic cells.

3. The likely diagnosis here is a breast abscess. These are very common in breast-feeding women, caused by (usually staphylococcal) infection of one or more mammary ducts, which may have become blocked. They respond well to oral antibiotics (e.g. flucloxacillin) and needle aspiration to remove pus. This may need to be repeated daily for several days until the infection is resolved. This woman should continue to breast feed, but using the other breast until this episode has settled. Milk from the infected breast should be expressed using a breast pump and discarded.

4. This emergency echocardiogram reveals:

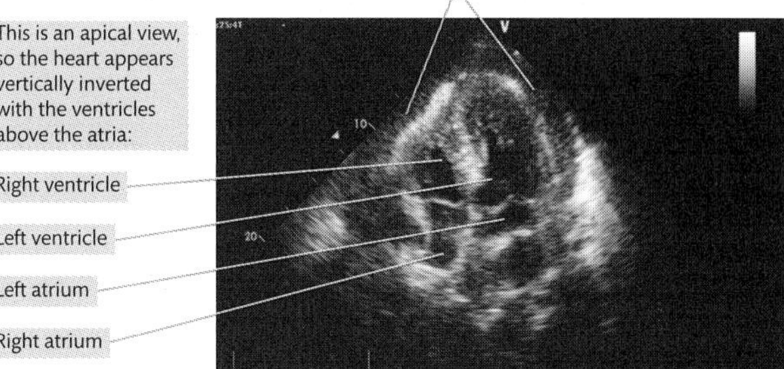

This emergency echocardiogram performed to investigate the cause of this woman's hypotension reveals evidence of a pericardial effusion. Although other causes are possible (e.g. sepsis), this effusion is likely to be the cause of her symptoms due to the tamponading effect of the fluid on the heart. Even in the presence of advanced malignant disease, pericardiocentesis (performed by an experienced doctor under ultrasound guidance, using a long pericardial catheter) is likely to be indicated to improve her symptoms.

This woman's problem list should focus on interventions that can be offered to improve her quality of life, with measures that will reduce suffering and which are acceptable for the patient. Involvement of the palliative care team is essential at this stage.

Problem	Likely cause	Management
Acute breathlessness	Malignant pericardial effusion	Pericardiocentesis and drain
Confusion	Hypotension. Possible cerebral metastasis	Drain effusion. If confusion persists, consider CT brain. Metastases may be suitable for palliative radiotherapy
Chest wall pain	Invasion of chest wall	Opioid analgesia (with laxatives and antiemetic). Possible palliative radiotherapy
Fungating breast cancer	Primary tumour	Palliative mastectomy could be considered if symptoms are severe and the patient is fit enough

5. The probable diagnosis here is fibrocystic breast disease, where local fibrosis and inflammation lead to pain and cyst formation. Because this may be hormone driven, the pain may be cyclical. Formation of multiple cysts leads the breasts to seem lumpy and uneven in size.

Breast cysts in women are common; single cysts are also common, and may cause considerable anxiety to women who discover them as lumps and are concerned about cancer. Characteristically, cysts are round, symmetrical, and smooth. They should be aspirated, generally yielding a yellow-green fluid. Cysts that fail to collapse fully should be investigated for a possible underlying cancer. Fibrocystic breast disease is treated by anti-inflammatory medication, cyst drainage, and possible hormonal treatment (e.g. the combined oral contraceptive pill).

All women are potentially at risk of developing breast cancer, including those with fibrocystic breast disease. Therefore, although this woman can be reassured that her lump is likely to be benign, triple assessment should still be undertaken if there is any doubt about the nature of this new lump.

Further reading

Guidelines: Scottish Intercollegiate Guidelines Network guidelines on managing breast cancer in women (http://www.sign.ac.uk/guidelines/fulltext/84/index.html)

OHCM: 604–605

Peripheral vascular disease

This section should be used to clerk patients with peripheral vascular disease, who may be managed as out-patients in vascular surgery clinics or receive interventional procedures (either endovascular or by open surgery), when they may be managed on a General or Vascular Surgery Ward.

Learning challenges

- What does the term 'arteriopath' refer to, and how might it guide the assessment of patients presenting with symptoms which might be suggestive of peripheral vascular disease?
- What common comorbidities are associated with peripheral vascular disease, and how might this affect fitness for surgery in patients in whom an operation is indicated?

History

Comment on

- Claudication (cramps in legs on walking)—distance walked before pain occurs
- Relief of pain on resting?
- Pain at night. How can the patient relieve this?
- Ulceration or other skin changes
- Other vascular disease
- Vascular risk factors

Examination

Well or unwell? Why?

Feet to face:

Vital signs: Temperature Blood pressure Pulse rate Respiratory rate O2 saturations

Clinical clues:

Cardiovascular:

1 2 1

Respiratory:

Abdominal:

Neurological:

Other:

Comment on

- General appearance of patient
- Heart rhythm, murmurs
- Abdominal aortic aneurysm
- Legs—colour, temperature, ulceration
- Peripheral pulses, pallor
- Buerger's test

Doppler probe

Comment on

- Assess for distal pulses
- Ankle:brachial pressure index

Colour duplex Doppler ultrasound

Comment on

- Patency and flow patterns through large vessels

Digital subtraction angiography/magnetic resonance angiography

Comment on

- Level and degree of obstruction
- Distal vascular patency

Abdominal ultrasound

Comment on

- Presence of aortic aneurysm
- Anteroposterior diameter
- Proximal extension

Blood tests

Comment on

- Renal function
- Haemoglobin
- Group and save/cross-match (if for surgery)

Evaluation

1. Has acute limb ischaemia been excluded?

2. Is the pain vascular in origin? Have other causes of pain in the leg been excluded?

3. What is the severity of the symptoms?

Grade	Symptoms	Ankle:brachial pressure index
Grade I	None	>0.9
Grade II	Claudication	0.4–0.9
Grade III	Rest pain	<0.4
Grade IV	Ulcers and gangrene	<0.4

Grades III and IV constitute critical limb ischaemia.

4. How can the patient's lifestyle and medical management be optimized?

Smoking cessation
Weight loss, exercise
Diabetic control
Blood pressure control
Aspirin and statin

5. Is surgery or endovascular intervention indicated? What procedure is most appropriate?

Questions

1. A 62-year-old man is referred to the vascular surgery out-patient clinic after complaining to his GP about pain in his legs. The pain is cramp-like and comes on in his calves when he walks approximately 200 m. When he rests for a minute or so, the pain settles, and he is able to continue walking. He is pain free at rest, can lie flat, and is comfortable at night. He has had no other medical problems in the past, and takes no medications regularly. He has smoked 20 cigarettes a day for 40 years. On examination his blood pressure is 165/75 mmHg and his capillary blood glucose is 8 mmol/L. His legs appear grossly normal, with normal strength and sensation throughout. There is no tenderness or swelling around any of the joints, and all have a good range of movements. Peripheral pulses can be felt in both groins, both popliteal arteries and both posterior tibial arteries. The dorsalis pedis pulses are absent bilaterally. His ankle:brachial pressure index is 0.7.

(1) What is the diagnosis?

(2) What other diagnoses should also potentially be made?

(3) How should this man be managed?

2. A 79-year-old woman is brought to the Emergency Department by ambulance complaining of sudden-onset pain and weakness in her right leg. It came on over several minutes whilst she was sitting in a chair, and there was no history of trauma. She describes the pain as initially tingling 'like pins and needles', before becoming more severe and persistent. Her previous medical history included an 'irregular heart beat', hypertension, and a stroke with good recovery of function. Her regular medications include aspirin, atorvastatin, digoxin, perindopril, and amlodipine. On examination she appears unwell and uncomfortable. Her pulse is fast (around 120 bpm) and irregular. Her right leg appears pale compared with the left with a bluish discoloration, is cool to touch, and is painful on palpation. No pulses are palpable below the femoral artery, though all pulses are palpable in the left leg. What is the diagnosis and correct management?

3. A patient with peripheral vascular disease has been under review in the vascular surgery out-patient clinic. He also suffers with diabetes mellitus and hypertension, and smokes 15 cigarettes a day. His vascular disease has been stable for many years with good medical management; however, for the past 6 months his claudication distance had noticeably decreased. He now reports pain is his left calf at rest–especially when lying flat, and he has resorted to sleeping upright in a chair. He reports being able to take only four or five steps before the pain in his left leg becomes excruciating. Three weeks before he stubbed his left great toe, and since then the wound has failed to heal and has developed into a superficial painful ulcer. No pulses can be palpated in the left leg below the femoral artery. When both legs are raised up to an angle of 45° above the bed and maintained there for 1 minute, the left leg becomes white, cool, and painful. When the patient then sits up and allows the legs to hang over the side of the bed, the left leg becomes red and hot for a few minutes before returning to its normal colour. An angiogram is arranged of the left leg (shown below).

(1) What does the angiogram show, and what management is indicated?

(2) What is the principle behind Buerger's test?

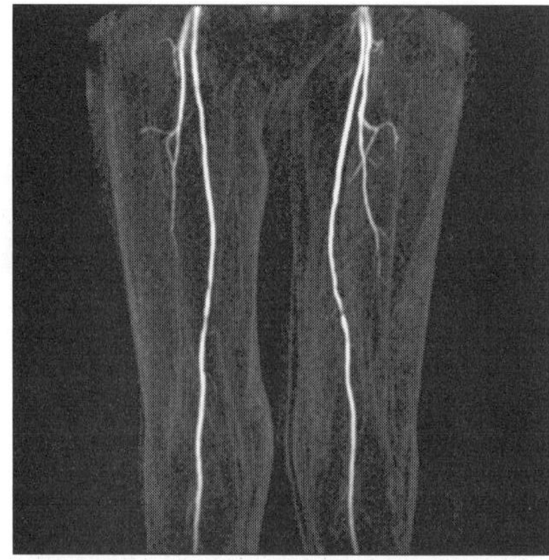

4. A patient with known severe peripheral vascular disease had balloon angioplasty and a metal stent inserted into her right superficial femoral artery 9 months ago because of symptoms of critical limb ischaemia. She experienced initial reduction in pain and was even able to walk several hundred metres before pain forced her to stop. However, her claudication distance has steadily decreased since, and for the past 3 weeks she has experienced rest pain again. She has also developed a severe necrotizing infection of her lateral two toes of the right foot with a deep ulcer, at the bottom of which bone can be felt when probed. She is admitted to hospital as an emergency and an angiogram is arranged, which reveals a patent superficial femoral artery (where she had previously been stented), but severe popliteal artery stenosis. Flow through collateral vessels was present and patent distal vessels were seen.

(1) What are the options for management of this woman

(2) Why is it crucial to make a decision about the viability of her ulcerated foot?

5. A 63-year-old man is rushed to the Emergency Department by ambulance after collapsing at work. He is alert and complaining of severe left-sided pain radiating to the back. His past medical history includes diverticular disease and ischaemic heart disease. Basic observations include temperature 36.3°C, heart rate 144 bpm, blood pressure 72/56 mmHg, and oxygen saturations of 97% on air. Two large-bore intravenous cannulae are inserted and a fast infusion of intravenous colloid is commenced. The patient is rushed to the CT scanner where the following image is obtained:

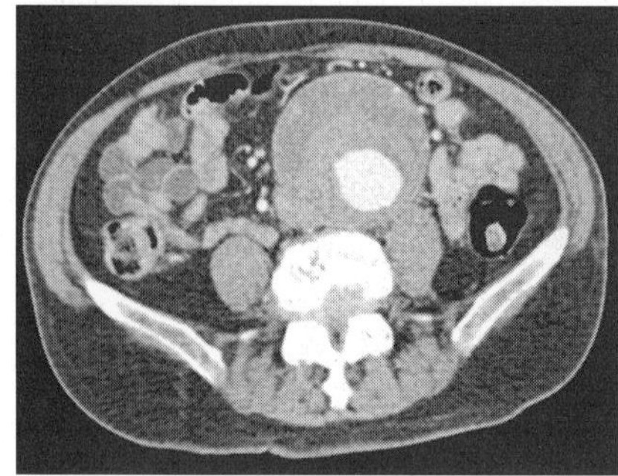

(1) What does it show?

(2) What is the emergency management?

Answers

1. The diagnosis for this man's leg pains here is intermittent claudication. This patient has classical symptoms of pain on exercise, which settles at rest. The absence of dorsalis pedis pulses is indicative of lower leg circulatory insufficiency. Other causes of pain in the legs on walking include arthritis of any cause (where the pain is felt in the joints, and generally begins immediately on moving), neurological pain (e.g. sciatica, where shooting pains are commonly felt down the posterior surface of the leg), or spinal stenosis (where a narrowing of the distal spinal cord causes ischaemia to the nerve roots on exercise—this may closely mimic claudication but the pain generally takes much longer to resolve on resting).

Other diagnoses which should be suspected in this man include hypertension and diabetes. Having developed one atherosclerotic disease, he is at increased risk of developing vascular disease in other organs, including heart disease, strokes, and renal vascular disease.

Of patients with claudication, around a third will get better with medical management, a third will remain the same, and a further third will deteriorate, with 10% going on to develop critical ischaemia. No surgical or endovascular interventions have shown a long-term benefit for claudication. Therefore the correct management for this man is medical. The patient should receive:

- advice on smoking cessation,
- encouragement to lose weight and exercise more,
- aspirin and a statin,
- referral to his GP for a glucose tolerance test, fasting lipid measurement, and repeat blood pressure measurement, with diabetic and antihypertensive medication prescribed as necessary.

2. This woman has acute limb ischaemia, which is a surgical emergency. Unless urgent surgical intervention is provided, the leg will suffer irreversible damage and become necrotic and gangrenous. The window for intervention is around 6 hours from the onset of symptoms. Much acute limb ischaemia occurs on the background of chronic peripheral vascular disease, from thrombus formation over a ruptured atherosclerotic plaque. However, a proportion are caused by emboli, usually of cardiac origin. This is likely in this patient who clearly has atrial fibrillation.

Acute limb ischaemia is a diagnosis that must not be missed. The characteristic signs are described by 'six Ps'. These features are:

- Pain
- Pallor
- Pulselessness
- Paralysis
- Paraesthesia
- Perishingly cold

Management is aimed at rapid reperfusion of the leg. A heparin infusion should be started and the vascular surgical team consulted. Often a surgical embolectomy is carried out, when the embolus is removed from within the artery by introducing a catheter through an open incision in the artery, passing it beyond the level of the occlusion, and withdrawing the catheter with the balloon inflated. Alternatives include thrombolysis, emergency stenting with radiological screening, and emergency bypass surgery.

3. This man has critical limb ischaemia, which is defined by rest pain lasting for more than 2 weeks or by the presence of end tissue disease (such as ulceration). The diagnosis is not surprising given his angiogram, which reveals:

Profunda femoris artery.

Superficial femoral arteries.

Two areas of moderate stenosis in the right superficial femoral artery.

The biggest abnormality is an area of almost complete occlusion of the left superficial femoral artery at the level of the mid-thigh. The area of stenosis is short and well defined, meaning that an endovascular approach may prove successful, with balloon angioplasty to dilate the vessel, and then possibly a stent to maintain patency of the vessel.

This man requires urgent revascularization. This may be attempted first using an endovascular approach, since the level of occlusion is clear. In this man's case, he was treated by balloon angioplasty and insertion of a reinforcing metal stent. An alternative in other patients would be bypass surgery, such as a femoral-popliteal bypass, where a vein removed from the leg is reversed in direction and attached above and below the blocked vessel to allow reperfusion.

Buerger's test is used to detect significant vascular disease. As the legs are elevated above the bed, the blood pressure in the legs is unable to overcome gravity and the leg becomes pale and drained of blood. On swinging the legs over the side of the bed, the leg is reperfused and a there is a reactive hyperaemia, where the leg turns red.

4. This woman initially requires treatment with intravenous antibiotics to treat the infection to her foot. This ulcer will not heal without vascular improvement, but even if this can be achieved the damage may already be very severe. If her toes are confirmed to be gangrenous they should be amputated. If there is severe deep tissue infection of the foot, a careful decision must be made, considering amputation at the level of the forefoot, ankle, or above or below the knee depending on the angiography results.

Distal arterial occlusions are difficult to treat with an endovascular approach, and the treatment of choice in this woman is an arterial bypass procedure. Various different bypass operations can be carried out. The most common is the femoral–popliteal bypass (to bypass an occluded section of superficial femoral artery). In proximal stenosis at the level of the iliac arteries, a femoral–femoral crossover can be performed to divert blood from the patent side to the non-patent side. An aorto-bifemoral ('trouser') graft may be used in bilateral iliac narrowing, and rarely long subcutaneous axillo-femoral grafts are used. In this woman the most appropriate operation will be a femoral–distal bypass, where a vein or synthetic graft is anastomosed to the patent proximal femoral artery and to the distal vessel of choice, for instance the anterior tibial artery.

5. The abdominal CT shows a large abdominal aortic aneurysm:

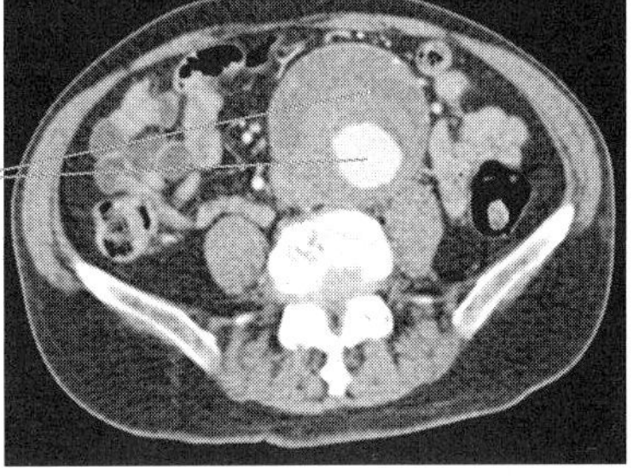

The main abnormality here is a very large abdominal aortic aneurysm, the diameter of which was measured at 7.5 cm. Note contrast medium in the lumen, surrounded by greyish atheroma in the vessel wall.

In the presence of sudden abdominal pain radiating to the back, and haemodynamic instability, this patient should be presumed to have a ruptured aneurysm and emergency vascular repair is indicated.

Repair may be performed via an endovascular approach or by open laparotomy. Aneurysms that rupture anteriorly (into the peritoneal cavity) are almost universally fatal. If an aneurysm ruptures posteriorly, the bleeding may be tamponaded due to the confines of the retroperitoneal cavity, and the patient may survive to the operating theatre.

Further reading

Guidelines: Scottish Intercollegiate Guidelines Network guidelines on managing peripheral vascular disease (http://www.sign.ac.uk/guidelines/fulltext/89/index.html)

OHCM: 656–659

Haematuria

This section should be used to clerk patients presenting with haematuria—either presenting acutely to the Emergency Department or being referred by their doctor for assessment in secondary care. They may be found on urology and general surgical wards or in the out-patient cystoscopy suite.

Learning challenges

- What are the different types of renal stone? How are they formed and what are the risk factors for developing each type?
- Apart from pain and discomfort, what are the complications of urinary retention?

History

Comment on

- Episodes of macroscopic haematuria
- Suprapubic or loin pain
- Irritant lower urinary tract symptoms—dysuria, frequency
- Obstructive lower urinary tract symptoms—hesitancy, dribble, retention
- General health, other conditions, weight loss
- Warfarin or other anticoagulants
- Long-term urinary catheter? Recently changed? Recent urological procedures?
- Previous occupational exposure to dyes or other toxic chemicals, smoking
- Foreign travel

Examination

Well or unwell? Why?

Feet to face:

Vital signs: Temperature | Blood pressure | Pulse rate | Respiratory rate | O2 saturations

Clinical clues:

Cardiovascular:

1 2 1

Respiratory:

Abdominal:

Neurological:

Other:

Comment on

- Haemodynamic stability
- Kidney dysfunction—blood pressure, peripheral oedema
- Acute urinary retention (secondary to clots)—palpable bladder?
- Abdominal or loin tenderness. Renal mass?
- Digital rectal examination—size and surface of prostate

Urine dipstick

Comment on

- Evidence of infection (nitrites and leucocytes)
- Evidence of glomerular damage (heavy proteinuria)

Blood tests

Comment on
- Haemoglobin
- Renal function
- Clotting

Urine cytology

Comment on
- Malignant cells

Abdominal ultrasound or intravenous urogram

Comment on
- Kidney tumours and cysts
- Stones
- Hydronephrosis, hydroureter

CT kidneys/ureters/bladder

Comment on
- Tumours
- Obstructing stones

Cystoscopy

Comment on
- Bladder tumours
- Cystitis

Evaluation

1. **What is the likeliest source of bleeding based on symptoms and examination findings?**

Cause	Symptoms, signs and results
Urinary tract infection	Dysuria, frequency, tenderness, leucocytes, and nitrites
Calculus	Colicky pain from loin to groin
Bladder tumour	Previous chemical/dye exposure, smoking, painless
Renal cell carcinoma	Fever, hypertension, loin mass, metastatic disease
Glomerulonephritis	Evidence of systemic disease (e.g. rash), risk factors, proteinuria

2. **Is there obstruction to urinary flow (from any cause)? Is kidney function threatened?**

3. **What investigations may be helpful to discover the source of the bleeding?**

4. **What is the definitive diagnosis?**

5. **Which treatment is most appropriate for this particular patient?**

Questions

1. A 62-year-old woman is referred urgently by her GP to the urology clinic at the local hospital after experiencing two episodes of painless haematuria. She is otherwise fit and healthy and has not noticed any urological symptoms or changes in weight. She is a life-long smoker and formerly worked in a petrol refinery. When she was seen in clinic, examination was unremarkable and urine dipstick analysis revealed microscopic haematuria with no protein, nitrites, or leucocytes present. Blood tests were within normal limits. Urine cytology revealed the presence of malignant cells, and so a flexible cystoscopy was carried out, which revealed a 3 cm sessile lesion in the superior dome of the bladder. A rigid cystoscopy was then carried out under general anaesthetic, during which the lesion was removed by diathermy. The patient returns the next week to clinic, and is told that histology showed a grade 2 transitional cell carcinoma which had invaded the muscle wall of the bladder. A CT scan revealed thickening of the bladder wall as expected, but did not reveal any evidence of distal spread.

(1) What are this woman's treatment options given her cancer has spread into the muscularis mucosa?

(2) Why do toxic chemicals cause urinary tract cancer?

2. A 28-year-old man attends the hospital Emergency Department with acute severe pain in his left loin. It began that afternoon and has been excruciatingly painful since. He cannot find a comfortable position and is writhing around on the bed. He has vomited twice. On examination he is apyrexial and haemodynamically stable. He is clearly in severe pain. Examination reveals a soft abdomen with no masses or bowel sounds, but tenderness in the left loin. Urine dipstick shows: protein +, blood +++, leucocytes –, nitrites –. Blood tests are unremarkable. An intravenous urogram is performed, and an abdominal X-ray performed 20 minutes after injection of contrast is shown below.

(1) Prescribe appropriate medication for this man using a sample drug chart downloaded from the Online Resource Centre.

(2) What does the IVU reveal, and what treatment is indicated?

(3) How is an IVU performed, and what are the risks associated with one?

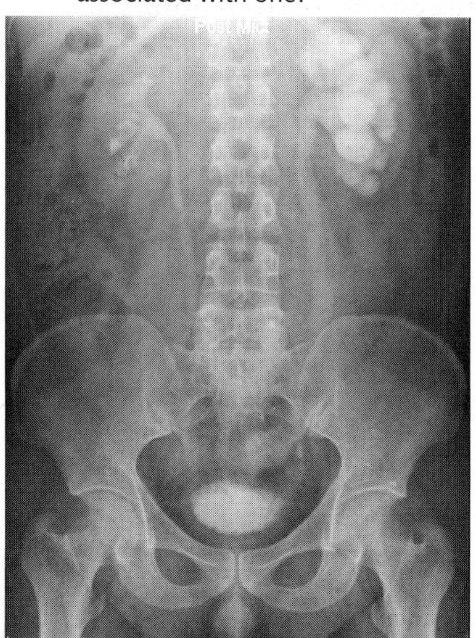

3. A 92-year-old man who lives in a residential home is admitted with abdominal pain and haematuria. He has a long-term urethral catheter *in situ* because of benign prostatic hypertrophy. He has suffered with episodes of haematuria for 2 months which have not been formally investigated because they were put down to trauma following catheter changes. This afternoon he began to pass blood through his catheter, but he has not now passed any blood or urine for several hours. On examination the patient is a frail elderly man with obvious lower abdominal discomfort. Initial observations are within normal limits except for a slight tachycardia (110 bpm). His abdomen is soft with lower abdominal tenderness over a palpably enlarged bladder. A urethral catheter is *in situ*, and the catheter bag contains a small amount (50 mL) of heavily blood-stained urine. Blood tests reveal urea 12.5 mmol/L and creatinine 156 μmol/L, both normal on previous hospital visits.

Why has this man developed pain, and what can be done to relieve the problem?

4. A 73-year-old man was diagnosed a month ago with cancer of the sigmoid colon. The cancer was found to be locally invasive on biopsy and CT and so he is being managed with chemotherapy and input from the palliative care team in the community. For the past week he has been complaining of a dull ache in his left loin. For the past 2 days his wife complains that he has been drowsy and confused, and has felt hot and sweaty, still complaining of worsening pain in the left loin. He has been opening his bowels normally each day. In the Emergency Department he is found to have evidence of sepsis (temperature 38.6°C, heart rate 122 bpm, blood pressure 87/55 mmHg). On examination he is drowsy but rousable (GCS 14/15), with a palpable and ballotable mass in his left loin, which is tender. The abdomen is soft. Urine dipstick reveals protein +, blood ++, nitrites + and leucocytes +++. Routine blood tests include urea 20.2 mmol/L, creatinine 235 μmol/L (both previously normal), CRP 187 mg/L, and white cell count 18.9×10^9/L. An urgent abdominal ultrasound scan is reported as showing left-sided hydronephrosis and hydroureter.

(1) What has happened to cause this man's acute illness?

(2) What emergency treatment is required?

Answers

1. Transitional cell carcinomas are the commonest form of urinary tract malignancy. The best chance of cure with early cancers comes if they can be completely excised by cystoscopic loop diathermy—this is possible if the cancer remains confined to the epithelium without evidence of deeper invasion (called 'carcinoma-in-situ'). Patients whose cancer can be resected fully in this way require regular screening since these tumours often recur.

If the cancer has invaded the muscularis mucosa, cure may still be possible but more radical surgery is required. The most common operation performed for this type of tumour is radical cystectomy with creation of an ileal conduit. Put simply, the whole bladder is removed, and then a portion of small intestine (ileum) is harvested (on its own blood supply) to create a new bladder, which empties through the abdominal wall in a similar way to an ileostomy. The two cut ends of the ureters are then connected to this replacement bladder, or 'ileal conduit'. Other complex procedures can be undertaken which preserve the patient's continence.

Transitional cell carcinoma is associated with exposure to toxic chemicals such as aromatic hydrocarbons found in dyes, petrol products, rubber, and soot. These chemicals can lead to bladder cancer because they are concentrated and held for long periods of time in the bladder, and have carcinogenic effects of the epithelium.

The other principal subtype of bladder cancer is squamous cell carcinoma, which is the commonest worldwide in association with chronic bladder inflammation caused by the eggs of the *Schistosoma haematobium* worm.

2. Renal colic can be excruciatingly painful and strong analgesia is necessary. Options include a strong non-steroidal anti-inflammatory, such as diclofenac, which is particularly effective when given via the rectal route. A strong opiate such as morphine may also be required. Drugs that relax smooth muscle (antispasmodics) such as buscopan may help to relieve symptoms. An antiemetic should also be prescribed. Below are four appropriate prescriptions for this man:

Date	Time	Drug	Dose	Route	Signature
08/02	1715	Diclofenac	100 mg	PR	DR
08/02	1715	Morphine	2.5–10 mg (titrate to pain)	IV	DR
08/02	1715	Metoclopramide	10 mg	IV	DR
08/02	1715	Buscopan	20 mg	IV	DR

This intravenous urogram reveals:

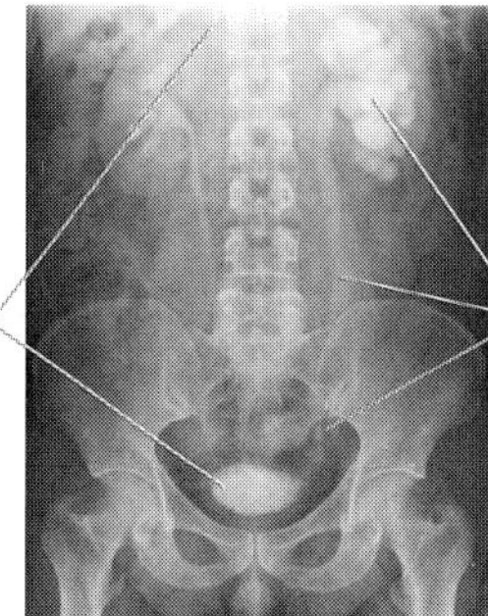

This is a post-micturition study, as shown not just by the label but also by a largely empty bladder. The right kidney and ureter are normal.

On the left side there is gross hydronephrosis and hydroureter (seen as a 'standing column' of fluid) - notice how the renal pelvis is enlarged and the calyces are clubbed. Notice too a stone in the distal ureter. Around 80% of renal stones are visible on x-ray, compared with only 10% of gallstones.

This is a urological emergency—this man is at risk of losing all function in his left kidney unless the ureteric obstruction can be relieved. There are two options for doing this. A reverse ureteric stent (called a 'JJ' stent) which bypasses the obstruction and allows urine to drain into the bladder can be placed using a cystoscope. Alternatively a percutaneous nephrostomy can be introduced into the renal pelvis via the posterior abdominal wall under ultrasound guidance. Either method will allow urine to drain, which should hopefully lead to resolution of the hydronephrosis and preservation of function in the left kidney. The stone itself may pass spontaneously (this is more likely to occur if the stone is <5 mm in diameter, and may be assisted by use of an alpha-adrenergic blocker such as tamsulosin). Larger stones may remain lodged in the ureter and require a surgical procedure or ultrasound lithotripsy to remove or fragment them.

A full IVU consists of three lower abdominal X-rays. The first is a plain film, after which intravenous contrast is given (through a peripheral cannula), and further X-rays are taken at 20 minutes and 2 hours after contrast is given. In the case of suspected renal colic, if no evidence of obstruction is seen then the patient can safely be discharged with the diagnosis of a small kidney stone which has passed spontaneously. These patients should be followed up in an out-patient clinic for further assessment to look for additional stones. The risks of giving intravenous contrast include allergic, asthmatic, or rarely anaphylactic reactions, and of precipitating acute renal failure—worse if renal function is already compromised by obstruction.

3. Blood clots are one of the commonest causes of acute urinary retention. Such clots may be large and completely block off a standard long-term urethral catheter. This is the likely cause of obstruction in any patient with haematuria who develops retention. The simplest solution to this problem is simply to change the catheter; however, the problem is likely to recur, because the bladder is probably full of blood clots. Instead, a large three-way irrigation catheter is introduced into the bladder. This has three lumens, one allowing the balloon at the end of the catheter to inflate to secure the catheter within the bladder, a second allowing water to be poured into the bladder to wash out all the clots, and a third large-bore lumen to allow urine and clots to drain out. This patient should be admitted to hospital and irrigation continued until the urine is running clear. A cystoscopy might be carried out to discover the cause of the bleeding.

4. The ultrasound here confirms ureteric obstruction—most likely caused by invasion or compression of the ureter by the sigmoid tumour. Ureteric obstruction leads to swelling of the kidney (hydronephrosis), with progressive destruction of the renal architecture and deterioration of renal function. Hydronephrotic kidneys are prone to infection, and given the evidence of sepsis in this man, and urine dipstick analysis suggesting a urinary source, this must be presumed to be what has happened. Hydronephrosis can be caused by anything that obstructs the outflow of urine, with common causes including ureteric or bladder transitional cell carcinoma, ureteric stones, and extrinsic compression by other structures.

This man has acute hydronephrosis, renal failure, and sepsis. He requires emergency intervention. He should be managed with fluid resuscitation to bring up his blood pressure, and appropriate antibiotics (such as gentamicin with the normal dose reduced because of his renal failure). He requires emergency drainage of the urine proximal to the obstruction. This can be achieved either via a percutaneous nephrostomy (where a catheter is passed into the renal pelvis through the skin of the back) or a retrograde ureteric stent (inserted into the ureter from below, using a cystoscope).

Further reading

Guidelines: Canadian guidelines or the management of asymptomatic microscopic haematuria in adults (http://www.ncbi.nlm.nih.gov/pmc/articles/PMC2645872/)

OHCM: 286, 640–643, 646–649

Prostate disease

This section should be used to clerk patients admitted acutely with symptoms of prostate disease, such as acute urinary retention or symptoms of metastatic prostate cancer. It can also be used to clerk patients being seen in urology out-patient clinics for assessment of the symptoms of prostate enlargement.

Learning challenges

- Why has the prostate-specific antigen proved such a controversial test, particularly in patients with no symptoms of prostate disease?
- It is estimated from autopsy studies that 80% of men over the age of 80 have prostate cancer. Why are only a comparatively small number of these diagnosed or treated for it?

History

Comment on

- Acute painful retention
- Frequency, hesitancy, poor stream, terminal dribble, nocturnal voiding
- Back pain, neurological symptoms in legs, bowel function
- Weight loss
- Bone pain
- Medications

Examination

Well or unwell? Why?

Feet to face:

Vital signs: Temperature | Blood pressure | Pulse rate | Respiratory rate | O2 saturations

Clinical clues:

Cardiovascular:

1 2 1

Respiratory:

Abdominal:

Neurological:

Other:

Comment on

- General: comfortable? Cachectic?
- Fluid balance
- Palpable bladder, suprapubic dullness to percussion and tenderness
- Groin lymphadenopathy
- Digital rectal examination: prostate size and surface; tenderness
- Perineal sensation

Bladder scan

Comment on

- Bladder volume
- Post-micturition residual volume

Blood tests

Comment on
- Renal function
- Prostate-specific antigen
- Calcium, alkaline phosphatase

Abdominal ultrasound

Comment on
- Kidney size and shape, hydronephrosis, hydroureter
- Masses

Transrectal ultrasound biopsy

Comment on
- Gross anatomy of prostate
- Histology, Gleason score

Pelvic MRI

Comment on
- Evidence of local invasion

Bone scan

Comment on
- Evidence of bony metastasis

Urodynamic studies

Evaluation

1. **Is this presentation an acute emergency?**

Evidence of:
- acute urinary retention (has cauda equina syndrome been excluded?)
- hydronephrosis
- renal failure

2. **Based on the initial presentation and examination, is this prostate likely to be benign or malignant?**

3. **If this patient has evidence of cancer, how advanced is it and how aggressive is it? What are the patient's wishes, and their life expectancy and level of functioning? What management is best?**

Localized disease (within prostate)	Potentially curable	Older patients: watchful waiting, treat symptoms, monitor PSA
		Younger patients: surgery, radiotherapy, or brachytherapy
Locally invasive disease	Incurable	Hormone therapy
Metastatic disease	Incurable	Hormone therapy, palliative radiotherapy

4. **How can troublesome urinary tract symptoms be addressed?**

Questions

1. An 87-year-old man presents to the Emergency Department with acute lower abdominal pain. The pain has been progressively more severe for the past 6 hours, during which time he has not passed any urine at all. He has never had anything like this before, though he has noticed for the previous few months that passing urine has been difficult, with the desire to pass urine frequently. He has had difficulty in starting to void and a urinary stream which is weak and continues to dribble at the end of the stream. He is otherwise well and has no active medical problems, his only medications being prophylactic calcium and vitamin D supplementation. His weight is stable. On examination he is extremely uncomfortable and restless. He is apyrexial, slightly tachycardic, and normotensive. On palpation, the abdomen is soft with marked suprapubic tenderness. A mass arising from the pelvis can be palpated, which reaches almost all the way to the umbilicus and which is dull to percussion. Digital rectal examination reveals a smoothly enlarged prostate which is not tender to touch. What are the management priorities:

- immediately,
- within the next few days,
- over the next few weeks?

2. A 56-year-old man is referred to the urology out-patient clinic after presenting to his GP complaining of problems in urinating. He finds that he needs to get up twice most nights to go to the toilet, and has noticed difficulty in initiating micturition as well as a poor urinary stream. These problems have been affecting him for the previous 3 months. His International Prostate Symptom Score is 22/35. He has no other symptoms, is in good health, takes no medications, and has not experienced any unexpected weight loss. Examination of the abdomen is normal, but digital rectal examination reveals a markedly enlarged prostate, the size of which the urologist estimates at around 60 g. The prostate has a smooth contour with a central groove. The patient's level of prostate specific antigen (PSA) is 3.2 ng/mL and his renal function and other blood tests are within normal ranges.

(1) What is the likely diagnosis? How likely is cancer?

(2) How is the International Prostate Symptom Score calculated?

(3) What medical and surgical options exist for managing this man?

3. Two patients are reviewed, one after the other, in the urology out-patient clinic. Both were referred to the clinic urgently because of lower urinary tract symptoms, a hard, irregular prostate on digital rectal examination, and a raised serum PSA level. Both had pelvic MRI scans which suggested cancer limited to the prostate gland, and both had transrectal ultrasound-guided prostate biopsies, with the histological reports for both revealing prostatic adenocarcinoma with a Gleason score of 4/10. The first patient is a fit and active 55-year-old man, and the second is a fit and active 85-year-old man.

(1) What treatment options may be appropriate for the first, younger patient? What different risks are associated with these?

(2) What treatment option may be appropriate for the second, older patient?

(3) How can the difference in approach be justified simply on the grounds of age?

4. A 62-year-old man attends his GP asking to have his level of serum PSA measured. He does not report any urinary symptoms and is generally in good health. He has no family history of prostate disease. One of his friends had recently been diagnosed with metastatic prostate cancer after a pathological fracture of his femur, having had no prostate symptoms, and this patient was concerned in case he could have similarly silent disease. His doctor informs him that using a cut-off of PSA >4.0 ng/mL (the generally accepted standard for screening) the sensitivity of this test is 86% and the specificity 33%.

(1) What do the terms sensitivity and specificity mean when referring to a screening test?

(2) What might be the risks for this man if he elects to have the tests?

Presentation

Presented to ______ Grade ______ Date ______

Signed

Answers

1. Acute urinary retention is a common presentation of prostate disease, requiring urgent attention which will bring immediate relief to a patient in great distress. The management priorities for this man are as below:

Immediate
Give analgesia, e.g. morphine Confirm the diagnosis of retention (if there is any doubt) with a bladder scan Insert a urinary catheter and ensure it is draining well. This should provide rapid relief for the patient Test the urine to look for signs of urinary tract infection Monitor urine output—after prolonged retention, there can often be a marked diuresis with several litres of urine passed each day. Intravenous fluids may need to be given to prevent dehydration
Next few days
Confirm the diagnosis of benign prostatic hypertrophy leading to retention. Rule out other common causes If the cause is benign prostatic hypertrophy, consider starting an alpha adrenoceptor antagonist (e.g. tamsulosin) and a 5-alpha-reductase inhibitor (e.g. finasteride) Attempt a trial without catheter (TWOC)—remove the catheter in the morning and ensure that the patient is passing urine later. After 6 hours, perform a bladder scan to exclude retention. Recatheterize if necessary
A few weeks later
Check how the patient is coping. Is he still suffering from symptoms of prostatism, or have the drugs reduced these? If the patient still has a catheter *in situ* (if they failed their trial without catheter), is a further trial in the community something worth trying? If the patient remains very symptomatic, is surgical prostate resection worth offering? How bad are their symptoms and how much do they affect their quality of life?

2. This man has benign prostatic hypertrophy. There are absolutely no features to suggest malignancy, with the patient being well, not losing weight, the prostate being smoothly enlarged, and the PSA being within 'normal' range. Although the PSA is a very imperfect screening test (see Question 4), a low level in this man is reassuring. If there was any doubt about malignancy in this patient then investigations to exclude cancer would include transrectal ultrasound and biopsy. An experienced urologist can estimate the degree of prostatic enlargement very accurately at palpation of the prostate on digital rectal examination.

This man has quite marked symptoms. The degree of prostatism experienced by a patient can be quantified using the International Prostate Symptom Score, in which the patient marks the severity of symptoms they experience for various factors (for instance, how often they pass urine during the night, or how often they have to strain hard to start to pass urine). This scoring system is well validated and produces a clear indication of how likely a patient is to require prostate surgery. A score above 20 constitutes severe symptoms.

This man should be managed initially with medications. Alpha adrenoceptor antagonists (such as tamsulosin) work by relaxing the alpha-1A receptors of the smooth muscle at the prostatic urethra. Their antiadrenergic effects may cause dizziness, hypotension, and fainting. 5-Alpha-reductase inhibitors (such as finasteride) are antiandrogens, preventing the conversion of testosterone to dihydrotestosterone, which results in overall involution of the prostate. A combination of tamsulosin and finasteride may produce considerable relief from the symptoms of prostatism without the need for surgery. If symptoms are not controlled medically then surgery may be required. The commonest operation performed for benign prostatic hypertrophy is transurethral resection of the prostate (TURP), though photocoagulation with lasers is now growing in popularity.

3. Many prostate cancers are very low grade (such as in these two patients—anything up to Gleason grade 6 is not aggressive). It will be many years before either of these men develops symptoms from metastatic or locally invasive disease. Guidelines suggest that patients with non-invasive disease should be managed aggressively if they have a life expectancy of more than 10 years. For many elderly men who develop low-grade prostate cancer, they will die from another cause not related to the cancer. Therefore for the 85-year-old man, rather than exposing him to the risks of surgery, it is better advised to adopt a policy of 'watchful waiting', with serial measurements of PSA. Sharp increases in PSA are seen if the tumour invades or becomes more malignant or metastatic and the decision to treat can then be reviewed.

The 55-year-old man is likely to have several more decades of life before him. The commonest treatment for non-invasive prostate cancer is surgery—often a transurethral prostatectomy. However, this has a number of possible unpleasant side-effects, including infection (prostatitis), impotence, and incontinence, which should be discussed with the patient. Radiotherapy is another accepted treatment, although this also has complications including radiation proctitis (anorectal bowel strictures that can cause obstruction), cystitis (bladder inflammation), and impotence. Brachytherapy is a newer treatment option where radioactive beads are inserted into the prostate under ultrasound guidance.

4. The sensitivity of a test is the proportion of patients with the disease who are picked up by the screening test. The inverse of the sensitivity is the false negative rate—so if 85% of patients with cancer are picked up by a positive PSA, 15% of patients with cancer will be falsely reassured. The specificity of a test deals with what a positive test actually means—what proportion of patients who test positive actually have prostate cancer. The inverse of this is the false positive rate. Here, of patients with a positive PSA, only 33% actually have prostate cancer; 67% are given a positive test despite the fact that they are healthy.

Dangers for this man exist with both a negative and a positive test. If he tests negative then he could be one of the 15% of patients who have prostate cancer (including in some cases high-grade cancers) who could be falsely reassured by a negative test. If he tests positive then he is similarly at risk. Although the odds are still 2:1 against his having cancer, he is likely to undergo a transrectal biopsy (carrying the risk of rectal bleeding, pain, incontinence, and infection), simply (in most cases) to investigate a spurious result. This patient should be counselled about the unreliability of PSA as a screening test and be encouraged not to have the test. PSA levels can be useful if extremely high (strongly suggesting malignancy) or if very low (suggesting the opposite). They are also useful in assessing disease progression and recurrence after surgery.

Further reading

Guidelines: NICE prostate cancer guidelines (http://guidance.nice.org.uk/CG58)

OHCM: 65, 644–647

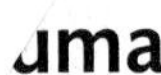

ʇma

This section should be used when observing a 'trauma call', where a team including surgeons, Emergency Department doctors, and anaesthetists rapidly assess, stabilize, diagnose, and begin definitive management of a seriously injured patient following trauma, beginning in the Emergency Department and progressing to theatre, ITU, or a General Surgical Ward as appropriate.

Learning challenges

- What is the trimodal distribution of deaths after major trauma and what strategies can be used to reduce deaths in each peak?
- What is 'permissive hypotension' and why is it used to treat shock in trauma but not for other forms of shock, e.g. septic shock?

Mechanism of injury

- As exact as possible, detailing possible injuries. For example, in road traffic collisions think about: speed of travel, damage to vehicle/lamppost etc., restraint with seat-belt, 'bulls-eye' to windscreen etc.

Airway and cervical spine

- Evidence of airway obstruction (e.g. apnoea, stridor, cyanosis, distortion of facial anatomy or blood in airway)
- Should they be in a surgical brace?
- Injuries suggestive of head/neck trauma? (e.g. bruising/bleeding/swelling to head or complaint of neck pain)
- Decreased level of consciousness secondary to cerebral hypoxia (Glasgow Coma Scale/AVPU)
- **Does this patient require intubation?**

Breathing

- Is the trachea central?
- Is the chest moving symmetrically? Are there bruises to the chest wall? Is there a penetrating thoracic injury?
- Is there bilateral air entry? Is this equal?
- An urgent portable 'trauma series' of X-rays should be performed, including chest X-ray and pelvic X-ray
- **Does this patient require chest drains or needle decompression?**

Circulation

- **Obtain intravenous access with two large-bore cannulae. Routine blood tests and cross match**
- What is the blood pressure and heart rate? Is the capillary refill time prolonged? Is there evidence of shock?
- Is there an obvious source of bleeding? (e.g. open femoral fracture)
- Is their vascular compromise to any limbs? (e.g. secondary to displaced fractures or penetrating trauma)
- Is there abdominal pathology? (e.g. penetrating injury, pain, distension)
- An eFAST (Extended Focused Assessment with Sonography for Trauma) ultrasound scan should be performed (usually by a radiologist or A&E doctor). Is there free fluid (blood) visualized in the abdomen?
- Is there an alternative source of circulatory compromise (e.g. pericardial tamponade, massive haemothorax, pelvic fracture with retroperitoneal bleeding)?
- **Fluid resuscitation** should be carefully considered, and generally reserved for massive haemorrhage, with blood (red packed cells and fresh frozen plasma) the fluid of choice to prevent trauma related coagulopathy
- **Does this patient require invasive haemorrhage control?** (e.g. immediate laparotomy for splenic/liver/bowel trauma or interventional radiology for angiographic embolization of pelvic vessels)
- **Is further imaging necessary** e.g. CT abdomen/pelvis?

Disability

- GCS
- Pupils—are they symmetric, reactive? (unilateral fixed dilated pupils suggest an ipsilateral intracranial haematoma with herniation of the brain until proven otherwise, and represent a neurosurgical emergency)
- Gross sensation and power in all four limbs
- Is there spinal tenderness or deformity? This should only be examined with a four-person 'log-roll', maintaining in-line spinal precautions
- **Does this patient require a CT head?** (see NICE Guidelines CG56 for useful guidance on investigations and management of head injury; http://www.nice.org.uk/CG056)
- **Should cervical spine immobilization be continued?** In the presence of a 'distracting' injury a cautious approach is mandatory, and imaging of the C-spine is frequently necessary prior to 'clinical clearance'

Exposure

- Undress the patient completely and assess for other injuries
- Maintain patient's body temperature; warm if necessary

Completion of the secondary survey must include:

- **AMPLE** history: **A**llergies; **M**edications; **P**revious medical history; **L**ast meal; **E**vent—what do they remember? This mnemonic serves as a reminder of the important features of a quick trauma history in the potentially unstable or deteriorating patient, and gives useful information for an anaesthetist should the patient require emergency surgery
- Head-to-toe examination including all orifices

Evaluation (after secondary survey)

1. **Has this patient responded to resuscitation? Do they require an urgent operation for control of haemorrhage?**

2. **What injuries has this patient sustained? What is the definitive treatment for each of these?**

Injury	Definitive management

3. **Can these injuries be treated at this hospital or is transfer to another hospital required?**

4. **Does this patient require significant rehabilitation?**

Questions

1. An 18-year-old woman is brought in after having been hit by a car while she was crossing the road late at night. The car driver had fled the scene, but the ambulance crew report that the car had subsequently been abandoned, and that the front windscreen was shattered with an external 'bulls-eye' pattern. The patient had been found at the side of the road. She had an initial GCS of 13/15 (E3/V4/M6). Her cervical spine has been immobilized in a rigid collar and is supported by blocks. Her airway is clear. Examination of her chest shows symmetrical movements, and good bilateral air entry. Her respiratory rate is 24 breaths/min and oxygen saturations are 97% on air. She has good peripheral pulses and is warm and well-perfused. Her BP is 115/67 mmHg, heart rate 88 bpm and temperature 36.4°C. Her abdomen is soft. Her chest X-ray, pelvis X-ray, and eFAST scan are all normal. Her pupils are equal in size at 4 mm and reactive to light. She is groaning incomprehensibly, opening her eyes in response to pain. and withdrawing her hand from painful stimulus.

(1) What is her level of consciousness according to the GCS and AVPU scoring systems?

(2) A decision is taken to transfer the patient to the radiology department for an urgent CT scan of her head and neck. What precautions need to be taken to ensure that her transfer and time in the scanner are safe?

2. A 25-year-old man is brought in by ambulance after being hit by a car. The mechanism of injury suggests blunt trauma to the left-hand side of the chest On arrival his GCS is 15 but he is too tachypnoeic to say more than a few words at a time. There is no stridor. Part of the left-hand side of his chest is moving paradoxically, being sucked in on inspiration and blown out on expiration. There are no breath sounds and a dull percussion note at the left base. Basic observations include respiratory rate 36 breaths/min, heart rate 114 bpm, blood pressure 94/52 mmHg, and oxygen saturations are 88% on high-flow oxygen via a non-rebreathe mask. A portable chest X-ray is ordered (shown below).

(1) What does it show and what are the next steps in his management?

(2) What other injuries should be considered?

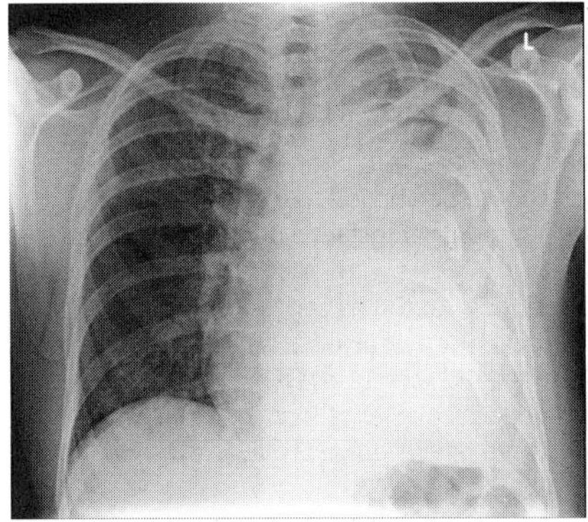

3. A 37-year-old man is rushed to hospital after a motorcycle injury. He had been travelling at approximately 25 miles per hour when a car pulled out in front of him. He was thrown over the car to land heavily on his head and left side. On arrival at hospital a primary survey is carried out, and reveals a GCS of 15, an uncompromised airway, good bilateral air entry with a respiratory rate of 22 breaths/min and saturations of 100% on oxygen (though significant tenderness was detected over the left lower rib-cage). Other observations included heart rate 98 bpm and blood pressure 128/88 mmHg. A chest X-ray is performed where left lower rib fractures are noted but the lungs fields are clear and there is no sign of intrathoracic bleeding. There is no injury seen to the cervical spine on X-ray. An eFAST scan is performed and is negative. The secondary survey is completed and no obvious injuries are apparent. The patient is given analgesia and transferred to a surgical ward to be monitored with hourly basic and neurological observations overnight, ahead of potential discharge the following day. Six hours later the on-call doctor is called to review the patient on the basis of a deterioration in their basic observations. The patient is still conscious but complaining of feeling faint and short of breath.

(1) Why is the patient deteriorating?

(2) How should the patient be investigated?

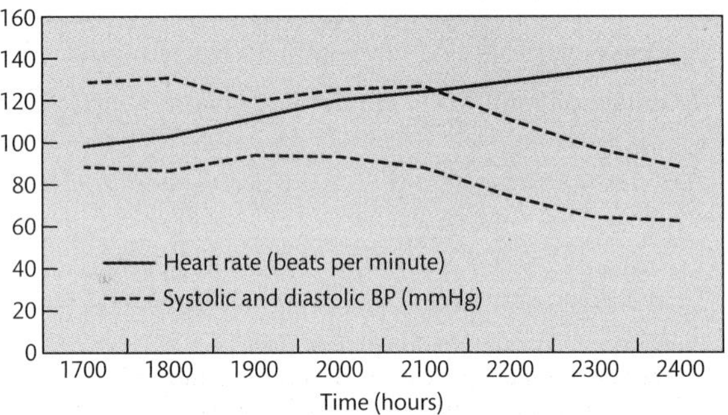

4. A 47-year-old man is brought in by paramedics after having been involved in a fight in a pub. He thinks he has been punched several times to the head, but denies any other injuries. He does not think he lost consciousness. He has vomited once in the presence of the paramedics. On examination he is somewhat drowsy but fully rousable, with a GCS of 14/15 (E4, V4, M6). He smells strongly of alcohol and is unkempt and malodorous. He is aggressive when disturbed, and does not comply with physical examination, but is noted to be significantly ataxic when he attempts to stand to urinate in the corner. He has a 3 cm laceration above the left eyebrow to which the paramedics have applied a compression bandage. He says that he wants to be left alone to sleep.

(1) How should head injury be assessed in a fully competent patient?

(2) What are the options for managing this man, who will not comply with physical examination?

5. A 19-year-old football player in brought in to the hospital's Emergency Department after damaging his left ankle in a tackle 30 minutes earlier. He is in severe pain which is not relieved by inhaled nitrous oxide ('Entonox'). Examination of the left lower leg reveals a large skin laceration running superiorly from the medial malleolus, through which exposed bone can be seen. The foot is held in a very awkward position, externally rotated, and with considerable swelling around the ankle joint. The left foot appears pale, and is cool to touch. The dorsalis pedis pulse is impalpable. A nurse asks whether you would like an urgent X-ray to be requested. What is your reply and how should you proceed?

Remember that you can find large-size, annotated versions of many of the X-rays and ECGs that appear in this book on the book's web site at www.oxfordtextbooks.co.uk/orc/randall/

Answers

1. This patient's GCS has reduced to 8 (E2,V2,M4), and on the AVPU scale (calculated on whether the patient is Alert, responsive to Voice or Pain, or is Unresponsive), she is at the level P. At this level of consciousness she is not able to protect her own airway, and an anaesthetist or A&E doctor should consider rapid sequence anaesthesia with placement of an endotracheal tube to protect her airway. This allows safe transfer for CT scan in a controlled manner, and safeguards the patient should there by any further reduction in level of consciousness whilst in transit. At a GCS of 8 or below, reflexes are lost which protect the patency of the patient's airway, meaning the patient is at risk of airway compromise and apnoea, and of aspiration. Endotracheal intubation should be performed with great care with in-line immobilization considering the possibility of cervical-spine injury.

The history here of a rapidly falling level of consciousness following significant head trauma makes a serious head injury likely, and this patient may require urgent neurosurgery (for instance, for decompression of an extradural haematoma). Given the 'distracting' head injury, she should have CT imaging performed of her spine as well, as further clinical assessment is limited with the patient anaesthetized and hence it will not be possible to rule out spinal injury.

2. The chest X-ray reveals:

The most obvious abnormality here is a large left-sided haemothorax. The appearances are the same as a pleural effusion, but the fluid is blood rather than exudate or transudate. If a haemothorax is massive (as here), then the trachea and mediastinum may be deviated to the opposite side.

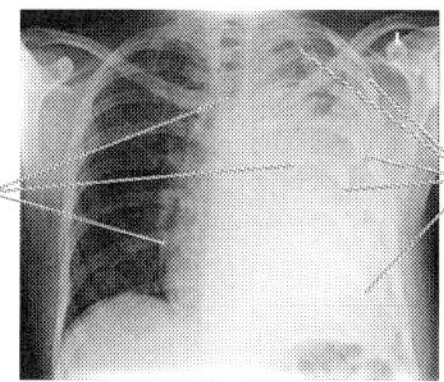

Note the number of broken ribs this patient has suffered. It is important to see that some of the ribs are broken in two places, which can form a 'flail segment' that moves paradoxically during respiration – pulled in during inspiration and pushed out during expiration, opposite to the rest of the chest wall.

His cardiovascular instability is caused by a combination of haemorrhagic shock, the reduction in intrathoracic volume and tensioning effect of the expanding bleed in his left hemithorax, and the effect of the flail chest on his respiratory mechanics. The first definitive intervention that this patient needs is the insertion of an intercostal drain, after which operative fixation of his flail segment may be necessary if significant respiratory compromise persists. Whilst preparations are made for insertion of the drain, he should have intravenous access with two large-bore cannulae, and blood should be sampled for routine bloods and cross-match of 4–8 units. Blood should be administered as resuscitation fluid to maintain his blood pressure and regain cardiovascular stability. Trauma fluid resuscitation in major haemorrhage aims to maintain an adequate blood pressure for cerebral perfusion, without such an increase as to disrupt important clots which are preventing further bleeding. A combination of packed red cells, platelets, fresh frozen plasma, and cryoprecipitate will be needed where massive transfusion is indicated, and trauma-related coagulopathy should be anticipated.

Insertion of a large-bore intercostal drain, under local anaesthetic, should not be delayed in this patient, and an improvement in the respiratory dynamics can be anticipated after insertion. A repeat X-ray should be performed to confirm the position of the drain. The drain is inserted through an incision in the fourth or fifth intercostal space in the mid-axillary line, and directed in the appropriate direction before secure suturing and dressing. In haemothorax the drain should be directed inferoposteriorly, and in pneumothorax it should be superoanterior. The drainage bottle should always be checked for a 'swinging' fluid level and this should be closely monitored.

In penetrating chest trauma (for instance, if this man had been stabbed instead of hit by a car), the important differential diagnoses leading to shock, cardiovascular instability, and cardiac arrest are tension pneumothorax, cardiac tamponade, and massive haemothorax from heart or great vessel injury. It may be necessary for an experienced emergency physician or surgeon to perform a life-saving thoracotomy and attempt to evacuate pericardial clot manually, or attempt to identify and repair a cardiac or great vessel injury. This procedure is clearly an extreme measure often carried out in patients who are periarrest or even during cardiac arrest, and consequently is associated with a poor outcome.

3. This patient's heart rate has been increasing steadily since admission, and now his blood pressure has begun to fall. In the context of trauma this is very suggestive of haemorrhage. Young people may compensate well even in major haemorrhage by increasing arteriolar tone (vasoconstriction) and by increasing cardiac output (through tachycardia). They may only decompensate (i.e. fail to maintain a normal blood pressure) once a significant amount of haemorrhage has occurred.

In this patient, and in view of the known left-sided rib injuries, several causes of deterioration should be considered. Examination of the chest and abdomen is likely to provide the most important information. If there is reduced air entry and dullness to percussion a haemothorax may be suspected. However, abdominal haemorrhage from a laceration to the spleen is far more likely in the presence of left lower rib injuries. Volume resuscitation with blood should be commenced, and urgent chest X-ray and abdominal ultrasound or CT should be arranged. Immediate intervention via laparotomy or angiography may be indicated.

There are five possible causes of life-threatening haemorrhage in humans: external bleeding from wounds, bleeding into the thorax (haemothorax), bleeding into the abdomen, bleeding into the pelvis (retroperitoneal), and bleeding into soft tissue compartments after long bone fracture.

4. Most head injuries are minor with no significant intracranial pathology. The NICE guidelines advise that CT should be performed immediately in adults with:

- GCS less than 13 on initial assessment in the Emergency Department
- GCS less than 15 at 2 hours after the injury on assessment in the Emergency Department
- Suspected open or depressed skull fracture
- Any sign of base of skull fracture (haemotympanum, 'panda' eyes, cerebrospinal fluid leakage from the ear or nose, Battle's sign)
- Post-traumatic seizure
- Focal neurological deficit
- More than one episode of vomiting
- Amnesia for events more than 30 minutes before impact

If there is a history of loss of consciousness the following patients should also receive CT scan:

- Age 65 years or older
- Coagulopathy (history of bleeding, clotting disorder, warfarin treatment)
- Dangerous mechanism of injury (a pedestrian or cyclist struck by a motor vehicle, an occupant ejected from a motor vehicle, or a fall from a height of greater than 1 m or five stairs)

Assessment of the intoxicated patient, as in this scenario, is a challenge to all Emergency Department doctors, and clinical judgement must be exercised. It is important to note that the alcoholic population may have a greater tendency for intracranial haemorrhage (especially subdural haemorrhage) because of coagulopathy secondary to liver dysfunction, poor platelet function, and chronic cerebral atrophy. If there is any suspicion of intracranial injury a CT scan must be performed. If the patient is considered low risk, a period of observation, and reassessment once sobriety has been achieved is mandatory.

5. Limb fractures or dislocations associated with compromise to distal blood supply represent a clinical emergency. There should be no delay in reducing this fracture–dislocation. The patient will need to be given strong analgesia, and may need sedation, e.g. with midazolam or ketamine. Firm traction should be applied to the foot, with an assistant applying counter-traction (for instance pulling upwards on a towel wrapped around the knee). The foot should be reduced into an anatomical position, or as close to this as can be achieved. This will invariably lead to spontaneous return of distal blood supply and the foot will become pink, warmer, and the pulses will become palpable. Traction should be maintained as a plaster of Paris 'backslab' is applied and allowed to set. X-ray should be performed to assess the reduction and the severity of the fracture.

This patient is likely to have suffered an open fracture–dislocation of the ankle. He will need an urgent orthopaedic review. Depending on the extent of contamination to the tissue, emergency debridement may be indicated. The fracture may need to be fixed and this can be done internally, or if there is a significant contamination, and subsequent risk of infection, with an external fixator. This patient should receive antibiotics, and his tetanus status should be checked.

Further reading

Guidelines: World Health Organization trauma guidelines (http://www.who.int/violence_injury_prevention/publications/services/guidelines_traumacare/en/index.html)

OHCM: 65, 644–647

Index

N

O

P

R

S

T

U

V

W